Prenatal Medicine

Prenatal Medicine

edited by

John M. G. van Vugt
VU University Medical Center
Amsterdam, The Netherlands

Lee P. Shulman
Feinberg School of Medicine
Northwestern University
Chicago, Illinois, U.S.A.

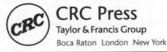

CRC Press
Taylor & Francis Group
Boca Raton London New York

CRC Press is an imprint of the
Taylor & Francis Group, an **informa** business

CRC Press
Taylor & Francis Group
6000 Broken Sound Parkway NW, Suite 300
Boca Raton, FL 33487-2742

First issued in paperback 2019

ISBN-13: 978-0-8247-2844-1 (hbk)
ISBN-13: 978-0-367-39071-6 (pbk)

Library of Congress Card Number 2006040301

Library of Congress Cataloging-in-Publication Data

Prenatal medicine / edited by John M. G. van Vugt, Lee P. Shulman
    p. ; cm.
  Includes bibliographical references and index.
  ISBN-13: 978-0-8247-2844-1 (hardcover : alk. paper)
  ISBN-10: 0-8247-2844-0 (hardcover : alk. paper)
  1. Prenatal diagnosis. 2. Genetic screening. 3. Fetus--Diseases--Diagnosis. I. Vugt, John M. G. van. II. Shulman, Lee P.
  [DNLM: 1. Prenatal Care. 2. Fetal Diseases--therapy. 3. Pregnancy Complications--therapy. 4. Prenatal Diagnosis. WQ 175 P9267 2006]

RG628.P744 2006
618.3'2075--dc22
                                                        2006040301

Visit the Taylor & Francis Web site at
http://www.taylorandfrancis.com

and the CRC Press Web site at
http://www.crcpress.com

"L'audace, l'audace, toujours l'audace."
The greatest honor and privilege bestowed on any person is the responsibility
to care for patients. This book is thus dedicated to those teachers, mentors,
and colleagues who helped us develop the requisite skills to provide that
care and to teach it to others; to our families (Suzanne, Laura, Becky,
and Andrew) who provided the foundation for our development as
people and physicians and love us for who we are and what we do;
and to our patients who honor us everyday with their trust and
expectations and challenge us to become better physicians
and human beings.

John M. G. van Vugt and Lee P. Shulman
Amsterdam and Chicago
2006

Foreword

In 1970, Henry L. Nadler and Albert B. Gerbie helped usher in the era of prenatal genetic diagnosis in their landmark paper "Role of amniocentesis in the interuterine detection of genetic disorders" (*N Engl J Med* 1970;282:596-9). Since that time, advances in genetics and perinatal medicine have occurred at an amazing pace, allowing physicians to detect and treat genetic disorders in utero with increasing success. There has also been an escalating demand by the public for translational medicine where discoveries in the laboratory are rapidly brought to the bedside. Although scientific breakthroughs in prenatal genetics have been nothing short of dazzling, we must always remember that the benefits they bring to pregnant women and their families is dependent upon the continuation of social attitudes and social support that made these developments possible.

Prenatal Medicine provides a succinct overview of prenatal genetic diagnosis and related topics. This text is particularly valuable because the authoritative contributors of each chapter have put into perspective massive amounts of research data material into clinically relevant information applicable to patient care. The safety and accuracy of state-of-the-art procedures and technologies are covered, including genetic amniocentesis, chorionic villus sampling, maternal serum screening for fetal genetic disorders, and high resolution and three-dimensional ultrasonography. Important topics related to prenatal diagnosis are addressed, including ethical and legal issues, prevention of labor, open fetal surgery, and fetal reduction and selective feticide. Exciting emerging areas of prenatal genetic diagnosis that will undoubtedly change the future of obstetrical care are considered, including fetal cells and DNA in maternal blood, new DNA technologies (e.g., multiplex ligation-dependent probe amplification and fluorescence in situ hybridization), and prenatal pharmaceutical therapy.

The editors of this text, John M. G. van Vugt and Lee P. Shulman, are internationally recognized leaders in prenatal genetic diagnosis, and each has contributed extensively to the literature of this field. Their gravitas and expertise are self-evident as they have carefully orchestrated and edited the contributed chapters into a coherent, cohesive, and highly informative text.

I wish to take this opportunity to add a few personal notes about the editors. I have known John M. G. van Vugt for more than ten years through the International Fetoscopy Work Group and the International Society for Prenatal Diagnosis.

His research in trophoblast cells and chromosome 21-encoded mRNA of placental origin in maternal blood, as well as ultrasonographic markers of fetal genetic disorders, has been pioneering in the quest for non-invasive prenatal diagnosis. He brings a balanced perspective and honesty to our discipline for which we should all be grateful. Finally, I would like to comment about Lee P. Shulman, a reproductive genetics fellow of long ago and an esteemed professional colleague and treasured friend for more than twenty years. His research has bridged prenatal genetic research with family planning and contraception to address the broader needs of women and their families. I know him to be a truly outstanding physician and clinical investigator who always has the best interests of his patients at heart. Lee is my comic relief, and I look forward to working with him each and every day.

Sherman Elias, M.D.
John J. Sciarra Professor and Chair
Northwestern University
Feinberg School of Medicine
Chicago, Illinois, U.S.A.

Preface

The goal of obstetrical care—regardless of all the medical, surgical, and technical advances of the past 50 years—still remains the delivery of healthy infants and the maintenance of good maternal health. Because those of us who practice obstetrics usually care for young, healthy women, this goal is one that is usually attained.

However, congenital and acquired maternal and fetal diseases are not uncommon complications during many pregnancies. Although maternal–fetal specialists and geneticists provide the care for those women with maternal conditions that can affect fetal or maternal well being or those women found to be carrying fetuses with congenital and acquired abnormalities, such complications can and do arise during the care of the ostensibly normal pregnancy. Indeed, lifestyle considerations such as nutritional status, maternal age, and an increasing recognition of specific genetic factors in the predisposition of fetal, newborn, and maternal conditions as a result of the Human Genome Project have considerably altered the delineation of low-risk and high-risk pregnancies.

Recognizing that such new and novel advances in our knowledge of maternal and fetal physiology have lead to profound changes in obstetrical management of low- and high-risk pregnancies, we sought to assemble a compilation of the state-of-the-art of prenatal care. We recognized, however, that such advances had led to considerably different approaches to incorporating this information into clinical practice. Therefore, to provide the most accurate presentations of the clinical applications of these novel advances, we utilized our rather disparate clinical and research experiences to recruit an international group of researchers and clinicians who could present an accurate overview of these advances as they apply to a variety of patients, clinical scenarios, and distinct communities of genetically and socially different peoples. We believe that presenting a wide and realistic spectrum of obstetrical practice and research is the best way for our colleagues to determine the best approaches for incorporating this information into their practices. In this way, *Prenatal Medicine* represents a unique and dynamic approach to the challenge of effectively incorporating novel and recent scientific information into the care of pregnant women worldwide.

Although many can agree on the scientific concepts that continue to change and improve our care of pregnant women and fetuses in all stages of pregnancy, one aspect that will assuredly divide clinicians is the legal and political differences that separate us. Whether the result of geographical boundary or personal conviction, these differences will continue to color and, at times, direct the care of women and their pregnancies. To this end, we also present different legal and political approaches to obstetrical care and seek to engage in dialogue that will hopefully spark lively discussion among colleagues and ultimately improve the care of all pregnant women.

We are indebted to the authors of the chapters, who not only provided outstanding reviews of their particular areas of expertise, but also serve as outstanding clinicians, teachers, mentors, and researchers. Their work improves the care of their patients, and through texts such as *Prenatal Medicine*, may improve the care of women far from their homes, offices, and communities.

The ongoing improvement in medical care relies on all practitioners to commit to lifelong learning. We hope that *Prenatal Medicine* will be a component of that commitment and serve as a resource and motivation for the appropriate incorporation of new and novel scientific advances that will improve the care of women and fetuses no matter where they live.

John M. G. van Vugt
Lee P. Shulman

Contents

Contributors

N. Scott Adzick The Center for Fetal Diagnosis and Treatment, The Children's Hospital of Philadelphia, The University of Pennsylvania School of Medicine, Philadelphia, Pennsylvania, U.S.A.

Gerard Barki Karl Storz Endoskope, Tuttlingen, Germany

Michael W. Bebbington The Center for Fetal Diagnosis and Treatment, The Children's Hospital of Philadelphia, The University of Pennsylvania School of Medicine, Philadelphia, Pennsylvania, U.S.A.

Mireille N. Bekker Department of Obstetrics and Gynecology, VU University Medical Center, Amsterdam, The Netherlands

Diana W. Bianchi Division of Genetics, Department of Pediatrics, Tufts-New England Medical Center, Boston, Massachusetts, U.S.A.

Caterina M. Bilardo Department of Obstetrics and Gynaecology, Academic Medical Centre, Amsterdam, The Netherlands

Jay J. Bringman Department of Obstetrics and Gynecology, University of Tennessee Health Sciences Center, Memphis, Tennessee, U.S.A.

David W. Britt Department of Obstetrics and Gynecology, Institute for Genetics and Fetal Medicine, St. Luke's-Roosevelt Hospital Center, New York, New York, U.S.A.

Joe Bruner Vanderbilt University Medical Center, Nashville, Tennessee, U.S.A.

Sabine Bueschle Karl Storz Endoskope, Tuttlingen, Germany

Simona Cicero Harris Birthright Research Centre for Fetal Medicine, Kings's College Hospital, Denmark Hill, London, U.K.

Doina Ciorica Department of Obstetrics and Gynecology, Institute for Genetics and Fetal Medicine, St. Luke's-Roosevelt Hospital Center, New York, New York, U.S.A.

Leeber Cohen   Department of Obstetrics and Gynecology, Division of Reproductive Genetics, Feinberg School of Medicine, Northwestern University, Chicago, Illinois, U.S.A.

Anna L. David   Department of Obstetrics and Gynaecology, Royal Free and University College London Medical School, London, U.K.

Pascal De Lagausie   Ecole de Chirurgie du Fer à Moulin (AP-HP), and Unité de Recherche EA3102, Paris, and Service de Chirurgie Pédiatrique, Hôpital la Timone, AP-HM, Marseille, France

W. J. B. Dennes   Centre for Fetal Care, Queen Charlotte's and Chelsea Hospital, Hammersmith Campus, London, U.K.

Jan Deprest   Department of Obstetrics and Gynaecology, University Hospitals Leuven, Leuven, Belgium

Roland Devlieger   Department of Obstetrics and Gynaecology, University Hospitals Leuven, Leuven, Belgium

Guido de Wert   Health Ethics and Philosophy, Faculty of Medicine, Maastricht University, Maastricht, The Netherlands

Marc Dommergues   Service de Gynécologie Obstétrique, Hôpital Pitié-Salpétrière, AP-HP and Université Paris VI, Paris, France

Wybo Dondorp   Health Ethics and Philosophy, Faculty of Medicine, Maastricht University, Maastricht, The Netherlands

Nanette Elster   Spence & Elster, P.C., Lincolnshire, Illinois, U.S.A.

Melanie A. J. Engels   Department of Obstetrics and Gynecology, VU University Medical Center, Amsterdam, The Netherlands

Mark I. Evans   Department of Obstetrics and Gynecology, Institute for Genetics and Fetal Medicine, St. Luke's-Roosevelt Hospital Center, New York, New York, U.S.A.

N. M. Fisk   Institute of Reproductive and Developmental Biology, Imperial College London and Queen Charlotte's and Chelsea Hospital, Hammersmith Campus, London, U.K.

John C. Fletcher[†]   Department of Obstetrics and Gynecology, Institute for Genetics and Fetal Medicine, St. Luke's-Roosevelt Hospital Center, New York, New York, U.S.A.

[†] Deceased.

Denis Gallot   Department of Obstetrics and Gynaecology, University Hospitals Leuven, Leuven, Belgium

Annegret Geipel   Department of Obstetrics and Prenatal Medicine, University of Bonn, Bonn, Germany

Ulrich Gembruch   Department of Obstetrics and Prenatal Medicine, University of Bonn, Bonn, Germany

Susan E. Gerber   Department of Obstetrics and Gynecology, Division of Maternal Fetal Medicine, Feinberg School of Medicine, Northwestern University, Chicago, Illinois, U.S.A.

Norman Ginsberg   Feinberg School of Medicine, Northwestern University, Chicago, Illinois, U.S.A.

Attie T. J. I. Go   Department of Obstetrics and Gynecology, VU University Medical Center, Amsterdam, The Netherlands

James D. Goldberg   San Francisco Perinatal Associates, San Francisco, California, U.S.A.

Eduardo Gratacos   Hospital Clinic, Barcelona, Spain

Jean Guibourdenche   Biochimie-Hormonologie, Hôpital Robert Debré (AP-HP), Paris, France

Monique C. Haak   Department of Obstetrics and Gynecology, VU University Medical Center, Amsterdam, The Netherlands

Pak Chung Ho   Department of Obstetrics and Gynecology, Queen Mary Hospital, Pokfulam, Hong Kong, Special Administrative Region, China

Jacques Jani   Department of Obstetrics and Gynaecology, University Hospitals Leuven, Leuven, Belgium

Kirby L. Johnson   Division of Genetics, Department of Pediatrics, Tufts-New England Medical Center, Boston, Massachusetts, U.S.A.

Mark P. Johnson   The Center for Fetal Diagnosis and Treatment, The Children's Hospital of Philadelphia, The University of Pennsylvania School of Medicine, Philadelphia, Pennsylvania, U.S.A.

Deborah Levine   Department of Radiology, Beth Israel Deaconess Medical Center, Boston, Massachusetts, U.S.A.

Liesbeth Lewi   Department of Obstetrics and Gynecology, University Hospitals Leuven, Leuven, Belgium

Dominique Luton   Département de Périnatologie, Maternité de l'Hôpital Robert Debré (AP-HP), and Université Paris VII (UFR Lariboisière Saint Louis), and, Unité de Recherche EA3102, Ecole de Chirurgie du Fer à Moulin (AP-HP), Paris, France

Kamlesh Madan   Department of Clinical Genetics, VU University Medical Center, Amsterdam, The Netherlands

Françoise Muller   Laboratoire de Biochimie Hormonale, Hôpital Robert Debré, Université Paris Ile-de-France-Ouest, Paris, France

Thomas J. Musci   San Francisco Perinatal Associates, San Francisco, California, U.S.A.

K. H. Nicolaides   Harris Birthright Research Centre for Fetal Medicine, King's College School of Medicine and Dentistry, London, U.K.

Dick Oepkes   Department of Obstetrics, Leiden University Medical Center, Leiden, The Netherlands

Cees B. M. Oudejans   Department of Clinical Chemistry, VU University Medical Center, Amsterdam, The Netherlands

Jean-François Oury   Département de Périnatologie, Maternité de l'Hôpital Robert Debré (AP-HP), and Université Paris VII (UFR Lariboisière Saint Louis), and Unité de Recherche EA3102, Paris, France

Eugene Pergament   Department of Obstetrics and Gynecology, Northwestern University, Chicago, Illinois, U.S.A.

T. Philipp   Department of Obstetrics and Gynecology, Danube Hospital, Vienna, Austria

Owen P. Phillips   Department of Obstetrics and Gynecology, University of Tennessee Health Sciences Center, Memphis, Tennessee, U.S.A.

Charles H. Rodeck   Department of Obstetrics and Gynaecology, Royal Free and University College London Medical School, London, U.K.

A. R. Rudnicka   Wolfson Institute of Preventive Medicine, Barts and the London Queen Mary's School of Medicine and Dentistry, Charterhouse Square, London, U.K.

Julien Saada   Département de Périnatologie, Maternité de l'Hôpital Robert Debré (AP-HP), and Ecole de Chirurgie du Fer à Moulin (AP-HP), Paris, and Fédération de Gynécologie-Obstétrique, Secteur Échographie et Diagnostic Anténatal, Hôpital Paule de Viguier, Toulouse, France

Lee P. Shulman   Department of Obstetrics and Gynecology, Division of Reproductive Genetics, Feinberg School of Medicine, Northwestern University, Chicago, Illinois, U.S.A.

Rosalinde J. M. Snijders Fetal Medicine Foundation Netherlands, Rotterdam, The Netherlands

J. D. Sonek Department of Obstetrics and Gynecology, Ohio State University, Columbus, Ohio, U.S.A.

Federico Spelzini Department of Obstetrics and Gynaecology, University Hospitals Leuven, Leuven, Belgium

Kevin Spencer Prenatal Screening Unit, Clinical Biochemistry Department, Harold Wood Hospital, Gubbins Lane, Romford, Esssex, U.K.

Ghislaine Sterkers Laboratoire d'Immunologie, Hôpital Robert Debré (AP-HP), Paris, France

Oi Shan Tang Department of Obstetrics and Gynecology, Queen Mary Hospital, Pokfulam, Hong Kong, Special Administrative Region, China

May Lee Tjoa Division of Genetics, Department of Pediatrics, Tufts-New England Medical Center, Boston, Massachusetts, U.S.A.

Phebe Nanine Adama van Scheltema Department of Obstetrics, Leiden University Medical Center, Leiden, The Netherlands

Dominique van Schoubroeck Department of Obstetrics and Gynaecology, University Hospitals Leuven, Leuven, Belgium

John M. G. van Vugt Department of Obstetrics and Gynecology, VU University Medical Center, Amsterdam, The Netherlands

Marc Vandevelde Department of Obstetrics and Gynaecology, University Hospitals Leuven, Leuven, Belgium

Edith Vuillard Département de Périnatologie, Maternité de l'Hôpital Robert Debré (AP-HP), Paris, France

N. J. Wald Wolfson Institute of Preventive Medicine, Barts and the London Queen Mary's School of Medicine and Dentistry, Charterhouse Square, London, U.K.

R. Douglas Wilson The Center for Fetal Diagnosis and Treatment, The Children's Hospital of Philadelphia, The University of Pennsylvania School of Medicine, Philadelphia, Pennsylvania, U.S.A.

1

First Trimester Serum Screening

Kevin Spencer
Prenatal Screening Unit, Clinical Biochemistry Department, Harold Wood Hospital, Gubbins Lane, Romford, Esssex, U.K.

INTRODUCTION

The natural frequency of chromosomal abnormalities at birth is around 6 cases per 1000 births among populations without any form of prenatal screening. The aneuploides represent the most frequent of these, with Down syndrome being the most common with a historical birth prevalence of 1 in 800. The other common autosomal trisomies include Edward's syndrome (trisomy 18) and Patau's syndrome (trisomy 13), occurring with historical birth incidences of 1 in 6500 and 1 in 12,500, respectively. The other group of aneuploides include the sex aneuploidies, such as Turner's syndrome (45x), Klinefelter syndrome (47xxy), and those with 47xyy, and the types I and II versions of triploidy.

The incidence of the major trisomies (13, 18, and 21) increases with maternal age, although for the sex aneuploidies and triploidy there is no increased incidence with maternal age (Fig. 1). As a consequence of the changing pattern of childbirth in recent years, with women postponing childbirth until later life, the resulting general prevalence of the age-related trisomies has increased and that for trisomy 21 has changed from 1 in 740 to 1 in 500 in a 23-year period (1).

Although the birth incidence of the major chromosomal abnormalities approaches 6 per 1000, the actual incidence at any one time in pregnancy varies due to the varying intrauterine lethality of the various conditions (2). This means that when screening women in early pregnancy, there is a significantly greater number of fetuses affected than at mid-gestation or at term. (Fig. 2).

The aim of prenatal screening programs is to identify a subgroup of women who may be at a higher risk of carrying a fetus with a chromosomal anomaly. This group could then be offered an invasive diagnostic test such as amniocentesis or chorionic villus sampling (CVS) followed by karyotyping of the fetal cells. Such invasive procedures themselves carry a potential fetal loss rate of 0.5–1% above the background fetal loss rate. At the same time, prenatal screening programs aim to provide information with which couples can make appropriate informed choices about reproductive decisions, rather than focusing on disabilities and their eradication (3).

Screening for Down syndrome (trisomy 21) over the past two decades has become an established part of obstetric practice in many developed countries,

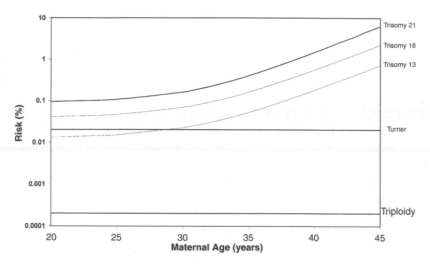

Figure 1 Variation of risk for various chromosomal anomalies with maternal age.

primarily through the use of maternal serum biochemical screening in the second trimester of pregnancy. In the second trimester, a range of maternal serum biochemical markers have been investigated, but routine screening has come to rely on the use of a combination of 2, 3, or 4 markers. The concentration of many of the biochemical markers varies with the duration of pregnancy. By expressing the observed concentration as a ratio of the median value observed in a normal pregnancy of the same gestation to obtain a multiple of the median (MoM), these gestational fluctuations are removed. The distributions of the MoM values in normal and Down pregnancies usually follow a gaussian distribution when the MoM is log transformed; however, with all markers there is a significant overlap of the two populations, but it is possible to establish from the gaussian distributions, the likelihood of any one result coming from the population of results associated with fetal Down syndrome. An individual patient-specific risk is then calculated by multiplying the a priori risk (usually based on maternal age) with the likelihood ratio. Unfortunately, no one individual marker alone has sufficient discriminatory power and a more efficient screening program can be achieved by combining information from

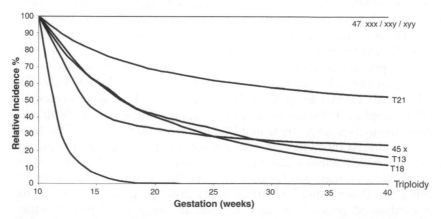

Figure 2 Gestational age-related risk for various chromosomal anomalies relative to the risk at 10 weeks. *Source*: From Ref. 2.

Table 1 Modeled Expected Detection Rates at a 5% False-Positive Rate Using a Variety of Combinations of Second-Trimester Biochemical Markers

Marker combination	Detection rate (%)
AFP, free β-hCG	63.2
AFP, free β-hCG, unconjugated estriol	66.8
AFP, free β-hCG, unconjugated estriol, inhibin A	72.1

Abbreviations: AFP, alpha-fetoprotein; β-hCG, β human chorionic gonadotropin.
Source: From Ref. 5.

more than one marker. The detailed mathematics of this multimarker approach is beyond the scope of this review but can be found in other publications (4). A summary of the modeled expected second trimester screening performance using various marker combinations (5) is shown in Table 1. Apart from Down syndrome, the only other major aneuploidy that is routinely screened for in some second trimester screening programs is Edward's syndrome (trisomy 18). In all other regards the biochemical patterns observed with the other aneuploidies are unremarkable—perhaps with the exception of triploidy types I and II (Table 2).

The past decade has seen a considerable focus on moving screening earlier into the first trimester. Earlier screening is anticipated to provide women with an earlier reassurance and, if termination of pregnancy is required, this can often be completed before fetal movements are evident. Also termination of pregnancy in the first trimester is safer than later in pregnancy (6). The fact that some Down syndrome pregnancies detected in the first trimester will be spontaneously lost before term is not a valid argument against early screening. For these women, it is important to have this information with regard to future reproductive decisions, so that a late miscarriage can be prevented.

A range of maternal serum biochemical markers has been investigated in both the first and second trimesters of pregnancy in normal and chromosomally abnormal pregnancies. Table 3 summarizes a meta-analysis of published cases with trisomies 13, 18, and 21 in the first trimester. For trisomy 21, of the markers of value in the second trimester, only the elevated free β human chorionic gonadotropin (β-hCG) is of any value in the first and second trimesters, and is reduced in both trimesters when trisomy 18 is present. The only other biochemical marker of value is the lowered levels of pregnancy-associated plasma protein A (PAPP-A) seen in cases with trisomies 13, 18, and 21. A guide to the scale of clinical effectiveness in discriminating normal

Table 2 Second Trimester Marker Patterns in Common Aneuploidies

Anomaly	HCG	AFP	UE3	Inhibin A
T21	High	Low	Low	High
T18	Low	Low	Low	Small decrease
T13	Normal	Small increase	Normal	Normal
Turner's	High/low +/− hydrops	Small decrease	Small decrease	High/low +/− hydrops
Other sex	Normal or high	Normal or high	Normal	
Triploidy I	High	High		
Triploidy II	Low	Normal		

Abbreviations: AFP, alpha-fetoprotein; HCG, human chorionic gonadotropin; UE3, unconjugated estriol.

Table 3 Meta-Analysis of Published Maternal Serum Biochemical Markers in Cases with Trisomies 21, 18, and 13 in the First Trimester

Serum marker	Trisomy 21		Trisomy 18		Trisomy 13	
	Median MoM	N	Median MoM	N	Median MoM	N
AFP	0.80	611	0.91	53	0.92	42
Total hCG	1.33	625	0.39	53	0.74	42
Unconjugated estriol	0.71	210				
Free β-hCG	1.98	846	0.27	126	0.51	45
Inhibin A	1.59	112	1.41	235	0.74	45
Free α-hCG	1.00	163				
CA125	1.14	34				
PAPP-A	0.45	777	0.20	119	0.25	42
SP1	0.86	246				
Activin	1.36	45	1.23	45		

Abbreviations: AFP, alpha-fetoprotein; hCG, human chorionic gonadotropin; PAPP-A, pregnancy-associated plasma protein A.

pregnancies and those affected by trisomy 21 can be obtained using the Mahalanobis distance (7), calculated from:

$$mean(unaffected) - mean(affected)/SD(unaffected)$$

where the mean and standard deviation (SD) are in the log domain (2). Table 4 summarizes this clinical effectiveness scale and includes, for comparison, the ultrasound marker nuchal translucency (NT) thickness, which is the single most prominent marker for fetal aneuploidy at the 11- to 14-week period.

FREE β-HCG

General Biology

Intact hCG is a 39.5 kDa dimeric glycoprotein of two different subunits. The α subunit is a 15 kDa protein identical to the common α subunits of the other pituitary

Table 4 Relative Clinical Effectiveness (Mahalanobis Distance) of Markers in Discriminating for Trisomy 21 in the First Trimester

Marker	Mahalanobis distance
NT	6.46
PAPP-A	2.08
Free β-hCG	1.45
Unconjugated estriol	0.68
Total/intact hCG	0.38
Dimeric inhibin A	0.35
AFP	0.23

Abbreviations: NT, nuchal translucency; PAPP-A, pregnancy-associated plasma protein A; hCG, human chorionic gonadotropin; AFP, alpha-fetoprotein.

glycoprotein hormone family. The 23 kDa β subunit of this family confers biological activity and there is an 80% sequence homology between the β subunits of luteinizing hormone and hCG. hCG synthesis occurs in the synctiotrophoblast of the placenta and involves an independent translation of the respective mRNAs for the α and β subunits. The β subunit is coded for by at least six genes on chromosome 19 while only one gene on chromosome 6 codes for the α subunit. Post-translational glycosylation of the subunits occurs before the subunits are released in the form of free α-hCG or free β-hCG along with the intact dimeric molecule. Control of secretion of the β subunit is thought to be the rate-limiting step in the production of the intact molecule and this is influenced in a positive way by cyclic adenosine monophosphate, insulin, calcium, interleukin-1, fibroblast growth factor, and placental gonadotropin-releasing hormone. Inhibitory influences include prolactin, progesterone, and inhibin.

In the placenta, maternal pregnancy serum, and urine, hCG is present in multiple related forms including degraded hCG molecules, hyper- and hypoglycosylated hCG, free subunits, and fragments (8). Urine is the major route for clearance of hCG from the circulation, with the major breakdown product β-core being produced within the kidney. The clearance half-life of the intact dimer is of the order of 24–36 hours, while the free subunits are more rapidly cleared in 2–5 hours. It is thought that the degradation process of intact hCG may involve peptide nicking of the β subunit at peptide linkages 47–48 (less frequently at 43–44 and 44–45) and that the nicked intact hCG is less stable than non-nicked hCG and rapidly dissociates to the free subunit, which is then cleared. In pregnancies affected by trisomy 21, there is some limited evidence that both the nicked forms of β-hCG and the hyperglycosylated forms may be increased in both maternal serum and urine.

Since free β-hCG is present in serum in a milieu of other hCG-related molecules in the first trimester, it is important to ensure that the assay that is used in clinical practice measures the component of interest and not any of the other potential species (8). In the first trimester it appears that only the free β-hCG subunit is of proven clinical value, and while assays should also measure the nicked and non-nicked form, cross-reactivity with the intact molecule may reduce the clinical discrimination.

Levels in Cases with T21, T18, T13, and Other Aneuploidies

In 1992, Spencer et al. (9) first reported that levels of free β-hCG were elevated in cases with trisomy 21 and subsequently many other studies have confirmed that levels approach 2 MoM, being slightly lower than the average value of 2.20 seen in the second trimester. The largest series to date (10) with 210 cases of trisomy 21 showed a median MoM of 2.15. In studies which have investigated total hCG, the median in the first trimester is considerably lower than that in the second trimester with a median of 1.33 compared to 2.06 in the second trimester (11).

In cases with trisomy 18, early studies (9) indicated that free β-hCG levels were reduced. Since then a number of studies have confirmed these findings with levels approaching 0.27 MoM (12), which is very close to the 0.33 average seen in the second trimester (13). Total hCG levels in cases with trisomy 18 are also reduced by a similar amount (14).

In cases with trisomy 13, the median free β-hCG MoM is decreased (15) to around 0.51 MoM, unlike in the second trimester, when levels are normal to slightly elevated (K. Spencer, unpublished). Total hCG is also reduced at the same time, albeit to a lesser extent than free β-hCG (14).

In cases with Turner's syndrome, free β-hCG levels are not particularly different from normal (1.11 MoM), as was the case in other cases with sex aneuploidy (16).

In cases with triploidy, free β-hCG levels are supra-elevated (8.04 MoM) in cases with triploidy type I (17) and to a lesser extent for total hCG (4.91). In triploidy type II, levels are dramatically reduced (0.18 MoM), as is total hCG (0.16).

PREGNANCY-ASSOCIATED PLASMA PROTEIN A

General Biology

PAPP-A is a large (800 kDa) dimeric zinc containing metalloglycoprotein synthesized by the syncytiotrophoblast tissue of the placenta in an initial pro-form approximately 80 amino acids longer than the mature subunit. Each mature subunit consists of 1547 amino acid residues, and in pregnancy serum, PAPP-A exists as a 2:2 complex with the pro-form of eosinophil major basic protein (ProMBP) (18). ProMBP also circulates bound to angiotensinogen, and this new complex can also bind complement 3dg. In pregnancy, ProMBP concentrations exceed PAPP-A by 10-fold. PAPP-A is encoded by a gene on the long arm of chromosome 9. Although the biological function of PAPP-A is not clearly defined, it has recently been shown to be an insulin-like growth factor 4 (IGF4) protease (19) and it is speculated that PAPP-A, therefore, may have some form of regulatory role in the growth of the fetus by controlling the amount of bioavailable IGF1 and IGF2.

Levels in Cases with T21, T18, T13, and Other Aneuploides

Brambati et al. (20) first observed that PAPP-A levels were reduced in cases with aneuploidy (including trisomy 21) during the early first trimester. Subsequently, many studies have been published which, although showing quite wide variation of median MoM, have confirmed that levels are on average reduced to around 0.45 MoM. The variation in median MoM from study to study can now be attributed to the temporal variation of marker levels, since in early first trimester studies, median levels of PAPP-A were very low (0.3), and in studies performed around 12–13 weeks, levels were higher (0.65) (10). This temporal variation also results in a loss of clinical discrimination for PAPP-A by the time one reaches the 17th week of gestation (21,22).

In cases with trisomy 18 in the first trimester, levels of PAPP-A are reduced (12) significantly with a median MoM from accumulated world series of 0.20. Unlike with trisomy 21, levels slightly reduce in the second trimester making PAPP-A a useful marker of trisomy 18 at this time (23,24).

In cases with trisomy 13 in the first trimester, levels of PAPP-A are also reduced (15) to around 0.25, making it difficult to discriminate between trisomies 13 and 18 because of the similar biochemical pattern (25).

In Turner's syndrome, PAPP-A levels are lower (0.49 MoM) in the first trimester, but for other sex aneuploides, levels are not significantly different (16).

In triploidy type I, PAPP-A levels are slightly decreased (0.75 MoM), while in type II, they are dramatically reduced to almost immeasurable levels (0.06 MoM) (17).

COMBINED MODELED DETECTION RATES

When used as a single marker in combination with maternal age, at a fixed 5% false-positive rate, the best estimates for detection of cases with trisomy 21 range from

42% to 46% for free β-hCG (10,26) and 48% to 52% for PAPP-A (10,26) for specimens collected between the 10- and 14-week period. When the two markers are combined together with maternal age, the detection rates increase to from 65% to 67%.

For trisomies 13 and 18, it is not possible to produce individual specific risks since the biochemical patterns and the NT patterns are quite similar; however, it is possible to provide a combined trisomy13/18 risk estimate (25). Modeling has shown that for a 0.3% false-positive rate, 95% of cases could be identified (25).

Temporal Variation

It has become evident over time that many markers show a different pattern of variation in cases with aneuploidy across the first and second trimester. Berry et al. (27) collected samples from 45 cases with trisomy 21 in the first and second trimesters. They showed that in these same patients the first trimester free β-hCG median was 1.99 compared with 2.79 in the second trimester. Similarly, for PAPP-A the corresponding values were 0.50 and 0.94 MoM. In the second trimester, Spencer and Macri (28–33) have demonstrated that median free β-hCG levels and detection rates for trisomy 21 are higher at around 14–16 weeks than at 17–19 weeks. A similar pattern was shown for free β-hCG in the first trimester when levels increased from 1.75 at 11 weeks to 2.25 at 13 weeks, and for PAPP-A, the levels increased from 0.44 at 11 weeks to 0.69 at 13 weeks (10). In a comprehensive analysis of data from between 700 and 1000 cases with trisomy 21 and over 100,000 unaffected pregnancies, Spencer et al. (21,22) have described in detail the temporal variation across the first and second trimesters for the markers alpha-fetoprotein (AFP), PAPP-A, free β-hCG, and total hCG. The result of this temporal variation is that the separation between normal pregnancies and those with trisomy 21 is changing all the time, and unless this is taken into account in the screening algorithm by using a variable separation model (21,22) rather than the constant median separation model assumed by Wald et al. (34–36), then significant errors in individual patient-specific risks can be created. The other feature of such temporal variation is that for individual markers, there are key measuring periods. For example PAPP-A is a better marker before 10 weeks, but free β-hCG is a better marker at around 12–14 weeks. The consequence of this opposing changing pattern is to some extent to balance detection rates so that across the 8- to 13-week window the variation is from 72.5% at 8 weeks to 62.6% at 13 weeks (22).

Temporal variation also exists for other aneuploidies. For example, in cases with trisomy 18, levels of PAPP-A are low in the first trimester and get progressively lower throughout the second trimester. Indeed for trisomy 18, PAPP-A is probably the best second trimester clinical discriminator, and a two-stage screening program has been proposed (23,24). In cases with trisomy 13, the low first trimester levels of free β-hCG increase such that by the 18th week, levels are elevated (K. Spencer, unpublished).

In order to compare detection rates between the first and second trimesters, it is necessary to allow for the intrauterine lethality of fetal aneuploidy between the two gestational periods. In the first trimester, there are more cases of trisomy 21, for example, than in the second trimester (Fig. 2). A statistical methodology for this has been developed by Dunstan and Nix (37), but this relies on having a suitable measure of the fetal loss rate in cases with trisomy 21 between the 12- and 16-week period. Typical fetal loss rates have been constructed from studies looking at the incidence of trisomy 21 at the time of CVS and the incidence at the time of amniocentesis (38). Unfortunately these data may well be biased because they are observations in a group which are largely of advanced maternal age (39), and it is known that advancing maternal age per se is a factor that increases fetal loss rates (40). Probably one of the more secure estimates of fetal loss is from the UK National Down Syndrome register, which collects data from all pre- and postnatally detected cases (41). Assuming a 75% second trimester detection rate, a detection rate would need to be 3.5% higher in the first trimester in order to be considered better. Clearly, first trimester maternal serum biochemistry and age together cannot achieve the detection rates of second trimester maternal serum biochemistry. Indeed it is questionable whether NT in conjunction with maternal age can achieve any better detection than first trimester maternal serum biochemistry. Fortunately, NT and maternal serum biochemical markers in the first trimester are not correlated (10), and a much more effective screening program can be obtained by combining both screening modalities together either in a one-stop clinic (OSCAR) (42–47) or delivered in a sequential screening program (48). The benefits of screening at the point of care (OSCAR) have been outlined (43,44).

MODELED AND ACHIEVABLE PERFORMANCE IN STUDIES OF MATERNAL SERUM BIOCHEMISTRY WITH NT

A retrospective study of 210 cases of trisomy 21 and approximately 1000 controls showed that the combined approach could achieve a detection rate of 89% for a 5% false-positive rate (10). Other studies using modeling or observed data have also shown that the combined approach can achieve detection rates of the order of 85% (26,48–53). In addition to cases with trisomy 21, combined screening can identify pregnancies complicated by trisomy 13 (15), trisomy 18 (12), Turner's syndrome and other sex aneuploidies (16), and triploidy types I and II (17). It is expected that 90% of these other chromosomal anomalies can be identified for an additional 1% false-positive rate.

In prospective screening in two OSCAR clinics over a 5-year period (46,47) that screened over 45,000 women, a detection rate of 92% (145/158) was achieved for trisomy 21 with a further 107 other aneuploidies identified for a total screen positive rate of 5.3% (44). Similarly, in a sequential prospective screening program (54), 93% of cases with trisomy 21 were identified with a false-positive rate of 5.9%, and 96% (25/26) of other anomalies identified for an overall false-positive rate of 6.3%.

SAMPLE COLLECTION CONDITIONS

Consideration should be given to preanalytical variables that can affect the maternal serum biochemical markers. Free β-hCG stability at room temperature was originally queried based on anecdotal evidence of the thermal degradation of intact hCG leading to elevated levels of the free β subunit. Accelerated thermal degradation studies have shown that serum intact hCG is stable for up to 70 hours at room temperature, although the free β-hCG levels can increase in whole blood after 36 hours at room temperature (55). Others have also shown that such limitations have no impact on screening performance (56–58). Provided samples are transported as serum, then stability is not an issue. We recommend to all our outlying hospitals and clients that serum samples should not take longer than 72 hours to reach the laboratory (unless sent refrigerated), and that whole blood should be with us within 36 hours. The transport of samples as whole blood filter paper spots has also been shown to be a reliable alternative (51,55).

Blood collection tube type is also known to influence measured PAPP-A levels (59). Samples collected as heparinized plasma and citrated plasma all had significantly lower values than samples collected as native serum, while those collected as ethylenediaminetetraacetic acid plasma had dramatically reduced levels. Levels of free β-hCG were not affected. Serum is thus the medium of choice for first trimester biochemical screening.

COVARIABLES

A range of factors is known to affect the biochemical marker levels and some of these factors may have a sufficiently large effect to warrant some form of correction. Correction for such variables aims to reduce the spread of the normal and affected populations, thus leading to a smaller overlap of the gaussian distributions and hence improvement in detection rate or reduction of false-positive rate. In many instances, although correcting for these covariables by themselves will have little impact on population detection rates, they can be quite significant for the individual and result in significantly different individual risks, which in turn may lead to different clinical interventions.

Gestational Age

Nearly all maternal serum marker levels vary with gestational age. As noted previously, comparison of levels at different gestations is achieved by conversion of the marker concentration to a MoM. However, the precision of this estimate depends upon the accuracy of the gestational estimate—whether this be derived from the last menstrual period or more preferably from an ultrasound assessment of fetal maturity. With the first trimester markers, free β-hCG levels rise to a peak at around 9 weeks and then fall, while PAPP-A levels increase in a fairly linear fashion (Fig. 3).

Maternal Weight

Maternal serum biochemical markers have a tendency to be lower than normal in women with maternal weights larger than normal and conversely tend to be higher

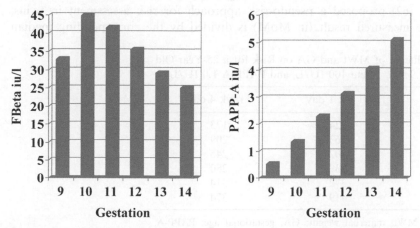

Figure 3   Gestational age variation of free β-hCG and PAPP-A in the first trimester.

than normal in women with lower than average maternal weight. This phenomenon is due to the fact that in women of larger weight the circulating blood volume is greater than normal, hence the placenta producing markers at the normal rate will result in the marker being diluted in a larger blood volume. In smaller women, with a lower blood volume, the effect is to concentrate the marker level. Correction for maternal weight can be made by dividing the result in MoM by the expected value for the weight based on a regression curve. Regression curves can be of two types, either a linear regression method (60) or a reciprocal regression procedure. In the first trimester both methods are seen to fit the data reasonably well, with perhaps the linear regression procedure having a slightly better fit to the data.

The importance to an individual of taking maternal weight into account is shown in Table 5, which also shows the importance of accurate dating in calculating risk. In most risk algorithms if no weight is given, the algorithm uses the average pregnancy population weight, which in Europe is around 69 kg. Thus, if the mother is 55 kg rather than 69 kg, the risk she will be given in this example is close to 1:280 when it should be 1:224, but if she were a 120-kg woman, then her risk should have been 1:419, changing her from high risk to low risk.

Multiple Pregnancy

Several complex issues are associated with screening for chromosomal anomalies in twin pregnancies, namely: how to interpret the marker values, the paucity of data in abnormal affected pregnancies when the fetuses are either concordant or discordant for an anomaly, the dilemmas regarding which invasive test to offer, the perceived increased risk of such procedures in twins, the technical difficulties of ensuring fetal tissue is obtained from each fetus, the need to ensure each fetus can be clearly differentiated at a later date, and finally, the difficulties of clinical management of fetal reduction and potential risk to the unaffected co-twin. These concerns form the basis of arguments that screening in twins poses such a serious clinical, ethical, and moral dilemma that it should be discouraged. Despite such reservations, screening programs for twin pregnancies have been successfully implemented in both the second and first trimesters, in units that have strong links with specialized fetal medicine centers (61).

The biochemical markers in twin pregnancies are on average twice that in normal singleton pregnancies. In a summary of the world literature, the median MoM PAPP-A in 707 cases was 1.826 and for free β-hCG was 2.035 from 825 cases (61). Wald et al. (62) proposed a pseudo-risk approach for risk assessment in twins, whereby the measured result (in MoM) is divided by the corresponding median

Table 5 Influence of MWt and GA on Risk for a 25-Year-Old with NT of 1.9 mm, FBeta 100 IU/L, and PAPP-A 1.0 IU/L

MWt (kg)	11 wk 1 day	11 wk 4 day
55	224	173
65	263	209
75	302	245
85	339	280
95	372	314
120	419	374

Abbreviations: MWt, maternal weight; GA, gestational age; PAPP-A, pregnancy-associated plasma protein A.

MoM value found in twin pregnancies and treating the risk calculation as for a singleton pregnancy. Although such an approach leads to lower detection rates in twins (compared to singleton pregnancies), it is thought to be a valuable procedure in the second trimester (63–65). In the first trimester it is predicted that adding in twin biochemistry correction will improve the detection rate by NT alone from 75% to 80%—some 10% less than achieved in singleton pregnancies (66). In prospective practice, this does seem to also be achievable (67,68). However, the median MoM twin-corrected free β-hCG was only 1.39 in 19 cases discordant for trisomy 21 while that for PAPP-A was 0.56 (61). When chorionicity or zygosity is considered, there does appear to be measurable differences in the marker levels, particularly for PAPP-A, which appear 10% lower in monochorionic twins (69). Further studies are needed to confirm these differences. It remains to be seen whether screening in twins in the first trimester is more widely accepted using ultrasound alone or ultrasound in combination with maternal serum biochemistry. Little data are available in higher order multiple pregnancies.

Insulin-Dependent Diabetes Mellitus

In the second trimester, women with insulin-dependent diabetes mellitus (IDDM) were shown to have reduced levels of AFP, and correction for this was considered appropriate by dividing the measured MoM by the median MoM observed in IDDM pregnancies. The validity of such correction is now questioned, since more recent data show that in women with IDDM, the difference is much smaller, and it has been suggested that this is because of improved diabetic control in patients over the past 25 years. For first trimester markers, there is very little evidence to support the need for correction. Levels of PAPP-A were shown to be reduced in IDDM mothers in one study (70) and in those with pre-existing or gestational diabetes free β-hCG was reduced by 20% and PAPP-A by 25% (71). In another smaller study (72), both free β-hCG and PAPP-A levels were 14% lower in women with gestational diabetes. If such reductions are confirmed in other studies, then it may be necessary to make correction in women with IDDM.

Fetal Sex

In the second trimester of pregnancy, free β-hCG levels are around 7% higher in women carrying a female fetus (73). In the first trimester, levels in normal pregnancies are 15% higher in the presence of a female fetus and 11% higher in the presence of female fetuses with trisomy 21, while PAPP-A levels were 10% and 13% higher (74). The potential impact of such changes would be a reduction in the detection rate in female fetuses of the order of 1–2% (74). To make correction for such sex differences would require an accurate method of sex determination at the 11- to 14-week scan, ultrasound at best can only provide a 75% level of accuracy at this time.

Assisted Conception

An important point to remember when estimating risks in in vitro fertilization (IVF) pregnancies is that in cases where a donor egg is used, the prior risk should be based on the maternal age of the donor at the time of egg collection rather than the recipient's age.

First trimester marker levels have been investigated in a few studies. The general consensus is that in IVF pregnancies, free β-hCG was increased by about 14% (75), while PAPP-A was reduced by some 8%, although other smaller studies have not confirmed this. In a small number of cases having intracytoplasmic sperm injection, PAPP-A levels were 20% lower. The overall impact of such changes has been estimated to increase the false-positive rate in the IVF group by around 1%. Further studies are needed to make secure correction factors by which to reduce the false-positive rate and potential invasive testing rate in this important group of individuals.

Ethnicity

When maternal weight is taken into account, in the second trimester it has been reported that free β-hCG levels are 12% higher in Afro-Caribbean women than in Caucasians, and in Asian and Oriental women, levels are also known to be higher. In the first trimester in one study (76), weight-corrected free β-hCG levels were 21% higher and PAPP-A 57% higher in Afro-Caribbean women than in Caucasians. In Asian women the levels were 4% higher for free β-hCG and 17% higher for PAPP-A. Such large differences, if confirmed in other studies and other ethnic groups, would seriously warrant correction. Watt et al. (77) have proposed a method of correcting for ethnicity in the second trimester which could be applied in the first trimester (76).

Smoking

In the second trimester of pregnancy, maternal cigarette smoking has been shown to influence the levels of maternal serum biochemical markers. In unaffected pregnancies, smoking is associated with a mean increase in serum AFP (4%) and inhibin A (45–62%) and a decrease in unconjugated estriol (3%), total hCG (24%), and free β-hCG. On the whole, the limited data in pregnancies with Down syndrome suggest a similar level of change. On the whole, correcting for smoking status by dividing the measured MoM by that found in a group of smokers results in a reduction in the false-positive rate of less than 1%. In the first trimester, preliminary data suggested that PAPP-A levels in smokers were reduced by 15% but were unaltered for free β-hCG in normal pregnancies (78) and were perhaps reduced by 13% in pregnancies with Down syndrome with PAPP-A being 6% higher (79). A much extended study of nearly 30,000 nonsmokers and 4000 smokers has shown that free β-hCG levels in unaffected pregnancies are reduced by 3% while PAPP-A is reduced by 18% (80). Furthermore, it has been demonstrated that this effect does not seem to be related to the number of cigarettes smoked (80). The false-positive rate when screening using first-trimester biochemistry and age alone or in combination with NT was shown to be 0.7–1.5% higher than in the nonsmoking group, and after correction the rates in the two groups were the same (80).

Gravidity/Parity

In the second trimester, free β-hCG levels are decreased by a small amount with an increasing number of pregnancies (gravidity) or an increasing number of births (parity), but the effect is so small as to not warrant correction (81). In the first trimester, it also appears that gravidity or parity is associated with a small but progressive increase in both free β-hCG and PAPP-A. None of these small changes are significant or warrant correction (82).

Vaginal Bleeding

The presence of vaginal bleeding in early pregnancy may complicate the interpretation of screening results, partly because vaginal bleeding is often related to unfavorable pregnancy outcome, and low levels of PAPP-A and increased levels of free β-hCG are known to be associated with such adverse events. In a study of 253 cases, which reached term and who had early vaginal bleeding, the median free β-hCG was significantly higher (9%) than in 2077 cases with no vaginal bleeding, but levels of PAPP-A were not significantly different (3% higher) (83). In a similar but unpublished analysis of 89 cases with early vaginal bleeding and 1047 without, no statistically significant difference was observed, but levels of free β-hCG were increased by 8% and PAPP-A was decreased by 5% (72, unpublished data therein).

Previous Pregnancy Results

In women who have an increased second trimester Down syndrome risk in a first pregnancy, there is a fivefold greater chance of them also having an increased risk in a second or subsequent pregnancy (84). Between pregnancies, there is a significant correlation between the same marker in a subsequent pregnancy, and such association suggests that there are additional maternal or genetic factors influencing the levels of the serum markers. In the first trimester, a significant between-pregnancy correlation for free β-hCG ($r = 0.3976$) and PAPP-A ($r = 0.4371$) has been shown (85,86). The end result is that women who have an increased first-trimester risk of Down syndrome are two to three times more likely to repeat this event in their next pregnancy (85,86). Although the impact of correcting for previous results is unlikely to have more than a 1% improvement in population detection rates, some have argued that correction would be worthwhile (87), and others proposed methods for taking previous results into account (88).

Previous Trisomy

The risk for trisomies in women who have had a previous pregnancy with a trisomy is higher than that expected on the basis of age alone. One estimate for women with a previous Down syndrome pregnancy is the addition of 0.75% to the maternal and gestational age-related risk for Down syndrome. Similar corrections also apply for trisomies 18 and 13 (89). However, this assumes that the marker distributions are the same in women with and without a family history of aneuploidy. A recently published study provides evidence that this may not be the case (90). In this study of 375 women with a previous aneuploidy (303 with Down syndrome, 63 with Edwards' syndrome, and 9 with Patau's syndrome), in a subsequent pregnancy free β-hCG was significantly increased (10%) as was PAPP-A (15%). In the series with Edwards' syndrome if anything the increase was greater (25%) than with those with Down syndrome. Such difference may require correction.

DETECTION RATE AND FALSE-POSITIVE RATE BY MATERNAL AGE

One factor that is often overlooked in screening programs is the fact that detection rates and false-positive rates vary considerably with maternal age. In younger women the detection rate using second-trimester screening falls quite dramatically,

Table 6 Detection Rate and False-Positive Rates for Trisomy 21 in the First Trimester Combined Program and the Second Trimester Triple Test Program

Maternal age (yr)	First trimester		Second trimester	
	False-positive rate (%)	Detection rate (%)	False-positive rate (%)	Detection rate (%)
20	78.8	2.3	44.7	3.2
25	80.6	2.9	47.5	3.8
30	83.8	4.0	56.0	6.1
35	89.7	8.7	73.8	15.8
38	93.9	15.9	85.5	28.6
40	96.1	24.4	91.6	40.9
44	98.8	47.1	98.1	70.0

as does the false-positive rate. Screening programs that quote only global detection and false-positive rates could be misleading to patients. When counseling women on the test and its results, these issues need to be considered (91). Two studies have used modeling to calculate expected detection rates and false-positive rates at various maternal ages using either the second-trimester triple-marker approach (91) or the combined ultrasound and biochemical approaches in the first trimester (92). Table 6 summarizes these data. The odds of an increased risk result being Down is 1 in 55 in the second trimester compared with 1 in 29 in the first trimester in general population terms.

ADVERSE OUTCOME

In second-trimester screening, there are conflicting views on the relationship between biochemical marker levels and the incidence of adverse outcomes such as preeclampsia, intrauterine growth restriction (IUGR), low birth weight, preterm delivery, and stillbirth (93). An increased free β-hCG may be associated with an increased incidence of preeclampsia, but when examined in the first trimester, levels were not elevated in cases developing preeclampsia (71). Low levels of PAPP-A, however, were found to be associated with subsequent miscarriage, the development of pregnancy-induced hypertension, and growth restriction, although the authors concluded that the sensitivity and specificity of these were low and were not useful predictors of adverse outcome. Other studies have also shown this association between low levels of PAPP-A and IUGR or low birth weight (94–97) and one has found no evidence of this (98).

POTENTIAL FUTURE DEVELOPMENTS

One new and exciting ultrasound marker of aneuploidy is the observation of an absent nasal bone at the 11- to 14-week scan. The initial studies found an absent nasal bone in about 70% of fetuses with trisomy 21 and in 0.5% of normal fetuses (99). The findings in this preliminary study were confirmed in other smaller studies (100). An extension of the original study in 430 cases with an abnormal karyotype confirmed that the nasal bone was absent in 67% of cases with trisomy 21 and in 2.8% of cases with a normal karyotype. However, there were some differences in incidence between different ethnic groups and a relationship between crown–rump length and NT (101). One way in which this marker may be used in the future is to incorporate it into the existing first-trimester scan as part of the combined ultrasound and biochemistry screening at 11–14 weeks. Preliminary studies have shown (102) that absent nasal bone is not significantly correlated with the biochemical markers. Modeling would suggest that a detection rate of 97% could be achieved at a 5% false-positive rate. Alternatively, if one wanted to focus on reducing the invasive testing rate, then at a 0.5% false-positive rate, the detection rate would still be 90%.

Other biochemical markers may have a role to play in the future. ADAM 12, a metalloprotease which cleaves IGF–binding proteins 3 and 5, has been recently shown to be such a potential new marker (103). In this one study, levels of ADAM 12 were 0.14 MoM in early first-trimester cases with Down syndrome, and a project detection rate using this marker alone with maternal age gave an 81.5% detection at a 3.2% false-positive rate, and combined with NT, PAPP-A, and free β-hCG, a detection rate of 94.1% at a 1.5% false-positive rate.

Another area of potential for the future is the developments associated with the isolation and quantitation of fetal DNA (104–106) or placental mRNA (107–110) in maternal serum/plasma. Whether such techniques become viable as alternatives to invasive diagnostic procedures or whether they may be used as adjuncts to existing ultrasound and biochemical screening techniques, remains to be established.

REFERENCES

1. Egan JF, Benn P, Borgida AF, Rodis JF, Campbell WA, Vintzileos AM. Efficacy of screening for fetal Down syndrome in the United States from 1974 to 1997. Obstet Gynecol 2000; 96:979–985.
2. Snijders RJM, Sebire NJ, Nicolaides KH. Maternal age and gestational age specific risks for chromosomal defects. Fetal Diagn Ther 1995; 10:356–357.
3. Royal College of Obstetricians and Gynaecologists. Recommendations arising from the 32nd Study Group: screening for Down syndrome in the first trimester. In: Grudzinskas JG, Ward RHT, eds. Screening for Down Syndrome in the First Trimester. London: RCOG Press, 1997:353–356.
4. Reynolds TM, Penney MD. The mathematical basis of multivariate risk screening: with special reference to screening for Down's syndrome associated pregnancy. Ann Clin Biochem 1990; 27:452–458.
5. Cuckle H. Time for a total shift to first trimester screening for Down's syndrome. Lancet 2001; 358:1658–1659.
6. Lawson HW, Frye A, Atrash HK, Smith JC, Shilman HB, Ramick M. Abortion mortality, United States, 1972–1987. Am J Obstet Gynecol 1994; 171:1365–1372.
7. Wright D, Reynolds T, Donovan C. Assessment of atypicality: an adjunct to screening for Down syndrome that facilitates detection of other chromosomal defects. Ann Clin Biochem 1993; 30:578–583.
8. Cole LA. Immunoassays of human chorionic gonadotropin, its free subunits, and metabolism. Clin Chem 1997; 43:2233–2243.
9. Spencer K, Macri JN, Aitken DA, Connor JM. Free beta hCG as a first trimester marker for fetal trisomy. Lancet 1992; 339:1480.
10. Spencer K, Souter V, Tul N, Snijders R, Nicolaides KH. A screening program for trisomy 21 at 10–14 weeks using fetal nuchal translucency, maternal serum free β-human

chorionic gonadotropin and pregnancy associated plasma protein-A. Ultrasound Obstet Gynecol 1999; 13:231–237.

11. Spencer K, Berry E, Crossley JA, Aitken DA, Nicolaides KH. Is maternal serum total hCG a marker of trisomy 21 in the first trimester of pregnancy? Prenat Diagn 2000; 20:635–639.

12. Tul N, Spencer K, Noble P, Chan C, Nicolaides K. Screening for trisomy 18 by fetal nuchal translucency and maternal serum free β-hCG and PAPP-A at 10–14 weeks of gestation. Prenat Diagn 1999; 19:1035–1042.

13. Spencer K, Mallard AS, Coombes EJ, Macri JN. Prenatal screening for trisomy 19 with free beta human chorionic gonadotropin as a marker. Br Med J 1993; 307:1455–1458.

14. Spencer K, Heath V, Flack N, Ong C, Nicolaides KH. First trimester maternal serum AFP and total hCG in aneuploides other than trisomy 21. Prenat Diagn 2000; 20:635–639.

15. Spencer K, Ong C, Skentou H, Liao AW, Nicolaides KH. Screening for trisomy 13 by fetal nuchal translucency and maternal serum free β-hCG and PAPP-A at 10–14 weeks of gestation. Prenat Diagn 2000; 20:411–416.

16. Spencer K, Tul N, Nicolaides KH. Maternal serum free β-hCG and PAPP-A in fetal sex chromosome defects in the first trimester. Prenat Diagn 2000; 20:390–394.

17. Spencer K, Liao AWJ, Skentou H, Cicero S, Nicolaides KH. Screening for triploidy by fetal nuchal translucency and maternal serum β-hCG and PAPP-A at 10–14 weeks of gestation. Prenat Diagn 2000; 20:495–499.

18. Oxvig C, Sand O, Kristensen T, Kristensen L, Sottrup-Jensen L. Isolation and characterisation of a circulating complex between human pregnancy associated plasma protein-A and proform of eosinophil major basic protein. Biochem Biophys Acta 1994; 1201:415–423.

19. Lawrence JB, Oxvig C, Overgaard MT, et al. The insulin-like growth factor (IGF)-dependent IGF binding protein-4 protease secreted by human fibroblasts is pregnancy associated plasma protein-A. Proc Natl Acad Sci USA 1999; 96:3149–3153.

20. Brambati B, Lanzani A, Tului L. Ultrasound and biochemical assessment of first trimester pregnancy. In: Chapman M, Grudzinskas JG, Chard T, eds. The Embryo: Normal and Abnormal Development and Growth. New York: Springer-Verlag, 1991:181–194.

21. Spencer K, Crossley JA, Aitken DA, Nix ABJ, Dunstan FDJ, Williams K. Temporal changes in maternal serum biochemical markers of trisomy 21 across the first and second trimester of pregnancy. Ann Clin Biochem 2002; 39:567–576.

22. Spencer K, Crossley JA, Aitken DA, Nix ABJ, Dunstan FDJ, Williams K. The effect of temporal variation in biochemical markers of trisomy 21 across the first and second trimesters of pregnancy on the estimation of individual patient specific risks and detection rates for Down's syndrome. Ann Clin Biochem 2003; 40:219–231.

23. Spencer K, Crossley JA, Green K, Worthington DJ, Brownbill K, Aitken DA. Second trimester levels of pregnancy associated plasma protein-A in cases of trisomy 18. Prenat Diagn 1999; 19:1127–1134.

24. Muller F, Sault C, Lemay C, Roussel-Mizon N, Forestier F, Frendo JL. Second trimester two step trisomy 18 screening using maternal serum markers. Prenat Diagn 2002; 22:605–608.

25. Spencer K, Nicolaides KH. A first trimester trisomy 13/trisomy 18 risk algorithm combining fetal nuchal translucency thickness, maternal serum free β-hCG and PAPP-A. Prenat Diagn 2002; 22:877–879.

26. Cuckle HS, van Lith JMM. Appropriate biochemical parameters in first trimester screening for Down syndrome. Prenat Diagn 1999; 19:505–512.

27. Berry E, Aitken DA, Crossley JA, Macri JN, Connor JM. Screening for Down syndrome: changes in marker levels and detection rates between first and second trimesters. Br J Obstet Gynaecol 1997; 104:811–817.

28. Macri JN, Kasturi RV, Krantz DA, et al. Maternal serum Down syndrome screening: free beta protein is a more effective marker than human chorionic gonadotropin. Am J Obstet Gynecol 1990; 163:1248–1253.

29. Spencer K, Macri JN. Early detection of Down's syndrome using free beta human chor-iogonadotropin. Ann Clin Biochem 1992; 29:349–350.

30. Spencer K, Coombes EJ, Mallard AS, Ward AM. Free beta human choriogonadotro-phin in Down's syndrome screening: a multicentre study of its role compared with other biochemical markers. Ann Clin Biochem 1992; 29:506–518.

31. Spencer K, Coombes EJ, Mallard AS, Ward AM. Use of free β-hCG in Down's syndrome screening. Ann Clin Biochem 1993; 30:515–518.

32. Spencer K, Macri JN, Anderson RW, et al. Dual analyte immunoassay in neural tube defect and Down's syndrome screening; results of a multicentre clinical trial. Ann Clin Biochem 1993; 30:394–401.

33. Spencer K. Second trimester prenatal screening for Down's syndrome using alpha-fetoprotein and free beta hCG: a seven year review. Br J Obstet Gynaecol 1999; 106: 1287–1293.

34. Wald NJ, Cuckle HS, Densem JW, et al. Maternal serum screening for Down's syndrome in early pregnancy. Br Med J 1988; 297:883–888.

35. Wald NJ, Kennard A, Hackshaw A, Mcguire A. Antenatal screening for Down's syndrome. Health Technol Assess 1998; 2(whole issue).

36. Wald NJ, Rodeck C, Hackshaw AK, Walters J, Chitty L, Mackinson AM. First tri-mester and second trimester antenatal screening for Down's syndrome: the results of the Serum, Urine and Ultrasound Screening Study (SURUSS). Health Technol Assess 2003; 7(whole issue).

37. Dunstan FDJ, Nix ABJ. Screening for Down's syndrome: the effect of test date on the detection rate. Ann Clin Biochem 1998; 35:57–61.

38. Bray IC, Wright DE. Estimating the spontaneous loss of Down syndrome fetuses between the time of chorionic villus sampling, amniocentesis and livebirth. Prenat Diagn 1998; 18:1045–1054.

39. Spencer K. What is the true fetal loss rate in pregnancies affected by trisomy 21 and how does this influence whether first trimester detection rates are superior to those in the sec-ond trimester? Prenat Diagn 2001; 21:788–789.

40. Andersen AMN, Wohlfart J, Christens P, Olsen J, Melbye M. Maternal age and fetal loss: population based register linkage study. Br Med J 2000; 320:1708–1712.

41. Morris JK, Wald NJ, Watt HC. Fetal loss in Down syndrome pregnancies. Prenat Diagn 1999; 19:142–145.

42. Spencer K. Near patient testing and Down's syndrome screening. Proc UK NEQAS 1998; 3:130.

43. Spencer K. Point of care screening for chromosomal anomalies in the first trimester of pregnancy. Clin Chem 2002; 48:403–404.

44. Spencer K. Screening at the point of care: Down syndrome—a case study. In: Price CP, St John A, Hicks JM, eds. Point of Care Testing. Washington: AACC Press, 2004: 333–339.

45. Spencer K, Spencer CE, Power M, Moakes A, Nicolaides KH. One stop clinic for assessment of risk for fetal anomalies: a report of the first year of prospective screening for chromosomal anomalies in the first trimester. Br J Obstet Gynaecol 2000; 107: 1271–1275.

46. Spencer K, Spencer CE, Power M, Dawson C, Nicolaides KH. Screening for chromo-somal abnormalities in the first trimester using ultrasound and maternal serum biochemistry in a one stop clinic: a review of three years prospective experience. Br J Obstet Gynaecol 2003; 110:281–286.

47. Bindra R, Heath V, Liao A, Spencer K, Nicolaides KH. One stop clinic for assessment of risk for trisomy 21 at 11–14 weeks: a prospective study of 15,030 pregnancies. Ultra-sound Obstet Gynecol 2002; 20:219–225.

48. Crossley JA, Aitken DA, Cameron AD, McBride E, Connor JM. Combined ultrasound and biochemical screening for Down's syndrome in the first trimester: a Scottish multi-centre study. Br J Obstet Gynaecol 2002; 109:667–676.

49. Wald NJ, Hackshaw AK. Combining ultrasound and biochemistry in first trimester screening for Down's syndrome. Prenat Diagn 1997; 17:821–829.

50. de Graaf IM, Prjkrt E, Bilardo CM, Leschot NJ, Cuckle HS, van Lith JMM. Early pregnancy screening for fetal aneuploidy with serum markers and nuchal translucency. Prenat Diagn 1999; 19:458–462.

51. Krantz DA, Hallahan TW, Orlandi F, Buchanan P, Larsen JW, Macri JN. First trimester Down syndrome screening using dried blood biochemistry and nuchal translucency. Obstet Gynecol 2000; 96:207–213.

52. Wapner R, Thom E, Simpson JL, et al. First trimester screening for trisomies 21 and 18. N Engl J Med 2003; 349:1405–1413.

53. Muller F, Benattar C, Audibert F, Roussel N, Dreux S, Cuckle H. First trimester screening for Down syndrome in France combining nuchal translucency measurement and biochemical markers. Prenat Diagn 2003; 23:833–836.

54. Stenhouse EJ, Crossley JA, Aitken DA, Brogan K, Cameron AD, Connor JM. First trimester combined ultrasound and biochemical screening for Down's syndrome in routine clinical practice. Prenat Diagn 2004; 24:774–780.

55. Spencer K, Macri JN, Carpenter P, Anderson R, Krantz DA. Stability of intact hCG in serum, liquid whole blood and dried whole blood filter paper spots and its impact on free beta hCG Down's syndrome screening. Clin Chem 1993; 39:1064–1068.

56. Cuckle HS, Jones RG. Maternal serum free beta human chorionic gonadotrophin level: the effect of sample transportation. Ann Clin Biochem 1994; 31:97–98.

57. Cuckle HS, Jones RG. Posting serum free beta human chorionic gonadotrophin testing. Prenat Diagn 1995; 15:879–880.

58. Muller F, Doche C, Ngo S, et al. Stability of free beta subunit in routine practice for trisomy 21 maternal serum screening. Prenat Diagn 1999; 19:85–86.

59. Spencer K. The influence of different sample collection types on the levels of markers used for Down's syndrome screening as measured by the Kryptor immunoassay system. Ann Clin Biochem 2003; 40:166–168.

60. Spencer K, Bindra R, Nicolaides KH. Maternal weight correction of maternal serum PAPP-A and free β-hCG MoM when screening for trisomy 21 in the first trimester of pregnancy. Prenat Diagn 2003; 23:851–855.

61. Spencer K. Non-invasive screening tests. In: Blickstein I, Keith L, eds. Multiple pregnancy: epidemiology, gestation and perinatal outcome. London: Parthenon, 2005:368–384.

62. Wald NJ, Cuckle HS, Wu T, George L. Maternal serum unconjugated estriol and human chorionic gonadotrophin levels in twin pregnancies: implications for screening for Down's syndrome. Br J Obstet Gynaecol 1991; 98:905–908.

63. Spencer K, Salonen R, Muller F. Down's syndrome screening in multiple pregnancies using α-fetoprotein and free β-hCG. Prenat Diagn 1994; 14:537–542.

64. Neveux LM, Palomaki GE, Knight GJ, Haddow JE. Multiple marker screening for Down syndrome in twin pregnancies. Prenat Diagn 1996; 16:29–35.

65. Muller F, Dreux S, Dupoizat H, et al. Second trimester Down syndrome maternal serum screening in twin pregnancies: impact of chorionicity. Prenat Diagn 2003; 23:331–335.

66. Spencer K. Screening for trisomy 21 in twin pregnancies in the first trimester using free β-hCG and PAPP-A, combined with fetal nuchal translucency thickness. Prenat Diagn 200; 20:91–95.

67. Spencer K, Nicolaides KH. First trimester prenatal diagnosis of trisomy 21 in discordant twins using fetal nuchal translucency thickness and maternal serum free β-hCG and PAPP-A. Prenat Diagn 2000; 20:683–684.

68. Spencer K, Nicolaides KH. Screening for trisomy 21 in twins using first trimester ultrasound and maternal serum biochemistry in a one stop clinic: a review of three years' experience. Br J Obstet Gynaecol 2003; 110:276–280.

69. Spencer K. Screening for trisomy 21 in twin pregnancies in the first trimester: does chorionicity impact on maternal serum free β-hCG or PAPP-A levels. Prenat Diagn 2001; 21:715–717.

70. Pedersen JF, Sorensen S, Molsted-Pedersen L. Serum levels of human placental lactogen, pregnancy associated plasma protein A and endometrial secretory protein PP14 in first trimester of diabetic pregnancy. Acta Obstet Gynecol Scand 1998; 77: 155–158.

71. Ong CYT, Liao AW, Spencer K, Munim S, Nicolaides KH. First trimester maternal serum β-human chorionic gonadotrophin and pregnancy associated plasma protein A as predictors of pregnancy complications. Br J Obstet Gynaecol 2000; 107:1265–1270.

72. Tul N, Pusenjak S, Osredkar J, Spencer K, Novak-Antolic Z. Predicting complications of pregnancy with first trimester maternal serum free β-hCG, PAPP-A and inhibin-A. Prenat Diagn 2003; 23:990–996.

73. Spencer K. The influence of fetal sex in screening for Down syndrome in the second trimester using AFP and free β-hCG. Prenat Diagn 2000; 20:648–651.

74. Spencer K, Ong CYT, Liao AWJ, Papademetriou D, Nicolaides KH. The influence of fetal sex in screening for trisomy 21 by fetal nuchal translucency, maternal serum free β-hCG and PAPP-A at 10–14 weeks of gestation. Prenat Diagn 2000; 20:673–675.

75. Liao AW, Heath V, Kametas N, Spencer K, Nicolaides KH. First trimester screening for trisomy 21 in singleton pregnancies achieved by assisted reproduction. Hum Reprod 2001; 16:1501–1504.

76. Spencer K, Ong CYT, Liao AWJ, Nicolaides KH. The influence of ethnic origin on first trimester biochemical markers of chromosomal abnormalities. Prenat Diagn 2000; 20:491–494.

77. Watt HC, Wald NJ, Smith D, Kennard A, Densem J. Effect of allowing for ethnic group in prenatal screening for Down's syndrome. Prenat Diagn 1996; 16:691–698.

78. Spencer K. The influence of smoking on maternal serum PAPP-A and free beta hCG levels in the first trimester of pregnancy. Prenat Diagn 1999; 19:1065–1066.

79. Spencer K, Ong CYT, Liao AWJ, Papademetriou D, Nicolaides KH. First trimester markers of trisomy 21 and the influence of maternal cigarette smoking status. Prenat Diagn 2000; 20:852–853.

80. Spencer K, Bindra R, Cacho AM, Nicolaides KH. The impact of correcting for smoking status when screening for chromosomal anomalies using maternal serum biochemistry and fetal nuchal translucency thickness in the first trimester of pregnancy. Prenat Diagn 2004; 24:169–173.

81. Spencer K, Ong CYT, Liao AWJ, Nicolaides KH. The influence of parity and gravidity on first trimester markers of chromosomal abnormality. Prenat Diagn 2000; 20:792–794.

82. Spencer K. The influence of gravidity on Down's syndrome screening with free beta hCG. Prenat Diagn 1995; 15:343–346.

83. De Baisio P, Canini S, Crovo A, Prefumo F, Venturini PL. Early vaginal bleeding and first trimester markers for Down syndrome. Prenat Diagn 2003; 23:470–473.

84. Spencer K. Between pregnancy biological variability of maternal serum alpha fetoprotein and free beta hCG: implications for Down syndrome screening in subsequent pregnancies. Prenat Diagn 1997; 17:39–45.

85. Spencer K. Between pregnancy biological variability of first trimester markers of Downs syndrome: implications for screening in subsequent pregnancies. Prenat Diagn 2001; 21:445–447.

86. Spencer K. Between pregnancy biological variability of first trimester markers of Down syndrome and the implications for screening in subsequent pregnancies: an issue revisited. Prenat Diagn 2002; 22:874–876.

87. Larsen SO, Christiansen M, Norgaard-Pedersen B. Inclusion of marker measurements from a previous pregnancy improves Down syndrome screening performance. Prenat Diagn 1998; 18:706–712.

88. Wald NJ, Huttly WJ, Rudnicka AR. Prenatal screening for Down syndrome: the problem of recurrent false-positives. Prenat Diagn 2004; 24:389–392.

89. Nicolaides KH, Sebire NJ, Snijders RJM. The 11–14 Week Scan. In: The Diagnosis of Fetal Abnormalities. London: Parthenon, 1999:11–13.

90. Cuckle HS, Spencer K, Nicolaides KH. Down's syndrome screening marker levels in women with a previous aneuploidy pregnancy. Prenat Diagn 2005; 25:47–50.

91. Reynolds TM, Nix AB, Dunstan FD, Dawson AJ. Age-specific detection and false positive rates: an aid to counseling in Down's syndrome risk screening. Obstet Gynecol 1993; 81:447–450.

92. Spencer K. Age related detection and false positive rates when screening for Down's syndrome in the first trimester using fetal nuchal translucency and maternal serum free β-hCG and PAPP-A. Br J Obstet Gynaecol 2001; 108:1043–1046.

93. Spencer K. Second trimester prenatal screening for Down syndrome and the relationship of maternal serum biochemical markers to pregnancy complication with adverse outcome. Prenat Diagn 2000; 20:652–656.

94. Pedersen JF, Sorensen S, Ruge S. Human placental lactogen and pregnancy associated plasma protein A in the first trimester and subsequent fetal growth. Acta Obstet Gynecol Scand 1995; 74:505–508.

95. Smith GCS, Stenhouse EJ, Crossley JA, Aitken DA, Cameron AD, Connor JM. Early pregnancy levels of pregnancy associated plasma protein A and the risk of intrauterine growth restriction, premature birth, preeclampsia, and stillbirth. J Clin Endocrinol Metab 2002; 87:1762–1767.

96. Smith GCS, Stenhouse EJ, Crossley JA, Aitken DA, Cameron AD, Connor JM. Early pregnancy origins of low birth weight. Nature 2002; 417:916.

97. Yaron Y, Heifetz S, Ochshorn Y, Lehavi O, Orr-Urteger A. Decreased first trimester PAPP-A is a predictor of adverse outcome. Prenat Diagn 2002; 22:778–782.

98. Morssink LP, Kornman LH, Hallahan TW, et al. Maternal serum levels of free beta-hCG and PAPP-A in the first trimester of pregnancy are not associated with subsequent fetal growth retardation or preterm delivery. Prenat Diagn 1998; 18:147–152.

99. Cicero S, Curcio P, Papegeorghiou A, Sonek J, Nicolaides KH. Absence of nasal bone in fetuses with trisomy 21 at 11–14 weeks of gestation: an observational study. Lancet 2001; 358:1665–1667.

100. Sonek J. Nasal bone evaluation with ultrasonography: a marker for fetal aneuploidy. Ultrasound Obstet Gynecol 2003; 22:11–15.

101. Cicero S, Longo D, Rembouskos G, Sacchini C, Nicolaides KH. Absent nasal bone at 11–14 weeks of gestation and chromosome defects. Ultrasound Obstet Gynecol 2003; 22:135–137.

102. Cicero S, Bindra R, Rembouskos G, Spencer K, Nicolaides KH. Integrated ultrasound and biochemical screening for trisomy 21 at 11–14 weeks. Prenat Diagn 2003; 23:306–310.

103. Laigaard J, Sorensen T, Frohlich C, et al. ADAM 12: a novel first-trimester maternal serum marker for Down syndrome. Prenat Diagn 2003; 23:1086–1091.

104. Lo YMD, Lau TK, Zhang J, et al. Increased fetal DNA concentrations in the plasma of pregnant women carrying fetuses with trisomy 21. Clin Chem 1999; 45:1747–1751.

105. Yan Zhong X, Burk MR, Troeger C, Jackson LR, Holsgreve W, Hahn S. Fetal DNA in maternal plasma is elevated in pregnancies with aneuploid fetuses. Prenat Diagn 2000; 20:795–798.

106. Spencer K, de Kok JB, Swinkels DW. Increased total cell-free DNA in the serum of pregnant women carrying a fetus affected by trisomy 21. Prenat Diagn 2003; 23:560–583.

107. Poon LL, Leung TN, Lau TK, Lo YMD. Presence of fetal mRNA in maternal plasma. Clin Chem 2000; 46:1832–1834.

108. Ng EKO, Tsui MBY, Lau TK, et al. mRNA of placental origin is readily detectable in maternal plasma. Proc Natl Acad Sci USA 2003; 100:4748–4753.

109. Oudejans CBM, Go ATJJ, Visser A, Mulders MAM, Westerman BA, Blankenstein MA, van Vugt JMG. Detection of chromosome 21 encoded mRNA of placental origin in maternal plasma. Clin Chem 2002; 49:1445–1449.

110. Ng EKO, El-Sheikhah A, Chiu RWK, et al. Evaluation of human chorionic gonadotropin β-subunit mRNA concentrations in maternal serum in aneuploidy pregnancies: a feasibility study. Clin Chem 2004; 50:1055–1057.

2

Maternal Serum Screening for Down Syndrome

Françoise Muller
Laboratoire de Biochimie Hormonale, Hôpital Robert Debré, Université Paris Ile-de-France-Ouest, Paris, France

Marc Dommergues
Service de Gynécologie Obstétrique, Hôpital Pitié-Salpêtrière, AP-HP and Université Paris VI, Paris, France

INTRODUCTION

Over recent years, an ever increasing number of pregnant women have undergone Down syndrome screening based either on maternal serum markers (MSM) or on ultrasound, and a considerable amount of scientific literature has been published on the subject. However, one should bear in mind that screening for Down syndrome is by no means mandatory. Many women do not wish to undergo prenatal screening for trisomy 21, and would not consider terminating the pregnancy of an affected baby. Although it is accepted that women should be made aware of the existence of screening, their ethical positions should be respected while offering MSM screening. Besides, it would be unfair to implement large-scale prenatal screening policies without also implementing voluntary policies facilitating the integration of trisomy 21–affected persons into society.

Down syndrome screening targets patients at increased risk of chromosomal abnormality. Unequivocal diagnosis is made by fetal karyotyping using samples of chorionic villi, amniotic cells or occasionally fetal blood. Till the mid-1980s, the only screening strategy was to offer amniocentesis to older women (35 or ≥38 years), since maternal age was the longest established chromosomal abnormality risk factor. Development of ultrasonography subsequently enabled detection of fetal malformations, thus opening the way to screening for chromosomal abnormalities in younger women. The identification of biochemical markers in maternal serum in the second trimester then extended Down syndrome screening to all pregnant women, regardless of their age and whether or not fetal malformations are visible by ultrasound.

PRINCIPLE

In maternal serum screening for Down syndrome, individual risk associated with age is corrected using a factor related to serum marker concentrations. The relation between MSM and Down syndrome was discovered fortuitously. In 1984, levels of maternal serum alpha-fetoprotein (AFP) were found to be lower in Down syndrome–affected pregnancies (1). In 1987 and 1988, hCG, its free β fraction, and unconjugated estriol (uE3) were also found to be valuable markers for Down syndrome (2–5). Various combinations of maternal age with one or more of these markers were suggested to improve their predictive value. In 1988, Wald proposed a risk calculation, which is now used in all software programs (6). Many other markers have been investigated since, but in practice the four original markers are widely used: total hCG, or free β-hCG, AFP, and/or uE3 (7) with on average, a fetal Down syndrome detection rate of 60%, for a 5% false-positive rate among women under 35 (7,8).

MATHEMATICAL BASIS OF THE CALCULATION OF DOWN SYNDROME RISK

Calculation of a mother's risk of a Down syndrome-affected pregnancy incorporates the age-related risk and the risk determined from serum marker levels. Several markers can be combined. It is also possible to take into account sonographic data such as nuchal translucency measurement, provided these factors are proven to be independent of one another

In practice, this risk is calculated using computer programs. The mathematical model is based on the comparison of two populations, one of women with a Down syndrome-affected pregnancy and another with a non-Down syndrome-affected child.

Establishing the Age-Related Risk

The age-related risk of delivering a baby affected by Down syndrome has been established by a number of observational studies (9). Using such age-related risk reference values in the computerized calculation of the trisomy 21–derived risk has the advantage of predicting the odds of delivering an affected liveborn. It has the disadvantage of underestimating the actual risk of bearing an affected child at the time of screening, due to the relatively high spontaneous fetal loss rate in trisomy 21–affected pregnancies. It is usually estimated that the risk of bearing an affected infant at midtrimester is 1.2-fold greater than the risk of delivering an affected liveborn (10). This has a practical consequence when choosing a cutoff. It is expected that a 1/250 cutoff taking into account the midtrimester risk is equivalent to a 1/300 cutoff when computing the risk at birth.

Multiple of Median

Levels of all serum markers vary during gestation. However, if expressed in multiple of median (MoM), the marker value no longer depends on gestational age. To express a serum marker value in MoM, a median value (or 50th percentile) must first be determined in a control population for various gestational ages. The median is more accurately defined when the number of controls is high. It is generally accepted that to establish MSM normal values, at least 300 patients are needed per week of gestation. The raw values for each marker are converted into MoM by dividing them by the median value at the same gestational age. Because serum markers expressed in MoMs follow a log normal distribution, their value is deemed low when under 0.5 MoM, high when above 2.5 MoM, and otherwise normal.

Likelihood Ratio

The likelihood ratio (Fig. 1) determined for each marker (expressed in MoM) is calculated based on the comparison of the distribution of a given marker in a control population and in a Down syndrome population. Maternal age-related risk is adjusted by multiplying it by the likelihood ratio determined for the marker, giving a new risk. If the markers are independent, the corresponding likelihood ratios can be multiplied.

A 1/300 to 1/250 risk cutoff is used in many countries to determine which patients should be offered amniocentesis.

Sensitivity, Specificity, and Positive Predictive Value

Down syndrome screening efficiency is assessed using two main criteria. Detection rate or sensitivity indicates the percentage of Down syndrome cases detected. Screen-positive rate (expressed in practice by 100-specificity) indicates the amniocentesis rate that would be produced by screening using a given risk cutoff. The false-positive rate is often used instead of the screen-positive rate, an approximation that is possible because of the low prevalence of Down syndrome. Screening efficiency is influenced by the choice of the cutoff used to decide whether to offer amniocentesis and maternal age distribution in the population.

In a given screening method, the detection rate and amniocentesis rate vary inversely and depend on the chosen cutoff. In patients under 35 years of age, a 1/250 cutoff allows a detection rate of 60% to 65%, at the cost of a 5% amniocentesis rate. If a 1/370 cutoff was used, the Down syndrome detection rate would be higher, but the number of resulting amniocenteses would also rise.

Because of the exponential increase in Down syndrome risk with maternal age, sensitivity and screen-positive rate are higher in older women (11).

Other criteria derived from the previous ones are used to define screening efficiency. Positive predictive value (PPV) is the percentage of infants with Down syndrome observed in women whose risk is above the cutoff. In practice, a balance is sought between the probability that amniocentesis will detect a chromosomal abnormality (PPV, approximately 1/100) and the risk of amniocentesis-related complications (iatrogenic risk, approximately 1/100 to 1/200) (12).

Theoretically, screening efficiency increases as more markers are tested. If the screen-positive rate is set at 5%, the detection rate ranges from 36% to 49% using a single marker combined with maternal age, but is 63% to 68% when four markers are used. However, variations in analytical efficiency for each marker may considerably attenuate this effect. For example, the coefficients of variation are around 5% for AFP, 3% for hCG or its free β-hCG fraction, but reach 10% to 20% for estriol. It may be preferable to use two well-controlled markers rather than four technically dubious ones.

Serum marker levels vary during pregnancy, particularly between 14 and 15 weeks of gestation: β-hCG falls from 25 ng/mL at 14 weeks to 18 ng/mL at 15 weeks; AFP rises from 22 to 27 IU/mL. For this reason, gestational age must be accurately determined by ultrasound (7).

FACTORS AFFECTING MSM LEVELS

Screening efficiency can be improved by taking into account factors that influence serum marker levels.

Maternal Weight

Concentrations of AFP, hCG, and uE3 vary with maternal weight. An increase of 20 kg reduces the level of AFP by approximately 17%, uE3 by 7%, and hCG

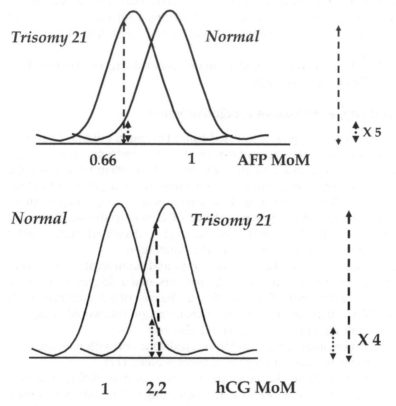

Figure 1 Distribution of maternal serum AFP and hCG (expressed in logarithm of MoM) in two groups of women, one with a Down syndrome–affected fetus, the other with an unaffected fetus. In the normal population, the median value is by definition equal to 1 MoM. In Down syndrome, AFP distribution is shifted toward low values and hCG distribution toward high values. In the example shown, the maternal serum concentrations were 0.66 MoM for AFP and 2.2 MoM for hCG. The software risk calculation is done by multiplying the age-related Down syndrome prevalence by the likelihood ratios generated by each marker. For a given value of a marker, the likelihood ratio is the ratio of the probability of having this concentration of marker while belonging to the trisomy 21–affected group to the probability of having the same concentration while belonging to the unaffected group. In the example, the likelihood ratio is 5 for AFP and 4 for hCG. If the patient is 20 years of age, the age-related risk is $1/1500$. Taking AFP alone into account, the patient's risk becomes $1/1500 \times 5 = 1/300$. Taking hCG alone into account, the risk becomes $1/1500 \times 4 = 1/375$. Taking into account AFP and hCG yields a risk of $1/1500 \times 4 \times 5 = 1/75$. Likelihood ratios derived from nonbiochemical markers, such as nuchal translucency measurement, can be incorporated into a similar calculation. *Abbreviations*: AFP, alpha-fetoprotein; MoM, multiple of median.

by 16% (13). All risk calculation software packages incorporate maternal weight in the risk calculation.

Diabetes

After adjustment for maternal weight, diabetes has no significant effect on serum markers (14).

Ethnic Background

Adjustment for maternal weight considerably reduces the impact of ethnic factors on serum markers (15,16). In some countries, such as France, ethnic background is not currently taken into account by calculation software.

Smoking

Smoking has a large impact on levels of hCG and free β-hCG (−18%) and a smaller effect (3–4%) on concentrations of AFP and estriol (17). The effect of smoking is independent of the number of cigarettes smoked, and is apparent from one cigarette a day. However, smoking is not yet taken into account by most software programs. The effect of passive smoking, on the other hand, is unknown.

Pregnancies Following Ovarian Stimulation or In Vitro Fertilization

A study of a large number of cases has shown that serum markers are unaffected in such pregnancies, in contrast to data reported in small study populations (18).

FACTORS INFLUENCING RISK CALCULATION

History of Down Syndrome

If the patient has had a previous Down syndrome pregnancy, performing an amniocentesis during subsequent pregnancies is a widely accepted policy, as the overall risk of recurrence is around 1% (19). However, the patient may wish to have a more precise evaluation of her risk prior to undergoing an invasive procedure. If the patient opts for MSM screening, this additional risk must be incorporated into the risk calculation, by altering the maternal age-related risk. An additional risk of 0.54% in the second trimester and 0.77% in the first is generally used (20).

This strategy is, however, not suitable when the history of Down syndrome is due to familial translocation, since the risk of transmission due to linkage disequilibrium is far greater than 1%.

Twin Pregnancies

Down syndrome screening cannot simply be applied to twin pregnancies since serum marker concentrations are physiologically higher. Furthermore, serum assays reflect the placental and fetal metabolism of both twins and this may limit screening sensitivity when only one fetus is affected by Down syndrome. Serum marker data are scarce for twin pregnancies with one or both fetuses affected. Marker concentrations in twins are "normalized" by dividing them by the median value defined for a control population of twin pregnancies. The normalized values are then entered in software programs calibrated for singleton pregnancies. The distribution of hCG varies with chorionicity, which should be taken into account to improve screening specificity

(21,22). In addition, Down syndrome screening in twin pregnancies is complicated by estimation of maternal age-related risk. Although in monozygotic twin pregnancies this risk is identical to that of singleton pregnancies, in dizygotic twin pregnancies (information unavailable prenatally: the chorionicity is known but not the zygosity) the risk of having at least one affected child is almost doubled compared with a singleton pregnancy (23). This theoretical risk is, however, not observed in study populations and is, therefore, not use in practice (24).

Despite all these limitations, if one considers predicting the "at least one affected twin event," maternal serum screening in twins may achieve a 54% detection rate with a screened positive rate of 8% (22). This is better than using maternal age alone, but not as good as what can be achieved based on first-trimester nuchal translucency measurement (25).

SERUM MARKERS AND SCREENING FOR OTHER ANOMALIES

Screening for Spina Bifida

Abnormally high maternal serum AFP is suggestive of open neural tube defects (NTD) including spina bifida and anencephaly, whose frequency varies with ethnic and geographical background. With a cutoff of 2.5 MoM, 1% of patients will have a serum AFP above this cutoff and the NTD detection rate will be 80%. Depending on the prevalence of NTD, a 1/25 to 1/50 PPV can be reached. Most software provides an NTD risk calculation. This risk may be underestimated when the patient's medical history and geographical background are not taken into account.

Once the patient is considered at risk for open NTD, the diagnostic strategy tends to be based on ultrasound. However, when fetal imaging remains inconclusive, amniocentesis can provide amniotic fluid for electrophoresis of cholinesterases.

Screening for Trisomy 18

AFP and hCG (or β-hCG) are simultaneously reduced to below 0.5 MoM in approximately 75% of trisomy 18–affected pregnancies. In such cases, ultrasonography should be used to search for morphological signs associated with trisomy 18 (26).

Other Risks

Other maternal or fetal diseases are associated with changes in serum markers, including pre-eclampsia (high hCG), fetal death (high AFP and/or low hCG), triploidy (very high hCG), Smith–Lemli–Opitz syndrome (low estriol). However, the markers for these diseases are of low specificity and cannot be used in practice (27–29).

QUALITY CONTROL AND SCREENING POLICIES

As for most laboratory assays, quality insurance procedures have been implemented for maternal serum screening. This includes internal quality control of assays generally provided by the manufacturers. In addition, an external quality control procedure is widely used as the U.K. NEQAS (30). The principle of this quality control designed for MSM screening consists of providing laboratories with selected sera and studying the interlaboratory agreement of the calculated risks and the distribution of the raw and MoM marker concentrations.

Screening policies vary greatly among countries and are usually based on hospitals or regions. In some countries such as France, stringent national screening policies are implemented.

THE EXAMPLE OF A NATIONAL SCREENING POLICY

In France, strict regulatory measures were put in place in January 1997 to govern MSM (31). The law stipulates that the gestational age at screening should range between 14 and 18 weeks, the pregnancy should be dated as accurately as possible, and a written informed consent is mandatory. Since doctors have been sued and condemned for not having informed pregnant women of the availability of MSM, it is widely accepted that this screening should be universally offered. MSM and subsequent fetal karyotyping are available free of charge. The MSM assay and risk calculation can only be performed by laboratories accredited by the ministry of health. Assay kits and software must be approved by a national health products safety agency. In addition to the quality controls mentioned above, each accredited laboratory must submit a yearly activity report to the ministry of health.

Using such a stringent national policy, the rate of patients electing to undergo MSM screening rose from 54% in 1997 to over 80% in 2004.

The major advantage of a standardized national policy is that it allows for large-scale evaluation of screening. For example, the national average Down syndrome detection rate has been shown to be of 70%, with a 6.5% amniocentesis rate based on a study of 854,902 patients (31). These good year-on-year results mean that great caution is exercised before making any methodological changes.

The drawback of such a standardized national policy is that any innovation, even minor or evidence-based, must be authorized by the national health agency following a long and complex procedure.

SECOND-TRIMESTER MSM RESULTS

Table 1 presents French data on MSM for Down syndrome (1997–2001). As in other countries, around 75% of laboratories assay two serum markers (AFP and hCG or β-hCG), whereas the remaining 25% use triple test screening, which includes the assay of estriol.

Patients Under 38 Years of Age

Between 1997 and 2001, 2,450,449 patients below 38 years of age chose to undergo maternal serum screening. Overall, 2332 cases of Down syndrome were diagnosed, either prenatally or at birth. Of these, 1676 were detected by MSM with an action threshold of 1/250, giving a detection rate of 72% and 159,334 patients had a calculated risk above 1/250, corresponding to a screened positive rate of 6.5%. The detection rate and the screened positive rate did not change between 1997 and 2001.

These results confirm that serum markers are more effective than maternal age alone, since their PPV of 1/95 is greater than that for maternal age 38, 39, or even 40 years (1/200). In other words, 95 amniocenteses are needed to detect one Down syndrome case by maternal serum screening, compared with 200 using maternal age alone.

Table 1 Cumulated Results for Maternal Serum Screening in France from 1997 to 2001

Patients < 38 years of age (singleton pregnancies)	
Total patients	2,450,449
Patients at risk (≥1/250)	159,334 (6.5%)
Total number of Down syndrome cases	2,332
Down syndrome cases in the at-risk group (1 ≥ 250)	1,676
Detection rate	71.9%
PPV	1/95
Patients ≥38 years of age (singleton pregnancies)	
Total patients	50,707
Patients at risk (≥1/250)	17,897 (35%)
Total number of Down syndrome cases	319
Down syndrome cases in the at-risk group (≥1/250)	304
Detection rate	95.3%
PPV	1/59

Abbreviation: PPV, positive predictive value.
Source: Data from medical laboratory technologists accredited for Down syndrome screening.

Patients Aged ≥38 Years

Serum markers can also be used in patients aged ≥38 years, who wish to avoid amniocentesis if they can be shown to be at low risk. Between 1997 and 2001, 20% ($n = 50,707$) of French pregnant women aged ≥38 years elected to undergo MSM. Only one-third of these patients had a risk >1/250. Amniocentesis was avoided in two-thirds of cases; however, a Down syndrome detection rate of 95% would still have been achieved (11,32).

CURRENT PROBLEMS IN DOWN SYNDROME SCREENING

Two aspects of screening need to be addressed. First, second-trimester MSM is performed relatively late in pregnancy (14–17 weeks of amenorrhea) and many women wish to have an earlier screening (33). Second, the risk calculated from second-trimester maternal serum screening is likely to be substantially overestimated in women who underwent first-trimester nuchal translucency screening.

First-Trimester Maternal Serum Screening

First-trimester screening for Down syndrome does not use the same markers as second-trimester screening, since total hCG, AFP, and estriol are less effective or ineffective before 14 weeks of gestation. Only free β-hCG is a good marker in both the first and second trimesters (34). Pregnancy-associated plasma protein A (PAPP-A), whose level is reduced in Down syndrome, can only be used before 14 weeks (35,36). Retrospective studies show that the most effective combination is PAPP-A plus free β-hCG, with a 60% detection rate and 5% amniocentesis rate (8). Quality control of these markers can be easily implemented (37).

Early screening for Down syndrome would enable diagnosis of chromosomal abnormality from 12 to 13 weeks, which has clear medical and psychological advantages. These advantages should nonetheless be balanced against technical considerations in fetal karyotyping. Before 15 weeks, amniocentesis carries an increased risk of fetal loss or rupture of the membranes and chorionic villi sampling (CVS) is preferable (38).

A meta-analysis including all available trials (39) shows that transabdominal CVS, when performed by very experienced operators, carries a risk of fetal loss similar (1.3-fold) to that of second-trimester amniocentesis.

This drawback of early diagnosis is counterbalanced by the fact that Down syndrome screening combining nuchal translucency and serum markers is highly specific and, therefore, assigns fewer patients to the at-risk group. However, generalization of first-trimester screening and prenatal diagnosis might necessitate additional medical training of doctors in performing CVS and of cytogeneticists for first-trimester methods. Another potential drawback of first-trimester Down syndrome screening is that it could not be used jointly with screening for spina bifida, since high maternal serum AFP is a good marker of neural tube closure defects, but is unusable before 14 weeks.

Sequential Screening

Three methods of screening for Down syndrome are available to most pregnant women in most industrialized countries: nuchal translucency measurement, second-trimester MSM, and second-trimester ultrasound. Considered separately, each method yields an amniocentesis rate of the order of magnitude of 5%, which seems reasonable. However, when these methods, which are deemed independent, are used sequentially on the same patients, almost 15% of women undergoing this multiple step screening will be offered amniocentesis (40).

Therefore, the results of first-trimester nuchal translucency and first- or second-trimester maternal markers should be analyzed together to produce a single integrated risk in order to maintain an acceptable screened positive rate (41–44). However, before considering the risk derived from nuchal translucency measurement, a specific quality insurance procedure is mandatory to ensure the quality of the measurement.

It is also possible to take into account second-trimester ultrasound markers to assess the risk of aneuploidy. For each "soft second-trimester ultrasound marker," estimations of a specific likelihood ratio have been published, and commercially available software is designed to incorporate MSM, first-trimester ultrasound, and second-trimester ultrasound to provide a single integrated risk assessment. However, there is no consensus regarding practical strategies of quality control of second-trimester ultrasound.

The best strategy in the short-term is probably to combine likelihood ratios derived from nuchal translucency measurement with MSM in the first and or second trimester. This can only be done if there is specific medical training in nuchal translucency measurement together with standardized quality control.

CONCLUSION

Prospective studies have shown that MSM detects at least 60% of Down syndrome-affected pregnancies, for a 5% amniocentesis rate. This screening strategy enables Down syndrome screening in younger women. Serum markers can also be used in patients aged 38 to 40 years, who wish to avoid unnecessary amniocentesis.

Maternal serum screening has been available free of charge in France since January 1997. Its use has spread rapidly in the general population and it has been applied to close to 80% of pregnancies since 1998. The aim now is to reduce the number of amniocentesis generated by currently available screening methods by performing a single–risk calculation combining nuchal translucency measurement with first- or second-trimester maternal serum screening.

REFERENCES

1. Merkatz IR, Nitowsky HM, Macri JN, Johnson WE. An association between low maternal serum alpha-fetoprotein and fetal chromosomal abnormalities. Am J Obstet Gynecol 1984; 148:886–894.
2. Bogart MH, Pandian MR, Jones OW. Abnormal maternal serum chorionic gonadotropin levels in pregnancies with fetal chromosome abnormalities. Prenat Diagn 1987; 7:623–630.
3. Canick JA, Knight GJ, Palomaki GE, Haddow JE, Cuckle HS, Wald NJ. Low second trimester maternal serum unconjugated oestriol in pregnancies with Down's syndrome. Br J Obstet Gynaecol 1988; 95:330–333.
4. Spencer K. Evaluation of an assay of the free beta-subunit of choriogonadotropin and its potential value in screening for Down's syndrome. Clin Chem 1991; 37:809–814.
5. Muller F, Aegerter P, Boué A. Prospective maternal serum human chorionic gonadotrophin screening for the risk of fetal chromosome anomalies and of subsequent fetal and neonatal deaths. Prenat Diagn 1993; 13:29–43.
6. Wald NJ, Cuckle HS, Densem JW, et al. Maternal serum screening for Down's syndrome in early pregnancy. Br Med J 1988; 297:883–887.
7. Wald NJ, Kennard A, Hackshaw A, McGuire A. Antenatal screening for Down's syndrome. J Med Screen 1997; 4:181–246.
8. Cuckle H. Biochemical screening for Down syndrome. Eur J Obstet Gynecol Reprod Biol 2000; 92:97–101 (review).
9. Morris JK, Wald NJ, Mutton DE, Alberman E. Comparison of models of maternal age-specific risk for Down syndrome live births. Prenat Diagn 2004; 24:1017–1018.
10. Snijders RJ, Sundberg K, Holzgreve W, Henry G, Nicolaides KH. Maternal age- and gestation-specific risk for trisomy 21. Ultrasound Obstet Gynecol 1999; 3:167–170.
11. Muller F, Thalabard JC, Ngo S, Dommergues M. Detection and false-positive rates of serum markers for Down syndrome screening according to maternal age in women over 35 years of age: a study of the agreement of 8 dedicated softwares. Prenat Diagn 2002; 22:350–353.
12. Muller F, Thibaud D, Poloce F, et al. Risk of amniocentesis in women screened positive for Down syndrome with second-trimester maternal serum markers. Prenat Diagn 2002; 22:1036–1039.
13. Watt HC, Wald NJ. Alternative methods of maternal weight adjustment in maternal serum screening for Down syndrome and neural tube defects. Prenat Diagn 1998; 18:842–845.
14. Kramer RL, Yaron Y, O'Brien JE, et al. Effect of adjustment of maternal serum alpha-fetoprotein levels in insulin-dependent diabetes mellitus. Am J Med Genet 1998; 75: 176–178.
15. O'Brien JE, Dvorin E, Drugan A, Johnson MP, Yaron Y, Evans MI. Race-ethnicity-specific variation in multiple-marker biochemical screening: alpha-fetoprotein, hCG, and estriol. Obstet Gynecol 1997; 89:355–358.
16. Muller F, Bussieres L, Pelissier MC, et al. Do racial differences exist in second-trimester maternal hCG levels? A study of 23,369 patients. Prenat Diagn 1994; 14:633–636.
17. Spencer K. The influence of smoking on maternal serum AFP and free beta hCG levels and the impact on screening for Down syndrome. Prenat Diagn 1998; 18:225–234.
18. Muller F, Dreux S, Lemeur A, et al. Medically assisted reproduction and second-trimester maternal serum marker screening for Down syndrome. Prenat Diagn 2003; 23: 1073–1076.

19. Carter CO, Pembury M. Risk of recurrence of Down syndrome. Lancet 1980; 8158:49.
20. Benn PA. Advances in prenatal screening for Down syndrome. I. General principles and second trimester testing. Clin Chim Acta 2002; 323:1–16 (review).
21. Spencer K, Salonen R, Muller F. Down's syndrome screening in multiple pregnancies using alpha-fetoprotein and free beta hCG. Prenat Diagn 1994; 14:537–542.
22. Muller F, Dreux S, Dupoizat H, et al. Second-trimester Down syndrome maternal serum screening in twin pregnancies: impact of chorionicity. Prenat Diagn 2003; 23:331–335.
23. Meyers C, Adam R, Dungan J, Prenger V. Aneuploidy in twin gestations: when is maternal age advanced? Obstet Gynecol 1997; 89:248–251.
24. Jamar M, Lemarchal C, Lemaire V, Koulischer L, Bours V. A low rate of trisomy 21 in twin-pregnancies: a cytogenetics retrospective study of 278 cases. Genet Couns 2003; 14:395–400.
25. Sebire NJ, Snijders RJ, Hughes K, Sepulveda W, Nicolaides KH. Screening for trisomy 21 in twin pregnancies by maternal age and fetal nuchal translucency thickness at 10–14 weeks of gestation. Br J Obstet Gynaecol 1996; 103:999–1003.
26. Muller F, Sault C, Lemay C, et al. Second trimester two-step trisomy 18 screening using maternal serum markers. Prenat Diagn 2002; 22:605–608.
27. Muller F, Savey L, Le Fiblec B, et al. Maternal serum human chorionic gonadotropin level at fifteen weeks is a predictor for preeclampsia. Am J Obstet Gynecol 1996; 175: 37–40.
28. Spencer K. Second-trimester prenatal screening for Down syndrome and the relationship of maternal serum biochemical markers to pregnancy complications with adverse outcome. Prenat Diagn 2000; 20:652–656.
29. Benn PA, Horne D, Briganti S, Greenstein RM. Prenatal diagnosis of diverse chromosome abnormalities in a population of patients identified by triple-marker testing as screen positive for Down syndrome. Am J Obstet Gynecol 1995; 173:496–501.
30. Knight GJ. Quality assessment of a prenatal screening program. Early Hum Dev 1996; 47(suppl):S49–S53 (review).
31. Muller F, Forestier F, Dingeon B. ABA Study Group. Second trimester trisomy 21 maternal serum marker screening. Results of a countrywide study of 854,902 patients. Prenat Diagn 2002; 22:925–929.
32. Muller F, Aegerter P, Ngo S, et al. Software for prenatal trisomy 21 risk calculation: comparative study of seven software packages. Clin Chem 1999; 8:1278–1280.
33. Spencer K, Aitken D. Factors affecting women's preference for type of prenatal screening test for chromosomal anomalies. Ultrasound Obstet Gynecol 2004; 24:735–739.
34. Macri JN, Spencer K, Aitken D, et al. First-trimester free beta (hCG) screening for Down syndrome. Prenat Diagn 1993; 13:557–562.
35. Muller F, Cuckle H, Teisner B, Grudzinskas JG. Serum PAPP-A levels are depressed in women with fetal Down syndrome in early pregnancy. Prenat Diagn 1993; 13:633–636.
36. Cuckle H, Lilford RJ, Teisner B, Holding S, Chard T, Grudzinskas JG. Pregnancy associated plasma protein A in Down's syndrome. Br Med J 1992; 305(6850):425.
37. Muller F, Benattar C, Audibert F, Roussel N, Dreux S, Cuckle H. First-trimester screening for Down syndrome in France combining fetal nuchal translucency measurement and biochemical markers. Prenat Diagn 2003; 23:833–836.
38. Smidt-Jensen S, Permin M, Philip J, et al. Randomised comparison of amniocentesis and transabdominal and transcervical chorionic villus sampling. Lancet 1992; 8830: 1237–1244.
39. Alfirevic Z, Sundberg K, Brigham S. Amniocentesis and chorionic villus sampling for prenatal diagnosis. Cochrane Database Syst Rev 2003; 3:CD 003252.
40. Thilaganathan B, Slack A, Wathen NC. Effect of first-trimester nuchal translucency on second-trimester maternal serum biochemical screening for Down's syndrome. Ultrasound Obstet Gynecol 1997; 10:261–264.
41. Nicolaides KH. Nuchal translucency and other first-trimester sonographic markers of chromosomal abnormalities. Am J Obstet Gynecol 2004; 191:45–67.

42. Rozenberg P, Malagrida L, Cuckle H, et al. Down's syndrome screening with nuchal translucency at 12(+0)–14(+0) weeks and maternal serum markers at 14(+1)–17(+0) weeks: a prospective study. Hum Reprod 2002; 17:1093–1098.
43. Audibert F, Dommergues M, Benattar C, Taieb J, Thalabard JC, Frydman R. Screening for Down syndrome using first-trimester ultrasound and second-trimester maternal serum markers in a low-risk population: a prospective longitudinal study. Ultrasound Obstet Gynecol 2001; 18:26–31.
44. Lam YH, Lee CP, Sin SY, et al. Comparison and integration of first trimester fetal nuchal translucency and second trimester maternal serum screening for fetal Down syndrome. Prenat Diagn 2002; 22:730–735.

3

Nuchal Translucency Screening

Caterina M. Bilardo
*Department of Obstetrics and Gynaecology, Academic Medical Centre,
Amsterdam, The Netherlands*

Rosalinde J. M. Snijders
Fetal Medicine Foundation Netherlands, Rotterdam, The Netherlands

INTRODUCTION

Down syndrome (DS) is the most frequent severe chromosomal anomaly in live
born infants, with a frequency of 1 in about 600 births. Its name originates from
the British physician Langdon Down who first described the syndrome in 1866
(1). The association of DS with maternal age was known from the beginning of
the 20th century. Since the 1970s, maternal age-based screening for DS has been
introduced in most developed countries. Invasive diagnostic procedures (amniocentesis and, chorion biopsies) were offered to all pregnant women above a certain age
threshold. Every country has variably set, from 35 years onward, the age limit for
offering DS screening, the choice in cutoff depending on public health, economic,
and/or social argumentations. Disadvantages of a maternal age-based selection
are (i) the high screen-positive rate—due to the increasing number of women postponing reproduction to a later phase in life, (ii) the low positive predictive value,
and (iii) the unfavorable ratio between detected DS cases and iatrogenic abortions
caused by the invasive diagnostic procedure. In fact, for each detected DS case
one healthy baby is lost as a consequence of the invasive procedures (2). Moreover,
as the majority of babies are still born from younger mothers, a screening strategy
based on maternal age only leads to the detection of about one-third of all DS cases.
Over the last decade, the need for a safer and more efficient screening strategy has
been a major challenge for researchers and health policy makers. In his *Observation
of an Ethnic Classification of Idiots*, Down described the typical features of affected
individuals as "... their skin appears to be too large for their bodies, the nose is
small and the face is flat..." One hundred and thirty years later, these features have
been proposed as, at the moment, the best available strategies for an early
ultrasound-based screening for DS. In this chapter, the various aspects and implications of first-trimester screening for chromosomal anomalies by nuchal translucency
(NT) measurement will be discussed.

33

METHODS OF SCREENING

Every woman has a risk that her fetus/baby is affected by a chromosomal defect. With the knowledge of the natural history of chromosomal anomalies, it is possible to calculate for every maternal age and gestational age the background risk of carrying a chromosomally abnormal fetus (3). When additional measurements are taken, measurement specific likelihood ratios are derived and these are applied to adjust the background risk. Based on these concepts new screening strategies have been developed. The first has been second trimester maternal serum screening (4). Since the late 1980s, the idea of an early and ultrasound-based screening strategy has become attractive, considering that many women undergo ultrasound examination from the early stages of pregnancy.

Nuchal Translucency

In 1990, Szabo first described the association between increased nuchal fluid in early gestation and trisomy 21 (5). A few years later, Nicolaides proposed NT screening as an early ultrasound screening strategy for chromosomal anomalies (6). Nuchal translucency, named in view of its ultrasound aspect, is a common feature observed in all fetuses between 10 and 14 weeks' gestation (7). Normal ranges for the measurement have been constructed (8). The measurement can be carried out transabdominally or transvaginally (9). Another relevant aspect is that in addition to being associated with chromosomal abnormality, increased NT is associated with perinatal death, major cardiac defects, and other structural defects, and has been reported to be associated with a number of genetic syndromes (10,11). The pathophysiology of a normal and increased NT is not yet fully understood. The anatomical substrate seems to be the presence of two rhomboidal cavities, symmetrically situated with respect to the sagittal plane and appearing at ultrasound investigation as a single black space, due to the lateral resolution of the ultrasound beam. The two spaces may be the superficial recesses of the jugular lymphatic sacs at a stage when they are not yet connected to the system. The connection occurs physiologically from 9 to 10 weeks onward and may be completed by 12 to 13 weeks (12). The pathophysiological background of an increased NT will be the subject of another chapter.

STUDIES ON NT SCREENING

Since the early 1990s, numerous studies on the association between fetal NT thickness and chromosomal anomalies have been published (13–16).

When it became clear that NT could be used as an early screening method for DS, studies have focused especially on aspects such as success rate in obtaining the measurement, and sensitivity of the screening method. Almost all studies have shown an association between trisomy 21 and increased NT in the late first trimester and early second trimester; however, the variation in reported performance was considerable due to variation in study design, population, gestational age, time assigned for the measurement, and cutoffs used to define an abnormal measurement. Table 1 presents studies with a great variation in the methodological approach in chronological order (17–26). Gestational age ranged from as early as 8 weeks up to 16 weeks. Success in obtaining the measurement ranged from 66% to 100%, false-positive rate (FPR) from 0.4% to 6.3%, and detection rate (DR) from 30% to 100%. Table 2 presents studies where the

Table 1 Studies Investigating the Value of NT Measurement as Screening Method for Chromosomal Anomalies and Showing a Great Variation in Methodology (Cutoff and Gestational Age Window)

Author	GA (wk)	N	Success rate measurement (%)	Used cutoff (mm)	FPR (%)	DR of trisomy 21 (%)
Bewley et al. (17)	$8–13^{+6}$	1704	66.1	3	6.2	33.3
Szabo et al. (18)	$9–12^{+6}$	3380	100	3	1.6	90
Kornman et al. (19)	$8–13^{+6}$	923	58.2	3	6.3	50
Haddow (26)	$9–15^{+6}$	4049	83	95th percentile	5	31
Economides (20)	$11–14^{+6}$	2256	100	95th percentile	0.4	75
Schuchter (25)	$10–12^{+6}$	9342	100	2.5	2.1	57.9
Wayda (23)	10–13	6841	100	2.5	4.1	100
Crossley (21)	$10–14^{+6}$	17,229	72.9	95th percentile	5	48.6
Rozenberg (24)	$12–14^{+6}$	6234	98.6	3	2.8	61.9
Wald (22)	$6–16^{+6}$	47,053	76.6	95th percentile	5	38.7

Abbreviations: GA, gestational age; FPR, false-positive rate; DR, detection rate; NT, nuchal translucency.

measurement has been performed in the same gestational age window (8,27–33). In spite of using different cutoffs for defining an abnormal measurement, the success rate has increased remarkably and the DR is about 75%.

The Role of the Fetal Medicine Foundation in Standardizing NT Screening

Since 1994, the Fetal Medicine Foundation (FMF) has played a crucial role in promoting a uniform measurement technique by holding courses aimed at teaching the principles of first-trimester ultrasound screening. The FMF provides certified ultrasonographers with a free software program that allows risk calculation based on the background risk (maternal age), NT measurement, and gestational age [crown–rump length (CRL)]. By combining these three parameters, it is possible to calculate for each fetus its individual risk of being affected by trisomy 21 (32). The license for the risk assessment is subject to renewal on a yearly basis. Condition for renewal is that the affiliated centers participate in an audit of their screening activities. This enables pooling of data and continuous evaluation of the technical skills. The

Table 2 Studies Investigating the Value of NT Measurement as Screening Method for Chromosomal Anomalies at the Same Gestational Age Window

Author	GA (wk)	N	Success rate measurement (%)	Used cutoff (mm)	FPR (%)	DR of trisomy 21 (%)
Pandya et al. (8)	$10–13^{+6}$	1763	100	2.5	3.4	75
Taipale et al. (27)	$10–13^{+6}$	6939	98.6	3	0.7	66.7
Pajkrt et al. (28,29)	$10–13^{+6}$	3614	100	3	4.2	69.6
Theodoropoulos et al. (31)	$10–13^{+6}$	3550	100	95th percentile	2.3	90.9
Schwarzler et al. (30)	$10–13^{+6}$	4523	100	2.5	2.7	66.7
Panburana et al. (32)	$10–13^{+6}$	2067	100	2.5	2.9	100

Abbreviations: GA, gestational age; FPR, false-positive rate; DR, detection rate; NT, nuchal translucency.

Table 3 Guidelines of the Fetal Medicine Foundation

- Ultrasound equipment of good quality with zoom, cineloop facility, and possibility of measuring in decimals of millimeters
- The measurement should be performed (preferably) transabdominally or vaginally
- The fetus has to be in a midsagittal plane with head in neutral position (not extended or flexed) (Fig. 1)
- The picture has to be magnified so that the fetus occupies 75% of the picture (every movement apart of the callipers should be equivalent to 0.1 mm) (Fig. 2)
- Distinction between amniotic membrane and fetal skin must be possible
- The callipers have to be placed on the maximal black thickness "on-to-on," which means on the white line at the limit of the black space (Fig. 2)

A few practical tips on how to obtain a good NT measurement:

a. As a general rule, the ultrasonographer should be patient and only be satisfied when the measurement is as good as possible
b. Fetal immobility: the woman can be asked to cough and, in case of no success, the scan should be repeated after a while (send her for a short walk)
c. Unfavorable fetal position (standing fetus): In this case the vaginal route should be tried
d. Impossibility to clearly visualize the nuchal area: the umbilical cord may be around the fetal neck preventing visualization of the optimal place to measure the NT (to verify this, turn color Doppler on). Avoid measuring too low (neck or upper back) as the measurement will be underestimated. Wait for a change in position or reschedule the scan for another day
e. In case there is an impression that the NT may be increased but a good measurement cannot be obtained, the nuchal area should be looked at in the transversal plane. This may confirm the presence of small septations. Wait then until a good sagittal measurement is obtained

---

Abbreviation: NT, nuchal translucency.

guidelines of the FMF are provided in Table 3. Examples of normal and enlarged NT and correct measurement techniques are provided in Figures 1–3. In 1998, a large multicenter study including 100,000 pregnancies based on the FMF criteria was published (34). When measurements are obtained according to the guidelines of the FMF, about 70% of fetuses with trisomy 21 have a measurement above the 95th percentile for gestational age. When risk calculation is used, it is expected that, in an unselected population, a risk cutoff of 1 in 300 will identify 75% of trisomy 21 fetuses for a 5% FPR. While the risk assessment focuses on trisomy 21, the group with a high risk of trisomy 21 is also known to contain the majority of other chromosomal defects (34).

Thanks to uniformity in the methodological approach, comparison of results of studies from different centers has become possible (Table 4) (34–40). DR is about 85% for an FPR of about 6%. A meta-analysis of studies reporting on NT as a screening method for chromosomal anomalies without description of used methodology reports a DR of 76% for an FPR of 6% (41).

Fetal Loss in Chromosomally Abnormal Pregnancies

It is known that chromosomally abnormal fetuses have a high spontaneous intrauterine lethality (3). About 40% to 50% of conceived DS fetuses will not end in live births. It is well known that chromosomally abnormal pregnancies relatively often result in spontaneous intrauterine loss. Therefore, if screening is applied in early pregnancy, it cannot be excluded that some degree of verification bias inflates the

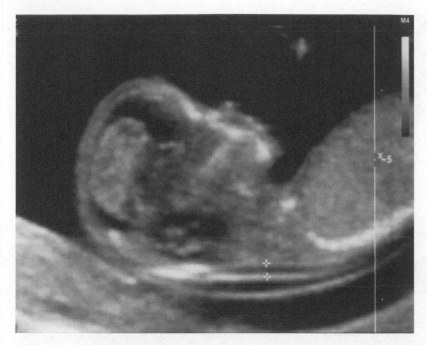

Figure 1 Correct fetal position to perform the NT measurement. *Abbreviation*: NT, nuchal translucency.

performance (3). The degree by which results are biased depends on the association between marker levels and spontaneous loss rate (41,42). In chromosomally normal fetuses increased NT is associated with an increased spontaneous fetal loss rate (43,44). However, in a study from Brasil the association between increased NT and intrauterine death in DS pregnancies seemed limited (45). Further studies are needed to assess to what extend NT thickness affects the chances of spontaneous loss. In the mean time, screening performances may be compared using the observed number of affected pregnancies and the expected number based on the maternal age and gestational age distribution of the population (34). Using this approach it is

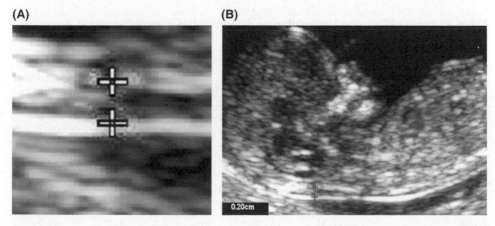

Figure 2 Example of a good NT measurement. Detail on callipers placement on the white lines. *Abbreviation*: NT, nuchal translucency.

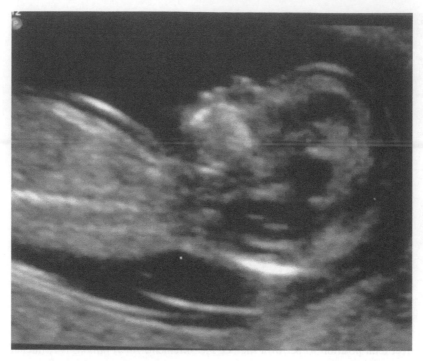

Figure 3 Example of a trisomy-21 fetus showing an extremely increased NT, generalized edema, and absent nasal bone. *Abbreviation*: NT, nuchal translucency.

estimated that screening based on fetal NT reduces the prevalance of DS among live born children by about 80% (34).

Quality Control of NT Measurements

The original FMF audit scheme entailed regular quantitative assessment of the distribution of NT measurements complemented by global qualitative examination of five randomly selected images (23). In a recently modified approach, the qualitative

Table 4 Studies Where the Methodological Approach Has Been Standardized According to the Guidelines of the FMF

Author	Mean maternal age	Population (N)	Cutoff	FPR (%)	DR of trisomy 21 (%)	DR of other chromosomal anomalies (%)
Snijders et al. (34)	31	96,127	1:300	8.3	82.2	77.8
Thilaganathan et al. (35)	29	9753	1:300	7.8	81	89.3
Gasiorek-Wiens et al. (38)	33	21,475	1:300	13	87.6	88.2
Zoppi et al. (36)	33	10,001	1:300	8.9	90.6	84.8
Brizot et al. (37)	28	2470	1:300	7.4	90	75
Chasen et al. (40)	33	2216	1:300	7.5	83.3	75
Prefumo et al. (39)	31	11,820	1:300	4.8	81.5	—
Total	31	153,862	1:300	8.3	85.2	82.2

Abbreviations: FPR, false-positive rate; DR, detection rate; FMF, Fetal Medicine Foundation.

assessment was objectified by a scoring system proposed by Herman et al. (46). Furthermore, it has been recommended that, at least in the training phase, video-taped examinations are evaluated to ensure that efforts are made to measure fetal NT, rather than the distance between the fetus and the amniotic membrane (47).

Two recent studies explored the efficacy of qualitative and quantitative approaches for monitoring performance of different operators in measuring NT. In both the studies, it is concluded that the quantitative approach is more practical than the qualitative assessment for monitoring on a large scale (47,48). In order to overcome the problem of difference in medians among operators and centers, Logghe proposed the use of center-specific medians (49).

Appropriate training and standardization of technique may limit intra-operator differences (50,51). Methods to enhance repeatability include the use of a PC based virtual ultrasound scanner (VirUS) or of ultrasound simulators. Results from studies that used these aids underline the importance of using standardized ultrasound settings and improving technical skills to achieve optimal repeatability (52,53). Methodological issues aimed at optimizing NT screening performance have been the subject of many articles published in the literature. In the calculation of risk for trisomy 21, two different approaches can be used: the delta (difference between obtained measurement and normal mean for gestation) or the multiple of the median (MoM) approach. The delta-NT approach appears more accurate than the NT-MoM approach (54). In case a nuchal scan must be planned based on the last menstrual period, the only optimal moment is at 12 to 13 weeks' gestation (55).

When the measurement is repeated twice in the 11 to 14 weeks' time frame, a considerable variation can be observed. About 20% of enlarged NT normalize at subsequent measurement. Although the chance of chromosomal anomalies is reduced in case of normalization, this is not invariably associated with a normal karyotype (56). Conversely, persistence or increase at subsequent measurement of the degree of enlargement worsens the prognosis (56,57).

Ethnic Origin

There is controversy as to the need for taking ethnic origin into account in interpre-tation of NT measurements. Jou et al. concluded that, given the small but statisti-cally significant differences, race-specific normative data should be used (58). Other authors concluded that it is acceptable to use one standard, as screen-positive rates in different groups are similar (59,60).

Three-Dimensional vs. Two-Dimensional Ultrasound

It has recently been suggested that three-dimensional (3-D) ultrasound may limit the time needed to obtain a reliable measurement and it may facilitate retrospective reas-sessment. Theoretically, stored volume data may be sliced in any desired plane, thus providing views of the nuchal region which could not be seen on a conventional 2-D scan. This would enable measurement of NT regardless of the fetal position, which could shorten examination time. In addition, by displaying three orthogonal planes at the same time, the use of 3-D ultrasound may ensure that the measurements are always performed in a true midsagittal plane.

Three recent studies reported that the difference between 2-D and 3-D mea-surements is small and the correlation is such that the same reference values can be used (61–63). Analysis of 3-D volumes demonstrated that the majority of 2-D measurements are not performed in a true midsagittal plane. Nevertheless, measurements obtained in the best 2-D view do not differ from measurements in a true mid-sagittal view to the degree that widespread introduction of 3-D ultrasound is warranted (61). The authors emphasize that 3-D measurements can only be performed successfully by examination of sagittal volumes that contain a clear view of the NT in the initial plane. When the fetus is lying in a position that precludes clear visualization of the nuchal fold, 3-D ultrasound is unlikely to be of help. Michailidis et al., in a study comparing usefulness of 2-D and 3-D ultrasound in examining fetal anatomy in the first trimester, also concluded that 2-D examination is preferable (64). In a comparison of 3-D transabdominal and 3-D transvaginal NT measurements, there were no significant differences. When 3-mm NT thickness was used as a cutoff level, however, there was a statistically significant overestimation of NT measurements by both 3-D transabdominal and 3-D transvaginal ultrasound (65).

INCREASED NT IN CHROMOSOMALLY NORMAL PREGNANCIES

An increased NT is found in 5% of karyotypically normal fetuses (32).

Although the vast majority of euploid fetuses with enlarged NT will be healthy, extra care must be taken in order to exclude pathological associations in these fetuses. In fact, an increased NT measurement has been found in association with a large number of developmental disorders such as structural defects and genetic syndromes (10,43,66). Moreover, an increased NT is also associated with hematological disorders, infections, and increased fetal and neonatal lethality (10,43,44,66). The rule is that the higher the degree of enlargement, the higher the chance of an abnormal outcome.

INCREASED NT AND PREGNANCY OUTCOME

In chromosomally normal pregnancies with increased NT and no visible structural anomalies, the rate of spontaneous abortion is increased (44). Souka et al. showed that in 1320 chromosomally normal fetuses with increased NT, 5.2% miscarried or died in utero, the majority by 15 weeks of gestation (43). Pajkrt showed an overall mortality of 4.1%, especially in early pregnancy, but some death also occurred later in pregnancy or in the neonatal period. When fetal NT is between 3.0 and 3.9 mm, the prevalence of spontaneous abortions is three times higher, and in those where the measurement is ≥4.0 mm, it is almost seven times higher than in pregnancies with NT measurements <3.0 mm (44).

In a large series of 4116 chromosomally normal fetuses with increased NT at 10 to 14 weeks of gestation, 94% resulted in live births; however, the chance of a live birth decreased as NT thickness increased (43). In another study in 6650 women who had attended first-trimester ultrasound assessment, the relative risk of adverse pregnancy outcome (spontaneous abortion, intrauterine death, or termination for fetal abnormality) was 4.7 and 12.2 times higher if the NT thickness was above the 95th and 99th percentile, respectively, when compared to fetuses with normal NT (67). A recent review has addressed the systematic work-up and counseling throughout pregnancies with increased NT and normal karyotype. Eleven studies reporting on the pregnancy outcome of 2128 fetuses with increased NT and normal karyotype (≥3 mm or ≥95th percentile) were included (68). Due to significant differences in study design, ranges rather than combined rates are provided. Overall, 70% to 90% fetuses had normal outcomes, 2.2% to 10.6% miscarried, and 0.5% to 15.8% ended in perinatal death. There was an overall rate of 0.5% to 12.7% neurodevelopmental problems, and 2.1% to 7.6% of the malformations remained undiagnosed before birth. The same author analyzed retrospectively pregnancy outcome in 168 euploid fetuses with increased NT (69). Of these, 38 (23%) had an adverse outcome: 11 (6%) had miscarriages, 14 (8%) were terminated because of fetal abnormalities detected on the prenatal scan, and 13 (7%) were found to have abnormalities postnatally. The odds ratios for adverse outcome were calculated using either NT-MoM or delta-NT approaches. Both methods were able to predict fetal outcome confidently. The authors suggested using a cutoff of either 2.0 MoM or delta-NT of 1.5 mm.

In view of the relatively high incidence of intrauterine demise in fetuses with increased NT, it is advisable to repeat the scan a few weeks after the measurement. A detailed two-step anomaly scan including midgestation fetal echocardiography should be part of perinatal management of pregnancies with increased fetal NT. It has been suggested that efforts for further surveillance should be confined to pregnancies where the NT thickness measures >3.5 mm (the 99th percentile). This would mean that a very large proportion of screen-positive couples (a mild increased NT thickness is the most frequent) can be confidently reassured on the fetal outcome once the karyotype is normal. In practice, we experience that parents with a screen-positive result need extra support and attention even after a normal karyotype (70).

Data on relevant family history and persistence of nuchal edema provide additional relevant information for planning pregnancy management.

However, it should be emphasized that increased NT per se does not constitute a fetal abnormality. Once a chromosome defect has been excluded, >85% of pregnancies with fetal NT <4.5 mm result in healthy live births; the rates for fetal NTs of 4.5–6.4 mm and >6.5 mm are about 75% and 45%, respectively (43,67,71,72).

INCREASED NT AND CARDIAC DEFECTS

With a prevalence of five to ten per 1000 at birth, heart defects are the most common congenital malformation. Traditional screening and selection of patients for detailed echocardiography relying upon anamnestic risk factors or use of teratogenic medications will only identify about 5% of affected cases (73). Prenatal screening for heart defects is performed in the second trimester by examination of the four-chamber–view, with or without assessment of the great vessels. This approach of the routine 20-week anomaly scan can be very effective, but the value of this screening technique for congenital heart defects is highly dependent on operator training and experience (74,75). Results from prospective studies that used this method of screening have been poor (76). It is, therefore, an appealing idea that the population could be screened for major cardiac defects by measuring NT at this early stage of pregnancy. Only fetuses with increased NT would have to be referred for detailed echocardiography in a specialized center. As the quality and resolution of ultrasound equipment have improved, earlier echocardiography will allow earlier diagnosis for parents, although further research on the sensitivity and specificity of these techniques is needed to determine whether decisions about terminating a pregnancy can safely be made at this stage (77–80). Haak et al. reported that in 96% of fetuses with increased NT, vaginal echocardiographic examination was successful (80). Huggon et al. successfully assessed the fetal heart by transabdominal ultrasound in 87% of the cases (79). Cardiac defects were identified in 60 fetuses. Validation of the scan findings was possible in 241 fetuses. Normal heart structure was confirmed in 204 fetuses, and previously unsuspected cardiac

Table 5 Studies Illustrating the Association Between Increased NT (95th and 99th Percentiles) and Major Congenital Heart Defects in Chromosomally Normal Fetuses

Author	Total population	CHD and NT ≥95th percentile[a] (%)	CHD and NT ≥99th percentile[b] (%)
Ghi et al. (82)	1319	4.5	7.0
Hiippala et al. (71)	—	—	7.6
Senat et al. (72)	—	—	6.7
Galindo et al. (83)	353	5.3	24
McAuliffe et al. (84)	263	4.9	10.7

[a] >3 mm or < 95th percentile.
[b] 3.5 mm.
Abbreviations: CHD, congenital heart defects; NT, nuchal translucency.

abnormalities were revealed in nine. Heart defects were verified in 28 fetuses, but five of these had important additional findings. There were false-positive findings in three fetuses.

Hyett has suggested that NT screening may also have the potential of acting as screening for critical cardiac defects (CHD) (81). Findings reported by the author indicated that offering echocardiography when fetal NT is increased might identify 56% of CHD. This has stimulated several investigators to further explore the potential of first-trimester screening for heart defects.

Results from recent studies confirm that in chromosomally normal fetuses with increased NT, the incidence of CHD is increased (Table 5) (71,72,82–84). All authors agree that in such cases specialized echocardiography is indicated. However, cohort-based studies report a considerable variation in observed prevalence of heart defects and in DR when increased NT is used as screening method (Table 6) (30,67,81,85–87). This may indicate that different groups use different diagnostic criteria, cases with extracardiac defects may have been excluded, and ascertainment may have been suboptimal (70). On the basis of presently available data, it seems unlikely that the percentage of serious heart defects that is detected through NT screening will be as high as expected on the basis of findings by Hyett et al. (81). A recent meta-analysis

Table 6 Cohort Studies in Chromosomally Normal Fetuses Reporting on Prevalence of Major Congenital Heart Defects and Detection Rate When the 95th and 99th Percentile for Fetal NT Are Used as a Cutoff for Screening

Author	N	NT >95th percentile	Number of MCHD	MCHD in NT >95th percentile
Hyett et al. (81)	29,154	1822 (6.3%)	50 (1.7/1000)	28 (56%)
Schwarzler et al. (30)	4500	110 (2.4%)	9 (2.0/1000)	1 (11.1%)
Mavrides et al. (85)	7339	258 (3.5%)	26 (3.5/1000)	4 (15.4%)
Michailidis et al. (67)	6498	219 (3.4%)	11 (2.0/1000)	4 (36.4%)
Orvos et al. (86)	4251		39 (9/1000)	18 (51%)[a]
Hafner et al. (87)	12,978	649 (5.0%)	27 (2.1/1000)	7 (25.9%)
Total	64,720	4.7%	2.5/1000	20%

[a] NT >3 mm.
Abbreviations: MCHD, major congenital heart defects; NT, nuchal translucency.

suggests that the sensitivity of increased NT for cardiac defects is about 30% (88). In data from our group on a low-risk cohort of 5000 pregnancies, the association between increased NT and CHD appeared even weaker (89). Differences in DRs may in part be due to differences in study design—the initial data were analyzed retrospectively, whereas the more recent studies were designed prospectively. NT measurement will not, replace traditional means of screening for major congenital cardiac disease, but does provide a useful adjunct to current methods of screening that have proven to be far from perfect (90).

Other Structural Anomalies and Genetic Syndromes

Findings from numerous studies indicate that an increased NT in chromosomally normal fetuses may be associated with serious additional structural anomalies or genetic defects (10,11,91). The list of structural anomalies and genetic syndromes that have been reported in association with increased NT is very long, but a true association has only been identified in a few cases and may act through one of the following mechanisms:

• cardiac dysfunction due to abnormalities of the heart or great vessels;
• venous congestion of the neck due to constriction of the body (e.g., in amnion rupture sequence), superior mediastinal compression (e.g., in diaphragmatic hernia), or narrow chest (e.g., skeletal dysplasia);
• failure of lymphatic drainage due to impaired or delayed development of the lymphatic system or impaired fetal movements (e.g., in neuromuscular disorders);
• altered composition of the subcutaneous connective tissue; and
• fetal hypoproteinemia.

Knowledge of possible underlying mechanisms is important in the planning of appropriate follow-up investigations and in counseling parents. In the majority of cases, the association may be purely coincidental.

Fetal Structural Defects Presenting with Increased NT at 11 to 14 Weeks

Fetal exomphalos can be identified from 11 weeks of gestation and has an increased prevalence in fetuses with increased NT. While exomphalos is usually associated with chromosomal abnormalities, such as trisomy 18, the prevalence remains increased in chromosomally normal fetuses with increased NT. Similarly, the prevalence of diaphragmatic hernia is significantly higher in a population of fetuses with increased NT. At later gestations, hemodynamic changes associated with diaphragmatic hernia mimic those seen with coarctation of the aorta. Pathological studies of the underlying mechanism of increased NT show that narrowing of the aortic isthmus is a common finding in fetuses with increased NT and similar hemodynamic changes, and therefore, may be occurring in these two groups. In a series of 19 cases of diaphragmatic hernia, seven (37%) had increased NT at 10 to 14 weeks and this included five of the six neonatal deaths due to pulmonary hypoplasia—NT thickness, therefore, may be a useful indicator for the prognosis of infants with this structural anomaly (92).

It is important that cases are reported where increased NT is found in association with rare syndromes or fetal anomalies. However, efforts should be made to clarify the exact underlying mechanism. For example, in two cases of Fanconi and

Blackfan–Diamond anemia, the most likely causes of increased NT were a cardiac defect and impaired cardiac function, respectively (93,94).

Increased NT and Genetic Syndromes

It is difficult to prove a strong association between genetic syndromes and increased NT as most syndromes have extremely low prevalence in the population, and we are, therefore, reliant on case reports rather than series (91). The prevalence of genetic syndromes and single gene disorders does, however, appear to be increased in fetuses with increased NT, being as high as 12.7% in one publication (11). It seems likely that syndromes such as Noonan's, where infants commonly have a webbed neck, are likely to have similar phenotypic expression in utero (95). Fetal akinesia deformation sequence has frequently been associated with increased NT, although the mechanism for this association is unclear (96). Many skeletal dysplasias appear to be associated with increased NT, and this may be due to the effects of mediastinal compression or differences in collagen expression. New case reports on the association of increased NT and structural or rare genetic defects are constantly published, and the list of anomalies detected in fetuses showing increased NT at 11 to 14 weeks increases daily (97–99). Based on our experience, it can be concluded that the role of NT measurement in genetic syndromes with a high recurrence (autosomal dominant or recessive) may be to alert parents, at a very early stage in pregnancy, to the likelihood of the fetus being affected.

Increased NT and Rare Chromosomal Anomalies

Apart from the known association of enlarged NT and trisomy 18, trisomy 13, and Turner syndrome (32), an increased NT is also found in association with rare chromosomal anomalies such us partial trisomies, trisomy 9, translocations, subtelomeric deletions, ring chromosomes, etc. (100–103).

Residual Risk After the 20-Week Scan

Although most mortality and morbidity associated with increased NT can be determined by the time of the 20-week scan, we should consider the residual risk of a fetal anomaly remaining undetected at this stage. Souka et al. found that in 980 cases of NT >3.5 mm, where no anomalies were found at the 20 week-scan, the residual risk of an adverse outcome was very small (2%)—including several cases of cardiac defects that were amenable to prenatal diagnosis (44). The risk of adverse outcome was significantly higher (18%) if nuchal edema or pericardial effusion was still recognizable at the time of the 20-week scan. In our experience, the residual risk of an anomaly being detected after birth when the 20-week scan is normal is about 3%. Giving accurate data about long-term outcome, and specifically the incidence of neurodevelopmental delay, is hampered by differences in the length of follow-up and method of data acquisition used by different study groups. The prevalence of neurodevelopmental delay ranges from 0% to 5.3% in studies with no formal pediatric evaluation (10,43,104,105). Another comparison of neurodevelopmental outcome between 89 infants who had had increased NT and 302 infants with normal findings at the 11 to 14 week scan found no significant difference between the two groups (106). This study included pediatric evaluation but follow-up ranged from 6 to 42 months and neurodevelopmental delay may not always be detected in the early stages of infancy. The most detailed report of neurodevelopmental outcome is provided by Hippala et al. who followed infants for 2.4 to 7.1 years and made a diagnosis of developmental delay in just one (2%) infant (72).

Increased NT, Pregnancy Complications, and Future Pregnancies

There seems to be an individual predisposition for a repeated isolated increased NT measurement at subsequent pregnancies (107). In pregnancies developing pregnancy-induced hypertension and preeclampsia, the finding of an enlarged NT early in pregnancy is more frequent than in normotensive pregnancies. Although increased NT cannot be considered as a marker for the subsequent development of preeclampsia, the association deserves further investigation (108).

Heart Function in Fetuses with Increased NT

Fetuses with DS have frequently associated cardiac defects. Hemodynamic disturbances are present already from early on in pregnancy. For instance, fetuses with DS often show tricuspidal regurgitation (109). A recent study that assessed by Doppler investigations the heart performance of normal fetuses with increased NT reported no change when compared with fetuses with normal NT (110). The conclusion was that important cardiac dysfunction could not be demonstrated in association with increased NT in normal or abnormal fetuses. This conclusion does not support a major role for cardiac functional abnormality in the development of NT. Conversely, a study performed at midgestation suggests that fetuses with increased NT showed diastolic dysfunction with decreased E/A ratios (111). Ductus venosus (DV) flow has been studied extensively in fetuses with increased NT. All studies agree that DV tends to show high pulsatility index for the veins (PIV) (resistance) and zero or reversed flow during the a-wave in fetuses with increased NT and chromosomal abnormalities. NT and DV together can improve the efficiency of screening for chromosomal anomalies. Sensitivities for DV alone vary between studies from 65% to 92% (112–115). Bilardo pointed out that one of the problems with DV studies is the poor reproducibility and the great intrafetal variation (113). In fact, 16% of fetuses with a normal NT also showed abnormal DV patterns, and mixed normal/abnormal patterns are also frequently encountered in chromosomally abnormal fetuses. Moreover, NT and DV are related and follow the same trend. This hampers combination of the two techniques in screening strategies (113).

Abnormal DV flow has also been observed in chromosomally normal fetuses with increased NT and heart defects (112,113). Bilardo and Favre observed cardiac defects in fetuses with enlarged NT, abnormal ductus flow and normal karyotype, in 26% and 30%, respectively (113,116). Haak found markedly changed DV velocities in fetuses with NT >95th percentile and with cardiac defects. As the type of cardiac defects found in these cases does not provide an explanation for the DV abnormality, the authors suggest that some other mechanisms seem to be involved (117). Assessment of DV blood flow velocimetry could improve the predictive capacity of NT alone for an underlying major cardiac defect (117).

Acceptance of NT Screening, Counseling, and Ethical Issues

As an increased NT measurement represents a visible fetal anomaly, many parents equate a high-risk result with fetal abnormality more readily than in the case of abnormal findings from maternal serum screening (118). However, the majority of fetuses with increased NT and a normal karyotype will have a normal outcome. This information together with a discussion about the plan for subsequent management should help them to continue the pregnancy with confidence and avoid choosing to terminate on the basis of an ultrasound marker rather than the identification of a fetal abnormality (71).

In many published studies on NT screening, the screen-positive rate is higher than the expected 5% due to overrepresentation of older women in the study populations. Women aged ≥35 years are traditionally informed that they should consider invasive testing because of their age-related risk. Against this background it can be speculated that the popularity of first-trimester screening among this group is inspired by the hope that the result will be reassuring enough to support a decision against invasive testing. In contrast, younger women may not feel the need to be reassured by a screening test, since they have been educated that they are at "low risk" based on their age alone.

The hypothesis that older women utilized screening to avoid invasive testing is supported by findings from an Italian study where uptake of screening and demand for invasive testing was evaluated. Zoppi reported that in 1999 virtually all women in their population who were ≥35 years opted for NT screening (36). The subgroup that went on to have invasive testing was significantly smaller (32%) than the proportion that opted for invasive testing prior to availability of screening. De Graaf assessed the knowledge of pregnant women about prenatal tests and asked them which method they would prefer (119). Overall, the women had limited knowledge of DS and the prenatal screening and diagnostic tests that are available. This finding is also supported by De Vigan (120). However, de Graaf indicated that, when informed, the majority of women expressed a clear preference for first-trimester screening, regardless of the rate of miscarriage of DS pregnancies between 10 and 15 weeks of gestation. Several authors stress that parents ought to be informed about the possible implications of NT screening *prior to assessment*. The aims of the scan should be fully explained, in addition to the choice to opt out of any screening tests (67,72). In practice, this approach has not been implemented in all centers. Williams assessed the dilemmas encountered in routine NT screening in a multidisciplinary discussion group. The authors reached the conclusion that, as a first step, resources should be allocated to train staff. In addition, further research needs to examine how resources should be used to ensure that all women are indeed fully informed. It is suggested that it would be preferable to separate "scanning" (to monitor the pregnancy) from "screening" (for fetal abnormality) (121).

Chasen stresses that NT is a reliable screening method when conducted according to accepted standards of quality. Offering NT screening to all women is an important autonomy-enhancing strategy and there is no compelling beneficence-based argument not to do this (122). In a study from The Netherlands, low-risk pregnant women were asked prior to any information to fill in questionnaires investigating their basic knowledge of screening and DS. After counseling and NT screening, their reactions to this screening method were also investigated. Women were able to understand the concept of screening and to appreciate the opportunity to undergo NT measurement. Also women who declined this screening test considered that Down syndrome screening should be offered to all pregnant women (123).

NT Screening in Pregnancies from Assisted Conception

Women who undergo assisted conception place greater value on the results of the ultrasound examination in their decision about invasive testing than women who get pregnant spontaneously. Due to the relative advanced maternal age in this group, a false positive result from ultrasound screening will be relatively common. Nevertheless, the age effect on the false positive rate is even stronger if the screening program would be based on midtrimester serum biochemistry (124,125).

NT Screening and Multiple Pregnancies

Sebire has studied the value of NT screening in twin pregnancies. In 448 twin pregnancies, the NT thickness was >95th percentile of the normal range of 7.3, including 88% of the trisomy 21. Increased translucency was also present in four fetuses with other chromosomal abnormalities. In the chromosomally normal twin pregnancies, the prevalence of increased NT was higher in fetuses from monochorionic (8.4%) than in dichorionic pregnancies (5.4%). In twin pregnancies, the sensitivity of fetal NT thickness in screening for trisomy 21 is similar to that in singleton pregnancies, but the specificity is lower because translucency is also increased in chromosomally normal monochorionic twin pregnancies (126).

In a paper from Spencer and Nicolaides, it was shown that the overall acceptance of first-trimester screening among women with twins was high (224/230 = 97%). The rate of detection of trisomy 21 was 75% (3/4). Uptake of invasive testing was 59%. First-trimester screening for trisomy 21 in twin pregnancies is both theoretically possible and practically achievable. The best performance is achieved by a combination of NT thickness and maternal serum biochemistry. However, when NT is normal and maternal serum is not, the attitudes of both the mother and health professionals suggest that greater reliance is placed on the NT thickness risk alone in the choice for the need of an invasive testing (127). Maymon stated that NT translucency measurement is among the best available and the most efficient screening method for multiple pregnancies. This sonographical method for screening enables specific identification of those fetuses at high risk of DS and other anomalies and, thus, contributes to a better outcome. Therefore, it should be systematically performed when fetal reduction in high-order multiple pregnancies is planned (124).

CONCLUSION

The finding that an early ultrasound feature, the NT, could be used as a screening method for chromosomal anomalies has been a major breakthrough in prenatal diagnosis. Standardization of the time when the ultrasound scans are performed has increased our knowledge on the pathophysiology of early pregnancy in singleton and multiple pregnancies. Even in the event that in the future other, more effective or non-invasive screening strategies may replace NT measurement, evaluation of this ultrasound marker will provide unique, unequalled information on the normal development of the human fetus.

REFERENCES

1. Down JL. Observations on an ethnic classification of idiots. Clin Lect Rep Lond Hosp 1866; 3:259–262.
2. Tabor A, Philip J, Madsen M, Bang J, Obel EB, Norgaard-Pedersen B. Randomised controlled trial of genetic amniocentesis in 4606 low-risk women. Lancet 1986; 1(8493):1287–1293.

3. Snijders RJ, Sundberg K, Holzgreve W, Henry G, Nicolaides KH. Maternal age- and gestation-specific risk for trisomy 21. Ultrasound Obstet Gynecol 1999; 13(3):167–170.
4. Wald N, Cuckle H, Royston P. Antenatal screening for Down's syndrome. Lancet 1988; 2(8624):1362.
5. Szabo J, Gellen J. Nuchal fluid accumulation in trisomy-21 detected by vaginosonography in first trimester. Lancet 1990; 336(8723):1133.
6. Nicolaides KH, Azar G, Byrne D, Mansur C, Marks K. Fetal nuchal translucency: ultrasound screening for chromosomal defects in first trimester of pregnancy. Br Med J 1992; 304:867–869.
7. Pajkrt E, Bilardo CM, van Lith JMM, Mol BWJ, Bleker OP. Nuchal translucency measurement in normal fetuses. Obstet Gynecol 1995; 86:994–997.
8. Pandya PP, Snijders RJ, Johnson SP, Dc Lourdes Brizot M, Nicolaides KH. Screening for fetal trisomies by maternal age and fetal nuchal translucency thickness at 10–14 weeks of gestation. Br J Obstet Gynaecol 1995; 102(12):957–962.
9. Braithwaite JM, Economides DL. The measurement of nuchal translucency with transabdominal and transvaginal sonography—success rates, repeatability and levels of agreement. Br J Radiol 1995; 68(811):720–723.
10. Souka AP, Snijders RJM, Novakov A, Soares W, Nicolaides KH. Defects and syndromes in chromosomally normal fetuses with increased nuchal translucency thickness at 10–14 weeks of gestation. Ultrasound Obstet Gynecol 1998; 11:391–400.
11. Bilardo CM, Muller MA, Paijkrt E. Outcome of fetuses with increased nuchal translucency. Curr Opin Obstet Gynecol 2001; 13:169–174.
12. Castelli E, Todros T, Mattutino G, Torre C, Panattoni G. Light and scanning electron microscope study of nuchal translucency in a normal fetus. Ultrasound Obstet Gynecol 2003; 21(5):514–516.
13. Johnson MP, Johnson A, Holzgreve W, et al. First-trimester simple hygroma: cause and outcome. Am J Obstet Gynecol 1993; 168(1, Pt 1):156–161.
14. Shulman LP, Emerson DS, Felker RE, Phillips OP, Simpson JL, Elias S. High frequency of cytogenetic abnormalities in fetuses with cystic hygroma diagnosed in the first trimester. Obstet Gynecol 1992; 80(1):80–82.
15. Ville Y, Lalondrelle C, Doumerc S, et al. First-trimester diagnosis of nuchal anomalies: significance and fetal outcome. Ultrasound Obstet Gynecol 1992; 2(5):314–316.
16. van Zalen-Sprock RM, van Vugt JM, van Geijn HP. First-trimester diagnosis of cystic hygroma—course and outcome. Am J Obstet Gynecol 1992; 167(1):94–98.
17. Bewley S, Roberts LJ, Mackinson AM, Rodeck CH. First trimester fetal nuchal translucency: problems with screening the general population. 2. Br J Obstet Gynaecol 1995; 102(5):386–388.
18. Szabo J, Gellen J, Szemere G. First-trimester ultrasound screening for fetal aneuploidies in women over 35 and under 35 years of age. Ultrasound Obstet Gynecol 1995; 5(3): 161–163.
19. Kornman LH, Morssink LP, Beekhuis JR, De Wolf BT, Heringa MP, Mantingh A. Nuchal translucency cannot be used as a screening test for chromosomal abnormalities in the first trimester of pregnancy in a routine ultrasound practice. Prenat Diagn 1996; 16(9):797–805.
20. Economides DL, Whitlow BJ, Kadir R, Lazanakis M, Verdin SM. First trimester sonographic detection of chromosomal abnormalities in an unselected population. Br J Obstet Gynaecol 1998; 105(1):58–62.
21. Crossley JA, Aitken DA, Cameron AD, McBride E, Connor JM. Combined ultrasound and biochemical screening for Down's syndrome in the first trimester: a Scottish multicentre study. Br J Obstet Gynaecol 2002; 109(6):667–676.
22. Wald NJ, Rodeck C, Hachshaw AK, Chitty L, Machinson AM. SURUSS Research Group: first and second trimester antenatal screening for Down's syndrome: the result of the serum, urine and ultrasound study (SURUSS). Health Technol Assess 2003; 7:1–77.

23. Wayda K, Kereszturi A, Orvos H, et al. Four years experience of first-trimester nuchal translucency screening for fetal aneuploidies with increasing regional availability. Acta Obstet Gynecol Scand 2001; 80(12):1104–1109.

24. Rozenberg P, Malagrida L, Cuckle H, et al. Down's syndrome screening with nuchal translucency at 12(+0)–14(+0) weeks and maternal serum markers at 14(+1)–17(+0) weeks: a prospective study. Hum Reprod 2002; 17(4):1093–1098.

25. Schuchter K, Hafner E, Stangl G, Ogris E, Philipp K. Sequential screening for trisomy 21 by nuchal translucency measurement in the first trimester and maternal serum biochemistry in the second trimester in a low-risk population. Ultrasound Obstet Gynecol 2001; 18:23–25.

26. Haddow JE, Palomaki GE, Knight GJ, Williams J, Miller WA, Johnson A. Screening of maternal serum for fetal Down's syndrome in the first trimester. N Engl J Med 1998; 338(14):955–961.

27. Taipale P, Hiilesmaa V, Salonen R, Ylostalo P. Increased nuchal translucency as a marker for fetal chromosomal defects. N Engl J Med 1997; 337(23):1654–1658.

28. Pajkrt E, van Lith JM, Mol BW, Bleker OP, Bilardo CM. Screening for Down's syndrome by fetal nuchal translucency measurement in a general obstetric population. Ultrasound Obstet Gynecol 1998; 12(3):163–169.

29. Pajkrt E, van Lith JM, Mol BW, Bleker OP, Bilardo CM. Screening for Down's syndrome by fetal nuchal translucency measurement in a high-risk population. Ultrasound Obstet Gynecol 1998; 12(3):156–162.

30. Schwarzler P, Carvalho JS, Senat MV, Masroor T, Campbell S, Ville Y. Screening for fetal aneuploidies and fetal cardiac abnormalities by nuchal translucency thickness measurement at 10–14 weeks of gestation as part of routine antenatal care in an unselected population. Br J Obstet Gynaecol 1999; 106(10):1029–1034.

31. Theodoropoulos P, Lolis D, Papageorgiou C, Papaioannou S, Plachouras N, Makrydimas G. Evaluation of first-trimester screening by fetal nuchal translucency and maternal age. Prenat Diagn 1998; 18(2):133–137.

32. Panburana P, Ajjimakorn S, Tungkajiwangoon P. First trimester Down's syndrome screening by nuchal translucency in a Thai population. Int J Gynaecol Obstet 2001; 75(3):311–312.

33. Roberts LJ, Bewley S, Mackinson AM, Rodeck CH. First trimester fetal nuchal translucency: problems with screening the general population. 1. Br J Obstet Gynaecol 1995; 102(5):381–385.

34. Snijders RJM, Noble P, Sebire N, Souka A, Nicolaides KH. UK multicentre project on assessment of risk of trisomy 21 by maternal age and fetal nuchal translucency thickness at 10–14 weeks of gestation. Lancet 1998; 351:343–346.

35. Thilaganathan B, Sairam S, Michailidis G, Wathen NC. First trimester nuchal translucency: effective routine screening for Down's syndrome. Br J Radiol 1999; 72(862):946–948.

36. Zoppi MA, Ibba RM, Floris M, Monni G. Fetal nuchal translucency screening in 12,495 pregnancies in Sardinia. Ultrasound Obstet Gynecol 2001; 18(6):649–651.

37. Brizot ML, Carvalho MH, Liao AW, Reis NS, Armbruster-Moraes E, Zugaib M. First-trimester screening for chromosomal abnormalities by fetal nuchal translucency in a Brazilian population. Ultrasound Obstet Gynecol 2001; 18(6):652–655.

38. Gasiorek-Wiens A, Tercanli S, Kozlowski P, et al. Screening for trisomy 21 by fetal nuchal translucency and maternal age: a multicenter project in Germany, Austria and Switzerland. Ultrasound Obstet Gynecol 2001; 18(6):645–648.

39. Prefumo F, Thilaganathan B. Agreement between predicted risk and prevalence of Down's syndrome in first trimester nuchal translucency screening. Prenat Diagn 2002; 22(10):917–918.

40. Chasen ST, Chasen ST, Sharma G, Kalish RB, Chervenak FA. First-trimester screening for aneuploidy with fetal nuchal translucency in a United States population. Ultrasound Obstet Gynecol 2003; 22(2):149–151.

41. Malone FD, D'Alton ME. Society for Maternal–Fetal Medicine. First-trimester sonographic screening for Down's syndrome. Obstet Gynecol 2003; 102(5, Pt 1): 1066–1079.

42. Mol BW, Lijmer JG, van der Meulen J, Pajkrt E, Bilardo CM, Bossuyt PM. Effect of study design on the association between nuchal translucency measurement and Down's syndrome. Obstet Gynecol 1999; 94(5, Pt 2):864–869.

43. Souka AP, Krampl E, Bakalis S, Heath V, Nicolaides KH. Outcome of pregnancy in chromosomally normal fetuses with increased nuchal translucency in the first trimester. Ultrasound Obstet Gynecol 2001; 18:9–17.

44. Pajkrt E, Mol BWJ, Bleker OP, Bilardo CM. Pregnancy outcome and nuchal translucency measurements in fetuses with a normal karyotype. Prenat Diagn 1999; 19: 1104–1108.

45. Pandya PP, Snijders RJ, Johnson S, Nicolaides KH. Natural history of trisomy 21 fetuses with increased nuchal translucency thickness. Ultrasound Obstet Gynecol 1995; 5(6):381–383.

46. Herman A, Dreazen E, Maymon R, Tovbin Y, Bukovsky I, Weinraub Z. Implementation of nuchal translucency image-scoring method during ongoing audit. Ultrasound Obstet Gynecol 1999; 14(6):388–389.

47. Snijders RJ, Thom EA, Zachary JM, et al. First-trimester trisomy screening: nuchal translucency measurement training and quality assurance to correct and unify technique. Ultrasound Obstet Gynecol 2002; 19(4):353–359.

48. Wojdemann KR, Christiansen M, Sundberg K, Larsen SO, Shalmi A, Tabor A. Quality assessment in prospective nuchal translucency screening for Down's syndrome. Ultrasound Obstet Gynecol 2001; 18(6):641–644.

49. Logghe H, Cuckle H, Sehmi I. Centre-specific ultrasound nuchal translucency medians needed for Down's syndrome screening. Prenat Diagn 2003; 23(5):389–392.

50. Edwards A, Mulvey S, Wallace EM. The effect of image size on nuchal translucency measurement. Prenat Diagn 2003; 23(4):284–286.

51. Gyselaers WJ, Vereecken AJ, Van Herck EJ, et al. Audit on nuchal translucency thickness measurements in Flanders, Belgium: a plea for methodological standardization. Ultrasound Obstet Gynecol 2004; 24(5):511–515.

52. Maul H, Scharf A, Baier P, et al. Ultrasound simulators: experience with the SonoTrainer and comparative review of other training systems. Ultrasound Obstet Gynecol 2004; 24(5):581–585.

53. Newey VR, Nassiri DK, Bhide A, Thilaganathan B. Nuchal translucency thickness measurement: repeatability using a virtual ultrasound scanner. Ultrasound Obstet Gynecol 2003; 21(6):596–601.

54. Spencer K, Bindra R, Nix AB, Heath V, Nicolaides KH. Delta-NT or NT MoM: which is the most appropriate method for calculating accurate patient-specific risks for trisomy 21 in the first trimester? Ultrasound Obstet Gynecol 2003; 22(2):142–148.

55. Mulvey S, Baker L, Edwards A, Oldham J, Shekleton P, Wallace EM. Optimising the timing for nuchal translucency measurement. Prenat Diagn 2002; 22(9):775–777.

56. Muller MA, Pajkrt E, Bleker OP, Bonsel GJ, Bilardo CM. Disappearance of enlarged nuchal translucency before 14 weeks' gestation: relationship with chromosomal abnormalities and pregnancy outcome. Ultrasound Obstet Gynecol 2004; 24(2):169–174.

57. Zoppi MA, Ibba RM, Floris M, Manca F, Axiana C, Monni G. Changes in nuchal translucency thickness in normal and abnormal karyotype fetuses. Br J Obstet Gynaecol 2003; 110(6):584–588.

58. Jou HJ, Wu SC, Li TC, Hsu HC, Tzeng CY, Hsieh FJ. Relationship between fetal nuchal translucency and crown–rump length in an Asian population. Ultrasound Obstet Gynecol 2001; 17(2):111–114.

59. Thilaganathan B, Khare M, Williams B, Wathen NC. Influence of ethnic origin on nuchal translucency screening for Down's syndrome. Ultrasound Obstet Gynecol 1998; 12:112–114.

60. Chen M, Hang Lam Y, Hoi Yin Tang M, et al. The effect of ethnic origin on nuchal translucency at 10–14 weeks of gestation. Prenat Diagn 2002; 22(7):576–578.

61. Paul C, Krampl E, Skentou C, Jurkovic D, Nicolaides KH. Measurement of fetal nuchal translucency thickness by three-dimensional ultrasound. Ultrasound Obstet Gynecol 2001; 18(5):481–484.

62. Eppel W, Worda C, Frigo P, Lee A. Three- versus two-dimensional ultrasound for nuchal translucency thickness measurements: comparison of feasibility. Prenat Diagn 2001; 21:596–601.

63. Clementschitsch G, Hasenohrl G, Schaffer H, Steiner H. Comparison between two- and three-dimensional ultrasound measurements of nuchal translucency. Ultrasound Obstet Gynecol 2001; 18(5):475–480.

64. Michailidis GD, Papageorgiou P, Economides DL. Assessment of fetal anatomy in the first trimester using two- and three-dimensional ultrasound. Br J Radiol 2002; 75(891):215–219.

65. Worda C, Radner G, Lee A, Eppel W. Three-dimensional ultrasound for nuchal translucency thickness measurements: comparison of transabdominal and transvaginal ultrasound. J Soc Gynecol Investig 2003; 10(6):361–365.

66. Bilardo CM, Pajkrt E, de Graaf I, Mol BW, Bleker OP. Outcome of fetuses with enlarged nuchal translucency and normal karyotype. Ultrasound Obstet Gynecol 1998; 11:401–406.

67. Michailidis GD, Economides DL. Nuchal translucency measurement and pregnancy outcome in karyotypically normal fetuses. Ultrasound Obstet Gynecol 2001; 17: 102–105.

68. Maymon R, Herman A. The clinical evaluation and pregnancy outcome of euploid fetuses with increased nuchal translucency. Clin Genet 2004; 66(5):426–436.

69. Maymon R, Tercanli S, Dreazen E, Sartorius G, Holzgreve W, Herman A. Comparison of pregnancy outcome of euploid fetuses with increased nuchal translucency (NT) expressed in NT MoM or delta-NT. Ultrasound Obstet Gynecol 2004; 23(5):477–481.

70. Bilardo CM. Increased nuchal translucency and normal karyotype: coping with uncertainty. Ultrasound Obstet Gynecol 2001; 17(2):99–110.

71. Hiippala A, Eronen M, Taipale P, Salonen R, Hiilesmaa V. Fetal nuchal translucency and normal chromosomes: a long-term follow-up study. Ultrasound Obstet Gynecol 2001; 18(1):18–22.

72. Senat MV, De Keersmaecker B, Audibert F, Montcharmont G, Frydman R, Ville Y. Pregnancy outcome in fetuses with increased nuchal translucency and normal karyotype. Prenat Diagn 2002; 22(5):345–349.

73. Maher JE, Colvin EV, Samdarshi TE, Owen J, Hauth JC. Fetal echocardiography in gravidas with historic risk factors for congenital heart disease. Am J Perinatol 1994; 11:334–336.

74. Sharland GK, Allan LD. Screening for congenital heart disease prenatally. Results of a 2 1/2-year study in the South East Thames Region. Br J Obstet Gynaecol 1992; 99: 220–225.

75. Rustico MA, Benettoni A, D'Ottavio G, et al. Fetal heart screening in low-risk pregnancies. Ultrasound Obstet Gynecol 1995; 6:313–319.

76. Levi S. Mass screening for fetal malformations: the Eurofetus study. Ultrasound Obstet Gynecol 2003; 22(6):555–558.

77. Carvalho JS, Moscoso G, Ville Y. First trimester transabdominal fetal echocardiography. Lancet 1998; 351:1023–1027.

78. Sharland G. First trimester transabdominal fetal echocardiography. Lancet 1998; 351:1662.

79. Huggon IC, Ghi T, Cook AC, Zosmer N, Allan LD, Nicolaides KH. Fetal cardiac abnormalities identified prior to 14 weeks' gestation. Ultrasound Obstet Gynecol 2002; 20(1):22–29.

80. Haak MC, van Vugt JM. Echocardiography in early pregnancy: review of literature. J Ultrasound Med 2003; 22(3):271–280.

81. Hyett JA, Perdu M, Sharland GK, Snijders RSM, Nicolaides KH. Screening for congenital heart disease with fetal nuchal translucency at 10–14 weeks of gestation. Br Med J 1999; 318:81–85.

82. Ghi T, Huggon IC, Zosmer N, Nicolaides KH. Incidence of major structural cardiac defects associated with increased nuchal translucency but normal karyotype. Ultrasound Obstet Gynecol 2001; 18(6):610–614.

83. Galindo A, Comas C, Martinez JM, et al. Cardiac defects in chromosomally normal fetuses with increased nuchal translucency at 10–14 weeks of gestation. J Matern Fetal Neonatal Med 2003; 13(3):163–170.

84. McAuliffe FM, Hornberger LK, Winsor S, Chitayat D, Chong K, Johnson JA. Fetal cardiac defects and increased nuchal translucency thickness: a prospective study. Am J Obstet Gynecol 2004; 191(4):1486–1490.

85. Mavrides E, Cobian-Sanchez F, Tekay A, et al. Limitations of using first-trimester nuchal translucency measurement in routine screening for major congenital heart defects. Ultrasound Obstet Gynecol 2001; 17(2):106–110.

86. Orvos H, Wayda K, Kozinszky Z, Katona M, Pal A, Szabo J. Increased nuchal translucency and congenital heart defects in euploid fetuses. The Szeged experience. Eur J Obstet Gynecol Reprod Biol 2002; 101(2):124–128.

87. Hafner E, Schuller T, Metzenbauer M, Schuchter K, Philipp K. Increased nuchal translucency and congenital heart defects in a low-risk population. Prenat Diagn 2003; 23(12):985–989.

88. Makrydimas G, Sotiriadis A, Ioannidis JPA. Screening performance of first-trimester nuchal translucency for major cardiac defects: a meta-analysis. Am J Obstet Gynecol 2003; 189(5):1330–1335.

89. Bilardo CM, Timmerman E, Muller MA, Clur SA. Nuchal translucency measurement as screening method for major congenital heart defects in low risk pregnancies. Ultrasound Obstet Gynecol 2004; 24(3):361.

90. Carvalho JS, Moscoso G, Tekay A, Campbell S, Thilaganathan B, Shinebourne EA. Clinical impact of first and early second trimester fetal echocardiography on high risk pregnancies. Heart 2004; 90(8):921–926.

91. Nicolaides KH, Sebire NJ, Snijders RJM. In: Nicolaides K, ed. The 11–14 Week Scan. Diploma in Fetal Medicine Series. New York: Parthenon Publishing, .

92. Sebire NJ, Snijders RJM, Davenport M, Greenough A, Nicolaides KH. Fetal nuchal translucency thickness at 10–14 weeks of gestation and congenital diaphragmatic hernia. Obstet Gynecol 1997; 90:943–947.

93. Tercanli S, Miny P, Siebert MS, Hosli D, Surbek DV, Holsgreve W. Fanconi anemia associated with increased nuchal translucency detected by first-trimester ultrasound. Ultrasound Obstet Gynecol 2001; 17:160–162.

94. Souka AP, Bower S, Geerts L, Huggon I, Nicolaides KH. Blackfan–Diamond anemia and dyserythropoietic anemia presenting with increased nuchal translucency at 12 weeks of gestation. Ultrasound Obstet Gynecol 2002; 20(2):197–199.

95. Achiron R, Heggesh J, Grisaru D, et al. Noonan syndrome: a cryptic condition in early gestation. Am J Med Genet 2000; 92:159–165.

96. Makrydimas G, Sotiriadis A, Papapanagiotou G, Tsopelas A, Lolis D. Fetal akinesia deformation sequence presenting with increased nuchal translucency in the first trimester of pregnancy. Fetal Diagn Ther 2004; 19(4):332–335.

97. Hyett JA. Increased nuchal translucency in fetuses with a normal karyotype. Prenat Diagn 2002; 22(10):864–868.

98. Laurichesse-Delmas H, Beaufrere AM, Martin A, Kaemmerlen AG, Dechelotte P, Lemery D. First-trimester features of Fowler syndrome (hydrocephaly–hydranencephaly proliferative vasculopathy). Ultrasound Obstet Gynecol 2002; 20(6):612–615.

99. Souka AP, Raymond FL, Mornet E, Geerts L, Nicolaides KH. Hypophosphatasia associated with increased nuchal translucency: a report of two affected pregnancies. Ultrasound Obstet Gynecol 2002; 20(3):294–295.

100. Rauch A, Beese M, Mayatepek E, et al. A novel 5q35.3 subtelomeric deletion syndrome. Am J Med Genet 2003; 121A(1):1–8.

101. Sepulveda W, Wimalasundera RC, Taylor MJ, Blunt S, Be C, De La Fuente S. Prenatal ultrasound findings in complete trisomy 9. Ultrasound Obstet Gynecol 2003; 22(5): 479–483.

102. Le Caignec C, Boceno M, Joubert M, et al. Prenatal diagnosis of a small supernumerary, XIST-negative, mosaic ring X chromosome identified by fluorescence in situ hybridization in an abnormal male fetus. Prenat Diagn 2003; 23(2):143–145.

103. Kim YM, Cho EH, Kim JM, Lee MH, Park SY, Ryu HM. Del(18p) syndrome with increased nuchal translucency in prenatal diagnosis. Prenat Diagn 2004; 24(3):161–164.

104. Cha'ban FK, Van Splunder P, Los FJ, Wladimiroff JW. Fetal outcome in nuchal translucency with emphasis on normal fetal karyotype. Prenat Diagn 1996; 16:537–541.

105. van Vugt JMG, Tinnemans BWS, Van Zalen-Sprock RM. Outcome and early childhood follow-up of chromosomally normal fetuses with increased nuchal translucency at 10–14 weeks' gestation. Ultrasound Obstet Gynecol 1998; 11:407–409.

106. Brady AF, Pandya PP, Yuksel B, Greenough A, Patton MA, Nicolaides KH. Outcome of chromosomally normal livebirths with increased fetal nuchal translucency at 10–14 weeks' gestation. J Med Genet 1998; 35:222–224.

107. Maymon R, Padoa A, Dreazen E, Herman A. Nuchal translucency measurements in consecutive normal pregnancies. Is there a predisposition to increased levels? Prenat Diagn 2002; 22(9):759–762.

108. Tsai MS, Lee FK, Cheng CC, Hwa KY, Cheong ML, She BQ. Association between fetal nuchal translucency thickness in first trimester and subsequent gestational hypertension and preeclampsia. Prenat Diagn 2002; 22(9):747–751.

109. Huggon IC, DeFigueiredo DB, Allan LD. Tricuspid regurgitation in the diagnosis of chromosomal anomalies in the fetus at 11–14 weeks of gestation. Heart 2003; 89(9):1071–1073.

110. Huggon IC, Turan O, Allan LD. Doppler assessment of cardiac function at 11–14 weeks' gestation in fetuses with normal and increased nuchal translucency. Ultrasound Obstet Gynecol 2004; 24(4):390–398.

111. Rizzo G, Muscatello A, Angelini E, Capponi A. Abnormal cardiac function in fetuses with increased nuchal translucency. Ultrasound Obstet Gynecol 2003; 21(6): 539–542.

112. Matias A, Gomes C, Flack N, Montenegro N, Nicolaides KH. Screening for chromosomal abnormalities at 10–14 weeks: the role of ductus venosus blood flow. Ultrasound Obstet Gynecol 1998; 12:380–384.

113. Bilardo CM, Muller MA, Zikulnig L, Schipper M, Hecher K. Ductus venosus studies in fetuses at high risk for chromosomal or heart abnormalities: relationship with nuchal translucency measurement and fetal outcome. Ultrasound Obstet Gynecol 2001; 17(4):288–294.

114. Mavrides E, Sairam S, Hollis B, Thilaganathan B. Screening for aneuploidy in the first trimester by assessment of blood flow in the ductus venosus. Br J Obstet Gynaecol 2002; 109:1015–1019.

115. Borrell A, Martinez JM, Serés A, Borobio V, Cararach V, Fortuny A. Ductus venosus assessment at the time of nuchal translucency measurement in the detection of fetal aneuploidy. Prenat Diagn 2003; 23:921–926.

116. Favre R, Cherif Y, Kohler M, et al. The role of fetal nuchal translucency and ductus venosus Doppler at 11–14 weeks of gestation in the detection of major congenital heart defects. Ultrasound Obstet Gynecol 2003; 21(3):239–243.

117. Haak MC, Twisk JW, Bartelings MM, Gittenberger-de Groot AC, van Vugt JM. Ductus venosus flow velocities in relation to the cardiac defects in first-trimester fetuses with enlarged nuchal translucency. Am J Obstet Gynecol 2003; 188(3):727–733.

118. Weinans MJ, Kooij L, Muller MA, Bilardo KM, Van Lith JM, Tymstra T. A comparison of the impact of screen-positive results obtained from ultrasound and biochemical

screening for Down's syndrome in the first trimester: a pilot study. Prenat Diagn 2004; 24(5):347–351.

119. De Graaf IM, Tijmstra T, Bleker OP, Van Lith JM. Womens' preference in Down's syndrome screening. Prenat Diagn 2002; 22(7):624–629.

120. De Vigan C, Vodovar V, Goujard J, Garel M, Vayssiere C, Goffinet F. Mothers' knowledge of screening for trisomy 21 in 1999: a survey in Paris maternity units. Eur J Obstet Gynecol Reprod Biol 2002; 104(1):14–20.

121. Williams C, Alderson P, Farsides B. Dilemmas encountered by health practitioners offering nuchal translucency screening: a qualitative case study. Prenat Diagn 2002; 22(3):216–220.

122. Chasen ST, Skupski DW. Ethical dimensions of nuchal translucency screening. Clin Perinatol 2003; 30(1):95 102.

123. Müller MA, Bleker OP, Bonsel GJ, Bilardo CM. Women's opinion on the offer and use of nuchal translucency screening for Down syndrome. Prenatal Diagn 2006; 26:105–111.

124. Maymon R, Jauniaux E. Down's syndrome screening in pregnancies after assisted reproductive techniques: an update. Reprod Biomed Online 2002; 4(3):285–293.

125. Geipel A, Berg C, Katalinic A, et al. Different preferences for prenatal diagnosis in pregnancies following assisted reproduction versus spontaneous conception. Reprod Biomed Online 2004; 8(1):119–124.

126. Sebire NJ, Snijders RJ, Hughes K, Sepulveda W, Nicolaides KH. Screening for trisomy 21 in twin pregnancies by maternal age and fetal nuchal translucency thickness at 10–14 weeks of gestation. Br J Obstet Gynaecol 1996; 103(10):999–1003.

127. Spencer K, Nicolaides KH. Screening for trisomy 21 in twins using first trimester ultrasound and maternal serum biochemistry in a one-stop clinic: a review of three years experience. Br J Obstet Gynaecol 2003; 110(3):276–280.

4

Nasal Bone in Screening for Trisomy 21

Simona Cicero
*Harris Birthright Research Centre for Fetal Medicine, King's College Hospital,
Denmark Hill, London, U.K.*

J. D. Sonek
Department of Obstetrics and Gynecology, Ohio State University, Columbus, Ohio, U.S.A.

K. H. Nicolaides
*Harris Birthright Research Centre for Fetal Medicine, King's College School of Medicine
and Dentistry, London, U.K.*

In 1866 Langdon Down noted that a common characteristic of patients with trisomy 21 is a small nose (1). In the last five years it has become possible to identify this feature during intrauterine life by ultrasonography (2,3). This chapter reviews the studies on the prenatal diagnosis of hypoplasia of the nasal bone and the incorporation of this marker in screening for trisomy 21.

DEVELOPMENT OF THE NASAL BONES

The nasal bones develop from collections of neural crest cells that migrate to the frontonasal region of the face. During the eighth week of gestation, initial centers of ossification of the nasal bone appear in the membrane covering the cartilaginous nasal capsule (4–7). The earliest developmental stage at which the nasal bone can be demonstrated histologically is when the fetal crown–rump length is 42 mm and radiologically when the crown–rump length is 50 mm (8). The nasal bones develop as two separate structures with a gap in between them, which closes with advancing gestation.

RADIOLOGIC EVIDENCE OF NASAL HYPOPLASIA IN TRISOMY 21

An anthropometric study in 105 patients with trisomy 21 at 7 months to 36 years of age reported that the nasal root depth was abnormally short in about 50% of cases (9). In four postmortem radiologic studies, in a combined total of 145 aborted fetuses with trisomy 21, there was absence of ossification of the nasal bone in 42 (28.9%) (Table 1) (10–13). In addition, one of the studies examined the length of the nasal bone and reported this to be very short in 11 of the 23 (47.8%) cases (10). These findings suggest that in fetuses with trisomy 21, the nasal bones are absent in about 30% of cases and if present they are short in about 45% of cases.

Table 1 Prevalence of Absence of Ossification of the Nasal Bone in Radiologic
Studies of Aborted Fetuses with Trisomy 21

Author	N	Gestation (wk)	Absent nasal bone
Keeling et al. (10)	31	12–24	8 (25.8%)
Stempfle et al. (11)	60	15–40	14 (23.3%)
Tuxen et al. (12)	33	14–25	10 (33.3%)
Larose et al. (13)	21	13–25	10 (47.6%)
Total	145		42 (28.9%)

ULTRASOUND EVIDENCE OF NASAL HYPOPLASIA IN TRISOMY 21

Technique for Evaluation of the Nasal Bone

The nasal bones are two distinct structures and they can be identified as such on ultrasound. In order for the evaluation to be valid, a strict set of rules needs to be followed (14,15). This is especially true during the 11–13^{+6} weeks' scan. The most important confounding variables are the presence of bony and cartilaginous structures within the fetal face other than the nasal bone and the fact that sonographically, the skin over the nasal bridge is quite echogenic in appearance, especially in the first trimester and the early part of the second trimester.

The fetus needs to be facing the ultrasound transducer and a midsagittal view of the fetal face should be obtained. At the 11–13^{+6} weeks scan, the magnification of the fetus should be such that the head and the thorax occupy the whole image. For the purpose of simply identifying whether the nasal bone is present or absent, the face of the transducer needs to be parallel to the longitudinal axis of the nasal bone and to the skin over the nasal bridge. If the nasal bone is viewed "on end" (0° or 180° angle of insonation with respect to the longitudinal axis of the nasal bone), it will appear to be artificially absent (Fig. 1). In order to measure the nasal bone in the second trimester, a slightly oblique angle (45° or 135°) will help to define the edges of the nasal bone more sharply (Fig. 2).

The following echogenic lines are important to identify: first, the skin over the nasal bridge, second, a line below it, which represents the nasal bone and is parallel to the nasal bridge skin, and third, an echogenic line, which is further away from the forehead than the nasal bridge and at a slightly higher level, which represents the skin over the nasal tip. The two parallel lines representing the skin over the nasal bridge and the nasal bone compose the so-called "equal sign." The line representing the nasal bone is thicker and more echogenic than the skin and usually contains a highly echogenic center (Fig. 3). Both qualities need to be kept in mind in order to identify the nasal bone accurately. Tilting the transducer from side to side also helps to differentiate the skin from the nasal bone. If the bottom part of the equal sign is missing, the nasal bone is considered to be absent (Fig. 4). Occasionally, a faint and slightly echogenic line, which probably represents the nasal cartilage, is seen within the nasal bridge. If this line is less echogenic than the skin or if only a small echogenic dot is seen, then the nasal bone is also considered to be absent or hypoplastic.

If the nasal bone is absent on ultrasound between 11 and 12 weeks, we recommend a repeat examination in one week. The result of the second examination should be the one used for risk evaluation. This approach reduces the false-positive rate.

The subtleties of the nasal bone evaluation, especially during the 11- to 14-week scan, require adequate training and experience before it can be accurately

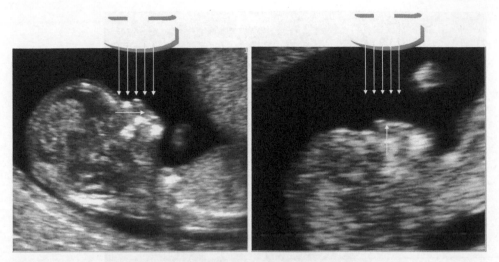

Figure 1   The best angle of insonation to assess the nasal bone in the first trimester is 90° to the longitudinal axis of the nasal bone (i.e., the beam of the ultrasound perpendicular to the longitudinal axis of the nasal bone) (*left*). Evaluation of the nasal bone should not be attempted with either a 0° or 180° angle of insonation (i.e., with the ultrasound beam parallel to the longitudinal axis of the nasal bone) (*right*).

employed. Cicero et al. studied the number of examinations required before sonographers became proficient in nasal bone evaluations (16). Fifteen sonographers, who were already trained to perform the 11- to 14-week scan, including the nuchal translucency (NT) measurement, were taught the technique of nasal bone evaluation.

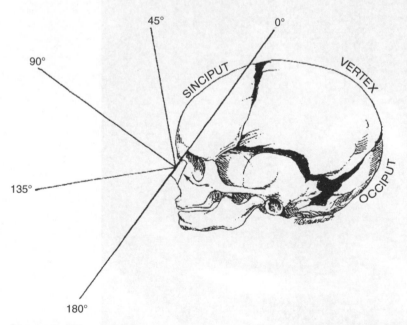

Figure 2   Diagrammatic representation of the bony structures of the fetal face with angles of insonation. *Source*: Adapted from O'Brien W, Cefalo R, Simpson J, eds. Obstetrics: Normal and Problem Pregnancies. 3rd ed. New York: Churchill Livingstone, 1996:393.

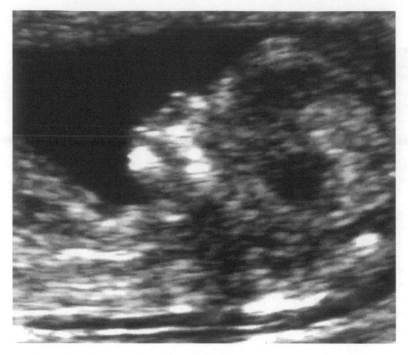

Figure 3 Fetal profile at 12 weeks of gestation in a normal fetus showing the nasal bone.

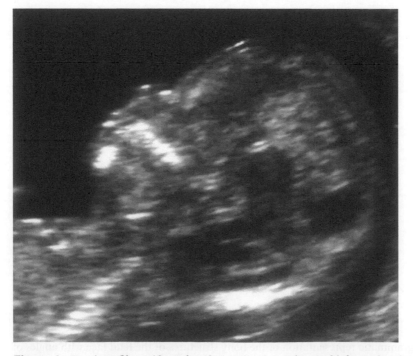

Figure 4 Fetal profile at 12 weeks of gestation in a trisomy-21 fetus showing absence of the nasal bone.

They found that the average number of studies required to achieve proficiency in nasal bone evaluation was 80 (40–120).

Three-Dimensional Ultrasound

Rembouscos et al. showed that three-dimensional (3-D) multiplanar imaging can be used to evaluate the fetal nasal bones at $11–13^{+6}$ weeks' gestation (17). However, in order to obtain a good quality volume, the same criteria as for optimal 2-D nasal bone assessment have to be met with the fetus being viewed in a midsagittal section facing the transducer and using the correct angle of insonation. Peralta et al. demonstrated that at $11–13^{+6}$ weeks a gap can be demonstrated between the nasal bones in about 20% of fetuses and that when the gap exceeds 0.6 mm, the nasal bones could not be visualized in a reconstructed perfectly midsagittal plane (18). This suggests that this distance is the limit of the lateral resolution of the ultrasound equipment. However, none of the fetuses were falsely diagnosed with nasal bone absence on 2-D ultrasound. This demonstrates that the presence of a gap does not increase the false-positive rate.

Benoit and Chaoui compared the 3-D and 2-D appearance of the nasal bone at 17–33 weeks (19). The nasal bone was present in all 18 euploid fetuses on 2-D ultrasound and all were found to have both nasal bones present on 3-D ultrasound. In the 20 fetuses with trisomy 21, nine had either an absent or hypoplastic nasal bone on 2-D ultrasound. The 3-D evaluation showed bilateral nasal bone absence in six fetuses and unilateral nasal bone absence in three. Goncalves et al. analyzed 3-D volumes of the nasal bone at 20–25 weeks. Nasal bone absence was detected in 9 of 26 (34.6%) fetuses with trisomy 21 and in 1 of 27 (3.7%) of the euploid fetuses (20).

Nasal Hypoplasia at 11–14 Weeks

Several studies have demonstrated a high association between absent nasal bone at $11–13^{+6}$ weeks and trisomy 21, as well as other chromosomal abnormalities. In the combined data from eight studies, the fetal profile was successfully examined in 98% of the cases (2,21–29). The nasal bone was absent in 185 of 15,048 (1.2%) chromosomally normal fetuses and in 282 of 412 (68.4%) of fetuses with trisomy 21 (Table 2). Absence of the nasal bone has also been reported in about 55% of fetuses with trisomy 18, 35% of those with trisomy 13, and 10% with Turner syndrome (28).

An important finding of the studies was that the incidence of absent nasal bone decreased with fetal crown–rump length, increased with fetal NT thickness, and was substantially higher in Afro-Caribbeans than in Caucasians (28). Consequently, in the calculation of likelihood ratios in screening for trisomy 21, adjustments must be made for these confounding factors.

The data of all studies have been contradicted by Malone et al. (30), who reported the results of a multicenter study, which included 6316 fetuses scanned at 10–14 weeks' gestation. Successful examination of the nasal bone was achieved in only 75.9% of the cases and the nasal bone was apparently present in all nine of their fetuses with trisomy 21. The most likely explanation for these findings is that their technique for assessment of the nasal bone was not consistent with that used by others.

Nasal Hypoplasia at 14–24 Weeks

Six studies have examined the fetal profile for absence of the nasal bone before genetic amniocentesis. In the combined data from these studies there was absence

Table 2 Summary of Studies Reporting on the Prevalence of Absent Nasal Bone in First-Trimester Fetuses with Trisomy 21

| | | Absent nasal bone ||
Author	Study	Normal, n (%)	Trisomy 21, n (%)
Cicero et al. (2)[a]	Pre-CVS	3/603 (0.5%)	43/59 (72.9%)
Otano et al. (21)	Pre-CVS	1/175 (0.6%)	3/5 (60.0%)
Zoppi et al. (22)	Screening	7/3,463 (0.2%)	19/27 (70.0%)
Orlandi et al. (23)	Screening	10/1,000 (1.0%)	10/15 (66.7%)
Viora et al. (24)	Screening	24/1,733 (1.4%)	8/10 (80.0%)
Senat et al. (25)	Retrospective	4/944 (0.4%)	3/4 (75%)
Wong et al. (26)	Pre-CVS	1/114 (0.9%)	2/3 (66.7%)
Cicero et al. (27)[a]	Pre-CVS	93/3,358 (2.8%)	162/242 (67%)
Cicero et al. (28)	Pre-CVS	129/5,223 (2.5%)	229/333 (68.8%)
Orlandi et al. (29)	Screening	9/2,396 (0.4%)	8/15 (53.3%)
Total		185/15,048 (1.2%)	282/412 (68.4%)

[a]Included in Cicero et al. (28).
Abbreviation: CVS, chorionic villous sampling.

of the nasal bone in 37% of the fetuses with trisomy 21 and in 1% of the chromosomally normal fetuses (Table 3) (19,31–35).

In addition, five studies have compared the length of the nasal bone in trisomy 21 and normal fetuses. In the combined data, the nasal bone was short in 46.3% of trisomy 21 and 2.8% of normal fetuses (Table 4) (31,32,35–37). When the data of the studies defining nasal hypoplasia as absent or short nasal bone are considered, there was nasal hypoplasia in 58% of trisomy 21 fetuses and in 2% of the normal fetuses (Figs. 5–7).

EXAMINATION OF THE NASAL BONE IN SCREENING FOR TRISOMY 21

First-Trimester Screening

Effective screening for trisomy 21 and all major chromosomal defects can be achieved at $11–13^{+6}$ weeks by a combination of maternal age, fetal NT thickness,

Table 3 Summary of Studies Reporting on the Prevalence of Absent Nasal Bone in Second-Trimester Fetuses with Trisomy 21

| | Gestation | Prevalence of absent nasal bone || Likelihood ratio ||
Study	(wk)	Trisomy 21	Normal	Positive	Negative
Bromley et al. (31)	15–20	6/16 (37.5%)	1/223 (0.4%)	93.8	0.63
Cicero et al. (32)	15–22	11/34 (32.4%)	6/982 (0.6%)	54.0	0.68
Vintzileos et al. (33)	18–20	12/29 (41.4%)	0/102 (0%)	—	—
Odibo et al. (34)	15–22	5/18 (27.8%)	14/583 (2.4%)	11.6	0.74
Tran et al. (35)	14–24	11/31 (35.5%)	1/136 (0.7%)	50.7	0.65
Benoit et al. (19)	17–33	9/20 (45.0%)	0/18 (0%)	—	—
Total		54/148 (36.5%)	22/2054 (1.1%)	33.2	0.64

Table 4 Summary of Studies Reporting on the Prevalence of Short or Absent Nasal Bone in Second-Trimester Fetuses with Trisomy 21

Study	Gestation (wk)	Abnormal nasal bone		
		Definition	Trisomy 21	Normal
Bromley et al. (31)	15–20	Short	5/10 (50.0%)	10/222 (4.5%)
		Absent or short	11/16 (68.8%)	11/223 (4.9%)
Cicero et al. (32)	15–22	Short	10/23 (43.5%)	6/976 (0.6%)
		Absent or short	21/34 (61.8%)	12/982 (1.2%)
Bunduki et al. (36)	16–24	Short	13/22 (59.1%)	82/1600 (5.1%)
Gamez et al. (37)	19–22	Short	5/5 (100%)	34/1899 (1.8%)
Tran et al. (35)	14–24	Short	4/20 (20.0%)	4/135 (3.0%)
		Absent or short	15/31 (48.4%)	5/136 (3.7%)
Total		Short	37/80 (46.3%)	136/4832 (2.8%)
		Absent or short	47/81 (58.0%)	28/1341 (2.1%)

and maternal serum–free β-human chorionic gonadotropin (β-hCG) and pregnancy-associated plasma protein-A (PAPP-A). Prospective screening studies have demonstrated that for a false-positive rate of 5%, the detection rate of trisomy 21 is about 90% (38,39). This compares favorably with the 30% detection rate achieved with screening by maternal age alone and the 60–70% detection rate by a combination of maternal age and second-trimester serum biochemistry.

A case–control study comprised of 100 trisomy 21 and 400 chromosomally normal singleton pregnancies at 11–13[+6] weeks of gestation found that the ultrasound finding of either the presence or absence of the nasal bone is independent of serum-free β-hCG and PAPP-A levels (40). Therefore, evaluation of the nasal bone can be added to the combination of NT and maternal serum–free β-hCG and PAPP-A measurements at 11–13[+6] weeks in screening for trisomy 21 to achieve a detection rate of 90%, with a substantial reduction in the false-positive rate.

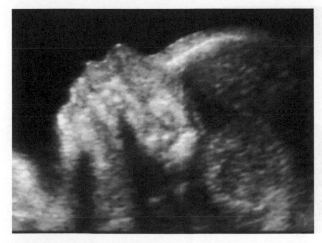

Figure 5 Fetal profile at 20 weeks of gestation in a trisomy-21 fetus showing absence of the nasal bone.

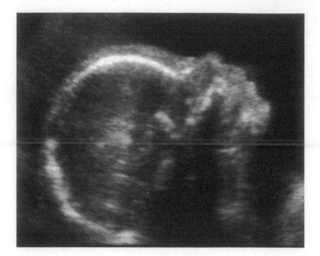

Figure 6 Fetal profile at 20 weeks of gestation in a trisomy-21 fetus showing nasal bone hypoplasia.

There are essentially two possible ways in which examination of the nasal bone can be incorporated into first-trimester screening. First, the nasal bone can be examined in all cases and the likelihood ratio for presence or absence of a visible bone can be multiplied by the estimated risk from maternal age, fetal NT, and maternal serum–free β-hCG and PAPP-A to derive a new integrated risk. Alternatively, since examination of the nasal bone can be difficult and requires extensive experience in first-trimester scanning, this examination is confined to a small subgroup of the patients (39). It was proposed that after combined fetal NT and maternal serum–free β-hCG and PAPP-A screening, patients are assigned into a high-risk category with a risk estimate of 1 in 100 or more, a low-risk category with a risk estimate of less than 1 in 1000, and an intermediate-risk category with a risk estimate of between 1 in 101 and 1 in 1000. Patients in the high-risk category are offered karyotyping by chorionic

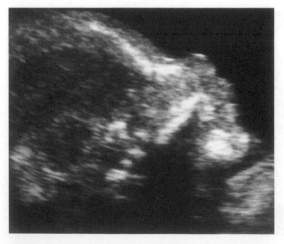

Figure 7 Fetal profile at 20 weeks of gestation in a normal fetus showing presence of the nasal bone.

villous sampling and those in the low-risk category are reassured that their fetus is unlikely to be chromosomally abnormal. The intermediate-risk category is offered nasal bone evaluation or one of the other novel screening tests, such as ductus venosus or tricuspid valve Doppler (41,42) at a center specializing in these procedures. If the nasal bone is absent, the patient is offered an invasive procedure and if the nasal bone is present, the patient is reassigned into the low-risk category and reassured. This approach achieves a detection rate of more than 90% and a false-positive rate of less than 3% (39).

Second-Trimester Screening

Trisomy 21 and other major chromosomal defects are associated with sonographically detectable major abnormalities or minor defects or markers. Systematic examination of the fetus for such major or minor defects led to the development of the so-called genetic sonogram. This is essentially applied in two situations. First, in women who, either through advanced maternal age or second-trimester biochemical screening, are considered to be at sufficiently high risk for chromosomal defects to necessitate the offer of amniocentesis. An increasing proportion of such women are reassured by the absence of any sonographically detectable defects and they choose to avoid having an amniocentesis. The second application of the genetic sonogram is in low-risk women. In such cases the presence of defects/markers increases the background maternal age–related risk for chromosomal defects. The methodology of adjusting the a priori maternal age-related or serum biochemistry-related risk by the findings of the genetic sonogram is essentially based on multiplying the a priori risk by the likelihood ratio for any given sonographic feature. The likelihood ratio is derived by dividing the prevalence of the defect in chromosomally abnormal fetuses by the prevalence in chromosomally normal fetuses (43).

In the combined data from two large series on a total of 350 trisomy 21 fetuses, a major anomaly or a minor defect was detected in about 75% of affected fetuses and in about 13% of the chromosomally normal controls (43–45). The respective prevalence in trisomy 21, prevalence in normals, and positive- and negative-likelihood ratios were 33.5%, 0.6%, 53.1, and 0.67 for increased nuchal fold thickness; 13.3%, 0.6%, 21.2, and 0.87 for echogenic bowel; 28.2%, 4.4%, 6.4, and 0.75 for intracardiac echogenic focus; 17.6%, 2.6%, 6.8, and 0.85 for mild hydronephrosis; and 41.4%, 5.2%, 7.9, and 0.62 for short femur.

On the basis of current evidence, the prevalence in trisomy 21, prevalence in normals, and positive- and negative-likelihood ratios for absent nasal bone are 36.5%, 1.1%, 33.2, and 0.64, and it, therefore, appears to be a more important marker than most of the other sonographic features. Since examination of the fetal profile is an inherent part of the genetic sonogram, assessment of the nasal bone will inevitably become a routine component of such a scan.

REFERENCES

1. Down LJ. Observations on an ethnic classification of idiots. Clin Lect Rep Lond Hosp 1866; 3:259–262.
2. Cicero S, Curcio P, Papageorghiou A, Sonek J, Nicolaides K. Absence of nasal bone in fetuses with trisomy 21 at 11–14 weeks of gestation: an observational study. Lancet 2001; 358:1665–1667.

3. Sonek J, Nicolaides K. Prenatal ultrasonographic diagnosis of nasal bone abnormalities in three fetuses with Down syndrome. Am J Obstet Gynecol 2002; 186:139–141.
4. Enlow DH. Facial Growth. 3rd ed. Philadelphia: WB Saunders, 1990.
5. Beck JC, Sie KCY. The growth and development of the nasal airway. Funct Reconstr Rhinoplasty 1999:257–262.
6. Larsen WJ. Human Embryology. 3rd ed. New York: Churchill Livingstone, 2001: 367–369.
7. Sperber GH. Craniofacial Embryology. 4th ed. London: Butterworths, Wright: 1989: 104–124.
8. Sandikcioglu M, Molsted K, Kjaer I. The prenatal development of the human nasal and vomeral bones. J Craniofac Genet Dev Biol 1994; 14:124–134.
9. Farkas LG, Katic MJ, Forrest CR, Litsas L. Surface anatomy of the face in Down's syndrome: linear and angular measurements in the craniofacial regions. J Craniofac Surg 2001; 12:373–379.
10. Keeling JW, Hansen BF, Kjaer I. Pattern of malformation in the axial skeleton in human trisomy 21 fetuses. Am J Med Genet 1997; 68:466–471.
11. Stempfle N, Huten Y, Fredouille C, Brisse H, Nessmann C. Skeletal abnormalities in fetuses with Down's syndrome: a radiologic postmortem study. Pediatr Radiol 1999; 29:682–688.
12. Tuxen A, Keeling JW, Reintoft I, Fischer Hansen B, Nolting D, Kjaer I. A histological and radiological investigation of the nasal bone in fetuses with Down syndrome. Ultrasound Obstet Gynecol 2003; 22:22–26.
13. Larose C, Massoc P, Hillion Y, Bernard JP, Ville Y. Comparison of fetal nasal bone assessment by ultrasound at 11–14 weeks and by postmortem X-ray in trisomy 21: a prospective observational study. Ultrasound Obstet Gynecol 2003; 22:27–30.
14. Bouley R, Sonek J. Fetal nasal bone: the technique. Down's Screen News 2003; 10:33–34.
15. Sonek JD, Cicero S. Ultrasound evaluation of the fetal nasal bone: the technique (an update). Down's Screen News 2004; 11:25.
16. Cicero S, Dezerega V, Andrade E, Scheier M, Nicolaides KH. Learning curve for sonographic examination of the fetal nasal bone at 11–14 weeks. Ultrasound Obstet Gynecol 2003; 22:135–137.
17. Rembouskos G, Cicero S, Longo D, Vandecruys H, Nicolaides KH. Assessment of the fetal nasal bone at 11–14 weeks of gestation by three-dimensional ultrasound. Ultrasound Obstet Gynecol 2004; 23:232–236.
18. Peralta CF, Falcon O, Wegrzyn P, Faro C, Nicolaides KH. Assessment of the gap between the fetal nasal bones at 11 to 13 + 6 weeks of gestation by three-dimensional ultrasound. Ultrasound Obstet Gynecol 2005; 25:464–467.
19. Benoit B, Chaoui R. Three-dimensional ultrasound with maximal mode rendering: a novel technique for the diagnosis of bilateral or unilateral absence or hypoplasia of nasal bones in second-trimester screening for Down syndrome. Ultrasound Obstet Gynecol 2005; 25:19–24.
20. Goncalves LF, Espinoza J, Lee W, et al. Phenotypic characteristics of absent and hypoplastic nasal bones in fetuses with Down syndrome: description by 3-dimensional ultrasonography and clinical significance. J Ultrasound Med 2004; 23:1619–1627.
21. Otano L, Aiello H, Igarzabal L, Matayoshi T, Gadow EC. Association between first trimester absence of fetal nasal bone on ultrasound and Down's syndrome. Prenat Diagn 2002; 22:930–932.
22. Zoppi MA, Ibba RM, Axiana C, Floris M, Manca F, Monni G. Absence of fetal nasal bone and aneuploidies at first-trimester nuchal translucency screening in unselected pregnancies. Prenat Diagn 2003; 23:496–500.
23. Orlandi F, Bilardo CM, Campogrande M, et al. Measurement of nasal bone length at 11–14 weeks of pregnancy and its potential role in Down syndrome risk assessment. Ultrasound Obstet Gynecol 2003; 22:36–39.

24. Viora E, Masturzo B, Errante G, Sciarrone A, Bastonero S, Campogrande M. Ultrasound evaluation of fetal nasal bone at 11–14 weeks in a consecutive series of 1906 fetuses. Prenat Diagn 2003; 23:784–787.

25. Senat MV, Bernard JP, Boulvain M, Ville Y. Intra- and interoperator variability in fetal nasal bone assessment at 11–14 weeks of gestation. Ultrasound Obstet Gynecol 2003; 22:138–141.

26. Wong SF, Choi H, Ho LC. Nasal bone hypoplasia: is it a common finding amongst chromosomally normal fetuses of southern Chinese women? Gynecol Obstet Invest 2003; 56:99–101.

27. Cicero S, Longo D, Rembouskos G, Sacchini C, Nicolaides KH. Absent nasal bone at 11–14 weeks of gestation and chromosomal defects. Ultrasound Obstet Gynecol 2003; 22:31–35.

28. Cicero S, Rembouskos G, Vandecruys H, Hogg M, Nicolaides KH. Likelihood ratio for Trisomy 21 in fetuses with absent nasal bone at the 11–14 weeks scan. Ultrasound Obstet Gynecol 2004; 23:218–223.

29. Orlandi F, Rossi C, Orlandi E, et al. First-trimester screening for trisomy-21 using a simplified method to assess the presence or absence of the fetal nasal bone. Am J Obstet Gynecol 2005; 192:1107–1111.

30. Malone FD, Ball RH, Nyberg DA, et al., for the FASTER Research Consortium. First-trimester nasal bone evaluation for aneuploidy in the general population. Obstet Gynecol 2004; 104:1222–1228.

31. Bromley B, Lieberman E, Shipp T, Benacerraf B. Fetal nasal bone length: a marker for Down syndrome in the second trimester. J Ultrasound Med 2002; 21:1387–1394.

32. Cicero S, Sonek J, McKenna D, Croom C, Johnson L, Nicolaides K. Nasal bone hypoplasia in fetuses with Trisomy 21. Ultrasound Obstet Gynecol 2003; 21:15–18.

33. Vintzileos A, Walters C, Yeo L. Absent nasal bone in the prenatal detection of fetuses with trisomy 21 in a high-risk population. Obstet Gynecol 2003; 101:905–908.

34. Odibo AO, Sehdev HM, Dunn L, McDonald R, Macones GA. The association between fetal nasal bone hyplasia and aneuploidy. Obstet Gynecol 2004; 104:1229–1233.

35. Tran L, Carr D, Mitsumori L, Uhrich S, Shields L. Second-trimester biparietal diameter/ nasal bone length ratio as an independent predictor of trisomy 21. J Ultrasound Med 2005; 24:805–810.

36. Bunduki V, Ruano J, Miguelez J, Yoshizaki C, Kahhale S, Zugaib M. Fetal bone length: reference range and clinical application in ultrasound screening for trisomy 21. Ultrasound Obstet Gynecol 2003; 21:156–160.

37. Gamez F, Ferreiro P, Salmean JM. Ultrasonographic measurement of fetal nasal bone in a low risk population at 19–22 gestational weeks. Ultrasound Obstet Gynecol 2003; 22:152–153.

38. Spencer K, Souter V, Tul N, Snijders R, Nicolaides KH. A screening program for trisomy 21 at 10–14 weeks using fetal nuchal translucency, maternal serum free beta-human chorionic gonadotropin and pregnancy-associated plasma protein-A. Ultrasound Obstet Gynecol 1999; 13:231–237.

39. Nicolaides KH, Spencer K, Avgidou K, Faiola S, Falcon O. Multicenter study of first-trimester screening for trisomy 21 in 75 821 pregnancies: results and estimation of the potential impact of individual risk-orientated two-stage first-trimester screening. Ultrasound Obstet Gynecol 2005; 25:221–226.

40. Cicero S, Bindra R, Rembouskos G, Spencer K, Nicolaides KH. Integrated ultrasound and biochemical screening for trisomy 21 using fetal nuchal translucency, absent fetal nasal bone, free beta-hCG and PAPP-A at 11 to 14 weeks. Prenat Diagn 2003; 23:306–310.

41. Matias A, Gomes C, Flack N, Montenegro N, Nicolaides KH. Screening for chromosomal abnormalities at 11–14 weeks: the role of ductus venosus flow. Ultrasound Obstet Gynecol 1998; 2:380–384.

42. Faiola S, Tsoi E, Huggon IC, Allan LD, Nicolaides KH. Likelihood ratio for trisomy 21 in fetuses with tricuspid regurgitation at the 11 to 13 + 6-week scan. Ultrasound Obstet Gynecol 2005; 26:22–27.
43. Nicolaides KH. Screening for chromosomal defects. Ultrasound Obstet Gynecol 2003; 21:313–321.
44. Nyberg DA, Souter VL, El-Bastawissi A, Young S, Luthhardt F, Luthy DA. Isolated sonographic markers for detection of fetal Down syndrome in the second trimester of pregnancy. J Ultrasound Med 2001; 20:1053–1063.
45. Bromley B, Lieberman E, Shipp TD, Benacerraf BR. The genetic sonogram. A method of risk assessment for Down syndrome in the second trimester. J Ultrasound Med 2002; 21:1087–1096.

5

Screening for Neural Tube Defects: Ultrasound and Serum Markers

Lee P. Shulman
Department of Obstetrics and Gynecology, Division of Reproductive Genetics,
Feinberg School of Medicine, Northwestern University, Chicago, Illinois, U.S.A.

INTRODUCTION

The detection of fetal neural tube defects (NTDs) in the second trimester has become a mainstay of noninvasive and invasive prenatal diagnosis for the past 30 years. NTDs are among the most common serious congenital malformations and are the result of the failure of the fetal NTD to close completely; the degree and location of the opening of the neural tube are key determinants of the severity of the defect. This chapter will review the current status of prenatal screening and detection of fetal NTDs.

CLASSIFICATION OF NTDs

Anencephaly is the most severe form of NTD and results from the failure of the anterior neural tube and overlying cranial bones to close and occurs at approximately 21–24 days of fetal development (Fig. 1). All cases of anencephaly are associated with abnormal development of the brain; this is what leads to the uniform lethality of this condition. Spina bifida, the most common form of NTD, is the result of the failed closure of a more caudal portion of the neural tube and occurs somewhat later than anencephaly, usually during the late third or early fourth week of fetal development (1). Spina bifida defects are further classified as myeloceles, meningoceles, or meningomyeloceles. Myeloceles are lesions in which neural tissue is exposed but without a herniation of the meninges; meningoceles are characterized by a herniation of the meninges and meningomyeloceles are a combination of both lesions (Fig. 2). However, myeloceles can result in severe disability or mortality despite not resulting from a more profound anatomical defect. Nonetheless, as meningomyeloceles involve the spinal cord and nerve roots, these defects are commonly associated with Arnold–Chiari malformations of the brain in which cranial contents are shifted caudally as a result of the spinal defect. Despite the neurological disruption associated with spina bifida, survival rates are considerably better than anencephaly, with a 5-year survival rate of approximately 85% (2).

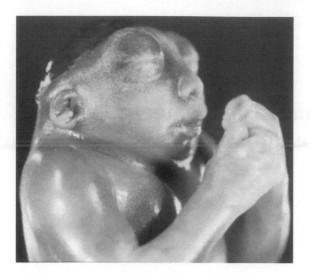

Figure 1 Stillbirth with anencephaly. Please note the prominence of the orbits with the lack of a formed cranial vault.

Almost all cases of anencephaly, as well as approximately 85% of cases of spina bifida, are characterized by open defects; such defects are either completely open or are covered by a thin membrane. Closed defects are covered by skin and are more difficult to prenatally detect than open defects. Although open defects are usually associated with a greater risk of handicap, closed NTDs can be associated with adverse pediatric outcomes. Anencephaly is invariably a lethal condition, whereas spina bifida is associated with a considerably lower incidence of mortality but a wide spectrum of morbidity including motor, bowel, and bladder dysfunction, and developmental delay (1).

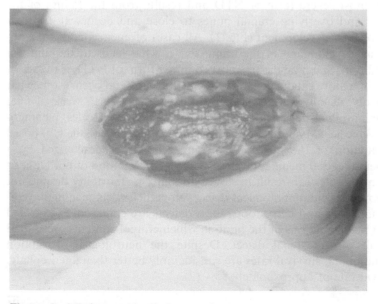

Figure 2 Meningomyelocele in a newborn.

Etiology and Prevalence of NTDs

Recent studies have demonstrated that a majority of NTDs can be prevented by adequate maternal intake of folic acid. This finding has been the seminal factor in developing approaches to reducing the incidence of NTDs. However, the strong association of folic acid and NTD incidence does not help delineate the etiologies of NTDs, as genetic and environmental causes of NTDs may similarly respond to folic acid supplementation. In addition, numerous other pathophysiologic states including chromosome abnormalities, mendelian disorders, and environmental exposures (e.g., drug, maternal disease, and toxic substances) have been shown to cause the remaining small percentage of NTD cases. To this end, it is critical to obtain the most accurate and complete diagnosis of a fetus or infant with a NTD as counseling for future pregnancies may be considerably altered if the NTD is a component of a particular syndrome rather than an isolated event (2).

NTDs are associated with many different causes (3) and accordingly, the incidences of NTDs are linked with patient ethnicity, geographic location, and associated syndromes. The highest rates in newborns have been reported in the United Kingdom (up to 1%) (4); the highest rates in North America are reported in the Appalachian region (1–2 per 10,000 livebirths) (5) and in Nova Scotia (6). In addition, high rates (approximately 1% of liveborns) have also been reported in China, Egypt, and India (7).

However, it is important to recognize that these high rates of NTDs have been decreasing for the past several decades. This decrease was initially associated with the increasing capability to accurately detect affected fetuses through the implementation of effective screening and diagnostic protocols to be reviewed in this chapter; more recently, the decline has also been associated with an increase in dietary folic acid intake that has reduced the incidence of NTDs in a primary fashion (3). Indeed, primary prevention of NTD by increased dietary folic acid intake through improved diet and supplementation (0.4 mg folic acid/day for all reproductive-aged women; 4.0 mg folic acid/day for women with a previous pregnancy affected with a NTD) is believed to account for approximately 50% of the decline (7). Declines in the incidence of NTDs have been observed in high- and low-frequency populations and may also be associated with long-term variations in the frequency of NTDs (4,6). Interestingly, Persad and colleagues (6) report that the type of and approach to folic acid supplementation may be important factors in the efficacy of folic acid to reduce the incidence of NTDs. In this study, the authors found that the recommendations for folic acid supplementation (0.4 mg/day) alone did not reduce the incidence of NTDs in Nova Scotia. Only after grains were fortified with folic acid was a substantial reduction in the incidence of NTDs observed.

The risk of recurrence for first-degree relatives of affected individuals with isolated NTDs is approximately 1 in 30 and for second-degree relatives is approximately 1 in 220 (7). However, Arata and colleagues reported that affected mothers may have only a 0.5–1.0% risk of having an affected offspring (8). Regardless, affected individuals and those with affected first- and second-degree relatives with NTDs are at increased risk for having offspring with NTDs.

ALPHA-FETOPROTEIN AND FETAL NTDs

The main sites of embryonic and fetal alpha-fetoprotein (AFP) production are the yolk sac and fetal liver (9). Certain fetal structural abnormalities such as NTDs and anterior abdominal wall defects such as omphalocele and gastroschisis lead to increased transudation of AFP into the amniotic fluid with subsequent passage into the maternal circulation. Accordingly, pregnancies affected by NTDs and certain other abnormalities are usually characterized by elevated levels of AFP in amniotic fluid and maternal serum. Accordingly, measurements of AFP in amniotic fluid and maternal serum can be used to confirm the presence of an abnormality and screen women for such structural abnormalities.

The screening for NTDs is primarily based on the measurement of AFP levels during the second trimester. Although optimal time for measuring maternal serum AFP (MSAFP) for identifying women at increased risk for carrying affected fetuses is 15–18 weeks' gestation, screening for fetal NTDs can reliably be accomplished from 15 to 20 weeks inclusive (10).

MSAFP screening is accomplished by establishing median values for serum levels of AFP at each gestational week to be included in the screening protocol. This is achieved by calculating the mean serum level of AFP of at least 100 unaffected cases at each gestational age. Once the median value for each gestational week has been calculated, prospective samples can be analyzed within the construct of the AFP screening paradigm and a value that describes the relative position of the sample's AFP measurement to the median value for that week can be assigned (9). This value is known as a "multiple of the median" or MoM. For example, if the median value of AFP at 18 weeks is 20 pg/mL, and a sample is found to have a concentration of 40 pg/mL, that value is reported as a 2.0 MoM. MSAFP values of unaffected and affected cases show classic gaussian curves; unfortunately, the curves of these two populations overlap, leading to some elevated levels being associated with normal pregnancies and some lower values of MSAFP being associated with affected pregnancies. The distribution of MSAFP values in affected pregnancies is higher (to the right) than the distribution of MSAFP values in unaffected pregnancies (11). As such, a threshold value is sought that maximizes the ability to detect women carrying affected fetuses, while minimizing the number of women who are "screen positive" but carrying unaffected fetuses. The threshold value for singleton pregnancies is 2.0–2.5 MoM and for twin pregnancies is 4.0–5.0 MoM (12); women with values higher than the threshold are at increased risk for fetal structural defects such as NTDs and are recommended for further evaluation (see the following text).

However, before a MoM value is reported, certain adjustments need to be performed in order to create a more effective screening protocol. MSAFP levels vary according to maternal weight; specifically, the greater the weight, the greater the tendency toward a lower MSAFP concentration as a result of the dilution of AFP in a greater blood volume (13). Accordingly, maternal weight is used to adjust the MSAFP MoM final value so as to reduce the variability of the AFP MoM distribution and increase the detection rate for open NTDs (14). Other adjustments that are routinely made to MSAFP measurements are based on factors unique to AFP physiology. Black African women have MSAFP levels that are 10–15% higher than non-Black women (15); failure to take this into account would lead to a considerable reduction in MSAFP screening efficacy in African women (14). Conversely, MSAFP levels in women who are insulin-dependent diabetics are approximately 20% reduced compared to nondiabetics (16). In addition, insulin-dependent diabetics have a higher frequency of fetuses with NTDs; accordingly, most programs utilize a "diabetic" correction as well as a lower threshold in diabetic women being screened for NTDs so as to assure maximal detection of affected fetuses in this high-risk group.

Some programs encourage the remeasurement of minimally elevated MSAFP values. The concept behind this is that a pathologic cause for the elevated level will continue to cause elevated measurements in subsequent evaluations. However, an elevated value not associated with fetal or maternal pathology may "regress to the mean" and be in the normal range upon retesting. In our program, the threshold for elevated MSAFP values is 2.5 MoM. All values between 2.5 and 3.0 MoM occurring before 18 weeks are reevaluated by a repeat MSAFP test. Such an approach should not be used for low values of MSAFP and other analytes as the distributions of affected and unaffected pregnancies overlap more than with NTD distributions; accordingly, remeasurement of values should not be used in situations where regression to the mean is likely to lead to a false-negative value. We also perform this retesting only before 18 weeks to ensure that appropriate counseling and testing can be offered in a timely fashion so that women are able to make informed decisions about pregnancy management.

In women who are found to have elevated MSAFP levels, certain diagnostic tests should be performed. First and foremost, a targeted ultrasound should be done upon learning of the elevated value. Several non-NTD–related conditions can account for elevated MSAFP values (1) and include:

1. Incorrect dates. If the screening was performed with the understanding that the woman was 16 weeks and was actually 20 weeks, then an elevated MSAFP value may have been calculated. In such cases, the more reliable gestational age assessment should be used to recalculate the MSAFP value; if the recalculation is below the threshold, then no further evaluation for elevated MSAFP needs to be pursued.
2. Multiple gestations. More than one fetus will produce considerably more AFP than a single fetus. Each fetus can be considered to be producing a "unit" of AFP, with multiple fetuses producing multiple "units" of AFP. Multifetal corrections can be made to determine whether MSAFP elevation for the multifetal pregnancy exists.
3. Fetal demise. Fetal demise can be associated with elevated or low levels of MSAFP.
4. Other fetal anomalies. In addition to NTDs and anterior abdominal wall defects, several other fetal anomalies can lead to elevated, and in some cases markedly elevated, levels of MSAFP. Congenital Finnish nephrosis is an autosomal recessive disorder caused by mutations in the *NPHS1* gene and associated with newborn renal failure and death if not treated. Renal transplantation is the only effective treatment for this condition. MSAFP and amniotic fluid AFP (AFAFP) values are usually markedly elevated (10–20 MoM) in this disorder. Other fetal renal and bladder conditions are associated with elevated MSAFP values and include obstructive uropathies and renal cysts. Nonrenal conditions associated with elevated MSAFP values include fetal teratomas, cutis aplasia, and epidermolysis bullosa.
5. Twin demise/multifetal reduction. The loss of a co-twin in a multiple pregnancy can be associated with elevated levels of MSAFP. In cases where iatrogenic or natural fetal reduction are known to have occurred prior to the time of MSAFP measurement, MSAFP should not be performed as values will likely be elevated regardless of the presence of a NTD.
6. Fetal chromosome and Mendelian disorders. Fetal chromosome and Mendelian abnormalities that are associated with elevated MSAFP levels

are those that result in phenotypes including structural changes that are associated with elevated MSAFP values. Examples are anterior abdominal wall defects in several aneuploidies and encephalocele in the autosomal recessive Meckel–Gruber syndrome.

7. Maternal conditions. Some maternal conditions can lead to elevated levels of MSAFP in the second trimester. Some malignancies are known to produce AFP and include hepatic cancer, germ cell tumors, and gastrointestinal tumors. Maternal viral hepatitis can also result in an elevated MSAFP value.

Ultrasound may or may not be able to detect the structural defect or pregnancy-related condition associated with the elevated MSAFP measurement. In cases where ultrasound has provided information concerning benign pregnancy-related conditions that have affected the MSAFP value (e.g., dates and fetal number), recalculation of the MSAFP value should be undertaken. Indeed, incorrect gestational dating is the most common cause for elevated MSAFP values (1). In those cases where ultrasound demonstrates fetal abnormality that has led to an elevated value, appropriate counseling should be provided. Such counseling should review the implications of the findings, review any further testing that would provide more information concerning etiology or prognosis, discuss pregnancy management options, and provide emotional support to the woman and her family.

In those cases in which ultrasound fails to provide meaningful information as to the cause of the elevated MSAFP value, counseling should again be provided (12). In this scenario, the counseling should review the screening outcome and review appropriate further testing that could detect fetal abnormalities. In most cases, this would involve the offering of amniocentesis to measure the AFAFP level, perform a cytogenetic analysis of fetal cells in the amniotic fluid, and possibly perform other testing such as detecting the presence of acetylcholinesterase (AChE) that could provide important information concerning the etiology of the elevated MSAFP value. Milunsky reported that only 779 (0.78%) of 100,000 AF samples screened for AFP had elevated ($\geq$5 SD) levels prior to 24 weeks' gestation. Almost two-thirds of these cases were associated with fetal NTDs or other serious structural defects (17). AChE is measured by an immunoassay using a monoclonal antibody and is found in amniotic fluid when there is a fetal lesion associated with exposed neural tissue. Accordingly, NTDs and anterior abdominal wall defects are associated with positive AChE findings in the amniotic fluid. However, false positives are not uncommon with AChE measurements, especially in amniotic fluid specimens obtained in the early second trimester and in the presence of fetal blood. As such, most laboratories only measure AChE when there is a markedly increased risk for fetal abnormality, such as an elevated AFAFP value or in a pregnancy at high risk for fetal structural abnormality. In all, the combination of MSAFP, AFAFP, and AChE, combined with targeted ultrasound, is a highly effective and specific approach to detecting fetal NTDs.

Nonetheless, a reason for the elevated MSAFP value may not be determined even after performing ultrasound and invasive diagnostic testing. In such cases, counseling should be provided that reviews all of the screening and diagnostic results, and the risk for adverse perinatal outcome should be assessed. Such pregnancies have been associated with a variety of adverse perinatal outcomes unassociated with NTDs or other fetal structural anomalies. Waller and colleagues (18) reported that women with unexplained elevated levels of MSAFP in the second trimester had a considerably increased chance of fetal death throughout their pregnancies. Morssink and colleagues (19) found an increased risk for small-for-gestational-age fetuses and preterm deliveries in women with unexplained elevated levels of MSAFP in the second trimester. Although no specific reason for this clinical correlation has been determined, a deficiency in the maternal–fetal placental barrier leading to increased transudation of AFP into the maternal compartment with a concomitant adverse effect on fetal wellbeing is considered to be a possible explanation. Unfortunately, no specific diagnostic evaluation of second- or third-trimester pregnancies with unexplained elevated MSAFP values has been shown to be effective in predicting adverse outcomes and allowing for timely intervention.

ULTRASONOGRAPHY TO DETECT FETAL NTDs

The central nervous system was one of the first fetal organ systems visualized by ultrasonography. Campbell and colleagues (20) described the ultrasonographic detection of the first previable case of anencephaly in 1972. Since then, the use of ultrasound to detect fetal central nervous system defects has been ongoing, and it has incorporated the varied advances in diagnostic ultrasonography. Despite the technical and experiential advances in diagnostic ultrasound, the main factor preventing midtrimester ultrasound from usurping the role of MSAFP screening in the detection of fetal NTDs is the subjectivity of the ultrasound examination. From the ultrasonographer to the woman being evaluated, too many variables keep ultrasonography from providing the consistent, cost-effective and broad spectrum screening for fetal NTDs that has been consistently demonstrated with MSAFP screening in a variety of clinical scenarios (21). Regardless, ultrasonography still plays a critical role in the detection of fetal NTDs, and this role will likely change with further advances in the technology of ultrasonography and in the training of health care professionals.

The ultrasonographic detection of fetal anencephaly is relatively straightforward and relies upon demonstrating the absence of the cranial vault (Fig. 3) (22).

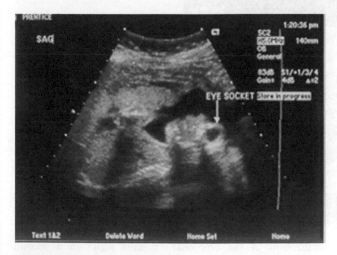

Figure 3 Ultrasonographic detection of fetal anencephaly in the third trimester. Please note the prominent orbit labeled as "eye socket."

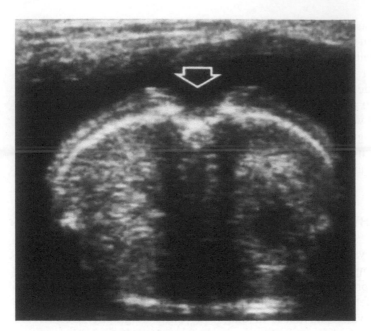

Figure 4 Ultrasonographic detection of open neural tube defect in the second trimester. Arrow points to the actual defect in the lumbar region.

Spinal NTDs are far more problematic, as visualizing the entire fetal spine is difficult in many cases, and the ultrasonographic visualization of a spinal NTD (Fig. 4) can be difficult even when the entire spine is amenable for ultrasound visualization.

The identification of fetal cranial markers has made the task of identifying an affected fetus possible without actually visualizing the specific defect of the fetal spine (22,23). Spinal defects typically lead to characteristic changes in the intracranial

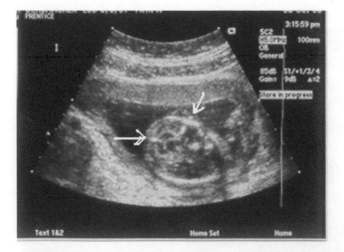

Figure 5 Ultrasonographic visualization of the cerebellar "banana sign" in a second trimester fetus with a lumbosacral neural tube defect. The arrows point to the banana-shaped cerebellum.

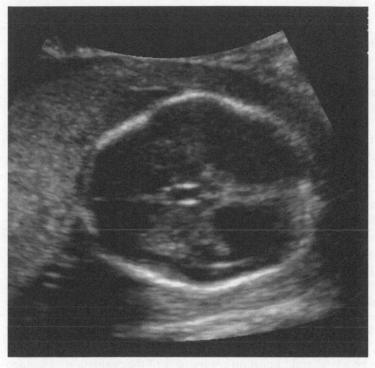

Figure 6 Ultrasonographic visualization of the "lemon" sign in a second-trimester fetus with an open spinal neural tube defect.

anatomy; specifically, displacement of the cerebellar vermis, fourth ventricle, and medulla oblongata occurs in some degree in virtually all cases of open spinal NTDs and in some closed NTDs. These changes are known as Arnold–Chiari malformation and result in the downward pull of the brain stem and the cerebellum through the foramen magnum. These alterations have also led to the ultrasound markers commonly referred to as the "fruit signs." The "banana" sign describes the shape of the cerebellar hemispheres after being impacted deep into the posterior fossa as a result of the aforementioned shifting of the intracranial contents (Fig. 5). The "lemon" sign refers to the puckering of the front cranial vault resulting from changes in ventricular shape and size (Fig. 6). Watson and colleagues (24) reported that the sensitivity of the fruit signs to identify open NTDs was approximately 99%; however, Pilu and Hobbins (22) confirm that the accuracy of the ultrasonographic diagnosis of fetal NTDs relies on the experience of the operator, the quality of the equipment, and the amount of time dedicated to the scan.

A good example of the inconsistencies of ultrasonography for the detection of fetal NTDs is found not in evaluations of referral centers, typically where the most experienced operators and the most advanced equipment is found, but rather by clinicians using ultrasound to screen low-risk populations. Levi and colleagues reported sensitivities of 30% and 40% in two studies (25,26) of low-risk women not utilizing MSAFP screening. The routine antenatal diagnostic imaging with ultrasound (RADIUS) trial (27) evaluated ultrasonography in conjunction with MSAFP screening and found a NTD detection sensitivity of 80%.

CONCLUSIONS

The advances in ultrasound over the past three decades will likely continue with improved capabilities to detect fetal structural abnormalities. Indeed, recent work (28–30) shows that ultrasound can be used in the late first and early second trimesters to effectively detect fetal structural abnormalities. However, larger comparative trials will be needed to assess the ability of early ultrasound to detect fetal structural defects.

Nonetheless, the technical advances in ultrasound including three- and four-dimensional capabilities and the use of new technologies (i.e., for prenatal assessment) such as magnetic resonance imaging (31,32) will continue to expand our opportunities to detect structural abnormalities in low- and high-risk pregnancies. However, excitement about these technological advances must be tempered with stark reality. In altering a prenatal screening or diagnostic paradigm, the cost-effectiveness of a new model must be a critical factor in determining whether the new protocol can or should replace existing clinical practice (33). In addition, the ability of a new screening protocol to consistently identify high-risk women must be thoroughly investigated. Also, screening protocols should be easy to implement, thus allowing a wide socioeconomic spectrum of individuals to benefit from these protocols.

For all these reasons, it appears unlikely that maternal serum screening will soon be replaced by ultrasound or another imaging technology. Ultrasound has been and will continue to be a vital and important component of the evaluation of women for fetal NTDs and for obstetrical care in general; indeed, it appears that our ability to detect fetal anomalies will continue to improve in the years ahead. However, the simplicity, consistency, and cost-effectiveness of MSAFP screening make it a valued screening protocol that will continue to be a part of routine obstetrical care worldwide for many years to come.

REFERENCES

1. Simpson JL, Elias S. Prenatal diagnosis of Mendelian disorders and neural tube defects. In: ed. Genetics in Obstetrics and Gynecology. 3rd ed. Philadelphia: Saunders, 2003: 405–411.
2. Milunsky A, Canick JA. Maternal serum screening for neural tube and other defects. In: Milunsky A, ed. Genetic Disorders and the Fetus: Diagnosis, Prevention and Treatment. 5th ed. Baltimore: The Johns Hopkins Press, 2004:719–722.
3. Shurtleff DB, Lemaire RJ. Epidemiology, etiologic factors, and prenatal diagnosis of open spinal dysraphism. Neurosurg Clin N Am 1995; 6:183–193.
4. Elwood JM, Elwood JH. Epidemiology of Anencephalus and Spina Bifida. New York: Oxford University Press, 1980.
5. Jorde LB, Fineman RM, Martin RA. Epidemiology of neural tube defects in Utah, 1940–1979. Am J Epidemiol 1984; 119:487.
6. Persad VL, Van Den Hof MC, Dube JM, et al. Incidence of open neural tube defects in Nova Scotia after folic acid fortification. Can Med Assoc J 2002; 167:241–245.
7. Shurtleff DB. Epidemiology of neural tube defects and folic acid. Cerebrospinal Fluid Res 2004; 1:5–10.
8. Arata M, Grover S, Dunne K, et al. Pregnancy outcome and complications in women with spina bifida. J Reprod Med 2000; 45:743–748.
9. Bahado-Singh RO, Sutton-Riley J. Biochemical screening for congenital defects. Obstet Gynecol Clin N Am 2004; 31:857–872.

10. Wald NJ, Cuckle H, Brock DJH, et al. Maternal serum alpha-fetoprotein measurement in antenatal screening for anencephaly and spina bifida in early pregnancy: report of the UK collaborative study on alpha-fetoprotein in relation to neural-tube defects. Lancet 1977; 1:1323.

11. Muller F. Prenatal biochemical screening for neural tube defects. Childs Nerv Syst 2003; 19:433–435.

12. Driscoll DA. Second trimester maternal serum screening for fetal open neural tube defects and aneuploidy. Gen Med 2004; 6:540–541.

13. Wald NJ, Cuckle H, Boreham J, et al. The effect of maternal weight on maternal serum alpha-fetoprotein levels. Br J Obstet Gynaecol 1980; 87:219.

14. Johnson AM, Palomaki GE, Haddow JE. Maternal serum alpha-fetoprotein levels in pregnancies among black and white women with fetal open spina bifida: a United States collaborative study. Am J Obstet Gynecol 1990; 162:328.

15. Benn PA, Clive JM, Collins R. Medians for second-trimester maternal serum α-fetoprotein, human chorionic gonadotropin and unconjugated estriol: differences between races or ethnic groups. Clin Chem 1997; 43:333.

16. Braunstein GD, Mills JL, Reed GF, et al. Comparison of serum placental protein hormone levels in diabetic and normal pregnancy. J Clin Endocrinol Metab 1989; 68:3.

17. Milunsky A, Canick JA. Maternal serum screening for neural tube and other defects. In: Milunsky A, ed. Genetic Disorders and the Fetus: Diagnosis, Prevention and Treatment. 5th ed. Baltimore: The Johns Hopkins Press, 2004.

18. Waller DK, Lustig LS, Cunningham GC, et al. Second-trimester maternal serum alpha-fetoprotein levels and the risk of subsequent fetal death. N Engl J Med 1991; 325:6.

19. Morssink LP, Kornman LH, Beekhuis JR, et al. Abnormal levels of maternal serum human chorionic gonadotropin and alpha-fetoprotein in the second trimester: relation to fetal weight and preterm delivery. Prenat Diagn 1995; 15:1041.

20. Campbell S, Johnstone FD, Holt EM, et al. Anencephaly: early ultrasonic diagnosis and active management. Lancet 1972; 2:1226–1227.

21. Strigini FAL, Carmignani A, Genazzani AR. Second trimester sonography and fetal spina bifida screening. Int J Gynecol Obstet 2003; 81:59–60.

22. Pilu G, Hobbins JC. Sonography of fetal cerebrospinal anomalies. Prenat Diagn 2002; 22:321–330.

23. Buisson O, De Keersmaecker B, Senat MV, et al. Sonographic diagnosis of spina bifida at 12 weeks: heading towards indirect signs. Ultrasound Obstet Gynecol 2002; 19: 290–292.

24. Watson WJ, Cheschier NC, Katz VL, et al. The role of ultrasound in evaluation of patients with elevated maternal serum alpha-fetoprotein: a review. Obstet Gynecol 1991; 78:123–128.

25. Levi S, Hijazi Y, Schaaps JP, et al. Sensitivity and specificity of routine antenatal screening for congenital anomalies by ultrasound: the Belgian multicentric study. Ultrasound Obstet Gynecol 1991; 1:102–110.

26. Levi S, Schaaps JP, De Havay P, et al. End-result of routine ultrasound screening for congenital anomalies: the Belgian Multicentric Study 1984–92. Ultrasound Obstet Gynecol 1995; 5:366–371.

27. Ewigman BG, Crane JP, Frigoletto FD, et al. Effect of prenatal ultrasound screening on perinatal outcome. N Engl J Med 1996; 329:821–827.

28. Fong KW, Toi A, Salem S, et al. Detection of fetal structural abnormalities with US during early pregnancy. Radiographics 2004; 24:157–174.

29. Souka AP, Pilalis A, Kavalakis Y, et al. Assessment of fetal anatomy at the 11–14-week ultrasound examination. Ultrasound Obstet Gynecol 2004; 24:730–734.

30. Timor-Tritsch IE, Bashiri A, Monteagudo A, et al. Qualified and trained sonographers in the US can perform early fetal anatomy scans between 11 and 14 weeks. Am J Obstet Gynecol 2004; 191:1247–1252.

31. Ertl-Wagner B, Lienemann A, Strauss A, et al. Fetal magnetic resonance imaging: indications, technique, anatomical considerations and a review of fetal abnormalities. Eur Radiol 2002; 12:1931–1940.
32. Aaronson OS, Nernanz-Schulman M, Bruner JP, et al. Myelomeningocele: prenatal evaluation-comparison between transabdominal US and MR imaging. Radiology 2003; 227:839–843.
33. Caughey A. Cost-effectiveness analysis of prenatal diagnosis: methodological issues and concerns. Gynecol Obstet Invest 2005; 60:11–18.

6

Antenatal Screening for Down Syndrome Using the Integrated Test

N. J. Wald and A. R. Rudnicka
Wolfson Institute of Preventive Medicine, Barts and the London Queen Mary's School of Medicine and Dentistry, Charterhouse Square, London, U.K.

INTRODUCTION

Antenatal screening for Down syndrome has advanced over the last two decades. In the early 1980s screening was based on maternal age alone. By the end of the 1980s second trimester serum markers were added to maternal age, so that at a 5% false-positive rate (FPR) over two-thirds of affected pregnancies could be identified compared with about one-third using age alone (1). By the 1990s tests using four serum markers in addition to maternal age were achieving detection rates (DRs) of about 75% for a 5% FPR (2) and first trimester screening markers, including nuchal translucency (NT) measurement and serum markers, were introduced. In 1999 the integration of screening markers across both trimesters into a single screening test improved screening performance compared with screening in either the first or second trimester alone. This integrated test merges first- and second-trimester markers into a single screening result, holding information collected in the first trimester (pregnancy-associated plasma protein A (PAPP-A) with or without NT) without immediate interpretation of the markers, until information from the second-trimester markers [alphafetoprotein (AFP), unconjugated estriol (uE$_3$), human chorionic gonadotrophin (hCG; either total or free β), and inhibin-A] was obtained. The integrated test could achieve DRs of about 85% for a 1% FPR (3,4). The test has now been introduced in a number of centers and found to be acceptable and effective in a multicenter international demonstration project.

In this chapter we consider the integrated test and the underlying screening issues under the headings (i) general principles, (ii) estimation of screening performance, (iii) screening performance of the integrated test compared with other tests, (iv) financial cost, (v) sequential screening policies, (vi) possible improvements in screening performance with the addition of an ultrasound fetal nasal bone examination, (vii) the integrated test in twin pregnancies, (viii) results from other studies, (ix) standardizing screening performance to about 17 weeks of pregnancy, (x) implementation of the integrated test, and (xi) conclusions. A glossary of terms to describe the main screening tests is given at the end of the chapter.

GENERAL PRINCIPLES

No marker currently used can discriminate completely between affected and unaffected pregnancies. The principle of multiple-marker screening is that screening using several markers together in a single test is more effective than using one marker alone or even several markers used as separate tests. Using markers in sequence, so that only women with a screen-positive result (that is, increased risk of Down syndrome) on one marker proceed to have another marker measured, provides no opportunity for other markers to "detect" affected pregnancies classified as screen-negative by the first markers. The most efficient method is to use all the markers simultaneously and combine the information. Each marker contributes to the overall discrimination between affected and unaffected pregnancies.

Maternal age is a screening marker and the same point applies. It is inefficient to classify women as positive or negative on the basis of maternal age alone (e.g., by offering women aged 35 years or more an amniocentesis) and restricting, for example, serum screening to younger women. This approach will inevitably have a higher FPR and, therefore, higher procedure-related fetal loss rate for a given DR than one in which serum screening is offered to all women. It also has significant effects for the individual; many older women who, on the basis of maternal age alone, might feel at high risk could, with the additional information from serum and ultrasound markers, learn that their risk was in fact very low, and so could avoid an invasive diagnostic procedure.

Treating first-trimester screening markers and second-trimester screening markers as separate tests is similarly inefficient. Identifying women as screen-positive using a first-trimester screening test and offering them a chorionic villus sampling (CVS) while leaving the remaining women to have a second-trimester test (rather than an integrated test) leads to a much larger FPR for a given DR, resulting in unnecessary fetal losses from the diagnostic test and is more expensive (4). Most, but not all, of the inefficiency can be overcome by adopting the universal maneuver of reusing the first-trimester markers together with second-trimester markers for women proceeding to the second-trimester screening. Any such stepwise (or sequential) approach is less discriminatory than performing the integrated test on all women. If the loss in screening performance is small, a sequential approach of reusing the first-trimester markers when the second-trimester markers are obtained may be an option.

ESTIMATION OF SCREENING PERFORMANCE

Screening performance is generally specified as a DR for a given FPR or the FPR for a given DR, which can be presented simply as DR_{FPR} or FPR_{DR}, respectively, so that, for example, DR_5 means the DR for a 5% FPR, and FPR_{85} means the FPR for an 85% DR.

The extent to which a test discriminates between affected and unaffected individuals is determined by knowledge of the relative frequency distributions of test values for affected and unaffected individuals, as shown in Figure 1. Figure 1 shows the distributions of three hypothetical screening markers in unaffected and affected populations. The horizontal scale is the value of the marker in arbitrary units. If we select a given FPR (e.g., 5%) we can plot a vertical line from the x-axis at the marker levels that place 5% of the unaffected population to the right of the line. The

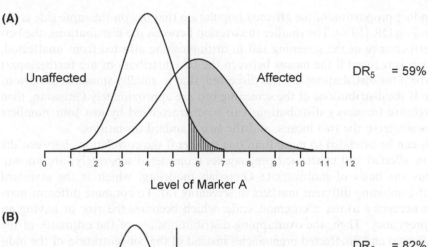

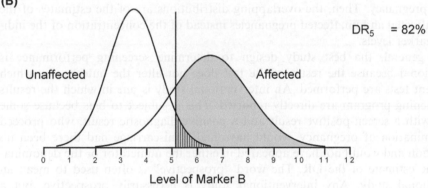

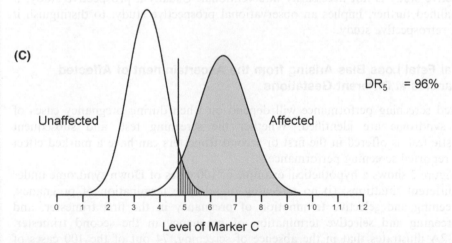

Figure 1 A hypothetical example of screening performance with a single marker. **(A)** It has a mean and standard deviation of 4.0 and 1.0, respectively, in the unaffected and 6.0 and 1.5 in affected individuals; at a 5% false-positive rate (FPR) the detection rate (DR) is 59%. If the mean were 3.5 instead of 4.0 in the unaffected and 6.5 instead of 6.0 in affected individuals (but the standard deviations unchanged), this would increase the DR to 82% **(B)** as a larger proportion of affected individuals are to the right-hand side of the risk cutoff line. If the standard deviation were reduced from 1.0 to 0.75 for unaffected and from 1.5 to 1.0 for affected individuals (but the means unchanged), this would increase DR further to 96% **(C)**.

corresponding proportion of the affected population that lies on the same side is the corresponding DR (59%). The smaller the overlap between the distributions, the better the performance of the screening test in distinguishing affected from unaffected. The overlap is reduced if the means between the two distributions are further apart (Fig. 1B) or if the distributions are less dispersed, that is, smaller standard deviations (Fig. 1C). If the distributions of the screening test are approximately Gaussian, then the two relative frequency distributions can be characterized by just four numbers (called parameters): the two means, and the two standard deviations.

This can be extended to more than one marker if the correlations between the markers in affected and unaffected pregnancies (considered separately) are known. This forms the basis of multivariate Gaussian modeling, which is the standard method of combining different markers in screening (5). To combine different markers, it is necessary to use a common scale, which becomes the risk of having an affected pregnancy. Then, the overlapping distributions are of the estimates of the risks in affected and unaffected pregnancies instead of the concentration of the individual marker levels.

In general, the best study design to determine screening performance is observational because the result of the test does not alter the outcome or which subsequent tests are performed. An interventional study is one in which the results of a screening program are directly reported. This is subject to bias because some women with a screen-positive result and a positive diagnostic result, who proceed to a termination of pregnancy, would have had a miscarriage had there been no intervention and would not have appeared in either the numerator or the denominator of the estimate of the DR. The word "prospective" is often used to mean an interventional study. Any interventional study is necessarily prospective, but a prospective study is not necessarily interventional. Usually a prospective study, if not qualified further, implies an observational prospective study, to distinguish it from a retrospective study.

General Fetal Loss Bias Arising from the Ascertainment of Affected Pregnancies at Different Gestations

Reported screening performance will depend on when during pregnancy cases of Down syndrome are identified. Whether the screening test, and subsequent diagnostic test, is offered in the first or second trimesters can have a marked effect on the reported screening performance.

Figure 2 shows a hypothetical example of 100 cases of Down syndrome under three different situations: (i) no screening or selective termination of pregnancy, (ii) screening and selective termination of pregnancy in the first trimester, and (iii) screening and selective termination of pregnancy in the second trimester. Figure 2A illustrates that in the absence of screening, 74 out of the 100 cases of Down syndrome in the first trimester would survive to the second trimester and 57 would survive to term (6); a fetal loss rate of 43% from the first trimester to term. Figure 2B and C illustrates what would happen if screening were performed in the first and second trimesters, respectively, with a test that had a "true" DR of 70%. In Figure 2B, where selective termination of pregnancy occurs in the first trimester, the total number of cases of Down syndrome that could be ascertained is $70 + 17$ given that the number of Down syndrome in 13 spontaneous abortions is not known, so the reported DR would be $70/(70 + 17) = 80\%$. An intervention study in which selective termination of pregnancies may occur will overestimate screening

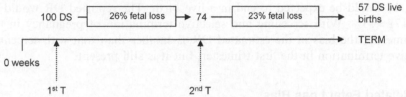

(A) No Screening or termination of pregnancy

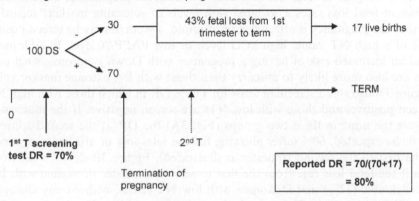

(B) Screening and selective termination of pregnancies in first trimester

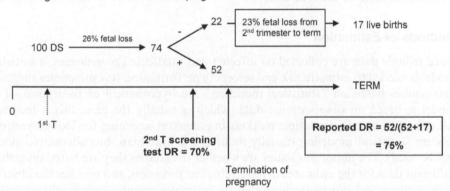

(C) Screening and selective termination of pregnancies in second trimester

Figure 2   The effect of general fetal loss bias on the estimated DR. *Abbreviations*: 1st T, first trimester; 2nd T, second trimester.

performance even if all false negatives that end in a live birth are ascertained. The bias in the estimation of the DR arises because the detected and missed cases of Down syndrome are identified at different times in pregnancy.

An adjustment for this "general fetal loss bias" can be made. For example, in Nicolaides et al. (7), 36 cases of Down syndrome were detected using first-trimester NT measurement with maternal age, and seven missed cases were identified at term (an apparent DR of 84%). Allowing for the 43% fetal loss between first trimester and term, the seven missed cases identified at term represent 12 in the first trimester. The DR corrected for the fetal loss bias is, therefore, $36/(36+12) = 75\%$.

Figure 2C illustrates screening in the second trimester. Of the 100 Down syndrome cases in the first trimester, 74 survive to the second trimester and undergo second trimester screening and 52 have screen-positive results. Of the 22 false negatives, 17 would be expected to end in a live birth. The reported DR would be $52/(52 + 17) = 75\%$. With screening and selective termination of pregnancy in the second trimester, the bias in the estimated DR is smaller than that with screening and selective termination in the first trimester, but it is still present.

Marker-Related Fetal Loss Bias

Apart from the general fetal loss that occurs in affected pregnancies there is also a difference in fetal loss rates associated with levels of screening markers regardless of whether the pregnancy is affected. For example, a woman may be screen positive because of a high NT value, high hCG level, or low PAPP-A level. In addition to being at an increased risk of having a pregnancy with Down syndrome, such pregnancies are also more likely to miscarry than those with less extreme marker values (4). Figure 3 illustrates a screening test with a 60% DR in which those with high NTs are screen positive, and those with low NTs are screen negative. If the miscarriage rates were the same in these two groups (Fig. 3A) the DR at the second trimester would be as expected, 60% (after allowing for the fetal loss of affected pregnancies from the first to the second trimester as illustrated). Figure 3B shows what would happen if the fetal loss rate from the first to second trimester in women with high NT were double (32%) that in women with low NT (16%), without any change to the overall fetal loss rate. The second-trimester DR would be 55% instead of 60%, an underestimate of the true DR.

Methods of Estimation

Once reliable data are collected on affected and unaffected pregnancies, a statistical model is needed to estimate risk and screening performance. It is sometimes suggested that studies based on "statistical modeling" are hypothetical or theoretical. If the model is based on observational data, which is usually the case, this is incorrect. All estimates based on multiple markers in antenatal screening for Down syndrome rely on statistical modeling (usually multivariate Gaussian, but alternative models can be used). The important issues are whether the studies they are based on provide sufficient data for the estimates to have sufficient precision, and whether the observed data fit the model satisfactorily so that the estimates are also sufficiently accurate.

One of two methods is usually used to estimate screening performance. They are set out in the Appendix (8). The study-specific method is easier to understand, but has drawbacks. It is based on every pregnancy in the study being allocated a risk of Down syndrome, selecting a risk cutoff level, and then counting the number of affected and unaffected pregnancies above the risk cutoff level to estimate the proportion above the cutoff, the former estimating the DR and the latter the FPR.

The second method, which can be called the general method is more complex but is preferable for two reasons: (i) it is much less dependent on the effects of chance affecting whether pregnancies (affected and unaffected) happen to be above a risk cutoff level, especially if the cutoff is extreme; it thus reduces an important source of imprecision that can only be avoided with the study-specific method if it is based on very large studies involving tens of thousands of unaffected pregnancies and many hundreds of affected pregnancies; (ii) the general method standardizes screening performance to a given maternal age distribution. This avoids bias that can arise, for example, if a study consists of pregnant women who are older than

(A)

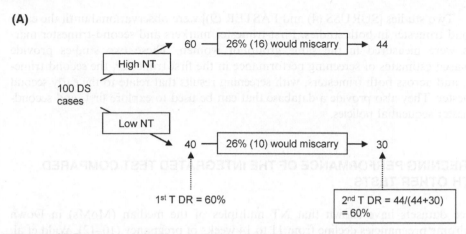

Reported DR not corrected for fetal loss= 60/(60+30) = 67%

(B)

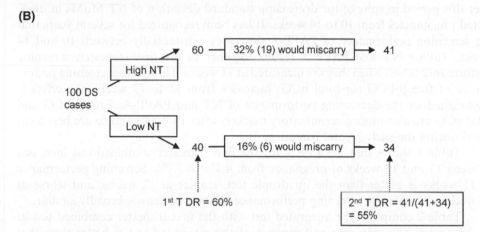

Reported DR not corrected for fetal loss = 60/(60+34) = 64%

Figure 3 Effect of marker-related fetal loss bias on the estimated DR (**A**) no marker related fetal loss bias, (**B**) pregnancies with high NT values have double the fetal loss rate compared with those with low NT values. Assumes complete ascertainment of screen negatives who do not miscarry and that the status of the screen negatives who miscarry is not known. *Abbreviations*: DR, detection rate; 1st T, first trimester; 2nd T, second trimester; NT, nuchal translucency.

pregnant women in general, which would overestimate the DR and FPR for a given risk cutoff because maternal age itself is a contributing factor to increasing risk.

Ideally, therefore, estimates of screening performance should be based on observational studies using the general method of estimating DR and FPR and, if possible, different tests should be compared by determining the distribution parameters of the screening markers in the same population of women. Second-trimester screening studies performed over 10 years ago were observational because they were carried out before screening became an established practice. As second-trimester screening is now standard medical practice, it is not possible to carry out an observational study in which all pregnancies proceed to term without screening, performing invasive diagnostic procedures, or terminating affected pregnancies. Few first-trimester screening studies have been observational.

Two studies [SURUSS (4) and FASTER (9)] were observational until the early second trimester in both studies. First-trimester markers and second-trimester markers were measured in the same group of women. These two studies provide unbiased estimates of screening performance in the first trimester, the second trimester, and across both trimesters, with screening results that relate to the early second trimester. They also provide a database that can be used to explore first- and second-trimester sequential policies.

SCREENING PERFORMANCE OF THE INTEGRATED TEST COMPARED WITH OTHER TESTS

Three datasets have shown that NT multiples of the median (MoMs) in Down syndrome pregnancies decline from 11 to 14 weeks of pregnancy (10–12). Wald et al. (11), using the SURUSS data, showed that this decreases NT screening performance over this period in spite of the decreasing standard deviation of NT MoMs in unaffected pregnancies from 10 to 14 weeks. It has been recognized for several years that the screening performance of PAPP-A decreases substantially between 10 and 14 weeks. Taking NT and PAPP-A results together in the first trimester, screening performance is best when they are measured at 11 weeks. Though the screening performance of free β-hCG (or total hCG) increases from 11 to 13 weeks, the effect is outweighed by the decreasing performance of NT and PAPP-A. Free β-hCG and total hCG are also more discriminatory markers after 13 weeks and so are best measured during the early second trimester.

Table 1 shows that the FPR_{85} for the first trimester combined test increases between 11 and 13 weeks of pregnancy from 4.3% to 7.7%. Screening performance at 11 weeks is better than the quadruple test, similar at 12 weeks, and worse at 13 weeks. Overall, the screening performance of the two tests is broadly similar.

Table 2 compares the integrated test with the first trimester combined test at 11–13 weeks. The screening performance of the integrated test is better than that of the combined test at all weeks and is higher at 11 weeks than at 12 or 13.

Table 3 shows a comparison of screening performance of the serum integrated test (that is, without NT measurement) with the first trimester combined test at 10–13 weeks. Estimates at 10 weeks are included since there are sufficient data relating to PAPP-A and free β-hCG at this time in pregnancy to provide reliable estimates (the 10 week estimate for the combined test is uncertain because of the lack of NT data at this time). The serum integrated test has a higher screening performance than the first trimester combined test at all gestational weeks and it is better at 11 weeks

Table 1 Comparison of First Trimester Combined Test (CT) and Second Trimester Quadruple Test

Week of gestation	FPR (%) for an 85% DR (FPR_{85})	Compared with Quadruple test ($FPR_{85} = 6.2\%$)
11	4.3	CT better
12	6.0	Similar
13	7.7	CT worse

Abbreviations: FPR, false-positive rate; DR, detection rate.
Source: From Ref. 4.

Table 2 Comparison of Screening Performance of Integrated Test with First Trimester Combined Test

| Week of gestation | FPR (%) for an 85% DR (FPR$_{85}$) | |
	Integrated test	Combined test
11	0.9	4.3
12	1.8	6.0
13	2.1	7.7

Abbreviations: FPR, false-positive rate; DR, detection rate.
Source: From Ref. 4.

than at 12 or 13. Compared with the combined test the serum integrated test achieves a 10–25% reduction in the FPR.

Figure 4 shows the FPR$_{85}$ for various screening tests estimated from SURUSS (tests that include first-trimester markers are measured at 11 weeks). Figure 5 shows the corresponding odds of being affected given a positive result (OAPR) and Figure 6 the corresponding number of procedure-related unaffected fetal losses per 100,000 women screened. Figure 7 shows receiver operator characteristic (ROC) (in which the DR is plotted against the FPR) curves for the main tests. Figure 8 shows the overlapping risk distributions for the main tests with cutoff set to yield a 3% FPR (i.e., DR$_3$). The improved screening performance of the integrated test compared with either the combined or the quadruple test is large and screening centers have started to offer this method of screening.

Results from SURUSS taken together with other studies show the importance of having week-specific screening means and standard deviations for the first trimester markers—something that is not critical in the second trimester. PAPP-A and NT are best measured at 11 weeks while all other markers are more discriminatory when measured in the second trimester. The integrated test takes advantage of the natural differences in the levels of the markers between affected and unaffected pregnancies at different stages of pregnancy, using each marker when the difference is greatest, thus optimizing discrimination between affected and unaffected pregnancies.

Variations of screening protocols that are suboptimal, for example, using inhibin-A as a first-trimester marker even though its discrimination at this time is poorer than at 14 or 15 weeks, are best avoided. Reporting partial results to women

Table 3 Comparison of Screening Performance of the Serum Integrated Test with the First Trimester Combined Test

| Week of gestation | FPR (%) for an 85% DR (FPR$_{85}$) | |
	Serum integrated test	Combined test
10	2.7	3.5
11	3.9	4.3
12	4.9	6.0
13	5.6	7.7

Abbreviations: FPR, false-positive rate; DR, detection rate.
Source: From Ref. 4.

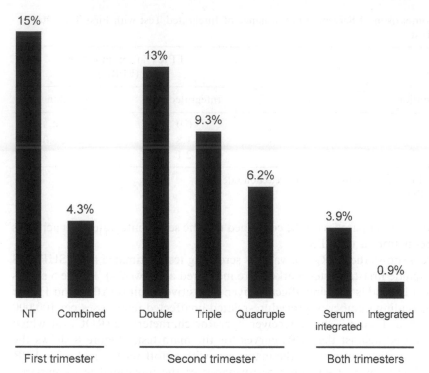

Figure 4 False-positive rate for an 85% detection rate according to screening test in the first trimester with first-trimester markers measured at 11 weeks and second-trimester markers at 14–22 weeks. *Source*: From Ref. 4.

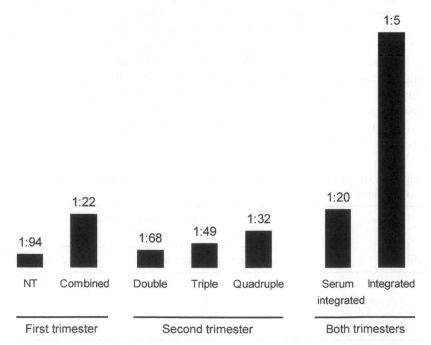

Figure 5 The odds of being affected given a positive result (OAPR) for the tests shown in Figure 4. *Source*: From Ref. 4.

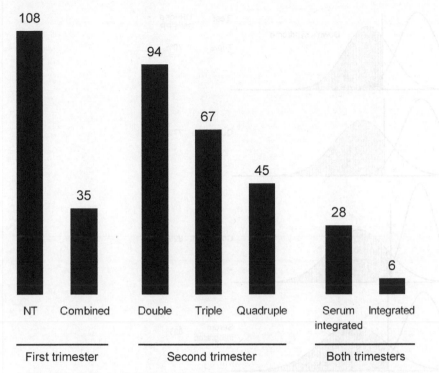

Figure 6 The number of procedure-related unaffected fetal losses in 100,000 women screened for the tests shown in Figures 4 and 5. *Source*: From Ref. 4.

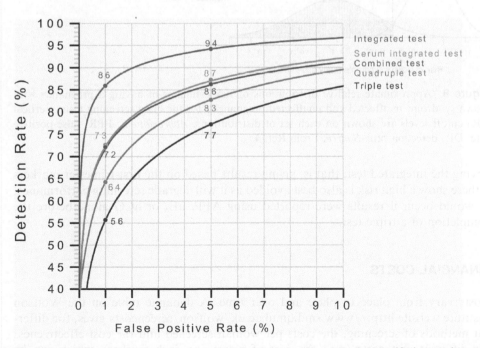

Figure 7 Down syndrome detection rates and false-positive rates for specified screening tests (ROC curves). *Abbreviation*: ROC curves, receiver operator characteristic curves. *Source*: From Ref. 4.

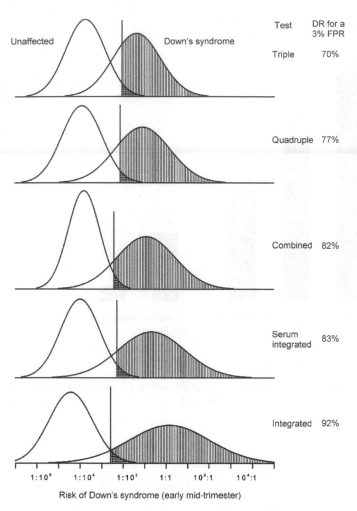

Figure 8 Approximate relative distributions of risk estimates of having a pregnancy with Down syndrome in affected and unaffected pregnancies for the main screening tests. Vertical DR$_3$ cutoff levels are shown on each set of distributions. *Abbreviations*: FPR, false-positive rate; DR, detection rate. *Source*: From Ref. 4.

having the integrated test, that is, giving results based on the first-trimester markers if these show a high risk is also best avoided as it will degrade screening performance, as would occur if results were reported using AFP, uE$_3$ or hCG alone before the completion of a triple test.

FINANCIAL COSTS

Costs vary from place to place and over time. A dynamic table on the Wolfson Institute website http://www.smd.qmul.ac.uk/wolfson/screencosts gives, for different methods of screening, the costs per woman screened and the cost-effectiveness for different unit costs (e.g., the cost of measuring each marker), which can be changed on the website.

SEQUENTIAL SCREENING POLICIES

Sequential screening is not the application of a single test but a series of tests, usually two, according to a specified protocol, for example, all women having a first-trimester test based on maternal age with NT and PAPP-A and screen negatives going on to have the integrated test. Provided a sequential screening policy does not lead to an excessively high FPR for a given DR (compared with the use of the integrated test on all women), it may be a valid screening option, but there will be trade-offs. An advantage is the detection of most affected pregnancies about 4 weeks earlier in pregnancy. The disadvantages include the implementation of a more complex screening protocol, which involves the estimation of more than one risk in the same pregnancy, which can cause confusion, and the termination of about 20% of affected pregnancies that would have miscarried naturally between the first and second trimesters of pregnancy. This last point is of some importance since the termination of an affected pregnancy is inevitably associated with doubt, anguish, and guilt. A miscarriage, though distressing, avoids this doubt and guilt.

Sequential screening is usually taken to mean performing a first-trimester test, then offering women with screen-positive results a diagnostic test, and rescreening remaining women 4 weeks later using an integrated test based on second-trimester markers with the reuse of the first-trimester markers. Such screening needs to be distinguished from having a separate second-trimester test (e.g., a quadruple test) without reusing the first-trimester markers—a practice that leads to a poor overall screening performance and should be avoided.

A variant of such a sequential approach is a method of screening called contingent screening (13). It is more complex because the first-trimester screening test separates women into three groups instead of two: a screen-positive group that is offered a diagnostic CVS, a screen-negative group that does not proceed for further measurements in the second trimester, and an intermediate, or pending, group that proceeds to an integrated test. Sequential screening and contingent screening can be formulated in a cost-effective way, though sequential screening is less cost-effective than either contingent screening or screening all women with the integrated test. Figure 9 shows the main nonfinancial points of comparison between the different methods. To maintain screening efficacy, the sequential approach requires that a very high cutoff level is set for the first test so that the FPR is no greater than about 0.5% or 1.0%. If the FPR of the first test is even a few percentage points higher, screening performance becomes markedly inferior relative to that achieved if all women had the integrated test. With contingent screening, most women do not have a second-trimester measurement. Three lower risk cutoffs are shown, 1 in 1000, 1 in 2000, and 1 in 3000, to define women as screen negative on the basis of the first-trimester test who would not, therefore, proceed to complete the integrated test. This means, however, that AFP measurement for neural tube defect screening is lost, which may be acceptable where routine first-trimester ultrasound examinations are offered in centers with sufficient expertise to ensure that spina bifida DRs are high. It probably would not be acceptable at centers where this cannot be assured. If blood is taken for an AFP measurement, it is little extra effort to measure the three other markers uE$_3$, hCG, and inhibin-A at the same time; thus, in effect, the policy would revert to sequential screening and then the principle concern is overall cost and the fact that about one in five terminations of pregnancy are unnecessary.

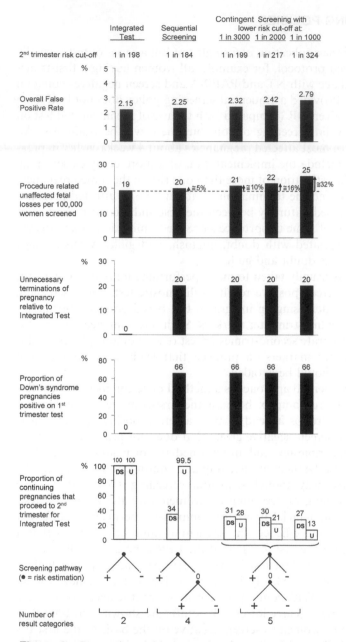

Figure 9 Comparison of integrated test, sequential screening, and contingent screening to achieve a 90% detection rate (false-positive rate of first trimester test NT, PAPP-A, and free β-hCG with maternal age set to 0.5% for sequential and contingent screening—risk cutoff 1 in 30) and first-trimester markers measured at 11 completed weeks. *Source*: From Wald NJ, Rudnicka AR, Bestwick JP. Prenatal Diagnosis (in press).

POSSIBLE IMPROVEMENTS IN SCREENING PERFORMANCE WITH THE ADDITION OF AN ULTRASOUND FETAL NASAL BONE EXAMINATION

The absence of a fetal nasal bone at the end of the first trimester of pregnancy is a marker of Down syndrome. Cicero and colleagues have estimated that the DR for this marker alone is about 70% for a FPR varying from about 0.5% to 2.5% (Table 4). It is a difficult examination to perform, requiring care and time on the part of the ultrasonographer. The addition of the examination can detect about two-thirds of the pregnancies that are missed by the combined test or the integrated test with an extra 0.5% FPR. It can, therefore, enhance the screening performance of both the tests. For example, assuming a 70% $DR_{0.5}$ for nasal bone examination, this would raise the DR of the combined or integrated test from 85% to about 95% with an increase in the FPR from 4.3% to 4.8% for the combined test and from 0.9% to 1.4% for the integrated test.

THE INTEGRATED TEST IN TWIN PREGNANCIES

Screening twin pregnancies poses a number of difficulties, the greatest of which is that in most affected pregnancies Down syndrome will affect one fetus and not the other. The question of selective feticide arises, with all the emotional and technical difficulties involved. There are also difficulties in terms of screening, because the ultrasound markers are specific to the fetus but the serum markers are specific to the pregnancy. A method has been described for combining ultrasound and serum-marker measurement so that all the measurements relate to the pregnancy (23). Serum-marker levels can be adjusted to allow for the increased levels observed in twin pregnancies and the risk estimate calculated as if the marker levels related to a singleton pregnancy. Such adjustments can ensure that the FPR in twin pregnancies is kept at an acceptably low level, similar to the rate expected in singleton pregnancies. The corresponding DR is uncertain, but is likely to be less than that achieved in singleton pregnancies for the same FPR. The risk estimate is also uncertain, and is best not reported.

RESULTS FROM OTHER STUDIES

In general, the results from SURUSS corroborate those obtained in most other studies, showing an approximate 85% DR for a 5% FPR for the combined test (87% DR for 5% FPR in Bindra et al. (24) after adjusting for fetal loss biases compared

Table 4 Summary of Studies on Nasal Bone Examinations

References	Study	Absent nasal bone	
		Normal, n (%)	Trisomy 21, n (%)
Cicero et al.[a] (14)	Pre-CVS	3/603 (0.5)	43/59 (72.9)
Otano et al. (15)	Pre-CVS	1/175 (0.6)	3/5 (60.0)
Zoppi et al. (16)	Screening	7/3,463 (0.2)	19/27 (70.0)
Orlandi et al. (17)	Screening	10/1,000 (1.0)	10/15 (66.7)
Viora et al. (18)	Screening	24/1,733 (1.4)	8/10 (80.0)
Senat et al. (19)	Retrospective	4/944 (0.4)	3/4 (75.0)
Wong et al. (20)	Pre-CVS	1/114 (0.9)	2/3 (66.7)
Cicero et al.[a] (21)	Pre-CVS	93/3,358 (2.8)	162/242 (67.0)
Cicero et al. (22)	Pre-CVS	129/5,223 (2.5)	229/333 (68.8)
Total		176/12,652 (1.4)	274/397 (69.0)

[a]Data included in Cicero et al. (13).
Source: From Ref. 13.

with an 83% DR for a 5% FPR in SURUSS). The BUN study (25) yielded somewhat lower estimates of the performance of the combined test. The SURUSS estimates for first-trimester screening indicate, as expected, a somewhat lower screening performance than most interventional studies (e.g., Bindra et al.). Second-trimester screening performance was, as expected, somewhat higher than estimates from previous studies because many previous second trimester studies were observational, but in SURUSS, intervention was offered after second-trimester screening was performed. A meta-analysis of second-trimester studies shows, for example, that free β-hCG levels in Down syndrome pregnancies are higher in interventional studies than in observational studies (Table 27 in the SURUSS report) indicating that screening performance will tend to appear better in the former than the latter. In SURUSS (4), the quadruple test yielded an 83% DR for a 5% FPR, compared with 76% from a study based on samples collected in Oxford before serum or ultrasound screening was introduced and which was observational throughout pregnancy.

The only other study similar in design to SURUSS is FASTER (9) and this has produced similar results (Fig. 10). FASTER excluded cystic hygroma, but this will not have a material effect on the DRs and FPRs because cystic hygroma is rare and is associated with a high risk of Down syndrome and other serious fetal abnormalities.

STANDARDIZING SCREENING PERFORMANCE TO ABOUT 17 WEEKS OF PREGNANCY

In the past it was appropriate to relate screening performance to Down syndrome livebirths, and hence to calculate the risk of a woman having an affected term pregnancy. Results from recent studies, notably those from SURUSS and FASTER,

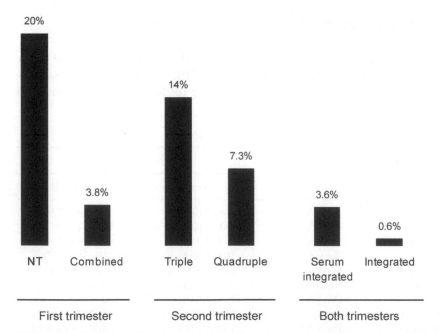

Figure 10 False-positive rate for an 85% detection rate according to screening test in the first trimester with first-trimester markers measured at 11 weeks and second-trimester markers at 14–22 weeks. *Source*: From Ref. 9.

cannot estimate either screening performance at term or the risk of having an affected term pregnancy because of intervention following the results of the early second-trimester screening tests. They will be subject to the general and the marker-related fetal loss bias from this point of pregnancy onward. While an adjustment can be made for the former, it cannot satisfactorily be done for marker-related bias. For this reason, risk estimates and screening performance necessarily have to relate to about 17 weeks of pregnancy rather than term.

IMPLEMENTATION OF THE INTEGRATED TEST

Six centers (two in Britain, two in Canada, one in Italy, and one in Portugal) participated in a demonstration project (the integrated risk screening or IRS project). By the end of March 2003, 23,814 women, including 54 who had pregnancies with Down syndrome, had been screened and completed their pregnancies. Some centers only offered the serum integrated test and some did not measure inhibin-A in the second trimester. Table 5 shows the DR for a fixed 3% FPR for four variants of the integrated test. All the available data from all women screened were used wherever possible, even if the women had been screened with a different variant. So, for example, a woman who had had the full integrated test could also be included in the table with the serum integrated test by ignoring the data on NT measurements. There were 11 affected pregnancies in women who had full integrated tests, and all were detected. All the tests had DRs that were close to those expected from the results in the SURUSS report, allowing for the ages of the women screened. Overall 3% of women in the demonstration project failed to complete the integrated test, often on account of a miscarriage between 11 and 15 weeks. Risk estimation was also accurate, in that the average predicted risk in each risk quintile group (classified according to quintile in affected pregnancies) was similar to the observed prevalence of Down syndrome in the same group: 1 in 1.2 compared with 1 in 2.3 in the high-risk group, 1 in 2.0 compared with 1 in 3 in the second, 1 in 6.5 compared with 1 in 1.97 in the third, 1 in 40 compared with 1 in 36 in the fourth, and 1 in 2700 compared with 1 in 2600 in the

Table 5 Observed and Expected Screening Performance for Four Variants of the Integrated Test at a 3% False-Positive Rate in 23,814 Pregnancies Screened in the Integrated Risk Screening (IRS) project

Screening test (all with maternal age)	Total Down syndrome pregnancies[a]	Down syndrome pregnancies detected	Early second-trimester detection rate (%)	
			Observed (95% CI)	Expected[b]
Full integrated test	11	11	100 (72–100)	90
Integrated without inhibin-A	44	36	82 (70–93)	87
Integrated without NT	18	16	89 (65–99)	80
Integrated without inhibin-A and NT	52	43	83 (72–93)	73

[a]Indicates the number of women with Down syndrome pregnancies (as a subset of the total of 54) in whom markers that make up the test specified were measured.
[b]By applying the distribution parameters reported in SURUSS to the age distribution of women screened in the IRS project.

lowest. The results of the demonstration project showed that screening for Down syndrome using the integrated test is feasible and can be introduced into medical practice, achieving DRs and FPRs similar to those expected from independent estimates.

CONCLUSIONS

Table 6 presents a simple summary of the efficacy and safety associated with currently generally recommended screening tests. Of these tests, the integrated test has the greatest efficacy, safety, and cost-effectiveness provided the costs of the individual components of each test are not excessive. Cost is generally not a concern with the serum markers, but there is a risk that the NT measurement could become expensive if it becomes an opportunity to perform a detailed ultrasound examination, which could lead to the examination costing US dollars 100 or more, instead of about US dollars 10. If NT measurement is not available, the serum integrated test is the next best screening method. For women who present for the first time in the second trimester of pregnancy, the quadruple test is the test of choice, and this has been confirmed in practice (26). For women who request a screening result before 14 weeks of pregnancy, the combined test is the best option. The addition of a nasal bone examination, if feasible, would increase the efficacy of screening using the combined test and the integrated test.

In sequential screening protocols, there is a 15–20% chance of needlessly terminating an affected pregnancy that would have aborted spontaneously. This is a serious adverse consequence, but one that is "hidden" because in an individual

Table 6 Efficacy and Safety of the Recommended Screening Tests (First-Trimester Markers Measured at 11 Completed Weeks)

		Efficacy		Safety
				Number of procedure related fetal losses per 100,000
Test		FPR (%) for an 85% DR	OAPR	
Offered routinely				
In general	Integrated	0.9	1:5	6
If NT not available[a]	Serum integrated	3.9 (2.7)	1:20 (1:14)	28 (19)
If first visit is in second trimester	Quadruple	6.2	1:32	45
Available but not offered routinely				
For women who request a first-trimester test	Combined	4.3	1:22	35

[a]Numbers in brackets relate to PAPP-A measured at 10 weeks instead of 11.
Abbreviations: FPR, false-positive rate; DR, detection rate; OAPR, odds of being affected given a positive result.
Source: From Ref. 27.

case, one cannot distinguish a terminated pregnancy that is destined to miscarry from one that would continue if the termination had not been performed. On the other hand, over 50% of affected pregnancies that would have been viable can be detected about 4 weeks earlier compared with an integrated test, which is a very "visible" benefit. The integrated test automatically includes an AFP measurement that is used to screen for open neural tube defects, which otherwise may not be done, and the quadruple test markers can be used to increase the ability to detect other serious abnormalities, such as trisomy 18.

The advantage of a sequential approach, namely an earlier diagnosis in most affected pregnancies, puts a premium on early decision making, which health professionals may rate more highly than patients. Patients may be more concerned about the worry associated with having a screen-positive result (or in the case of contingent screening, a pending result), with the increased chance of losing a healthy pregnancy from the invasive diagnostic test or with the possibility of having a needless termination. In a study performed by Bishop et al. (28), the views of 253 women being screened and 94 healthcare professionals were compared. It was concluded that "while pregnant women and health care professionals share similar relative values regarding optimal prenatal tests, health care professionals place a higher value on earlier tests. This may result in screening policies that over weight timing in the selection of a test to the relative neglect of tests associated with lower miscarriage rates and higher DR but conducted later in pregnancy" (28).

Weighing the trade-offs is complex, but unlike the management of individual patients who present with particular problems as is usual in clinical practice, screening practice cannot be effectively carried out by offering women an individual menu of screening options from which they can make a personal choice. The process would become too complicated, unpredictable, and costly.

It is necessary for health services to offer women the screening test (or tests) that are judged to be cost-effective and have the highest efficacy and safety that can be provided and afforded, and to do so in a cost-effective way, not a multiplicity of options. However, variations in what is actually provided should of course be considered, respecting the preferences of individual women. In this way, there need not be a bewildering set of options presented to women (29). What is offered can be clear, simple, and uniform, but what is done may vary to accommodate the preferences, wishes, and concerns of the individual women being screened.

ACKNOWLEDGMENTS

We thank Karen Wald, M Campogrande, M Perona, S Castedo, C Rodeck, A Summers, and P Wyatt for their contribution to the IRS project, Kia Abdullah for work on the figures, Simon Rish, Alicja Rudnicka, and Wayne Huttly for comments on the manuscript.

Disclosure of Interest: Nicholas Wald holds a patent interest on the Integrated test.

GLOSSARY

AFP	Alphafetoprotein
uE_3	Unconjugated estriol
hCG	Human chorionic gonadotrophin
PAPP-A	Pregnancy-associated plasma protein A
NT	Nuchal translucency. An ultrasound measurement of the width of an area of translucency at the back of the fetal neck early in pregnancy
CVS	Chorionic villus sampling
FPR	False-positive rate. The proportion of women with unaffected pregnancies who have positive results
DR	Detection rate. The proportion of women with Down syndrome (affected) pregnancies who have positive results
MoM	Multiple of the median among unaffected pregnancies
OAPR	Odds of being affected given a positive result. True positives to false positives
Double test	Second trimester test based on the measurement of AFP and hCG (either free β-hCG or total hCG), together with maternal age
Triple test	Second trimester test based on the measurement of AFP, uE_3, and hCG (either total hCG or free β-hCG) (or total hCG) together with maternal age
Quadruple test	Second trimester test based on the measurement of AFP, uE_3, free β-hCG (or total hCG), and inhibin-A together with maternal age
Combined test	First trimester test based on combining nuchal translucency measurement with free β-hCG (or total hCG) Pregnancy-associated plasma protein A (PAPP-A) and maternal age
Integrated test	The integration of measurements performed at different times of pregnancy into a single test result. Unless otherwise qualified, "Integrated test" refers to the integration of NT measurement and PAPP-A in the first trimester with the quadruple test markers in the second
Serum integrated test	A variant of the integrated test (without NT using PAPP-A in the first trimester and the quadruple test markers in the second trimester)
Cutoff level	The level chosen to define a positive result and distinguish it from a negative result. With a single marker this will be a specified level of the marker. With tests based on a combination of markers it will be a risk estimate
Affected pregnancy	A pregnancy affected with Down syndrome
Unaffected pregnancy	A pregnancy without a chromosomal defect
True positive	Affected pregnancy with a positive test result
False positive	Unaffected pregnancy with a positive test result

REFERENCES

1. Wald NJ, Cuckle HS, Densem JW, et al. Maternal serum screening for Down syndrome in early pregnancy. Br Med J 1988; 297:883–887.
2. Wald NJ, Densem JW, Smith D, Klee GG. Four-marker serum screening for Down's syndrome. Prenat Diagn 1994; 14:707–716.
3. Wald NJ, Watt HC, Hackshaw AK. Integrated screening for Down's syndrome based on tests performed during the first and second trimesters. N Engl J Med 1999; 341:461–467.
4. Wald NJ, Rodeck C, Hackshaw AK, Walters J, Chitty L, Mackinson AM. First and second trimester antenatal screening for Down's syndrome: the results of the Serum, Urine and Ultrasound Screening Study (SURUSS). Health Technol Assess 2003; 7(1).
5. Wald N, Hackshaw A. Tests using multiple markers. In: Wald NJ, Leck I, eds. Antenatal Neonatal Screening. 2nd ed. Oxford: Oxford University Press, 2000:23–57.
6. Morris JK, Wald NJ, Watt, HC. Fetal loss in Down syndrome pregnancies. Prenat Diagn 1999; 19:142–145.
7. Nicolaides KH, Sebire NJ, Snijders RJ, Johnson S. Down's syndrome screening in the UK. Lancet 1996; 347:906–907.
8. Wald N, Rudnicka A: (Accessed 4, April 2006 at, http://www.smd.qmul/wolfson/screeningperformance).
9. Malone FD, Canick JA, Ball RH, et al. First- and Second-Trimester Evaluation of Risk (FASTER) Research consortium. First-trimester or second-trimester screening, or both, for Down's syndrome. N Engl J Med 2005; 353:2001–2011.
10. Spencer K, Bindra R, Nix ABJ, Heath V, Nicolaides KH. Delta-NT or NT MoM: which is the most appropriate method for calculating accurate patient-specific risks for trisomy 21 in the first trimester? Ultrasound Obstet Gynaecol 2003; 22:142–148.
11. Wald N, Rodeck C, Rudnicka A, Hackshaw A. Nuchal translucency and gestational age. Prenat Diagn 2004; 24:150–153.
12. Aiello H, Otano L, Igarzabal L, Gadow EC. Nuchal translucency and gestational age. Prenat Diagn 2004; 24:748–749.
13. Wright D, Bradbury I, Benn P, Cuckle H, Ritchie K. Contingent screening for Down syndrome is an efficient alternative to non-disclosure sequential screening. Prenat Diagn 2004; 24(10):762–766.
14. Cicero S, Curcio P, Papageorghious A, Sonek J, Nicolaides KH. Absence of nasal bone in fetuses with trisomy 21 at 11–14 weeks of gestation: an observational study. Lancet 2001; 358:1665–1667.
15. Otano L, Aiello H, Igarzabal L, Matayoshi T, Gadow EC. Association between first trimester absence of fetal nasal bone on ultrasound and Down's syndrome. Prenat Diagn 2002; 22:930–932.
16. Zoppi MA, Ibba RM, Axinan C, Floris M, Manca F, Monni G. Absence of fetal nasal bone and aneuploidies at first trimester nuchal translucency screening in unselected pregnancies. Prenat Diagn 2003; 23:496–500.
17. Orlandi F, Bilardo CM, Campogrande M, et al. Measurement of nasal bone length at 11–14 weeks of pregnancy and its potential role in Down syndrome risk assessment. Ultrasound Obstet Gynecol 2003; 23:36–39.
18. Viora E, Masturzo B, Errante G, Sciarrone A, Bastonero S, Campogrande M. Ultrasound evaluation of fetal nasal bone at 11 to 14 weeks in a consecutive series of 1906 fetuses. Prenat Diagn 2003; 23:784–787.
19. Senat MV, Bernard JP, Boulvain M, Ville Y. Intra- and interoperator variability in fetal nasal bone assessment at 11–14 weeks of gestation. Ultrasound Obstet Gynecol 2003; 22:138–141.
20. Wong SF, Choi H, Ho LC. Nasal bone hypoplasia: is it a common finding amongst chromosomally normal fetuses of southern Chinese women? Gynecol Obstet Invest 2003; 56:99–101.

21. Cicero S, Longo D, Rembouskos G, Sacchini C, Nicolaides KH. Absent nasal bone at 11–14 weeks of gestation and chromosomal defects. Ultrasound Obstet Gynecol 2003; 22:31–35.

22. Cicero S, Rembouskos G, Vandecruys H, Hogg M, Nicolaides KH. Likelihood ratio for trisomy 21 in fetuses with absent nasal bone at the 11–14 week scan. Ultrasound Obstet Gynecol 2004; 23:218–223.

23. Wald NJ, Rish S, Hackshaw AK. Combining nuchal translucency and serum markers in prenatal screening for Down syndrome in twin pregnancies. Prenat Diagn 2003; 23: 588–592.

24. Bindra R, Heath V, Liao A, Spencer K, Nicolaides KH. One-stop clinic for assessment of risk for trisomy 21 at 11–14 weeks: a prospective study of 15,030 pregnancies. Ultrasound Obstet Gynecol 2002; 20:219–225.

25. Wapner R, Thom E, Simpson JL, et al. First-trimester screening for trisomies 21 and 18. N Engl J Med 2003; 349(15):1405–1413.

26. Wald NJ, Huttly WJ, Hackshaw AK. Antenatal screening for Down's syndrome with the quadruple test. Lancet 2003; 361:835–836.

27. Wald NJ, Rodeck C, Hackshaw AK, Rudnicka A. SURUSS in Perspective Br J Obstet Gynaecol 2004; 111:521–531.

28. Bishop AJ, Marteau TM, Armstrong D, et al. Women and health care professionals' preferences for Down's syndrome screening tests: a conjoint analysis study. Br J Obstet Gynaecol 2004; 111:775–779.

29. Mennuti MT, Driscoll DA. Screening for Down's syndrome—too many choices? N Engl J Med 2003; 349:1471–1473.

APPENDIX

Antenatal Screening for Down Syndrome
Determining screening performance (detection rates and false positive rates)

Start with:-
i) Sample of pregnant women with data on maternal age, gestational age, levels of the screening markers and outcome of pregnancy
ii) A study that reports the age-specific birth prevalence of Down syndrome

$\downarrow$

Convert marker levels into MoMs

$\downarrow$

Determine the means, Standard deviations, correlation coefficients
for the logarithm of marker MoMs for affected and unaffected pregnancies

$\downarrow$

The screening markers are shown to have acceptable Guassian distributions, which can be used to determine likelihood ratios for the study sample or for a standard population

Study Specific Method

Determine likelihood ratios (LRs) using multivariate Gaussian modelling for each woman in the study

$\downarrow$

LRs are then applied to the age specific risks of Down Syndrome to obtain the risk of Down syndrome for each pregnancy. (The likelihood ratio is the ratio of the proportion of affected and unaffected pregnancies with a particular combination of marker levels)

$\downarrow$

For a given risk cut-off the detection rate (DR) and false positive rate (FPR) are determined, respectively, by the proportion of Down syndrome and unaffected pregnancies with risks equal to or above the risk cut-off. These proportions are obtained by counting the number of Down syndrome pregnancies and unaffected pregnancies that have a risk estimate equal to or greater than the risk cut-off, and dividing by the total number of Down syndrome and unaffected pregnancies, respectively.

$\downarrow$

Similarly, the DR for a given FPR can be determined by counting. For example, the DR for a 5% FPR is determined by counting the proportion of Down Syndrome pregnancies that have a risk estimate equal to or greater than the risk estimate at the 95th centile of unaffected pregnancies. Alternatively, the same can be done by determining the risk cut-off for a given DR and then determining the FPR for that DR.

General Method

Apply the age specific risk of Down syndrome to a standard population of maternities (e.g. England & Wales 1996-98) to give the expected number of Down syndrome pregnancies and unaffected pregnancies at each year of age

$\downarrow$

From the multivariate Gaussian distribution of screening markers LRs are obtained from the ratio of the heights of these distributions for combinations of the screening markers in specified intervals, usually about 100 intervals per marker covering a wide range of values (say +/-4 Standard deviations).These LRs are then applied to the affected and unaffected pregnancies at each year of age to give risks for the resulting marker combinations.

$\downarrow$

In addition, the proportion of Down syndrome and the proportion of unaffected pregnancies within each of the specified intervals of the screening markers is estimated from the corresponding area under the multivariate Gaussian distributions in Down syndrome and unaffected pregnancies respectively.

$\downarrow$

For a given risk cut-off the detection rate (DR) and false positive rate (FPR) are determined, respectively, by the proportion of Down syndrome and unaffected pregnancies with risks equal to or above the risk cut-off. These proportions are obtained by summing the proportions of Down syndrome and unaffected pregnancies, with risks equal to or higher than the risk cut-off, across all maternal ages and screening marker categories.

$\downarrow$

Similarly, the above step can be repeated by determining the risk cut off corresponding to a given DR and then summing the proportions of the unaffected pregnancies with risks equal to or higher than the risk cut off to estimate the FPR for that DR. Alternatively the same can be done by determining the risk-cut-off for a given FPR and then determining the DR for that FPR.

Advantages
Intuitive

Each woman in a particular study is assigned a risk and a
the proportions of affected and unaffected pregnancies
exceeding different risk cut-offs are determined by counting
the women in the study

Advantages
Overcomes the problems of differences in maternal age
distribution between studies

Minimizes imprecision in estimating DRs and FPRs
because estimates of the proportions in the tails of the risk
distributions are less subject to random sampling error

Disadvantages
The resulting proportions (DRs and FPRs) are dependent
on the age distribution of women in the study sample so the
results are not generalizable

Estimates of DRs (and FPRs) are imprecise due to the
small number of pregnancies, especially, Down syndrome
pregnancies in a given study

Disadvantages
Less intuitive

The two methods are similar, but the Study Specific Method calculates each woman's likelihood ratio for her particular MoM
combination while the General Method uses the *distributions* of likelihood ratios derived from the *distributions* of MoM
values and then applies these likelihood ratios to each year of maternal age in a distribution of pregnancies (affected and
unaffected) in any given population.

The general method is the standard and preferred method for estimating DRs and FPRs. The Study Specific method is only
reliable in very large studies based on several hundred affected pregnancies and tens of thousands of unaffected
pregnancies and even then is still applicable only to the particular age distribution of women in the study.

A variant of the general approach is to use the Monte Carlo simulation instead of determining the area under the multivariate
gaussion distributions, as set out below.

Monte Carlo Simulation

Apply the age-specific birth prevalence of Down syndrome to a standard population of maternities (e.g. England & Wales
1996-98) to give the number of Down syndrome pregnancies and the number of unaffected pregnancies expected at each
year of age

↓

Assign each pregnancy a MoM value for each marker (this simulates the marker values that would be found in a large
population of affected and unaffected pregnancies) by drawing values at random from the corresponding Gaussian
distribution of marker levels, according to whether the pregnancy is affected or unaffected.

↓

Determine the likelihood ratio (LR) for each woman using the same procedure as for the Study Specific Method and the
General Method

↓

Apply the LR to the age specific risks to obtain the risk of Down syndrome for each pregnancy.

↓

Determine the detection rate (DR) for a given false positive rate (FPR) by counting as for the Study Specific Method

January 2004

7

Genetic Ultrasound Scan—Second Trimester

Annegret Geipel and Ulrich Gembruch
Department of Obstetrics and Prenatal Medicine, University of Bonn, Bonn, Germany

INTRODUCTION

During the last decades, various studies have described characteristic sonographically detectable features of most chromosomal abnormalities. In the first trimester, increased nuchal translucency thickness is a common sonographic finding of major aneuploidies. Risk evaluation by maternal age and measurement of nuchal translucency has emerged as a highly effective screening method with detection rates of 70% to 80% for autosomal trisomies, for a screen positive rate of 5% (1–3). In addition, the sonographic demonstration of the presence of a nasal bone allows a further decrease of the calculated individual risk (4).

With the widespread use of this sophisticated screening technique, the prevalence of trisomic fetuses in later pregnancy is now markedly reduced. Since screening strategies may differ from country to country and some women may prefer second rather than first trimester ultrasound screening, the approach of targeted second trimester evaluation should not be neglected. In the second trimester, each chromosomal disorder manifests its own phenotypic expression. This includes a variety of major malformations as described for trisomy 18, trisomy 13, and triploidy or more subtle changes as characteristic for trisomy 21. An increasing list of nonspecific sonographic findings, so-called "markers" or minor abnormalities, each of different significance, has been proposed to screen for chromosomal defects in the second trimester. These markers are most frequently found in normal pregnancies and as an isolated finding they are rarely associated with any adverse outcome. Sensitivity and specificity of Down syndrome (DS) screening are increased by use of multiple markers in combination, rather than one sole finding. The second trimester genetic scan includes a targeted search for fetal structural abnormalities, abnormal fetal biometry, and other sonographic findings suggestive of fetal aneuploidy. This method of risk assessment can be used to either identify fetuses at high risk for aneuploidy or to decrease the background risk in a pregnancy without markers present.

TRISOMY 21 (DOWN SYNDROME)

The estimated prevalence of Down syndrome ranges from about 1 in 500 to 1 in 700 at birth. The risk increases with maternal age and decreases with advancing gestation. The prevalence of trisomy 21 in the first trimester and in the early second trimester is about 30% to 43% and 21% to 23% higher than the prevalence at birth, respectively (5,6). Therefore, the risk of a 35-year-old woman, carrying a baby with DS is about 1 in 200 at 12 weeks, 1 in 270 at 20 weeks, and 1 in 360 at 40 weeks (2).

A number of referral centers with expertise in targeted ultrasound examination report sonographic abnormalities in 60–90% of second trimester fetuses with DS in selected high-risk patients, with a false-positive rate of 5–15% (7–11). However, the prenatal detection rate in unselected populations is much lower (12–14).

Sonographic findings are commonly described as structural defects (major abnormalities) and minor abnormalities (marker) (Table 1). A wide variety of ultrasound markers have been associated with fetal DS during the second trimester (7,15–23). The most frequently reported findings in fetuses with trisomy 21 include thickened nuchal fold, shortened long bones (humerus, femur), hyperechogenic bowel, renal pyelectasis, and intracardiac hyperechogenic foci. Other markers, such as small ears, clinodactyly with hypoplasia of the middle phalanx of the fifth digit, sandalfoot and cerebellar hypoplasia, and intermammarian distance have not been generally incorporated in the list of sonographic markers. More recently, nasal bone hypoplasia, larger iliac wing angle and shortened fingers have been added to this list (10,24–28). Systematic evaluation of these multiple markers is commonly referred to as a second trimester genetic sonogram. As the list of sonographic markers is growing, there is a good chance of identifying at least one marker by routine ultrasound. Extrapolation of the data collected on selected high-risk populations to low-risk women seems problematic, as the positive predictive value of each marker will be much lower (29).

Structural Defects

Congenital malformations associated with DS are less frequent than with trisomy 18 or trisomy 13 and will be identified in about 20% to 30% of fetuses (7,8,11,20, 25,30,40). These anomalies include heart defects, fetal hydrops, ventriculomegaly, duodenal atresia, and short fingers, among others (Fig. 1A–D). Heart defects represent the most common anomaly, but there is a widely differing detection rate in the second trimester. In a targeted echocardiography study, Paladini et al. reported a 56% incidence of congenital heart disease in fetuses with known DS, which was an atrioventricular septal defect (AVSD) in 44% of cases. Conversely, 53% of cases with AVSD and normal visceral situs were associated with DS (31). DeVore reported cardiac abnormalities in 76% of fetuses with DS, including structural and functional (tricuspid regurgitation, pericardial effusion) findings (9).

Nasal Bone Hypoplasia

Absence of the nasal bone has been proposed as a new marker for DS in the first trimester. The authors reported that at 11 to 14 weeks' gestation the nasal bone was not visible by ultrasound examination in about 70% of fetuses with DS and in less than 1% of chromosomally normal fetuses (4). Recently, this marker has been evaluated in second trimester high-risk pregnancies as well (10,25,27,32). In the studies of Bromley and Vintzileos, an absent nasal bone yielded detection rates of 37–41% for

Table 1 Sonographic Abnormalities Frequently Observed in Second-Trimester Fetuses with Trisomy

Sonographic abnormalities	Trisomy 21[a]	Trisomy 18[b]	Trisomy 13[c]
Head/central nervous system	10–30% Ventriculomegaly Brachycephaly	50–80% Choroid plexus cyst Strawberry-shaped head Abnormal cerebellum and spina bifida	40–60% Holoprosencephaly
Face	40–50% Nasal bone hypoplasia Flat facial profile	20% Micrognathia Cleft lip and palate	40–50% Hypotelorism/cyclopia Proboscis, one nostril, median cleft
Nuchal thickening	40–50%	15–20%	20–30%
Cardiac	10–50% AVSD, Fallot, VSD echogenic intracardiac focus	40–90% Outlet defects (VSD, Fallot) AVSD	50–60% Outlet defects (VSD, DORV, Fallot, TAC)
Urinary system	10–20% Hydronephrosis	<10%	30–40% Echogenic, enlarged kidneys
Gastrointestinal	10–20% Hyperechogenic bowel	20–40% Omphalocele	15–20% Omphalocele
Extremities	25–40% Short humerus/femur	70–90% Clenched fingers Rocker-bottom-feet	30–40% Polydactyly
Umbilical cord		15–40% Single umbilical artery Umbilical cord cyst	15–30% Single umbilical artery
IUGR	<10%	30–50%	30–50%

[a]According to Rotmensch et al. (30), Paladini et al. (31), Nyberg et al. (17), Bromley et al. (20), Bunduki et al. (32), Cicero et al. (25), and Hansmann (23).
[b]According to Shields et al. (33), DeVore (34), Tongsong et al. (35), and Bronsteen et al. (36).
[c]According to Lehmann et al. (37), Isaksen et al. (38), and Tongsong et al. (39).
Abbreviations: AVSD, atrioventricular septal defect; VSD, ventricular septal defect; DORV, double outlet right ventricle; TAC, truncus arteriosus communis; IUGR, intrauterine growth restriction.

DS with false-positive rates less than 1%. An absent nasal bone conferred a likelihood ratio of 83 for fetal DS (10). Cicero et al. (25) further reported absence of nasal bone or hypoplastic nasal bone (shorter than 2.5 mm) in 62% of fetuses with DS compared to 1.2% of chromosomally normal fetuses. They found ethnic variations in nasal bone length: in the chromosomally normal group nasal bone hypoplasia was present in 0.5% of Caucasians but in 8.8% of Afro-Caribbeans (25). These preliminary data suggest that hypoplastic nasal bone may be a powerful marker of fetal DS that should be integrated in the second trimester genetic sonogram.

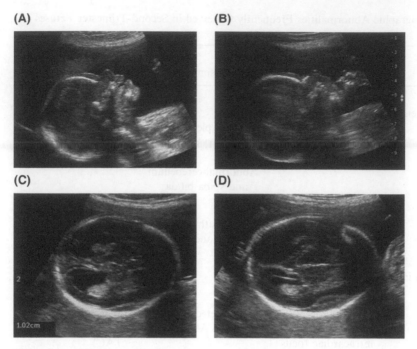

Figure 1 (A–D) Twin pregnancy at 21 weeks' gestation. Absent nasal bone, mild ventriculo-megaly, and brachycephaly in the fetus with Down syndrome (*left side*). Normal facial profile and ventricles in the euploid fetus (*right side*).

Nuchal Thickness

The thickened nuchal fold was the first sonographic marker for the detection of second trimester fetuses with DS (41). Since that time it has remained one of the most sensitive and specific second trimester markers for the detection of trisomy 21 (42,43). The correct measurement is performed at the level of the posterior fossa, by placing the calipers from the outside of the occipital bone to the outer edge of the skin. There is a slight increase in the nuchal thickness between 14 and 20 weeks of gestation. However, most centers use a single cutoff such as ≥5 or ≥6 mm, yielding an overall sensitivity of about 40% for the detection of DS (7,10,16,17,20). As an iso-lated marker, nuchal fold thickening increases the risk for fetal DS 11–17-fold (17,42). In a study of low-risk women <35 years, a thickened nuchal fold resulted in a 33% incidence of DS (44). This means that women of any age experience—in the presence of a thickened nuchal fold—a considerable increase in the risk of fetal DS. It is premature to speculate on the detection rates that could be achieved in the second trimester by combining nasal bone hypoplasia and nuchal thickness as the single most sensitive markers for trisomy 21.

Long Bone Biometry

A characteristic of individuals with DS is short stature, and second trimester fetuses with DS tend to have mildly shorter humeral and femoral length than chromo-somally normal fetuses of comparable gestational age (45–49). This finding will be evident in about 40% to 50% of fetuses with DS (20). There is considerable overlap between affected and normal fetuses and also some variation with gestational age and ethnic background (50–54). To define long bone shortening, most centers compare the actually measured length to the expected length, either based on biparietal diameter or gestational age (18,55). Humerus length may be relatively more shortened than femur length and therefore slightly more specific (17,20). In the presence of a short humeral length as an isolated marker, the a priori risk will increase five- to sixfold (17,20,42). A short femur is one of the most sensitive markers for DS; however, it is also one of the least specific. As an isolated finding, it was not found to be statistically associated with trisomy 21 (17,20). The combination of the humerus and femur length measurements resulted in an improved specificity (56,57).

Iliac Angle

The pelvic bone in neonates with DS is distinct from that of normal infants, with typically wide, flared, and flatted iliac wings due to an increased angle between them. This feature can be demonstrated sonographically already in utero, in a transverse view of the fetal pelvis. However, there have been variable findings in recent second trimester studies with mean iliac angles of 60–75° and 75–105° in euploid and DS fetuses, respectively (24,58–60). A recent study has also demonstrated that the iliac angle is dependent on fetal position (26).

Hyperechogenic Bowel

Echogenic bowel, defined as small bowel equally echogenic than bone, has been associated with congenital infections, cystic fibrosis, chromosomal abnormalities, severe intrauterine growth restriction, and bowel obstruction but also with digestion of blood (61–67). Nyberg et al. reported a prevalence of 0.8% of second trimester hyperechogenic bowel, compared with 14.5% in fetuses with DS (68). Hyperechogenic bowel as an isolated marker will increase the likelihood of fetal DS six- to sevenfold (17,42).

Echogenic Intracardiac Focus

An echogenic intracardiac focus (EIF) (synonyms are white spot, golf ball, hyperechogenic papillary muscle) represents a small bright echo seen within the cardiac

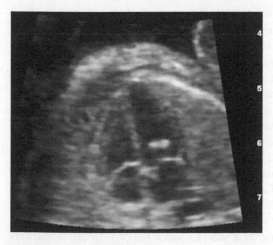

Figure 2   Double echogenic intracardiac focus in the left ventricle.

ventricles (Fig. 2). Bettelheim et al. (69) reported this finding in 96% in the left ventricle, in 3.3% in both ventricles, and in 0.7% in the right ventricle. The echogenity should be similar to that of bone. In pathological studies, EIF correlates with mineralization of the papillary muscle and chordae tendinae (70). Cardiac echogenic foci do not seem to be associated with structural cardiac abnormalities (71,72).

An EIF is a common finding during the second trimester and is reported in 2–5% of normal fetuses (17,73–75). The frequency of EIF in the left ventricle decreases with advancing gestation (76). The prevalence appears to be significantly higher among Asian populations (77). Multiple studies done on high-risk patients have established an association between EIF and fetal DS (8,17,20,73,78,79). However, because of the low sensitivity and specificity of this marker, its usefulness as an isolated marker remains controversial. In the absence of other sonographic findings, EIF increases the likelihood of fetal DS only 1.4–1.9-fold (17,20). Therefore, the majority of studies of isolated EIF in low-risk patients rejects an increased risk for trisomy 21 (74,80–82).

Pyelectasis

Mild dilatation of the fetal renal pelvis is a common finding in the second trimester and is found in about 3% of fetuses (19). Pyelectasis has been defined as an antero-posterior diameter of the renal pelvis of ≥ 4 mm at 16 to 20 weeks, and of ≥ 5 mm at 20 to 30 weeks (83). Other centers use gestational age-independent thresholds of 3–4 mm (7,11,16,19). Fetal pyelectasis may fluctuate during the course of examination, depending on the degree of fetal bladder filling and also micturition (84,85). Male fetuses are more commonly affected (86). In most cases, mild pyelectasis presents a normal variant, not associated with postpartal renal abnormalities (87).

Mild dilatation of the renal pelvis has been reported in 15% to 25% of fetuses with DS (23,83). Considering the relatively high false-positive rate, isolated pyelectasis increases the risk for fetal DS only marginally over the age-related baseline risk (1.5–1.9-fold) (17,20,42). In the low-risk population, mild pyelectasis is generally not considered as an indication for invasive testing (88–90).

Risk Assessment for Fetal Down Syndrome—The Genetic Sonogram

The genetic scan (synonym: "genetic sonography") is a clinical approach for adjusting the risk of aneuploidy based on the presence or absence of sonographic findings. The actual frequency of a single marker will vary with the type and number of markers sought as well with gestational age and ethnic groups. Nyberg et al. reported an isolated marker in 11.3% of high-risk pregnancies with a panel of six sonographic markers used (nuchal thickening, hyperechoic bowel, shortened femur or humerus, EIF, pyelectasis). If the presence of a sole marker is considered a positive test result, this will lead to a high false-positive rate. Table 2 presents the calculated likelihood ratios for isolated markers of fetal Down syndrome. Only a thickened nuchal fold, short humerus, hyperechoic bowel, and a major defect were shown to have sufficiently high likelihood ratios for DS. The same should be true for the hypoplastic or absent nasal bone. In contrast, the presence of a short femur, renal pyelectasis, and echogenic intracardiac focus grouped as a single marker increases the likelihood for DS just marginally, therefore not considerably changing the DS risk among low-risk patients.

Benacerraf et al. suggested the use of a scoring index (21,56). Isolated markers received weighted points (2 points each: nuchal fold, major anomaly, absent nasal

Table 2 Likelihood Ratios for Isolated Markers and Fetal Down Syndrome

	LR (95% CI)		
Marker	Nyberg et al. (17)	Smith-Bindmann et al. (42)	Bromley et al. (20)
Nuchal thickening	11 (5.5–22)	17 (8–38)	NC
Short humerus	5.1 (1.6–16.5)	7.5 (4.7–12)	5.8 (1–34)
Short femur	1.5 (0.8–2.8)	2.7 (1.2–6)	1.2 (0.5–2.7)
Hyperechoic bowel	6.7 (2.7–16.8)	6.1 (3–12.6)	NC
Pyelectasis	1.5 (0.6–3.6)	1.9 (0.7–5.1)	1.5 (0.6–4.3)
Echogenic intracardiac focus	1.8 (1–3)	2.8 (1.5–5.5)	1.4 (0.6–4.3)
Major defect	NC	NC	3.3 (1–10.8)

Abbreviations: CI, confidence interval; NC, not calculated; LR, likelihood ratios.

bone; 1 point each: short humerus or femur, pyelectasis, hyperechogenic bowel, EIF, choroid plexus cyst) and were added to a final score. With a positive threshold of ≥ 2 they were able to identify 81% of fetuses with DS, with a 4.4% false-positive rate. By this scoring system, the detection rate for trisomy 18 and 13 was 100% (56). An alternative method to the scoring index has been proposed by Nyberg et al., using the model of age-adjusted ultrasound risk assessment (8). In general, the risk of fetal aneuploidy increases as the number of abnormalities detected increases (Table 3). If more than one marker is identified, the likelihood ratios can be multiplied. In the study of Bromley et al. (20), the presence of any 1, 2, or 3 markers resulted in a likelihood ratio of 1.9, 6.2, and 80, respectively, for the presence of fetal DS.

A normal ultrasound scan is increasingly used for risk reduction in patients otherwise considered at high risk (advanced maternal age, abnormal serum screening). If there is no abnormality present, this confers a 70% to 80% risk reduction from the a priori risk (17,20,22,91). Over the years, there has been an increasing proportion of high-risk women who use this information in their decision of whether or not to undergo invasive testing. Offering genetic sonography services may clinically lead to a 61% to 68% reduction rate of genetic amniocentesis (22,92,93).

TRISOMY 18 (EDWARD SYNDROME)

After DS, trisomy 18 is the second most common autosomal trisomy and has a reported incidence of 1 in 3000 to 1 in 8000 (94,95). The prognosis of fetuses with trisomy 18 is uniformly poor and median survival in live births is 5 days (95).

Table 3 Likelihood Ratios of 0, 1, 2, or 3 Markers and Fetal Down Syndrome

	LR	
No. of markers	Nyberg et al. (17)	Bromley et al. (20)
0	0.36	0.2
1	2.0	1.9
2	9.7	6.2
≥ 3	115.2	80

Abbreviation: LR, likelihood ratios.

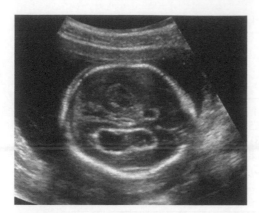

Figure 3 Strawberry-shaped head and large choroid plexus cyst in trisomy 18.

Most fetuses with trisomy 18 have multiple abnormalities and 80% to 90% are detected sonographically in centers with expertise (33–36). Therefore, the "genetic sonogram" should be more sensitive for trisomy 18 detection than for Down syndrome. Bronsteen et al. demonstrated an increasing detection rate with advancing gestational age (67% at 15–16 weeks to 100% at 19–24 weeks) (36). The most characteristic syndromal patterns involve the central nervous system, the limbs, and the cardiac system (Table 1). Typical sonographic findings include choroid plexus cysts, a strawberry-shaped head, and cisterna magna abnormalities (Fig. 3). Further characteristics of fetuses with trisomy 18 are major cardiac malformations (ventricular septal defects, conotruncal defects, atrioventricular septal defects), clenched fingers, radial defects, spina bifida aperta and clubbed or rocker-bottom feet. They may also have micrognathia, omphalocele, and umbilical cord abnormalities (33–36).

Fetal growth restriction is a common finding. The prevalence increases with gestational age from about 30% in the early second trimester to 90% in the third trimester (33,96). Severe fetal growth restriction in combination with polyhydramnios in a third trimester fetus should prompt a detailed search for associated malformations, since infants with trisomy 18 do not benefit from altered perinatal management.

Approximately 1% to 2% of normal fetuses are diagnosed with choroid plexus cysts (CPCs) on second trimester ultrasound examinations (36). In the presence of additional sonographic abnormalities, the association to fetal aneuploidy, especially trisomy 18 is undisputed. When fetal CPCs are the sole abnormality, the risk of fetal aneuploidy and the indication for karyotyping remain controversial (97–102). Meta-analyses of prospective studies of unselected populations with apparently isolated CPCs revealed likelihood ratios of having trisomy 18 between 7 and 14 (98,100,101). Neither complexity nor bilaterality of the cysts was found to be a predictor of aneuploidy (97). These data suggest that in fetuses with isolated CPC, the risk of trisomy 18 is rather low (approximately 1/350 to 1/550) and justification for universal karyotyping is not supported (97,98).

TRISOMY 13 (PATAU SYNDROME)

Trisomy 13 is the least common among of the three major autosomal trisomies that occur in liveborn children. This is attributable to the high intrauterine lethality.

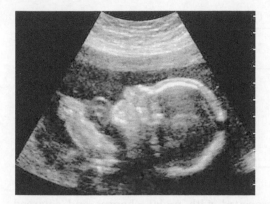

Figure 4   Abnormal facial profile (median cleft) in trisomy 13.

The incidence is estimated at about 1 in 5000 to 1 in 10,000 births (94,95). The median survival time for live born fetuses with trisomy 13 is 2.5 days and long-term survival is rather uncommon (95).

Fetuses with trisomy 13 present with a cluster of characteristic sonographic abnormalities (Table 1). The sonographic detection in the second trimester approaches 90% in experienced hands (37,39), but might be lower in unselected populations (14,95). The most frequently observed abnormalities include holoprosencephaly with and without associated facial defects (hypotelorism, cyclopia, ethmocephaly, cebocephaly, proboscis, single nostril, median clefts), cardiac defects, omphalocele, polydactyly (primarily of the hands), enlarged hyperechogenic kidneys and neural tube defects (Fig. 4) (37–39,103).

The three characteristic features in Meckel–Gruber-syndrome—postaxial polydactyly, occipital encephalocele, and enlarged hyperechogenic multicystic kidneys—overlap with the syndromal pattern in trisomy 13. In contrast to fetuses with trisomy 13 however, the majority of fetuses with Meckel–Gruber syndrome present with severe oligohydramnios or anhydramnios early in the second trimester. To definitively distinguish between the two diagnoses, fetal karyotyping is required. This is important despite the lethal condition in both, as Meckel–Gruber syndrome in an autosomal recessive disease with a 25% recurrence risk in affected families.

TRIPLOIDY

Triploidy (69 XXX; 69 XXY; 69 XYY) is one of the most frequent chromosomal anomalies in early pregnancy abortions (104). The prevalence of triploidy in the mid-second trimester is about 1 in 5000 pregnancies and only a few fetuses survive to term (105). Fetal survival seems to be influenced by the sex chromosomes. In the second and third trimester, XXX-cases are most frequently seen (65–85%) and XXY in the remainder, whereas the XYY-karyotype is an absolute rarity (106–109).

The most striking sonographic sign in the second trimester is an early onset severe asymmetrical growth restriction. Whereas the head appears slightly smaller than appropriate for gestational age, the fetal abdomen and the extremities, however, are extremely growth-restricted. Oligohydramnios and placentomegaly are common features too (Table 4). The parent of origin of the extra chromosomal set is thought to determine whether the fetus or the placenta is primarily affected.

Table 4 Ultrasound Findings in Cases of Triploidy

	Jauniaux et al. (107)	Rijhsinghani et al. (108)	Mittal et al. (110)	Blaicher et al. (109)
Number of cases (N)	70	17	20	13
Gestational age (weeks)	13–29	17–30	14–31	18–34
Fetal growth restriction	50 (71%)	12 (71%)	11 (55%)	11 (85%)
Placentomegaly	20 (29%)	7 (41%)	11 (55%)	2 (15%)
Oligohydramnios	31 (44%)	10 (59%)	12 (60%)	8 (62%)
Fetal anomalies	65 (93%)	12 (71%)	14 (70%)	9 (69%)

Paternal contribution (diandric) is associated with molar changes and enlarged placenta, consistent with partial mole (Fig. 5). In case of maternal origin (digynic) severe fetal growth restriction with oligohydramnios and a normal placenta is frequently seen.

Structural fetal defects are observed antenatally in 70% to 90% of cases. The central nervous system (ventriculomegaly, Dandy–Walker malformation, agenesis of the corpus callosum) is commonly affected. Other sonographic abnormalities seen in triploidy include facial dysmorphism (micrognathia), limb anomalies (syndactyly, clinodactyly, talipes), congenital heart defects, pericardial effusion, neural tube defects, and renal malformations (107–110). However, in the presence of oligohydramnios and an abnormal fetal position the antenatal diagnosis of minor lesions may be limited.

Unlike other chromosomal abnormalities, triploidy may also affect the mother with prenatal complications in up to 53% of patients. Obstetric complications frequently observed include first and second trimester vaginal bleeding, severe hyperemesis gravidarum, enlarged multicystic ovaries, ovarian hyperstimulation syndrome, and early onset preeclampsia (107,111). In a series of 17 second trimester pregnancies complicated by triploidy, the risk of developing preeclampsia or gestational hypertension was 35%. All those cases were associated with placentomegaly and markedly elevated serum hCG (108).

As for other lethal conditions, it is important to make the correct diagnosis of triploidy in utero, as those fetuses do not benefit from aggressive perinatal management.

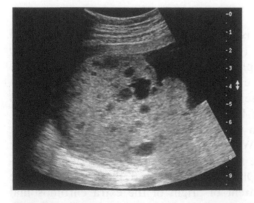

Figure 5 Molar placental structure in triploidy.

TURNER SYNDROME

Turner syndrome is a relatively common chromosomal disorder, caused by complete or partial X monosomy in some or all cells. More than 90% of the conceptions are aborted spontaneously and the estimated frequency among liveborn females is about 1/2500 (112). Clinical features of the syndrome include short stature, webbing of the neck, ovarian dysfunction, and cardiovascular abnormalities. The most useful tool in prenatal diagnosis is ultrasonography. Typical signs in this syndrome include huge septated cystic hygroma of the neck, increased nuchal translucency, cardiac defects, and renal malformations (38,113–115).

A recent evaluation of the prenatal diagnosis of Turner syndrome from 19 European registries reported on 125 cases (116). Sixty-seven percent of cases were detected prenatally by ultrasound examination due to the presence of congenital defects. The mean gestational age at detection was 19 weeks, 90.5% were diagnosed before 24 weeks, and 18% during the first trimester. The most frequent sonographic abnormalities were cystic hygroma (59.5%) and hydrops fetalis (19%). In this study, the most frequent karyotype was 45,X in 82% and different types of mosaicisms in the remainder. There was a significantly higher rate of congenital defects in 45,X karyotypes (63.7%) than in mosaicism cases (38.1%).

Although resolution of cystic hygroma and fetal hydrops has been described throughout gestation, they are commonly predictors of unfavorable outcome (113–115). Gravholt et al., in their study of 100 cases, observed a significantly higher probability of a mosaic karyotype fetus surviving than a 45,X fetus reaching term (117).

A congenital heart defect is found in about 30% of postnatal cases of Turner syndrome. Left-sided obstructive defects predominate, especially bicuspid aortic valve and coarctation of the aorta (118). There is a higher incidence of structural heart disease in those cases that are diagnosed (compared to those after birth) during fetal live (113–115). Surerus et al. reported cardiac malformations in 62% (33/53) of fetuses with Turner syndrome investigated in the first and mid-second trimester. Coarctation of the aorta (45%) and hypoplastic left heart syndrome (13%) were the most common diagnoses. A markedly increased nuchal translucency was frequently associated (47/53) (115). Narrowing of the aortic arch has been frequently described in smaller series in first and early second trimester, with hygroma colli and/or hydrops fetalis present in all cases (113,114). Berdahl et al. reported an 11-fold higher incidence of coarctation in infants with Turner syndrome and a web neck than in those with a normal neck (119). This observation may be explained by the Clark's hypothesis, which speculates that severe aortic coarctation is caused by an increased pressure in the surrounding lymphatic vessels resulting from primary lymphatic obstruction (120).

REFERENCES

1. Snijders RJM, Noble P, Sebire N, Souka A, Nicolaides K. UK multi-center project on assessment of risk of trisomy 21 by maternal age and fetal nuchal translucency thickness at 10–14 weeks of gestation. Lancet 1998; 352:343–346.
2. Nicolaides KH. Screening for chromosomal defects. Ultrasound Obstet Gynecol 2003; 21:313–321.
3. Nicolaides KH. Nuchal translucency and other first-trimester sonographic markers of chromosomal abnormalities. Am J Obstet Gynecol 2004; 191:45–67.

4. Cicero S, Papageorghiou A, Sonek J, Nicolaides K. Absence of nasal bone in fetuses with trisomy 21 at 11–14 weeks of gestation: an observational study. Lancet 2001; 358:1665–1667.

5. Morris JK, Wald NJ, Watt HC. Fetal loss in Down's syndrome pregnancies. Prenat Diagn 1999; 19:142–145.

6. Snijders RJM, Sundberg K, Holzgreve W, Henry G, Nicolaides KH. Maternal age- and gestation-specific risk for trisomy 21. Ultrasound Obstet Gynecol 1999; 13:167–170.

7. Vintzileos AM, Cambell WA, Guzman ER, Smulian JC, Mclean DA, Ananth CV. Second-trimester ultrasound markers for detection of trisomy 21: which markers are best? Obstet Gynecol 1997; 89:941–944.

8. Nyberg DA, Luthy DA, Resta RG, Nyberg BC, Williams MA. Age-adjusted ultrasound risk assessment for fetal Down's syndrome during the second trimester: description of the method and analysis of 142 cases. Ultrasound Obstet Gynecol 1998; 12:8–14.

9. DeVore GR. Trisomy 21: 91% detection rate using second-trimester ultrasound markers. Ultrasound Obstet Gynecol 2000; 16:133–141.

10. Bromley B, Liebermann E, Shipp TD, Benacerraf BR. Fetal nose bone length a marker for Down's syndrome in the second trimester. J Ultrasound Med 2002; 21:1387–1394.

11. Hobbins JC, Lezotte DC, Persutte WH, et al. An 8-center study to evaluate the utility of midterm genetic sonograms among high-risk pregnancies. J Ultrasound Med 2003; 22:33–38.

12. Stoll C, Dott B, Alembik Y, Roth MP. Evaluation of routine prenatal ultrasound examination in detecting fetal chromosomal abnormalities in a low risk population. Hum Genet 1993; 91:37–41.

13. Jorgensen FS, Valentin L, Salvesen KA, et al. MULTISCAN—a Scandinavian multicenter second trimester obstetric ultrasound and serum screening study. Acta Obstet Gynecol Scand 1999; 78:501–510.

14. De Vigan C, Baena N, Cariati E, Clementi M, Stoll C and the EUROSCAN Working Group. Contribution of ultrasonographic examination to the prenatal detection of chromosomal abnormalities in 19 centres across Europe. Ann Genet 2001; 44:209–217.

15. Benacerraf BR. The second-trimester fetus with Down's syndrome: detection using sonographic features. Ultrasound Obstet Gynecol 1996; 7:147–155.

16. Vergani P, Locatelli A, Picolli MG, et al. Best second trimester sonographic markers for the detection of trisomy 21. J Ultrasound Med 1999; 18:469–473.

17. Nyberg DA, Souter VL, El-Bastawissi A, et al. Isolated sonographic markers for detection of fetal Down's syndrome in the second trimester of pregnancy. J Ultrasound Med 2001; 20:1053–1063.

18. Nyberg DA, Souter VL. Sonographic markers of fetal trisomies: second trimester. J Ultrasound Med 2001; 20:655–674.

19. Nyberg DA, Souter VL. Use of genetic sonography for adjusting the risk for fetal Down's syndrome. Semin Perinatol 2003; 27:130–144.

20. Bromley B, Lieberman E, Shipp TD, Benacerraf BR. The genetic sonogram: a method of risk assessment for Down's syndrome in the second trimester. J Ultrasound Med 2002; 21:1087–1096.

21. Bromley B, Benacerraf BR. The genetic sonogram scoring index. Semin Perinatol 2003; 27:124–129.

22. Yeo L, Vintzileos AM. The use of genetic sonography to reduce the need for amniocentesis in women at high-risk for Down's syndrome. Semin Perinatol 2003; 27:152–159.

23. Hansmann M. Trisomy 21 in the mid trimester; sonographic phenotyping of the fetus is the key. Ultrasound Obstet Gynecol 2004; 23:531–534.

24. Belics Z, Beke A, Csabay L, Szabo I, Papp Z. Sonographic measurement of the fetal iliac angle in trisomy 21 and 13. Fetal Diagn Ther 2003; 18:47–50.

25. Cicero S, Sonek JD, Mckennas DS, Croom CS, Johnson LJ, Nicolaides KH. Nasal bone hypoplasia in trisomy 21 at 15–33 weeks gestation. Ultrasound Obstet Gynecol 2003; 21:15–18.

26. Massez A, Rypens F, Metens T, Donner C, Avni FE. The iliac angle: a sonographic marker of trisomy 21 during the midtrimester: dependency of fetal lying? Eur Radiol 2003; 13:2075–2081.

27. Vintzileos A, Walters C, Yeo L. Absent nasal bone in the prenatal detection of fetuses with trisomy 21 in a high-risk population. Obstet Gynecol 2003; 101:905–908.

28. Maymon R, Tovbin Y, Dreazen E, Weinraub Z, Hermann A. All five digits of the hands of fetuses with Down's syndrome are short. Ultrasound Obstet Gynecol 2004; 23:557–560.

29. Benacerraf BR. Should sonographic screening for fetal Down's syndrome be applied to low risk women? Ultrasound Obstet Gynecol 2000; 15:451–455.

30. Rotmensch S, Liberati M, Bronshtein M, et al. Prenatal sonographic findings in 187 fetuses with Down's syndrome. Prenat Diagn 1997; 17:1001–1009.

31. Paladini D, Tartaglione A, Agangi A, et al. The association between congenital heart disease and Down's syndrome in prenatal life. Ultrasound Obstet Gynecol 2000; 15: 104–108.

32. Bunduki V, Ruano R, Miguelez J, Yoshizaki CT, Kahhale S, Zugaib M. Fetal nasal bone length; reference range and clinical application in ultrasound screening for trisomy 21. Ultrasound Obstet Gynecol 2003; 21:156–160.

33. Shields LE, Carpenter LA, Smith KM, Nghiem HV. Ultrasonographic diagnosis of trisomy 18: is it practical in the early second trimester? J Ultrasound Med 1998; 17: 327–331.

34. DeVore GR. Second trimester ultrasonography may identify 77 to 97% of fetuses with trisomy 18. J Ultrasound Med 2000; 19:565–576.

35. Tongsong T, Sirichotiyakul S, Wanapirak C, Chanprapaph P. Sonographic features of trisomy 18 at midpregnancy. Obstet Gynecol 2002; 28:245–250.

36. Bronsteen R, Lee W, Vettraino IM, Huang R, Comstock CH. Second-trimester sonography and trisomy 18. J Ultrasound Med 2004; 23:233–240.

37. Lehman CD, Nyberg DA, Winter TC, Kapur RP, Resta RG, Luthy DA. Trisomy 13 syndrome: prenatal US findings in a review of 33 cases. Radiology 1995; 194:217–222.

38. Isaksen CV, Eik-Nes SH, Blaas HG, Torp SH, Van der Hagen CB, Ormerod E. A correlative study of prenatal ultrasound and post-mortem findings in fetuses and infants with an abnormal karyotype. Ultrasound Obstet Gynecol 2000; 16:37–45.

39. Tongsong T, Sirichotiyakul S, Wanapirak C, Chanprapaph P. Sonographic features of trisomy 13 at midpregnancy. Obstet Gynecol 2002; 76:143–148.

40. Snijders RJM, Nicolaides KH. Ultrasound Markers for Fetal Chromosome Defects. Carnforth: Parthenon Publishing, 1996.

41. Benacerraf B, Barss VA, Laboda LA. A sonographic sign for the detection in the second trimester of the fetus with Down's syndrome. Am J Obstet Gynecol 1985; 151:1078–1079.

42. Smith-Bindmann R, Hosmer W, Feldstein VA, Deeks JJ, Goldberg JD. Second-trimester ultrasound to detect fetuses with Down's syndrome. J Am Med Assoc 2001; 285:1044–1055.

43. Benacerraf BR. The signifiance of the nuchal fold in the second trimester fetus. Prenatal Diagn 2002; 22:798–801.

44. Benacerraf BR, Laboda LA, Frigoletto FD. Thickened nuchal fold in fetuses not at risk for aneuploidy. Radiology 1992; 184:239–242.

45. FitzSimmons J, Droste S, Shepard TH, Pascoe-Mason J, Chinn AM, Rack LA. Long-bone growth in fetuses with Down's syndrome. Am J Obstet Gynecol 1989; 161:1174–1177.

46. Benacerraf BR, Neuberg D, Frigoletto FD Jr. Humeral shortening in second-trimester fetuses with Down's syndrome. Obstet Gynecol 1991; 77:223–227.

47. Nyberg DA, Resta RG, Luthy DA, Hickok DE, Williams MA. Humerus and femur length shortening in the detection of Down's syndrome. Am J Obstet Gynecol 1993; 168:534–538.

48. Vintzileos AM, Egan JF, Smulian JC, Campbell WA, Guzman ER. Adjusting the risk for trisomy 21 by a simple ultrasound method using fetal long-bone biometry. Obstet Gynecol 1996; 87:953–958.

49. Vergani P, Locatelli A, Piccoli MG, et al. Critical reappraisal of the utility of sonographic fetal femur length in the prediction of trisomy 21. Prenat Diagn 2000; 20: 210–214.

50. Snijders RJ, Platt LD, Greene N, Carlson D, Krakow D, Gregory K. Femur length and trisomy 21: impact of gestational age on screening efficiency. Ultrasound Obstet Gynecol 2000; 16:142–145.

51. Pierce BT, Hancock EG, Kovac CM, Napolitano PG, Hume RF Jr, Calhoun BC. Influence of gestational age and maternal height on fetal femur length calculations. Obstet Gynecol 2001; 97:742–746.

52. Shipp TD, Bromley B, Mascola M, Benacerraf B. Variation in fetal femur length with respect to maternal race. J Ultrasound Med 2001; 20:141–144.

53. Kovac CM, Brown JA, Apodaca CC, et al. Maternal ethnicity and variation of fetal femur length calculations when screening for Down's syndrome. J Ultrasound Med 2002; 21:719–722.

54. Borgida AF, Zelop C, Deroche M, Bolnick A, Egan JF. Down's syndrome screening using race-specific femur length. Am J Obstet Gynecol 2003; 189:977–979.

55. Shipp TD, Benacerraf BR. Second trimester ultrasound screening for chromosomal abnormalities. Prenat Diagn 2002; 22:296–307.

56. Benacerraf BR, Neuberg D, Bromley B, Frigoletto FD. Sonographic scoring index for prenatal detection of chromosomal abnormalities. J Ultrasound Med 1992; 11:449–458.

57. Johnson MP, Michaelson JE, Barr M Jr, et al. Combining humerus and femur length for improved ultrasonographic identification of pregnancies at increased risk for trisomy 21. Am J Obstet Gynecol 1995; 172:1229–1235.

58. Kliewer MA, Hertzberg BS, Freed KS, et al. Dysmorphologic features of the fetal pelvis in Down's syndrome: prenatal sonographic depiction and diagnostic implications of the iliac angle. Radiology 1996; 201:681–684.

59. Bork MD, Egan JFX, Cusick W, Borgida AF, Campbell WA, Rodis JF. Iliac wing angle as a marker for trisomy 21 in the second trimester. Obstet Gynecol 1997; 89: 734–737.

60. Shipp TD, Bromley B, Lieberman E, Benacerraf BR. The iliac angle as a sonographic marker for Down's syndrome in second-trimester fetuses. Obstet Gynecol 1997; 89:446–450.

61. Bromley B, Doubilet P, Frigoletto FD Jr, Krauss C, Estroff JA, Benacerraf BR. Is fetal hyperechogenic bowel on second trimester sonogram an indication for amniocentesis? Obstet Gynecol 1994; 83:647–651

62. MacGregor SN, Tamura R, Sabbagha R, Brenhofer JK, Kambich MP, Pergament E. Isolated hyperechoic fetal bowel: significance and implications for management. Am J Obstet Gynecol 1995; 173:1254–1258.

63. Peters MT, Lowe TW, Carpenter A, Kole S. Prenatal diagnosis of congenital cytomegalovirus infection with abnormal screen results and hyperechoic fetal bowel. Am J Obstet Gynecol 1995; 173:953–954.

64. Irish MS, Ragi JM, Karamanoukian H, Borowitz DS, Schmidt D, Glick PL. Prenatal diagnosis of the fetus with cystic fibrosis and meconium ileus. Pediatr Surg Int 1997; 12:434–436.

65. Font GE, Solari M. Prenatal diagnosis of bowel obstruction initially manifested as isolated hyperechoic bowel. J Ultrasound Med 1998; 17:721–723.

66. Stipoljev F, Sertic J, Kos M, et al. Incidence of chromosomopathies and cystic fibrosis mutations in second trimester fetuses with isolated hyperechoic bowel. J Matern Fetal Med 1999; 8:44–47.

67. Simon-Bouy B, Muller F, the French Collaborative Group. Hyperechogenic fetal bowel and Down's syndrome. Results of a French collaborative study based on 680 prospective cases. Prenat Diagn 2002; 22:189–192.

68. Nyberg DA, Resta RG, Mahony BS, et al. Fetal hyperechogenic bowel and Down syndromc. Ultrasound Obstet Gynecol 1993; 3:330–333.

69. Bettelheim D, Deutinger J, Bernaschek G. The value of echogenic foci ("golfballs") in the fetal heart as a marker of chromosomal abnormalities. Ultrasound Obstet Gynecol 1999; 14:98–100.

70. Roberts DJ, Genest D. Cardiac histologic pathology characteristic of trisomies 13 and 21. Hum Pathol 1992; 23:1130–1140.

71. Wolman I, Jaffa A, Geva E, et al. Intracardiac echogenic focus: no apparent association with structural cardiac abnormality. Fetal Diagn Ther 2000; 15:216–218.

72. Wax JR, Mather J, Steinfeld JD, Ingardia CJ. Fetal intracardiac echogenic foci: current understanding and clinical significance. Obstet Gynecol Surv 2000; 55:303–311.

73. Bromley B, Lieberman E, Laboda L, Benacerraf BR. Echogenic intracardiac focus: a sonographic sign for fetal Down's syndrome. Obstet Gynecol 1995; 86:998–1001.

74. Anderson N, Jyoti R. Relationship of isolated fetal intracardiac echogenic focus of trisomy 21 mid-trimester sonogram in women younger than 35 years. Ultrasound Obstet Gynecol 2003; 21:354–358.

75. Sotiriadis A, Makrydimas G, Ioannidis JP. Diagnostic performance of intracardiac echogenic foci for Down's syndrome: a meta-analysis. Obstet Gynecol 2003; 101: 1009–1016.

76. Achiron R, Lipitz S, Gabbay U, Yagel S. Prenatal ultrasonographic diagnosis of fetal heart echogenic foci: no correlation with Down's syndrome. Obstet Gynecol 1997; 89:945–948.

77. Shipp TD, Bromley B, Lieberman E, Benacerraf BR. The frequency of the detection of fetal echogenic intracardiac foci with respect to maternal race. Ultrasound Obstet Gynecol 2000; 15:460–462.

78. Bromley B, Lieberman E, Shipp TD, Richardson M, Benacerraf BR. Significance of an echogenic intracardiac focus in fetuses at high and low risk for aneuploidy. J Ultrasound Med 1998; 17:127–131.

79. Wax JR, Philput C. Fetal intracardiac echogenic foci: does it matter which ventricle? J Ultrasound Med 1998; 17:141–144.

80. Caughey AB, Lyell DJ, Filly RA, Washington AE, Norton ME. The impact of the use of the isolated echogenic intracardiac focus as a screen for Down's syndrome in women under the age of 35 years. Am J Obstet Gynecol 2001; 185:1021–1027.

81. Coco C, Jeanty P, Jeanty C. An isolated echogenic heart focus is not an indication for amniocentesis in unselected patients. J Ultrasound Med 2004; 23:489–496.

82. Lamont RF, Havutcu E, Salgia S, Adinkra P, Nicholl R. The association between isolated fetal echogenic cardiac foci on second-trimester ultrasound scan and trisomy 21 in low-risk unselected women. Ultrasound Obstet Gynecol 2004; 23:346–351.

83. Benacerraf BR, Mandell J, Estroff JA, Harlow BL, Frigoletto FD Jr. Fetal pyelectasis: a possible association with Down's syndrome. Obstet Gynecol 1990; 76:58–60.

84. Petrikovsky BM, Cuomo MI, Schneider EP, Wyse LI, Cohen HL, Lesser M. Isolated fetal hydronephrosis: beware the effect of bladder filling. Prenat Diagn 1995; 15: 827–829.

85. Damen-Elias HAM, Stigter RH, De Jong TPVM, Visser GHA. Variability in dilatation of the fetal pelvis during a bladder filling cycle. Ultrasound Obstet Gynecol 2004; 24: 750–755.

86. Wilson RD, Lynch S, Lessoway VA. Fetal pyelectasis: comparison of postnatal renal pathology with unilateral and bilateral pyelectasis. Prenat Diagn 1997; 17:451–455.

87. John U, Kahler C, Schulz S, Mentzel HJ, Vogt S, Misselwitz J. The impact of fetal renal pelvic diameter on postnatal outcome. Prenat Diagn 2004; 24:591–595.

88. Thompson MO, Thilaganathan B. Effect of routine screening for Down's syndrome on the significance of isolated fetal hydronephrosis. Br J Obstet Gynaecol 1998; 105: 860–864.

89. Chudleigh PM, Chitty LS, Pembrey M, Campbell S. The association of aneuploidy and mild fetal pyelectasis in an unselected population: the results of a multicenter study. Ultrasound Obstet Gynecol 2001; 17:197–202.

90. Havutcu AE, Nikolopoulos G, Adinkra P, Lamont RF. The association between fetal pyelectasis on second trimester ultrasound scan and aneuploidy among 25586 low risk unselected women. Prenat Diagn 2002; 22:1201–1206.

91. Vintzileos AM, Guzman ER, Smulian JC, Yeo L, Scorca WE, Knuppel RA. Down's syndrome risk estimation after normal genetic sonography. Am J Obstet Gynecol 2002; 187:1226–1229.

92. Pinette MG, Garrett J, Salvo A, et al. Normal mid trimester (17–20 weeks) genetic sonogram decreases amniocentesis rate in a high-risk population. J Ultrasound Med 2001; 20:639–644.

93. Rosen DJ, Kedar I, Amiel A, et al. A negative second trimester triple test and absence of specific ultrasonographic markers may decrease the need for genetic amniocentesis in advanced maternal age by 60%. Prenat Diagn 2002; 22:59–63.

94. Jones ICL. Smith's Recognizable Patterns of Human Malformations. 5th ed. Philadelphia, PA: WB Saunders Co., 1997:18–19.

95. Parker MJ, Budd JLS, Draper ES, Young ID. Trisomy 13 and trisomy 18 in a defined population: epidemiological, genetic and prenatal observations. Prenat Diagn 2003; 23: 856–860.

96. Nyberg DA, Kramer D, Resta RG, et al. Prenatal sonographic findings of trisomy 18: review of 47 cases. J Ultrasound Med 1993; 12:103–113.

97. Gross SJ, Shulman LP, Tolley EA, et al. Isolated fetal choroid plexus cysts and trisomy 18: a review and metaanalysis. Am J Obstet Gynecol 1995; 172:83–87.

98. Gupta JK, Khan KS, Thornton JG, Lilford RJ. Management of fetal choroid plexus cysts. Br J Obstet Gynaecol 1997; 104:881–886.

99. Chitty LS, Chudleigh P, Wright E, Campbell S, Pembrey M. The significance of choroid plexus cysts in an unselected population: results of a multicenter study. Ultrasound Obstet Gynecol 1998; 12:391–397.

100. Yoder PR, Sabbagha RE, Gross SJ, Zelop CM. The second-trimester fetus with isolated choroid plexus cysts: a meta-analysis of risk of trisomies 18 and 21. Obstet Gynecol 1999; 93:869–872.

101. Ghidini A, Strobelt N, Locatelli A, Mariani E, Piccoli MG, Vergani P. Isolated fetal choroid plexus cysts: role of ultrasonography in establishment of the risk of trisomy 18. Am J Obstet Gynecol 2000; 182:972–977.

102. Bird LM, Dixson B, Masser-Frye D, et al. Choroid plexus cysts in the mid-trimester fetus—practical application suggests superiority of an individualized risk method of counseling for trisomy 18. Prenat Diagn 2002; 22:792–797.

103. Blaas HG, Eriksson AG, Salvesen KA, et al. Brains and faces in holoprosencephaly: pre- and postnatal description of 30 cases. Ultrasound Obstet Gynecol 2002; 19:24–38.

104. Szulman AE, Philippe E, Boue JG, Goue A. Human triploidy: association with partial hydatidiform moles and nonmolar conceptuses. Hum Pathol 1981; 12:1016–1021.

105. Fergusson-Smith MA, Yates JRW. Maternal age specific rates for chromosomal aberrations and factors influencing them: report of a collaborative European study on 52,965 amniocenteses. Prenat Diag 1984; 4:5–44.

106. Doshi N, Surti U, Szulman AE. Morphologic anomalies in triploid liveborn fetuses. Hum Reprod 1983; 14:716–723.

107. Jauniaux E, Brown R, Rodeck C, Kypros HN. Prenatal diagnosis of triploidy during the second trimester of pregnancy. Obstet Gynecol 1996; 88:983–989.

108. Rijhsinghani A, Yankowitz J, Strauss RA, Kuller JA, Patil S, Williamson RA. Risk of preeclampsia in second-trimester triploid pregnancies. Obstet Gynecol 1997; 90:884–888.

109. Blaicher W, Ulm B, Ulm MR, Hengstschlager M, Deutinger J, Bernaschek G. Dandy-Walker malformation as sonographic marker for fetal triploidy. Ultraschall Med 2002; 81:129–134.

110. Mittal TK, Vujanic GM, Morrissey BM, Jones A. Triploidy: antenatal sonographic features with post-mortem correlation. Prenat Diag 1998; 18:1253–1262.

111. Ludwig M, Gembruch U, Bauer O, Diedrich K. Ovarian hyperstimulation syndrome (OHSS) in a spontaneous pregnancy with fetal and placental triploidy: information about the general pathophysiology of OHSS. Hum Reprod 1998; 13:2082–2087.

112. Hsu LYF. Prenatal diagnosis of chromosomal abnormalities through amniocentesis. In: Milunsky A, ed. Genetic Disorders and the Fetus. Baltimore, MD: Johns Hopkins University Press, 1998:179–248.

113. Gembruch U, Baschat AA, Knöpfle G, Hansmann M. Results of chromosomal analysis in fetuses with cardiac anomalies as diagnosed by first- and early second-trimester echocardiography. Ultrasound Obstet Gynecol 1997; 10:391–396.

114. Bronshtein M, Zimmer EZ, Blazer S. A characteristic cluster of fetal sonographic markers that are predictive of fetal Turner syndrome in early pregnancy. Am J Obstet Gynecol 2003; 188:1016–1020.

115. Surerus E, Huggon IC, Allan LD. Turner's syndrome in fetal life. Ultrasound Obstet Gynecol 2003; 22:264–267.

116. Baena N, De Vigan C, Cariati E, et al. Turner syndrome: evaluation of prenatal diagnosis in 19 European registries. Am J Med Genet 2004; 129A:16–20.

117. Gravholt Ch, Juul S, Naeraa RW, Hansen J. Prenatal and postnatal prevalence of Turner's syndrome: a registry study. Br Med J 1996; 312:16–21.

118. Saenger P, Wikland KA, Conway GS, et al. Recommendations for the diagnosis and management of Turner syndrome. J Clin Endocrinol Metab 2001; 86:3061–3069.

119. Berdahl LD, Wenstrom KD, Hanson JW. Web neck anomaly and its association with congenital heart defects. Am J Med Genet 1995; 56:304–307.

120. Clark EB. Neck web and congenital heart defects: a pathogenic association in 45 XO Turner syndrome? Teratology 1984; 29:355–361.

8

Fetal Cells in Maternal Blood: Diagnostic and Therapeutic Implications

May Lee Tjoa, Kirby L. Johnson, and Diana W. Bianchi
Division of Genetics, Department of Pediatrics, Tufts-New England Medical Center, Boston, Massachusetts, U.S.A.

INTRODUCTION

It is now a well-established fact that fetal cells are present in the maternal circulation. The first evidence that fetal cells exist outside the fetoplacental unit was demonstrated in 1893 by Schmorl, who described the presence of trophoblast sprouts in the lungs of women who died of eclampsia (1). With the advent of sensitive molecular techniques, this finding has now been confirmed on numerous occasions. In 1969, Walknowska published a landmark study showing the detection of cells bearing a Y-chromosome in the blood of women carrying a male fetus (2). Since this report, the potential applications of using circulating fetal cells in prenatal screening have been researched extensively. Fetal cells represent a unique source of fetal DNA and RNA that can be used for the detection of fetal chromosomal aneuploidies and single gene disorders. In addition, new studies show that the fetoplacental unit is not as distinctly separate from the mother as was previously thought. In every pregnancy, there is trafficking of maternal and fetal cells and cell-free nucleic acids to and from the fetoplacental unit, respectively. Under normal circumstances, very few fetal cells enter the maternal bloodstream. However, in the case of many fetal or placental disorders, including aneuploidy or preeclampsia, an abnormally high number of fetal cells are present in the maternal circulation. Current data suggest that fetomaternal trafficking is a reflection not only of fetal health but also of placental development and pregnancy well-being. New evidence shows that the persistence of fetal cells in maternal tissues after delivery plays a role in subsequent maternal health. This chapter will discuss the role of circulating fetal cells in prenatal diagnosis and the relationship between abnormal fetomaternal trafficking of cells and the occurrence of disease in the woman both during gestation and postpartum.

FETAL CELLS IN MATERNAL BLOOD FOR NONINVASIVE
PRENATAL DIAGNOSIS

The utilization of prenatal diagnosis by expectant couples has increased substantially over the last three decades. This trend will only continue to increase as more women delay childbearing until an advanced maternal age and family sizes decrease, leading to a greater emphasis on the expectation of "normality" for each child. For prenatal diagnosis of trisomy 21 and other chromosomal abnormalities, the current standard of care in the United States and Europe is to offer prenatal diagnosis via amniocentesis or chorionic villus sampling (CVS) to pregnant women who will be >35 years of age at delivery. Although this group of women has an overall increased risk of bearing a child with Down syndrome, most babies with Down syndrome are actually born to women <35 years. The latter group is not generally offered invasive prenatal diagnosis, as the risk of pregnancy loss following the procedure is greater than the risk of Down syndrome in the fetus.

During the past 20 years, the development of novel noninvasive screening methods that allow accurate diagnosis of a fetal genetic disorder without the risk of miscarriage inherent in invasive procedures has been a focus of obstetric research. Both second-trimester maternal serum screening and nuchal translucency (NT) measurements have been successfully incorporated into routine obstetric care (3,4). The triple test consisting of measurement of human chorionic gonadotrophin (hCG), estriol, and alpha-fetoprotein levels with comparison to population standards detects up to 70% of trisomy 21 cases with a 5% false-positive rate (5). Addition of another marker, inhibin A, raises the sensitivity of the test (6). First-trimester screening of pregnancy-associated plasma protein A (PAPP-A) and beta-hCG combined with NT measurements is as effective as the second-trimester screening (7). These noninvasive tests estimate the chance of fetal trisomy 21 based on parameters including maternal age, weight, race, diabetes status, and gestational age, without the additional risk of pregnancy loss. Integration of first- and second-trimester screening markers and NT measurements yields a better screening performance than a single-trimester screening only (8). The results of the serum, urine, and ultrasound screening study show that integration of the two tests yields an 85% detection rate with a 1.2% false-positive rate, provided that NT measurements were obtained for nearly all pregnancies and PAPP-A is measured at 10 weeks of gestation (9). The clinical benefit of the so-called "integrated test" lies in the fact that the false-positive rate is decreased substantially compared to first- or second-trimester screening alone; therefore, fewer women would need to undergo an invasive diagnostic procedure. However, the numbers given after a test are solely mathematical calculations and are unable to give a definite diagnosis. Women who have a test result indicating a risk greater than 1:250 of having a child affected with Down syndrome are offered amniocentesis.

It is in this context that the use of circulating fetal cells as a noninvasive method for prenatal diagnosis should be placed. Although Schmorl published his work in the late 19th century, the presence of fetal cells outside the fetoplacental unit could not be confirmed until the development of molecular techniques. The application of techniques such as fluorescent in situ hybridization (FISH) (10,11), fluorescent activated cell sorting (FACS) (12–14), and polymerase chain reaction (PCR) (15,16) made it possible to isolate and identify fetal cells in the maternal circulation based on either their physical characteristics or specific fetal DNA sequences. A major advantage of using circulating fetal cells over other noninvasive prenatal screening methods is that fetal cells can give specific information regarding chromosome or single gene abnormalities. Maternal blood is easily obtained by venipuncture. Hypothetically, successful isolation and analysis of fetal cells from the maternal circulation could be implemented as a primary screen to help reduce the number of false-positive results found by the other noninvasive tests. Likewise, fetal cells could also be used in a diagnostic manner to study numerical chromosomal abnormalities or single gene disorders.

Various strategies have been employed to isolate fetal cells from the maternal circulation. The isolation techniques applied most frequently are separation of blood on a density gradient, followed by an additional fetal cell purification step using magnetic activated cell sorting (MACS) (17–20). MACS involves the selective depletion of maternal cells or enrichment of fetal cells using magnetic beads coated with specific antibodies. Immunocytochemistry is subsequently performed to physically identify fetal cells, and FISH analysis with chromosome-specific probes is used to determine the fetal karyotype (Fig. 1). Fetal cell identification can be performed using fetal cell-specific antibodies such as gamma globin, which recognizes fetal nucleated erythroblasts (21–24), or HLA-G, which recognizes fetal trophoblast cells (20,25). The most common chromosome-specific probes used are those that recognize chromosomes X, Y, 13, 18, and 21. Results are then compared to those found by the gold standard: metaphase karyotype performed on amniotic cells or chorionic villi. One model system uses blood samples from women who have undergone elective termination, which can lead to fetomaternal hemorrhage. An elevated number of fetal cells are released into the maternal circulation following termination,

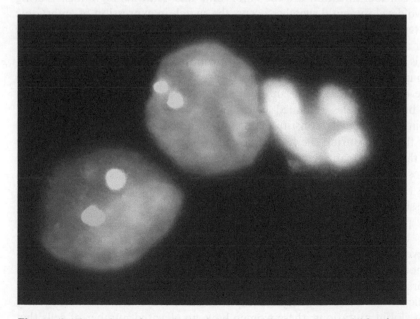

Figure 1 Detection of a male fetal NRBC (*left*) in a maternal blood sample using FISH probes specific for the X chromosome (*dark gray*) and Y chromosome (*light gray*). The image also shows a maternal cell in the middle (two *light gray signals*). The cell on the right has no FISH signals and its morphology resembles that of an apoptotic cell. The image was taken at 1000× magnification. *Abbreviations*: NRBC, nucleated red blood cells; FISH, fluorescent in situ hybridization. (*See color insert.*)

which in turn can potentially be used to test the application of fetal cell isolation and identification techniques (26,27). Other isolation methods that have been applied to the identification of fetal cells following density centrifugation are FACS, micromanipulation (28), and charge flow separation (29).

Target Cells

Nucleated Red Blood Cells

Research on circulating fetal cells is primarily focused on cell types that are differentiated into nucleated red blood cells (NRBCs) or trophoblast cells. Both of these cell types are representative of the full fetal genome, have morphologically distinguishing features, and are present in the maternal circulation at an early stage of gestation. Much emphasis has been placed on the use of NRBCs as a potential tool for noninvasive prenatal diagnosis. One of the most successfully used antibodies to identify NRBCs is directed against the transferrin receptor, CD71. Erythroblasts express this antigen on their cell surfaces from the burst-forming units during the erythroid stage (30). Although a small population of maternal cells also expresses CD71, most cells recovered from maternal blood on the basis of CD71 expression have been determined to be fetal by cytogenetic studies (31). In 1990, NRBCs were flow-sorted based on CD71 expression. Following isolation, fetal hemoglobin was detected in the CD71-positive cells by the Kleihauer–Betke technique, confirming the fetal origin of these cells (15).

The only other cell surface markers that have been consistently successfully used for fetal cell identification are the embryonic and fetal hemoglobins. During pregnancy two developmental switches occur, the switch in expression of embryonic hemoglobin (epsilon hemoglobin) to fetal hemoglobin (gamma globin) during the first trimester and to adult hemoglobin (beta hemoglobin) at birth (32). Embryonic hemoglobin is expressed during a very narrow window of time during early pregnancy, limiting the application of this marker to primitive erythroblasts. Fetal NRBCs have been identified using antibodies directed against epsilon hemoglobin in maternal blood samples obtained before week 14 of pregnancy (23,33). The epsilon globin–positive cells constitute the population of primitive erythroblasts produced by the fetus during the first trimester of pregnancy. Choolani et al. have shown that the general antigenic properties of these primitive erythroblasts are similar to those of definite gamma globin–expressing erythroblasts, including adult erythroblasts (34). The main difference between primitive and mature erythroblasts is the expression of CD71 by mature erythroblasts, which is not or is weakly expressed by primitive erythroblasts. Gamma globin, in contrast, is expressed by fetal NRBCs throughout the second and third trimesters of pregnancy, albeit at decreasing levels (35). Erythroblasts in umbilical cord blood express gamma globin (22,36). Although a small population of maternal cells expresses gamma globin (36–39), in practice most gamma globin–positive cells have been shown to be fetal by cytogenetic studies (40). The major exception seems to be in women who carry alpha or beta globin mutations; these women have an elevated number of cells that express gamma globin.

Other antibodies that are effective for the identification of fetal NRBCs are those directed against glycophorin A (GPA) (18,34,41) and the thrombospondin receptor (CD36) (18,42). The antibody that has been used most commonly to deplete maternal cells is directed against the leukocyte common antigen, CD45 (14,43,44), but antibodies directed against the lipopolysaccharide receptor, CD14 (45), and the IgG-receptor, CD32 (46) have also been used for this purpose.

Trophoblast Cells

Like NRBCs, trophoblast cells have a unique morphology, which make them easy to recognize among maternal blood cells. During the first weeks of pregnancy, cytotrophoblast stem cells differentiate into extravillous trophoblast cells, which in turn migrate into the maternal endometrium during the first and early second trimesters of pregnancy. The extravillous trophoblast cells specifically target toward the maternal spiral arteries, which initiates a transformation of the vessels by deposition of fibrinoid and a partial loss of their muscular layer (47–49). The end result of trophoblast invasion is the establishment of the uteroplacental circulation that is responsible for the transport of oxygen and nutrients to the growing fetus. Trophoblast cells may enter the maternal circulation during the migratory process since Y chromosome–specific sequences in maternal blood have been reported to be present as early as five weeks of gestation, before the fetal circulation has been established (50,51). Another mechanism by which fetal material, including trophoblast cells, enters the maternal bloodstream is placental apoptosis. Van Wijk et al. were able to show the presence of apoptotic fetal cells in the plasma of pregnant women (52). The demonstration that elevated levels of circulating fetal cells have been found in the blood of women with preeclampsia supports the theory that apoptosis allows entry of fetal trophoblast cells into the maternal bloodstream (53,54). There is also increased placental apoptosis in the placentas of preeclamptic pregnancies (55,56). Whether trophoblast cells are already in an apoptotic state upon entering the maternal bloodstream or whether they become apoptotic while circulating is currently unknown.

Although trophoblast cells were the first fetal cell type to be reported in maternal tissue (1), many investigators have been unable to isolate large numbers of trophoblast cells from the maternal blood. It is likely that the maternal pulmonary circulation effectively removes most trophoblast cells as they pass through the maternal lungs despite the reported presence of syncytiotrophoblasts in the maternal circulation until delivery, implying that migration or shedding of trophoblastic material is a continuous phenomenon during pregnancy (57).

Isolation and identification of trophoblast cells have largely been hampered by the lack of a suitable antibody. Mueller et al. tested 6800 candidate antibodies, of which only two were able to successfully isolate fetal cells (58). Durrant et al. used antibody 340 to isolate both cytotrophoblasts and syncytiotrophoblasts (59). Extravillous trophoblast cells have been identified by nonradioactive in situ hybridization using a probe directed against the ASCL2 gene (11) and by immunocytochemistry using a monoclonal antibody directed against HLA-G (20). Based on the observation that there is no unique trophoblast-specific antibody that positively identifies all circulating trophoblast cells, and the very low number of trophoblast cells detected in the maternal circulation during pregnancy, most research on this particular cell type is not being actively pursued.

Leukocytes

Fetal leukocytes were the first fetal cell type to be successfully isolated. In the report by Walknowska et al., Y-chromosomal material was present in mitogen-stimulated lymphocytes obtained from pregnant women carrying a male fetus (2). Herzenberg et al. used HLA-A2 antibody to flow-sort fetal HLA-A2+ cells from women who were HLA-A2 negative (12). In another publication, fetal gender and HLA type were successfully predicted using fetal leukocytes (60). Despite these initially promising results, clinical application of fetal leukocytes for prenatal diagnosis is considered too impractical due to the fact that HLA typing must be performed prior to the experimental procedures. The HLA gene is considerably polymorphic, making antibody selection challenging. Moreover, fetal leukocytes are not morphologically distinct from their maternal counterparts, making the identification of these cells more difficult. Finally, the presence of fetal lymphocytes in the maternal circulation up to decades postpartum has been demonstrated (61). This causes relative uncertainty whether the isolated fetal lymphocytes are indeed specific to the ongoing pregnancy or whether they remain from previous pregnancy.

Numbers of Circulating Fetal Cells During Pregnancy

Although novel molecular techniques with high sensitivity to analyze the fetal genome have been developed, to date no group has been able to isolate and identify fetal cells from the maternal circulation on a large scale. There is no dispute about the presence of small numbers of circulating fetal cells. The major obstacle to the development of prenatal diagnosis based on circulating fetal cells in maternal blood is the relative rarity of these cells. Approximately one to six fetal cells are present per milliliter of maternal blood (62). There is some controversy as to whether there is a relationship between the number of circulating fetal cells and gestational age. Bianchi et al. were unable to detect fetal DNA in maternal blood samples based on transferrin receptor expression after 16 weeks gestation (63). More recently, Lim et al. showed a decrease in the mean number of circulating fetal trophoblast cells and NRBCs with increasing gestational age (64). Although this decrease was not statistically significant, it does lead to a decrease in mean percentage purity, making it more challenging to accurately diagnose fetal chromosomal abnormalities during the third trimester. In contrast, Ariga et al. found increasing numbers of fetal cells in the maternal circulation with increasing gestational age. Fetal cells were rapidly cleared from the maternal circulation following delivery (65).

Interestingly, there is a significantly increased number of circulating fetal cells in the case of fetal aneuploidy. In a study published by Bianchi et al., a total of 230 peripheral whole blood samples were used for fetal cell analysis (66). Thirty-one of the samples were obtained from women carrying a male fetus with trisomy 21. Quantitative PCR amplification of a sequence present on the long arm of the Y-chromosome was performed. In the cases of fetal trisomy 21, there was a sixfold elevation in the mean number of male fetal-cell DNA genome equivalents as compared to women carrying a euploid male fetus. This difference was significant ($P = 0.001$) . Since then, other groups have reproduced this finding using MACS or FACS for fetal cell isolation followed by FISH. Aneuploidy affects placental anatomy, which potentially allows fetal cells to leak more easily into the maternal circulation than if the fetus were normal. Trisomy 21 is also associated with an early deficit or delay in syncytiotrophoblast formation, accompanied by a decrease in the excretion of hCG and other placental proteins (67). This may be a definitive explanation as to why more fetal cells are released into the maternal circulation. The evidence to date suggests that a dysfunctional placental barrier plays a role in fetomaternal trafficking of cells.

Significantly, higher numbers of fetal cells have also been detected in the peripheral blood of women both prior to and during clinical manifestations of preeclampsia (53,68,69). Preeclampsia is a systemic disorder of pregnancy, characterized by hypertension and proteinuria. One of the possible underlying causes of pree-clampsia is placental hypoxia, probably due to defective trophoblast invasion and subsequent maternal spiral artery conversion (70,71). As in the case of trisomy 21, the evidence points to a dysfunctional placenta, or more specifically, dysfunctional trophoblasts, as a causative factor in the increased number of fetal cells present in maternal blood. The measurement of the number of fetal cells present in a maternal blood sample may prove to be a useful screening tool to determine which pregnancies are at risk of fetal aneuploidy or preeclampsia.

Fetal Cells for Noninvasive Prenatal Diagnosis: Current Clinical Status

Based on promising scientific literature, the National Institutes of Health initiated a multicenter clinical evaluation, known as the NIFTY (*N*ational *I*nstitute of Child Health and Human Development *F*etal Cell Isolation S*t*ud*y*) trial in 1994. The primary aim of the study was to evaluate the use of circulating fetal cells to detect male gender compared to results found at CVS or amniocentesis; the secondary aim was to evaluate the use of circulating fetal cells to detect fetal chromosomal abnormalities. The first results of the NIFTY trial were published in 2002 (72). Fetal gender could be correctly identified in 41.4% of the cases. In the cases of a known fetal aneuploidy, the aneuploidy was detected in 74.4% by using circulating fetal cells. Most of the cytogenetic results in cases from the NIFTY trial were performed on a single isolated fetal cell.

Current research on fetal cells in the maternal circulation is focused on improving isolation and identification techniques. New methods include isolation by size of epithelial tumor cells (ISET) method, in which trophoblast cells are isolated from maternal blood by filtering the blood samples through a polycarbonate membrane (73). Using ISET, one group was able to isolate one to seven fetal cells from 2 mL of blood obtained from women carrying a male fetus (74). Moreover, these isolated cells could be analyzed by FISH (74) and also used to determine whether the fetus was affected by spinal muscular atrophy by PCR and gene sequencing (75). Bischoff et al. used a non-MACS–based enrichment procedure to isolate fetal cells from maternal blood samples. In this study, fetal progenitor cells were enriched by labeling the samples with a RosetteSep^{TM} progenitor antibody cocktail that removes mature hematopoietic cells or by depleting maternal leukocytes using a RosetteSep CD45 antibody cocktail. Following the labeling, density centrifugation over a Ficoll gradient was performed to remove the undesirable cells (76). Despite the new techniques, the recovery of intact fetal cells from the maternal circulation remains very low. Bischoff et al., for example, were able to detect an average of two to three fetal progenitor cells after RosetteSep enrichment from 20 to 30 mL of maternal blood (76). The technical difficulties encountered today have not really changed when compared to the ones encountered a decade ago. For this form of noninvasive prenatal diagnosis of aneuploidy to be considered clinically useful, a nearly 100% accurate diagnosis must be made in every reported case. Based on its current status, it is unlikely that circulating fetal cells will be used for noninvasive prenatal diagnosis of fetal aneuploidy within the next several years, unless a major advance in fetal cell isolation techniques occurs.

While it may be feasible to use circulating fetal cells for prenatal diagnosis, the rarity and fragility of these cells is also a major obstacle to the clinical implementation of this procedure. There has been a shift from studying fetal cells in maternal blood to studying cell-free fetal (CFF) nucleic acids in maternal circulation as potential tools for noninvasive prenatal diagnosis (77). One of the major advantages of using CFF-DNA in maternal plasma rather than whole fetal cells is the relative abundance of fetal DNA. CFF-DNA can be isolated rapidly and efficiently from maternal plasma samples compared to fetal cells. CFF-RNA has also been detected in the maternal circulation during pregnancy (78,79). Despite the fragility of RNA, its presence in the maternal bloodstream opens up new opportunities to study fetal genetic abnormalities, genes that are involved in fetal and placental development, and possibly, indicate which pregnancies are at risk for diseases such as preeclampsia.

FETAL CELL MICROCHIMERISM

The postpartum existence of fetal cells in the maternal circulation was initially demonstrated in the 1970s. Two studies were published during this decade showing the existence of male fetal lymphocytes by cytogenetic analysis in maternal blood for up to five years after delivery (80,81). Other studies have made use of PCR amplification of the Y chromosome to detect the long-term circulation of fetal cells in maternal blood. The results were often inconsistent, probably due to the fact that no enrichment techniques were used prior to the PCR. By selectively enriching fetal cells by flow sorting for the CD34+ antigen, Bianchi et al., showed that male hematopoietic progenitor cells can persist in maternal blood postdelivery for up to 27 years (61). The women recruited for this study had no history of blood transfusion, thereby eliminating the possibility that the male cells were acquired otherwise. It was surprising that not all of the fetal cells are degraded after the pregnancy has ended. Using PCR, male DNA was also found to be present in the peripheral blood of women who had undergone elective first trimester termination of pregnancy (82). A transfusion of fetal material, including fetal cells, to the maternal circulation probably occurs as a result of the termination procedure. The potential for development of fetal cell microchimerism is not confined to those women who gave birth to a live infant.

Fetal Cell Microchimerism and Maternal Disease

Speculation exists regarding the role of fetal cell microchimerism and its association with development of disease in the postpartum woman. Two different hypotheses have been proposed. The first hypothesis suggests that fetal cells may cause a graft versus host reaction. There is a higher incidence of autoimmune disease in women than in men, especially after their childbearing years. Several years ago, Nelson and colleagues studied the occurrence of fetal cell microchimerism in female scleroderma patients who had given birth to a male child. The results of this study suggested that persisting fetal cells might play a role in the pathogenesis of scleroderma (83,84). A blinded study was able to demonstrate the presence of significantly higher amounts of male fetal cell DNA equivalents in the peripheral blood of female scleroderma patients as compared to healthy controls (83). All of the women who participated in the study had given birth to at least one son previously. Figure 2 shows images of male fetal cell microchimerism present in ovarian tissue obtained from a woman with adenocarcinoma and adrenal gland obtained postmortem from a female scleroderma patient. Using both FISH and PCR analysis, Artlett et al. were able to demonstrate the presence of Y-chromosome material in peripheral blood and

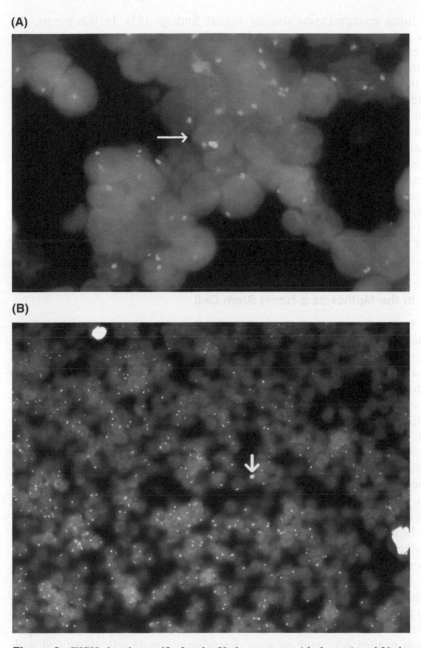

Figure 2 FISH signals specific for the X chromosome (*dark gray*) and Y chromosome (*light gray*) in nuclei from (**A**) ovary section, 1000× magnification, and (**B**) adrenal gland section, 400× magnification. The white arrows indicate the position of the male cells in the tissue sections. The sections were obtained from two different women, one of whom had adenocarcinoma (**A**), the other woman had died of complications of scleroderma (**B**) and both had given birth to a son previously. *Abbreviation*: FISH, fluorescent in situ hybridization. (*See color insert.*)

skin biopsies taken from scleroderma patients who had given birth to a son (85). In another study, fetal cell microchimerism was detected by FISH in various tissues obtained postmortem from women with scleroderma (86). A case report involving tissue specimens obtained postmortem from a woman who died of complications of systemic lupus erythematosus showed similar findings (87). In this report, the woman had given birth to two male children. Cells containing a Y chromosome, therefore presumably fetal by origin, were detected in all affected organs and spleen but not in unaffected organs.

    None of these studies, however, was able to precisely ascertain a role for fetal cells in maternal disease pathogenesis or progression. In the study published by Klintschar et al., microchimerism was studied in thyroid tissue obtained from women with Hashimoto's disease (88). All women who showed signs of autoimmune disease had had significantly more children than those women who had no microchimerism. Although speculative, this indicates that fetal cell microchimerism might not be an exclusively etiological mechanism triggering an autoimmune response. Furthermore, a certain amount of fetal cell microchimerism is also found in healthy women who have given birth to a son. In fact, fetal cell microchimerism has also been detected in tissues from women who suffer from nonautoimmune diseases such as hepatitis C (89), thyroid adenoma (90), and cervical cancer (91).

Fetal Cells in the Mother as a Novel Stem Cell

The second hypothesis proposes that fetal cell microchimerism is actually helpful instead of harmful. In the study by Cha et al., male cells were observed in cervical cancer patients but not in the positive controls (healthy women who had given birth to a male child) or in the negative controls (healthy women who had given birth to female children) (91). Lack of male cells in the latter group suggests that exposure to semen does not result in microchimerism. Based on immunophenotyping, nearly half of the microchimeric cells are hematopoietic in origin and a quarter are epithelial in origin. Migration of fetal progenitor cells to the cervix might occur in response to the presence of cancerous tissue. These cells would then target specifically to the squamous cell layer of the cervix where they differentiate into epithelial cells. There is neither sufficient evidence in this particular study to suggest that these fetal cells actually play a role in carcinogenesis, nor is their evidence pointing to a role in tissue repair or cell repopulation in case of cancer. However, the phenomenon of microchimerism may be more common than previously thought and should be investigated in relation to other forms of cancer specific to women.

    In order to fully understand the role of microchimerism in maternal disease, it is necessary to identify the source of microchimeric cells. New research from our group has demonstrated that pregnancy results in the transfer of fetal cells with multilineage potential to the mother (92). Tissue samples from various organs were obtained from women who had given birth to a son and compared to tissue samples obtained from women who had no sons. Surprisingly, male cells, identified with Y-chromosome markers, could also express epithelial, hepatic, or leukocyte markers depending on the tissue source where they were found. These intriguing results point to a role of fetal cells as possible "stem cells," or pregnancy-associated progenitor cells (PAPCs), that can subsequently be recruited to areas of maternal tissue inflammation or damage, possibly even years following pregnancy. It is also possible that the fetal cells that enter the maternal circulation during pregnancy are already in a differentiated state and are able to remain dormant in maternal organs. To try to answer some of these biologically interesting questions, animal models are being developed that can be used to study the source of microchimeric cells and their role in specific types of disease.

SUMMARY

Trafficking of fetal cells and fetal nucleic acids is a phenomenon that occurs through-out gestation. Initially, it was thought that fetal cells isolated from the maternal circulation could be used as tools for noninvasive prenatal diagnosis of fetal chromo-somal abnormalities or single gene disorders. Many techniques were applied to try to isolate and identify fetal cells from the maternal bloodstream. The recovery of fetal cells was at best very low and accurate identification of these cells was challenging due to the lack of specific antibodies. Despite the technological advances that have been made in molecular analysis during the past two decades, fetal cell isolation and identification remain two major obstacles that must be overcome in order to use circulating fetal cells for prenatal diagnosis in a clinical setting. Current research is concentrated on the isolation of fetal nucleic acids from the maternal circulation for prenatal diagnosis, diagnosis of pregnancy complications such as preeclampsia, and the study of placental and fetal development.

However, the presence of intact fetal cells in the maternal bloodstream and maternal organs, even years following delivery, has led to the hypothesis that every woman who has been pregnant becomes a chimera. Fetal cell microchimerism has been demonstrated in women who have given birth to a son, but it is likely that the same phenomenon also occurs in women who have had daughters. The role of fetal cell microchimerism in the postpartum health of women is unknown. Fetal cells may trigger immunological responses in the parous woman, leading to the develop-ment of autoimmune disease. Various studies have shown the presence of male cells, presumably fetal by origin, in the affected organs of women suffering from autoim-mune disease. It is also possible that fetal cells may act as stem cells, lying dormant in maternal organs for years, until they are recruited and specifically target toward inflamed or injured tissues. New data showing that fetal cells have the capability to differentiate into various cell types supports the possibility that these cells have "stem cell" like qualities; they have been named PAPCs. Pregnancy may thus be a novel source of undifferentiated stem cells for the mother that can aid her own immunological defense mechanisms when organ or tissue injury or inflammation occurs, even years following delivery. Future studies will indicate what the source of these PAPCs are, what their role in general maternal health is, and whether the postpartum persistence of fetal cells is either beneficial or harmful to the mother. Although speculative, the transfer of fetal cells to the mother may provide clues as to why women generally have a longer lifespan than men.

REFERENCES

1. Schmorl G. Pathologisch-anatomische untersuchungen uber puerperaleklampsia. Leipzig (Germany): Vogel, 1893.
2. Walknowska J, Conte FA, Grumbach MM. Practical and theoretical implications of fetal–maternal lymphocyte transfer. Lancet 1969; 1:1119–1122.
3. Herman A, Weinraub Z, Dreazen E, et al. Combined first trimester nuchal translucency and second trimester biochemical screening tests among normal pregnancies. Prenat Diagn 2000; 20:781–784.
4. Michailidis GD, Spencer K, Economides DL. The use of nuchal translucency measure-ment and second trimester biochemical markers in screening for Down's syndrome. Br J Obstet Gynecol 2001; 108:1047–1052.

5. Wald NJ, Cuckle HS, Densem JW, et al. Maternal serum screening for Down's syndrome in early pregnancy. Br Med J 1988; 297:883–887.

6. Benn PA, Fang M, Egan JF, Horne D, Collins R. Incorporation of inhibin-A in second-trimester screening for Down syndrome. Obstet Gynecol 2003; 101:451–454.

7. Wapner R, Thom E, Simpson JL, et al. First-trimester screening for trisomies 21 and 18. N Engl J Med 2003; 349:1405–1413.

8. Wald NJ, Watt HC, Hackshaw AK. Integrated screening for Down's syndrome on the basis of tests performed during the first and second trimesters. N Engl J Med 1999; 341:461–467.

9. Wald NJ, Rodeck C, Hackshaw AK, Walters J, Chitty L, Mackinson AM. First and second trimester antenatal screening for Down's syndrome: the results of the Serum, Urine and Ultrasound Screening Study (SURUSS). Health Technol Assess 2003; 7:1–77.

10. Bianchi DW, Mahr A, Zickwolf GK, Houseal TW, Flint AF, Klinger KW. Detection of fetal cells with 47,XY,+21 karyotype in maternal peripheral blood. Hum Genet 1992; 90:368–370.

11. van Wijk IJ, van Vugt JM, Konst AA, Mulders MA, Nieuwint AW, Oudejans CB. Multi-parameter in situ analysis of trophoblast cells in mixed cell populations by combined DNA and RNA in situ hybridization. J Histochem Cytochem 1995; 43:709–714.

12. Herzenberg LA, Bianchi DW, Schroder J, Cann HM, Iverson GM. Fetal cells in the blood of pregnant women: detection and enrichment by fluorescence-activated cell sorting. Proc Natl Acad Sci USA 1979; 76:1453–1455.

13. Wang JY, Zhen DK, Falco VM, et al. Fetal nucleated erythrocyte recovery: fluorescence activated cell sorting-based positive selection using anti-gamma globin versus magnetic activated cell sorting using anti-CD45 depletion and anti-gamma globin positive selection. Cytometry 2000; 39:224–230.

14. Bianchi DW, Klinger KW, Vadnais TJ, et al. Development of a model system to compare cell separation methods for the isolation of fetal cells from maternal blood. Prenat Diagn 1996; 16:289–298.

15. Bianchi DW, Flint AF, Pizzimenti MF, Knoll JH, Latt SA. Isolation of fetal DNA from nucleated erythrocytes in maternal blood. Proc Natl Acad Sci USA 1990; 87:3279–3283.

16. van Wijk IJ, van Vugt JM, Mulders MA, Konst AA, Weima SM, Oudejans CB. Enrichment of fetal trophoblast cells from the maternal peripheral blood followed by detection of fetal deoxyribonucleic acid with a nested X/Y polymerase chain reaction. Am J Obstet Gynecol 1996; 174:871–878.

17. Durrant LG, Martin WL, McDowall KM, Liu DT. Isolation of fetal trophoblasts and nucleated erythrocytes from the peripheral blood of pregnant women for prenatal diagnosis of fetal aneuploides. Early Hum Dev 1996; 47(Suppl):S79–S83.

18. Troeger C, Holzgreve W, Hahn S. A comparison of different density gradients and anti-bodies for enrichment of fetal erythroblasts by MACS. Prenat Diagn 1999; 19:521–526.

19. Smits G, Holzgreve W, Hahn S. An examination of different Percoll density gradients and magnetic activated cell sorting (MACS) for the enrichment of fetal erythroblasts from maternal blood. Arch Gynecol Obstet 2000; 263:160–163.

20. van Wijk IJ, Griffioen S, Tjoa ML, et al. HLA-G expression in trophoblast cells circulating in maternal peripheral blood during early pregnancy. Am J Obstet Gynecol 2001; 184:991–997.

21. Oosterwijk JC, Mesker WE, Ouwerkerk-van VM, et al. Development of a preparation and staining method for fetal erythroblasts in maternal blood: simultaneous immunocytochemical staining and FISH analysis. Cytometry 1998; 32:170–177.

22. Mesker WE, Ouwerkerk-van Velzen MC, Oosterwijk JC, et al. Two-colour immunocytochemical staining of gamma (gamma) and epsilon (epsilon) type haemoglobin in fetal red cells. Prenat Diagn 1998; 18:1131–1137.

23. Al-Mufti R, Hambley H, Farzaneh F, Nicolaides KH. Distribution of fetal and embryonic hemoglobins in fetal erythroblasts enriched from maternal blood. Haematologica 2001; 86:357–362.

24. Larsen RD, Schonau A, Thisted M, et al. Detection of gamma-globin mRNA in fetal nucleated red blood cells by PNA fluorescence in situ hybridization. Prenat Diagn 2003; 23:52–59.
25. van Wijk IJ, de Hoon AC, Griffioen S, et al. Identification of triploid trophoblast cells in peripheral blood of a woman with a partial hydatidiform molar pregnancy. Prenat Diagn 2001; 21:1142–1145.
26. Bianchi DW, Farina A, Weber W, et al. Significant fetal–maternal hemorrhage after termination of pregnancy: implications for development of fetal cell microchimerism. Am J Obstet Gynecol 2001; 184:703–706.
27. Wataganara T, LeShane ES, Chen AY, et al. Plasma gamma-globin gene expression suggests that fetal hematopoietic cells contribute to the pool of circulating cell-free fetal nucleic acids during pregnancy. Clin Chem 2004; 50:689–693.
28. Ikawa K, Yamafuji K, Ukita T, Kuwabara S, Igarashi T, Takabayashi H. Fetal DNA diagnosis from maternal blood: PEP-TaqMan PCR analysis of a single nucleated erythrocyte (NRBC). Ann NY Acad Sci 2001; 945:153–155.
29. Wachtel SS, Sammons D, Manley M, et al. Fetal cells in maternal blood: recovery by charge flow separation. Hum Genet 1996; 98:162–166.
30. Loken MR, Shah VO, Dattilio KL, Civin CI. Flow cytometric analysis of human bone marrow: I. Normal erythroid development. Blood 1987; 69:255–263.
31. Ganshirt D, Smeets FW, Dohr A, et al. Enrichment of fetal nucleated red blood cells from the maternal circulation for prenatal diagnosis: experiences with triple density gradient and MACS based on more than 600 cases. Fetal Diagn Ther 1998; 13:276–286.
32. Olivieri NF. Fetal erythropoiesis and the diagnosis and treatment of hemoglobin disorders in the fetus and child. Semin Perinatol 1997; 21:63–69.
33. Choolani M, O'Donnell H, Campagnoli C, et al. Simultaneous fetal cell identification and diagnosis by epsilon-globin chain immunophenotyping and chromosomal fluorescence in situ hybridization. Blood 2001; 98:554–557.
34. Choolani M, O'Donoghue K, Talbert D, et al. Characterization of first trimester fetal erythroblasts for non-invasive prenatal diagnosis. Mol Hum Reprod 2003; 9:227–235.
35. Al-Mufti R, Hambley H, Farzaneh F, Nicolaides KH. Fetal erythroblasts in maternal blood in relation to gestational age. J Matern Fetal Neonatal Med 2003; 14:392–397.
36. Lau ET, Kwok YK, Chui DH, Wong HS, Luo HY, Tang MH. Embryonic and fetal globins are expressed in adult erythroid progenitor cells and in erythroid cell cultures. Prenat Diagn 2001; 21:529–539.
37. Pembrey ME, Weatherall DJ, Clegg JB. Maternal synthesis of haemoglobin F in pregnancy. Lancet 1973; 1:1350–1354.
38. Hogh AM, Hviid TV, Christensen B, et al. Zeta-, epsilon-, and gamma-globin mRNA in blood samples and CD71(+) cell fractions from fetuses and from pregnant and nonpregnant women, with special attention to identification of fetal erythroblasts. Clin Chem 2001; 47:645–653.
39. Christensen B, Philip J, Lykke-Hansen L, Kolvraa S. Sensitivity and specificity of the identification of fetal cells in maternal blood by combined staining with antibodies against beta-, gamma- and epsilon-globin chains. Fetal Diagn Ther 2003; 18:479–484.
40. Zheng YL, DeMaria M, Zhen D, Vadnais TJ, Bianchi DW. Flow sorting of fetal erythroblasts using intracytoplasmic anti-fetal haemoglobin: preliminary observations on maternal samples. Prenat Diagn 1995; 15:897–905.
41. Al-Mufti R, Hambley H, Farzaneh F, Nicolaides KH. Assessment of efficacy of cell separation techniques used in the enrichment of foetal erythroblasts from maternal blood: triple density gradient vs. single density gradient. Clin Lab Haematol 2004; 26:123–128.
42. Bianchi DW, Zickwolf GK, Yih MC, et al. Erythroid-specific antibodies enhance detection of fetal nucleated erythrocytes in maternal blood. Prenat Diagn 1993; 13:293–300.
43. Lewis DE, Schober W, Murrell S, et al. Rare event selection of fetal nucleated erythrocytes in maternal blood by flow cytometry. Cytometry 1996; 23:218–227.

44. Samura O, Sekizawa A, Zhen DK, Falco VM, Bianchi DW. Comparison of fetal cell recovery from maternal blood using a high density gradient for the initial separation step: 1.090 versus 1.119 g/ml. Prenat Diagn 2000; 20:281–286.

45. Reading JP, Huffman JL, Wu JC, et al. Nucleated erythrocytes in maternal blood: quantity and quality of fetal cells in enriched populations. Hum Reprod 1995; 10:2510–2515.

46. Ferguson-Smith MA, Zheng YL, Carter NP. Simultaneous immunophenotyping and FISH on fetal cells from maternal blood. Ann NY Acad Sci 1994; 731:73–79.

47. Pijnenborg R, Dixon G, Robertson WB, Brosens I. Trophoblastic invasion of human decidua from 8 to 18 weeks of pregnancy. Placenta 1980; 1:3–19.

48. Pijnenborg R, Bland JM, Robertson WB, Brosens I. Uteroplacental arterial changes related to interstitial trophoblast migration in early human pregnancy. Placenta 1983; 4:397–413.

49. Kaufmann P, Black S, Huppertz B. Endovascular trophoblast invasion: implications for the pathogenesis of intrauterine growth retardation and pre-eclampsia. Biol Reprod 2003; 69:1–7.

50. Thomas MR, Williamson R, Craft I, Yazdani N, Rodeck CH. Y chromosome sequence DNA amplified from peripheral blood of women in early pregnancy. Lancet 1994; 343:413–414.

51. Thomas MR, Tutschek B, Frost A, et al. The time of appearance and disappearance of fetal DNA from the maternal circulation. Prenat Diagn 1995; 15:641–646.

52. van Wijk IJ, de Hoon AC, Jurhawan R, et al. Detection of apoptotic fetal cells in plasma of pregnant women. Clin Chem 2000; 46:729–731.

53. Holzgreve W, Li JJ, Steinborn A, et al. Elevation in erythroblast count in maternal blood before the onset of preeclampsia. Am J Obstet Gynecol 2001; 184:165–168.

54. Jansen MW, Korver-Hakkennes K, van Leenen D, et al. Significantly higher number of fetal cells in the maternal circulation of women with pre-eclampsia. Prenat Diagn 2001; 21:1022–1026.

55. DiFederico E, Genbacev O, Fisher SJ. Preeclampsia is associated with widespread apoptosis of placental cytotrophoblasts within the uterine wall. Am J Pathol 1999; 155: 293–301.

56. Ishihara N, Matsuo H, Murakoshi H, Laoag-Fernandez JB, Samoto T, Maruo T. Increased apoptosis in the syncytiotrophoblast in human term placentas complicated by either preeclampsia or intrauterine growth retardation. Am J Obstet Gynecol 2002; 186:158–166.

57. Douglas GW, Thomas L, Carr M, Cullen NM, Morris R. Trophoblast in the circulating blood during pregnancy. Am J Obstet Gynecol 1959; 78:958–973.

58. Mueller UW, Hawes CS, Wright AE, et al. Isolation of fetal trophoblast cells from peripheral blood of pregnant women. Lancet 1990; 336:197–200.

59. Durrant LG, McDowell KM, Holmes RA, Liu DT. Screening of monoclonal antibodies recognizing oncofetal antigens for isolation of trophoblasts from maternal blood for prenatal diagnosis. Prenat Diagn 1994; 14:131–140.

60. Iverson GM, Bianchi DW, Cann HM, Herzenberg LA. Detection and isolation of fetal cells from maternal blood using the flourescence-activated cell sorter (FACS). Prenat Diagn 1981; 1:61–73.

61. Bianchi DW, Zickwolf GK, Weil GJ, Sylvester S, DeMaria MA. Male fetal progenitor cells persist in maternal blood for as long as 27 years postpartum. Proc Natl Acad Sci USA 1996; 93:705–708.

62. Krabchi K, Gros-Louis F, Yan J, et al. Quantification of all fetal nucleated cells in maternal blood between the 18th and 22nd weeks of pregnancy using molecular cytogenetic techniques. Clin Genet 2001; 60:145–150.

63. Bianchi DW, Stewart JE, Garber MF, Lucotte G, Flint AF. Possible effect of gestational age on the detection of fetal nucleated erythrocytes in maternal blood. Prenat Diagn 1991; 11:523–528.

64. Lim TH, Tan AS, Goh VH. Relationship between gestational age and frequency of fetal trophoblasts and nucleated erythrocytes in maternal peripheral blood. Prenat Diagn 2001; 21:14–21.

65. Ariga H, Ohto H, Busch MP, et al. Kinetics of fetal cellular and cell-free DNA in the maternal circulation during and after pregnancy: implications for noninvasive prenatal diagnosis. Transfusion 2001; 41:1524–1530.

66. Bianchi DW, Williams JM, Sullivan LM, Hanson FW, Klinger KW, Shuber AP. PCR quantitation of fetal cells in maternal blood in normal and aneuploid pregnancies. Am J Hum Genet 1997; 61:822–829.

67. Frendo JL, Vidaud M, Guibourdenche J, et al. Defect of villous cytotrophoblast differentiation into syncytiotrophoblast in Down's syndrome. J Clin Endocrinol Metab 2000; 85:3700–3707.

68. Holzgreve W, Ghezzi F, Di NE, Ganshirt D, Maymon E, Hahn S. Disturbed feto-maternal cell traffic in preeclampsia. Obstet Gynecol 1998; 91:669–672.

69. Al-Mufti R, Hambley H, Albaiges G, Lees C, Nicolaides KH. Increased fetal erythroblasts in women who subsequently develop pre-eclampsia. Hum Reprod 2000; 15:1624–1628.

70. Pijnenborg R, Anthony J, Davey DA, et al. Placental bed spiral arteries in the hypertensive disorders of pregnancy. Br J Obstet Gynaecol 1991; 98:648–655.

71. Zhou Y, Damsky CH, Fisher SJ. Preeclampsia is associated with failure of human cytotrophoblasts to mimic a vascular adhesion phenotype. One cause of defective endovascular invasion in this syndrome? J Clin Invest 1997; 99:s2152–s2164.

72. Bianchi DW, Simpson JL, Jackson LG, et al. Fetal gender and aneuploidy detection using fetal cells in maternal blood: analysis of NIFTY I data. National Institute of Child Health and Development Fetal Cell Isolation Study. Prenat Diagn 2002; 22:609–615.

73. Vona G, Sabile A, Louha M, et al. Isolation by size of epithelial tumor cells: a new method for the immunomorphological and molecular characterization of circulating tumor cells. Am J Pathol 2000; 156:57–63.

74. Vona G, Beroud C, Benachi A, et al. Enrichment, immunomorphological, and genetic characterization of fetal cells circulating in maternal blood. Am J Pathol 2002; 160:51–58.

75. Beroud C, Karliova M, Bonnefont JP, et al. Prenatal diagnosis of spinal muscular atrophy by genetic analysis of circulating fetal cells. Lancet 2003; 361:1013–1014.

76. Bischoff FZ, Marquez-Do DA, Martinez DI, et al. Intact fetal cell isolation from maternal blood: improved isolation using a simple whole blood progenitor cell enrichment approach (RosetteSep). Clin Genet 2003; 63:483–489.

77. Chiu RW, Lo YM. Recent developments in fetal DNA in maternal plasma. Ann NY Acad Sci 2004; 1022:100–104.

78. Poon LL, Leung TN, Lau TK, Lo YM. Circulating fetal RNA in maternal plasma. Ann NY Acad Sci 2001; 945:207–210.

79. Ng EK, Tsui NB, Lau TK, et al. mRNA of placental origin is readily detectable in maternal plasma. Proc Natl Acad Sci USA 2003; 100:4748–4753.

80. Schroder J, Tiilikainen A, De lC. Fetal leukocytes in the maternal circulation after delivery. I. Cytological aspects. Transplantation 1974; 17:346–354.

81. Ciaranfi A, Curchod A, Odartchenko N. [Post-partum survival of fetal lymphocytes in the maternal blood]. Schweiz Med Wochenschr 1977; 107:134–138.

82. Wataganara T, Chen AY, LeShane ES, et al. Cell-free fetal DNA levels in maternal plasma after elective first-trimester termination of pregnancy. Fertil Steril 2004; 81:638–644.

83. Nelson JL, Furst DE, Maloney S, et al. Microchimerism and HLA-compatible relationships of pregnancy in scleroderma. Lancet 1998; 351:559–562.

84. Evans PC, Lambert N, Maloney S, et al. Long-term fetal microchimerism in peripheral blood mononuclear cell subsets in healthy women and women with scleroderma. Blood 1999; 93:2033–2037.

85. Artlett CM, Smith JB, Jimenez SA. Identification of fetal DNA and cells in skin lesions from women with systemic sclerosis. N Engl J Med 1998; 338:1186–1191.
86. Johnson KL, Nelson JL, Furst DE, et al. Fetal cell microchimerism in tissue from multiple sites in women with systemic sclerosis. Arthritis Rheum 2001; 44:1848–1854.
87. Johnson KL, McAlindon TE, Mulcahy E, Bianchi DW. Microchimerism in a female patient with systemic lupus erythematosus. Arthritis Rheum 2001; 44:2107–2111.
88. Klintschar M, Schwaiger P, Mannweiler S, Regauer S, Kleiber M. Evidence of fetal microchimerism in Hashimoto's thyroiditis. J Clin Endocrinol Metab 2001; 86:2494–2498.
89. Johnson KL, Samura O, Nelson JL, McDonnell M, Bianchi DW. Significant fetal cell microchimerism in a nontransfused woman with hepatitis C: evidence of long-term survival and expansion. Hepatology 2002; 36(5):1295–1297.
90. Srivatsa B, Srivatsa S, Johnson KL, Samura O, Lee SL, Bianchi DW. Microchimerism of presumed fetal origin in thyroid specimens from women: a case-control study. Lancet 2001; 358:2034–2038.
91. Cha D, Khosrotehrani K, Kim Y, Stroh H, Bianchi DW, Johnson KL. Cervical cancer and microchimerism. Obstet Gynecol 2003; 102:774–781.
92. Khosrotehrani K, Johnson KL, Cha DH, Salomon RN, Bianchi DW. Transfer of fetal cells with multilineage potential to maternal tissue. J Am Med Assoc 2004; 292:75–80.

9

Fetal DNA and mRNA in Maternal Plasma

Attie T. J. I. Go and John M. G. van Vugt
*Department of Obstetrics and Gynecology, VU University Medical Center,
Amsterdam, The Netherlands*

Cees B. M. Oudejans
*Department of Clinical Chemistry, VU University Medical Center, Amsterdam,
The Netherlands*

FETAL NUCLEIC ACIDS IN MATERNAL CIRCULATION

Introduction

For prenatal diagnosis of genetic disorders of the fetus like aneuploidy or inherited genetic diseases, invasive procedures are required to obtain informative fetal cells. As these invasive procedures, i.e., amniocentesis and chorionic villus sampling, have an intrinsic risk of fetal loss by the technique being invasive, it is considered a big challenge to develop a *noninvasive* test with identical diagnostic possibilities and specificities. The presence and detectability of fetal cells in maternal blood was seen as the entrance to a new era of noninvasive prenatal diagnosis. For instance, trophoblast studies demonstrated fetal DNA to be present among maternal cells in early pregnancy in the cellular fraction with densities characteristic of trophoblast. Fetal sex was predicted correctly in 91.7% of the cases in weeks 9–13 of pregnancy by the polymerase chain reaction (PCR) for X- and Y-chromosome–specific sequences after analysis of the cellular fraction enriched for fetal cells (1). In addition, immunostaining (human leukocyte antigen-G) combined with fluorescent in situ hybridization (XY) confirmed the existence and detectability of trophoblast cells in the maternal blood (2).

However, the rarity of fetal cells, both of extraembryonic (trophoblasts) and embryonic origin (nucleated red blood cells, NRBCs) in the maternal circulation and the elaborate techniques necessary to enrich and identify these cells prevented a breakthrough with widespread clinical use (3). Despite its high specificity (when fetal cells are identified, their fetal origin can be scored reliably), the sensitivity remains low. Fetal cells cannot be found in all pregnant samples or are found in numbers too low to permit reliable clinical implementation. The latter features prevented their introduction and use in a routine clinical setting. The finding of cell-*free* fetal DNA in *plasma* and *serum* of pregnant women as first demonstrated by Lo et al. (4) revitalized and redirected the pursuit of noninvasive prenatal diagnosis. Circulating fetal nucleic acids, both genomic DNA and messenger RNA (mRNA), can be obtained from pregnant plasma and serum in amounts much higher and by methods less elaborate than the amounts obtained and methods used for fetal DNA from the cellular fractions. Moreover, fetal mRNA can be obtained from maternal plasma as well.

This review focuses on the cellular origin, biological features, and clinical potentials of the cell-free fetal nucleic acids, both DNA and mRNA, present in maternal plasma and serum during pregnancy.

FETAL DNA

Biology of Circulating DNA

Circulating Fetal DNA During Pregnancy

Fetal DNA is present in maternal blood in a high background of maternal DNA. Lo et al. started with the use of the most obvious difference between maternally and paternally derived genetic material, the Y chromosome. The Y chromosome is present if the fetus is male. With the PCR technique, amplification of a single-gene copy sequence (DYS 14) from the Y chromosome was performed. By this technique, 80% of the male pregnancies were correctly identified (4). All the female-bearing pregnancies were negative for the Y sequence. These findings were confirmed by others (5–7). The mean concentration of fetal DNA in plasma is about 11 times higher in late gestation than in early gestation. In early pregnancy, fetal DNA in maternal plasma constitutes a mean of 3.4% (range 0.39–11.9%) of the total amount of DNA, which includes maternal DNA. In late pregnancy, the mean is 6.2% (range 2.33–11.4%). This is about 21 times higher than the amount of fetal DNA found in the cellular fraction in maternal blood at the same gestational age (8), even despite enrichment of these fractions for fetal cells. This clearly indicated one important advantage of cell-free fetal DNA over cellular DNA. Fetal, i.e., male, DNA can be detected in maternal plasma as early as 32 days of gestation and can be detected consistently after 52 days of gestation, both by quantitative (real-time) or semiquantitative (conventional) PCR amplification (6,9). This demonstrates the second advantage if fetal DNA is to be used for clinical diagnosis: detection becomes possible within or before the same time window as currently employed for invasive prenatal diagnosis. By analysis of serial blood samples from women pregnant after in vitro fertilization or intrauterine insemination, the earliest detection of Y-chromosome–specific SRY sequences was at five weeks and two days. By 10 weeks of gestational age, the correct fetal sex can be detected in all patients. In pregnancies ending in a miscarriage, SRY cannot be detected (10). In the first trimester, the calculated increase of the amount of fetal DNA is about 4.2 genome equivalents/mL/wk (9). In the late third trimester, there is an interindividual variation in fetal DNA concentration. The median concentration is 74 genome equivalents/mL (range 53–141). Serial sampling in late trimester shows a mean increase of 29.3% with each week. There is no statistically significant correlation between β-globin concentration and gestational age. β-Globin sequences in maternal plasma represent the total amount of extracted DNA, both maternal and fetal (11).

Information about fluctuation of DNA and fetal DNA levels within an individual is scarce. Zhong et al. analyzed blood samples taken on three consecutive days from healthy males, healthy females, and 16 healthy pregnant women with uncomplicated pregnancies between 9 and 42 weeks of gestation. The total amount of free circulatory DNA in pregnant and nonpregnant individuals fluctuates with a range of 1.3- to 130-fold. The concentration of male fetal DNA in the 10 pregnant women carrying a male fetus is less with a mean difference of 2.2-fold (range 1.4–4.5). The variation in the amount of circulatory fetal DNA occurred independent of the variation in the quantity of maternal DNA. It can be concluded, therefore, that the release of fetal versus maternal DNA is not coupled (12). This reflects their different origin, biological clearance, or other factors.

Size distribution of DNA and fetal DNA has also been studied. The median percentage of plasma DNA with sizes >201 bp was 57% for pregnant women and 14% for nonpregnant women. The median percentage of fetal-derived DNA (SRY gene) with sizes >193 and >313 bp was 20% and 0%, respectively, in maternal plasma. Fetal DNA molecules are, therefore, shorter than maternal DNA molecules. On the other hand, the DNA fragments in the plasma of pregnant women are significantly longer than those in the plasma of nonpregnant women (13). Similar results were found in another study, where the potential advantage of size separation was explored. Theoretically, selection or enrichment could permit easier analysis of both paternally and maternally inherited DNA polymorphisms. But a solid determination of fetal ploidy by determination of paternally and maternally inherited polymorphic markers was not yet possible with the method used (14).

Methods to increase the percentage of free fetal DNA in maternal serum and plasma have been described. The addition of formaldehyde to maternal blood samples has been claimed to increase yield of fetal DNA. By stabilization of the cell membranes, the percentage of maternal cell lysis is decreased, and thereby, the amount of free maternal DNA leaking into the plasma. As such, the relative percentage of free fetal DNA increases. The absolute percentage remains the same. This addition seems to have a positive effect in samples shipped overnight (15). A yet unpublished study, with samples shipped overnight, also supports this hypothesis (A. Benachi, unpublished). No difference in fetal DNA concentration was observed in the sample groups with or without addition of ethylenediaminetetraacetic acid (EDTA) and with or without addition of formaldehyde. The total DNA concentration decreased dramatically when the sample was treated with formaldehyde ($P < 0.0001$). So, the proportion of fetal DNA increased in samples collected in tubes containing formaldehyde. It can be concluded that formaldehyde increases the percentage of free fetal DNA in maternal plasma or serum by inhibiting cell lysis. It might well be possible that addition of formaldehyde is an advantage if transport between venapuncture and samples processing takes more time.

Circulating Fetal DNA After Pregnancy

If to be used reliably for clinical applications, it is crucial that fetal DNA disappears from the circulation after delivery with no carryover and persistence into subsequent pregnancies. In the first publication, female-bearing pregnancies tested negative although these women gave birth to sons in the past. This was a good indication. Detailed analysis on the clearance of fetal DNA from maternal plasma showed that the calculated mean half-life was 16.3 minutes (range 4–30 minutes). One day after delivery, no fetal DNA could be detected in the samples from 12 women (16). This was confirmed by Rijnders et al. who studied 120 women who either had delivered previously or were childless. All women were nonpregnant at the time of analysis. Of these, 64 women had previously given birth to one or more sons and 43 were childless. From the latter, five had abortions or extrauterine pregnancies. The rest only gave birth to daughters. This cohort, therefore, consisted of a representative study set of females. In all cases, no SRY sequences were found by PCR in the DNA isolated from plasma (17). These results were confirmed by Smid et al. (18) and Benachi et al. (19).

Therefore, the majority of studies show absence of long-time persistence of fetal DNA in maternal plasma, except for one study. Invernizzi et al. showed the presence of fetal DNA in maternal plasma decades after pregnancy (20). Lambert et al. reported the presence of fetal DNA in 36% of the nonpregnant women who previously gave birth to a son, but filtration studies showed that this DNA was not cell-free (21). Smid hypothesizes that the centrifugation protocol of Invernizzi et al. led to fetal SRY amplification originating from fetal cells remaining in the supernatant after centrifugation. For fetal nucleated cells, it is known that specific subsets can be detected years after delivery (22) and can settle and survive in specific maternal tissues. These persistent cells (pregnancy-associated progenitor cells) are unique in nature, possess stem cell properties, and share phenotypic characteristics with lymphoid cells. Details on these intriguing cells are explained in Chapter 8.

Clearance from the Circulation

The mechanism underlying clearance of fetal DNA from plasma is unknown. The kidney and liver are logical candidates to play a role in this process. Studies on renal clearance show conflicting results. In two studies, Y-chromosome–specific sequences could be detected in a number of urine samples (first trimester) of pregnant women carrying a male fetus. Botezatu et al. could detect Y-chromosome–specific sequences in urine of 8 of 10 pregnant women carrying a male fetus. Controls, i.e., pregnant women carrying a female fetus were all negative (23). Al-Yatama et al. found in 38% of the samples a positive result (24). Li et al. studied urine of normal pregnant women and of women with preeclampsia and HELLP (hemolysis, elevated liver enzymes, low platelets) syndrome in the third trimester and could not detect fetal DNA (25). Maternal plasma and urine samples were collected in the third trimester from 20 pregnant women. Eighteen of them had an unremarkable pregnant history and delivered healthy babies. Two had manifest HELLP syndrome with proteinuria of at least 5 g on a 24-hour urine collection. Urinary DNA was examined by Y-chromosome–specific nested PCR or real-time PCR (RT-PCR). No fetal DNA could be detected in maternal urine—not even in those pregnancies affected by HELLP syndrome although copious quantities of cell-free DNA were present in maternal plasma. Total cell-free DNA in maternal urine was measured using RT-PCR assay for GAPDH (glyceraldehyde-3-phosphate dehydrogenase) gene; no differences in quantity were found between normal pregnancies and pregnancies complicated by HELLP syndrome.

Clearance of fetal DNA after delivery has been found impaired in patients with preeclampsia. Median half-life was 114 minutes in patients with preeclampsia and 28 minutes in controls. Six hours after delivery, fetal DNA was not detectable anymore in the majority of the controls but still present (median 208 genome equivalents/mL) in all of the preeclampsia cases. Preeclampsia is a multisystem disorder associated with damage and dysfunction of many organ systems, including liver and kidney. Organ damage is likely to induce the observed abnormalities in fetal DNA clearance (26). The liver as a detoxification organ might play a role, but there is no direct proof of this hypothesis. Indirect evidence of the involvement of the liver is indicated by the study of Nelson who reported an impaired fetal DNA clearance in a case with acute fatty liver disease in pregnancy. Fetal DNA remained detectable until 11 days after delivery (27).

Source and Mechanism of Release

Where fetal DNA in maternal plasma comes from is still an enigma. After delivery, fetal DNA from maternal plasma is cleared rapidly, mean half-life of 16.3 minutes (16).

This result together with the fact that fetal DNA can be detected in all stages of pregnancy indicates that fetal DNA is liberated in large quantities into the maternal circulation as long as the placenta and/or fetus is present, while clearance by the maternal system is a constant process (28).

Because the fetal DNA is not immediately degraded and can be readily amplified from plasma and serum, it has been suggested that the circulating DNA is protected within apoptotic bodies. As possible sources, hematopoietic cells, trophoblasts, and direct fetomaternal transfer of DNA molecules have been suggested. Of these, the placenta is the most logical source for several reasons. The placenta is large, has abundant cellular activity, is the first organ formed, and is in direct contact with maternal blood. In a case of placenta increta, a small part of the placenta remained adherent to the uterus. Postpartum monitoring showed that fetal DNA was detectable until 10 weeks after delivery (29). Recently, an interesting case has been published. In a pregnant woman carrying a male pregnancy, the SRY gene was absent in maternal serum despite male genitalia being seen at ultrasound. The karyotype was 45,X after direct trophoblast culture and 45,X/46,Xidic (Yp) after culture and in all fetal tissues studied. This confined placenta mosaicism with Y chromosomal sequences, present in all fetal tissues but absent in cytotrophoblast and maternal serum, indicates that free fetal DNA originates from trophoblast cells (30). Secondly, an interesting study on the time of appearance of fetal DNA in maternal plasma has recently been published. Fetal SRY gene sequences were measured in serum samples of 22 women who conceived using artificial reproductive technology. In male pregnancies, the SRY gene was found as early as day 18 following embryo transfer in a twin gestation, day 22 following embryo transfer in a singleton gestation, and by day 37 in all 10 women pregnant with a male fetus (31). The definitive fetoplacental circulation is not established until days 28–30 postconception. In another study, SRY gene was detectable from 35 days of gestation (about 23 days after conception). Eighty percent of the study subjects had detectable fetal DNA in their blood at a gestational age of 49 days. The appearance of fetal DNA in the maternal circulation prior to the establishment of fetoplacental circulation once again indicates that the trophoblast is the most important source, and in first trimester probably the only source (10). The finding of placental-specific mRNA molecules in maternal plasma further support the hypothesis that the placenta is the main source (32) as is discussed later. Fetal NRBCs might contribute at least after the first trimester but the amount of DNA from these cells in maternal blood is less than the amount of cell-free fetal DNA (8). There are about 19 nucleated fetal cells in 16 mL of maternal blood (33). Apoptosis of fetal NRBCs has been studied using a technique called TdT-mediated dUTP nick end labeling (TUNEL). A significant number, 42.7%, of nucleated erythrocytes were undergoing apoptosis in maternal blood at the time of sampling (34). On the contrary, fetal DNA levels were significantly elevated in preterm labor (35) without any incremental increase in fetal NRBCs (36). So fetal hematopoietic cells add to the total amount of DNA, but are not the main source.

Clinical Applications (Fig. 1)

Gender-Dependent Approaches (Fig. 1)

Fetal Gender Assessment.   In pregnancies at risk for congenital adrenal hyperplasia or X-linked recessive diseases like hemophilia, determination of the sex of the fetus is a common indication to perform an invasive procedure. In congenital

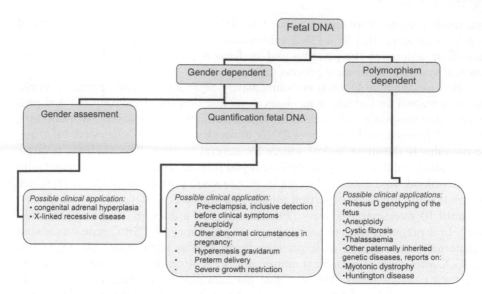

Figure 1 Overview of clinical applications of fetal DNA in maternal plasma, grouped by fetal DNA characteristics.

adrenal hyperplasia, a female fetus is at risk for virilization. By giving the mother dexamethasone as early as possible, virilization of an eventually affected fetus can be prevented. If the pregnancy concerns a male fetus, dexamethasone can be stopped, because male fetuses are not at risk in utero. So, in 50% of the cases dexamethasone is started unnecessarily and an invasive procedure can be avoided in male fetus–carrying pregnancies. In X-linked recessive diseases, it is the other way around. Female fetus–carrying pregnancies are not at risk (37). Using the Y single-copy gene sequence DYS 14 to identify fetal DNA in maternal plasma and serum (4) for fetal sex determination, 95–100% of male and 100% of female fetuses were correctly identified (5–7,38–40). These good results justify clinical application, especially for congenital adrenal hyperplasia. Rijnders et al. propose starting treatment with dexamethasone and testing from five weeks of gestational age onward with serial testing up to 11 weeks or until male DNA is detected. In male fetuses, dexamethasone treatment can be stopped with invasive tests becoming unnecessary. As long as no male DNA is detected, dexamethasone treatment should be continued except when karyotype analysis of fetal chorionic villi shows the fetus is an unaffected female (38). Unnecessary invasive procedures and the related risk of miscarriage can be avoided by reliable identification of the fetus not at risk, in this case the males.

Quantification of Fetal DNA

1. *Preeclampsia*: In pregnancies complicated by preeclampsia, levels of circulating fetal DNA are significantly (5–10 times) higher than in normotensive pregnancies (41,42). This increase is correlated with severity, the amounts are higher if the preeclampsia is more severe or complicated by the HELLP syndrome (42,43). Total DNA is also elevated in plasma of pregnant women with preeclampsia (42).

   Elevation of cell-free fetal DNA before the onset of preeclampsia has also been studied. Prior to the onset of clinical presentation of preeclampsia, an increased concentration of maternal plasma fetal DNA can be detected in second trimester, in one study even in early second trimester in susceptible subjects (44). However, there was an overlap in fetal DNA concentrations between the preeclamptic and control groups (44–47). Levine et al. reported a two-stage elevation in a group of 120 preeclampsia cases and 120 matched controls. At stage 1 (17–28 weeks of gestation) and stage 2 (within three weeks of the onset of preeclampsia), fetal DNA was elevated compared to controls. Before 17 weeks of gestation, no difference could be found between both groups. Among cases there were differences in the amount of fetal DNA according to the disease severity, gestational age, and the presence of a small-for-gestational age infant (48). Early identification of women at risk for developing severe preeclampsia is important for close monitoring and if preventive treatments are available. But as long as the overlap between normal pregnancies and pregnancies complicated by preeclampsia is high, neither early detection nor prediction is feasible in individual patients.

In patients with preeclampsia, clearance is impaired (29). The underlying mechanism, like the origin of fetal DNA, is unclear, but it can be due to increased liberation of fetal DNA in the maternal circulation and/or reduced clearance of circulating DNA from maternal blood. Increased liberation can be a result of increased degradation of cells, by necrosis or apoptosis. The amount of fetal DNA can increase because of placental hypoxia, the amount of maternal DNA, and as such total DNA because of endothelial damage of the maternal vessels. Both conditions are present in preeclampsia. However, placental dysfunction is not unique for preeclampsia.

2. *Aneuploidy*: Although not found in all studies, there seems to be an indication that fetal DNA levels in maternal plasma and serum are higher in trisomy 21 pregnancies compared to euploid pregnancies. Experienced research groups found significantly higher concentrations of fetal DNA in plasma of pregnant women carrying a male fetus with trisomy 21. In the study of Lo et al., the median cell-free fetal DNA in women carrying trisomy 21 fetuses was 2.96-fold higher than that of women carrying euploid fetuses in the Hong Kong group (49). In samples collected in Boston but measured in Hong Kong, a 1.97-fold increase was found (49). The group of Zhong et al. confirmed these findings. In this study, trisomies 13 and 18 were also studied. In the trisomy 13 cases (4), the concentration was also significantly higher, but in the trisomy 18 group (7), no significant difference was found between cases and controls (50). When archived maternal serum was analyzed, a 1.7-fold higher level of cell-free fetal DNA compared with matched controls was found (51). It is remarkable that clinically used markers for Down syndrome of placental origin such as human chorionic gonadotropin (hCG) and inhibin-A are also elevated about twice the value of euploid pregnancies. It is possible that the observed elevation of fetal DNA levels reflects a similar biologic pathway. Like hCG and inhibin-A, the median concentration of fetal DNA seems to be higher, but there is an important overlap with the normal range. If the analyzed values are expressed as multiples of the median (MoM), test performance can be determined as a screening marker for Down syndrome. Fetal DNA alone was calculated to give a 21% detection rate at a 5% false-positive rate (52). When added to second-trimester quadruple marker screening, fetal DNA increased the estimated detection rate from 81% to 86% at a 5% false-positive rate (52). For comparison, total hCG alone in maternal serum is calculated to give a detection rate of 53% at a false-positive rate of 5%, inhibin-A 59% at a detection rate of 5% (53). Yet, the calculated test performance of fetal DNA is not very impressive.

In two studies, no difference in fetal DNA concentration could be found between cases and controls (54,55). Hromadnikova measured DNA levels in maternal plasma in the early second trimester using RT-PCR and using SRY and β-globin genes as markers (54). The median fetal DNA levels in women carrying a Down syndrome fetus ($n = 11$) and the controls ($n = 13$) were 23.3 and 24.5 genome equivalents/mL. Total median DNA levels in cases and controls were also not significantly different (54). Ohashi used maternal serum in the early second trimester (55). He included five male Down syndrome pregnancies and 55 male controls with normal karyotype. Mean concentration of fetal DNA in maternal serum of the controls was 31.5 and 23.5 copies/mL in the cases. No significant differences in the concentration of fetal DNA were found (55).

3. *Other abnormal circumstances in pregnancy*: In several pregnancy-associated complications, like hyperemesis gravidarum, preterm delivery, severe growth restriction, a case of polyhydramnios (56), and invasive placenta, increased levels of fetal DNA in maternal plasma compared to normal pregnancies have been described. In patients with hyperemesis gravidarum, the median concentration of fetal DNA in plasma of cases was higher than in controls (57). If subdivided according to severity, a relationship was found. The more severe the hyperemesis gravidarum, the higher the concentration of fetal DNA (58). In patients with preterm delivery not reacting to tocolytic therapy, the median concentration of fetal DNA was significantly higher compared to normal pregnancies. In cases of threatened preterm labor, for which tocolytical therapy was started and the delivery was postponed to term, no difference was found in fetal DNA between cases and controls (35). Reports on the levels of cell-free fetal DNA in the plasma of pregnant women with severe fetal growth restriction are conflicting. Sekizawa et al. could not demonstrate an increase in fetal DNA level (59). Caramelli et al. found significantly higher levels of fetal DNA, with an MoM of 2.16, in the (sub)group with an abnormal Doppler waveform in the uterine artery and growth restriction (60). In a few cases with placenta previa, a significantly higher concentration of fetal DNA was observed; in two cases of placenta increta the concentrations were even higher. In one case, a piece of placenta could not be removed. The concentration of fetal DNA during delivery was very high, 1104 genome equivalents/mL (61). Fetal DNA was detected until 10 weeks after delivery, whereas plasma β subunit of human placental chorionic gonadotropin (βhCG) could not be detected by 11 days postpartum (29).

In special circumstances like twin pregnancies and external cephalic version near term, higher levels of fetal DNA were also reported (62). In twin pregnancies with two male fetuses, higher levels of SRY-gene were measured compared to twin pregnancies with one male and one female. Chorionicity in male–male pregnancies did not result in different levels (63).

Considerations

In the above-mentioned approach, quantitative RT-PCR for the SRY- or DYS14-gene on the Y chromosome was used as a model system representative of fetal DNA. In earlier studies, this approach proved to be reliable and technically feasible (7,8,10,39,40). In pathological circumstances like preeclampsia, or special circumstances like twin pregnancies, the measured levels of fetal DNA were higher in cases than in controls, often with a considerable overlap. Elevated levels of fetal DNA in maternal plasma are a nonspecific indication of pathological processes in pregnancy. Most of these pathological conditions are known to be placenta-related. The overlap

of fetal DNA levels between uncomplicated pregnancies and pregnancies with pathological circumstances is considerable in nearly all studies. This makes discrimination
between normal and abnormal situations difficult. Especially if fetal DNA is considered as a marker for aneuploidy, the calculated test performance is poor.

Another important disadvantage is that the use of SRY- or DYS14-gene is
gender dependent and so only applicable to 50% of the pregnancies. This limitation
makes this method unsuitable for clinical application.

Polymorphism-Dependent Approaches

In contrast, detection of fetal-derived paternally inherited X-chromosome polymorphisms in maternal plasma can be used as a gender-independent marker allowing
positive identification of fetal DNA in all pregnancies. The technique applied for this
purpose was detection of highly polymorphic short tandem repeats (STRs). The use
of five STR polymorphisms increased the chance that a fetomaternal pair would be
informative for sequences unique to the fetus by being derived from the father.
Among the 25 pairs of samples of women carrying a female fetus, 76% were informative for at least one STR marker (64). In this feasibility study, the possibility of
this approach was clearly demonstrated. Other possible applications like rhesus D
(RHD) genotyping and genetic disorders such as recessive autosomal single-gene disorders were studied. The studies on several specific genetic disorders (mentioned later
in the text) are case reports or contain small numbers of patients. They mainly
demonstrate that identification in maternal plasma is possible, but their value in
clinical practice must still be proven.

Rhesus D Genotyping of the Fetus

In this approach, the genotypic difference between an RHD-negative pregnant
woman and her eventually RHD-positive fetus is used. The RHD gene is absent
in an RHD-negative individual and present in an RHD-positive individual. If the
RHD gene is detectable in maternal blood, it must originate from the RHD-positive
fetus. An RHD-negative woman with a heterozygote RHD partner has a 50%
change of carrying an RHD-positive fetus. If she develops antibodies, the risk of
hemolytic disease of the neonate increases, with a possible adverse pregnancy outcome. The present strategy consists of screening RHD-negative women for alloimmunization. If she has antibodies, the partner will be checked for the specific
blood group genotype. If he is positive, the pregnancy will be monitored closely.
Invasive procedures might be carried out to obtain fetal genetic material for prenatal
testing of the blood group genotype to identify fetuses at risk. This invasive procedure carries a risk of miscarriage and has an increased risk of fetomaternal hemorrhage (65). The great advantage of a noninvasive way to genotype the fetus is that
these risks are avoided. Another advantage is that immunoprophylaxis can be given
on indication. Since there is a shortage of anti-D, it would be better to give it only to
pregnancies at risk. The detection of fetal RHD-specific sequences in maternal
plasma has been studied extensively. With the use of RT-PCR technology, the fetal
RHD status can be determined correctly from early second to third trimester with a
sensitivity of 100% and a specificity of 96.6–100% (66–69). The only exception concerned a false-positive case where the fetus had a variant RHD gene, most likely an
RHD φ gene (67). In an early study, seven out of nine first-trimester samples were
concordant with the outcome after birth. Two RHD-positive fetuses were false

negative (66). Clinical implementation of fetal RHD genotyping in maternal plasma is clearly indicated, and is the preferred method of choice, as demonstrated recently by screening of a large cohort (70).

Aneuploidies

In cases of paternally inherited fetal aneuploidy, prenatal detection is possible using fetal DNA in maternal plasma. In this technique, polymorphic markers outside the Y chromosome are used. This is only possible in the presence of a fully known paternal balanced translocation. This technique has been applied successfully in a case with fetal distal 3p trisomy and 7q36 deletion, resulting from a paternal t(3;7) reciprocal translocation (71). In another case, three consecutive pregnancies of one mother were followed. The father had a balanced reciprocal translocation between the long arm of chromosome 10 and the short arm of chromosome 22. Analysis of fetal DNA in maternal plasma successfully demonstrated the presence of a balanced or unbalanced translocation in the fetuses (72).

Cystic Fibrosis

Cystic fibrosis is an autosomal recessive disorder and can be caused by different mutations in the CFTR gene. A child is affected if mutations are inherited from both parents. Detection of a paternally inherited cystic fibrosis mutation has been demonstrated successfully in maternal plasma at a gestational age of 13 weeks. Single PCR amplification of the Q890X mutation was used. In that case, the fetus was carrier of the paternal mutation (73). In another study, the D1152H mutation was identified correctly by allele-specific PCR despite the presence of an excess of the corresponding wild-type sequence. Reliability of the assay was tested up to 300 ng of DNA. Of the 10 controls, nine were tested negative, one positive. This false-positive sample stood six days before processing. The amount of wild-type genomic DNA in the PCR exceeds 300 ng, which is abnormally high and seems to be the result of lysis of intact cells. It appears that 300 ng is close to the limit of the assay, and analysis of samples containing amounts of DNA exceeding this limit is not reliable. The quantity of other samples was <300 ng (74). Population-based studies are necessary to study test performances, like sensitivity and specificity. If the mutation of the father is found in maternal plasma, an invasive procedure is still necessary to be sure if the fetus is affected or not. In case of a negative result, the invasive procedure can be canceled. The fetus can be a carrier of the maternal mutation but will not be affected itself.

Thalassemia

β-Thalassemia is a common autosomal recessive single-gene disorder that can cause severe anemia. The disease is caused by mutations in the β-globin gene. One of these mutations, namely the deletion of four nucleotides (–CTTT) at codons 41/42, has been studied. First, the specificity and sensitivity of the allele-specific assay was investigated and confirmed by subjecting plasma, buffy coat, and amniotic fluid samples from 100 pregnancies to screening for the mutation. Subsequently, the assay was applied for prenatal testing of eight fetuses at risk for β-thalassemia major. The aim was to exclude fetal inheritance of the paternally transmitted codon 41/42. The fetal genotype was completely concordant with conventional analysis and β-thalassemia major could be excluded in two of the pregnancies noninvasively (75). New techniques appear very useful for this and related purposes. MassARRAY system was used to develop a new protocol, termed single-allele base extension reaction (SABER).

The approach was applied to exclude the fetal inheritance of the four most common South Asian β-thalassemia mutations in at-risk pregnancies between 7 and 21 weeks of gestation. Fetal genotypes were correctly predicted in all cases studied. Fetal haploid analysis based on a single-nucleotide polymorphism linked to the β-globin locus, HBB, in maternal plasma was also achieved (76). Development of such systems might help clinical implementation.

Detection of fetal β^E-globin gene in maternal plasma was evaluated as a noninvasive strategy for the most common β-thalassemic condition among the South Asian population. Nested PCR method was followed by the MnL 1 restriction analysis. Of the five pregnant women examined, three were correctly identified (77).

Other Paternally Inherited Genetic Diseases

Prenatal diagnosis of myotonic dystrophy, an autosomal dominant disorder, was reported using fetal DNA in maternal plasma. The blood was sampled at 10 weeks of gestational age (78). In another case, a Huntington disease unaffected fetus was successfully diagnosed by testing fetal DNA in maternal plasma. The blood was sampled at 13 weeks of gestational age. In both cases, it was essential to perform an analysis of parental DNA to know the size of paternal and maternal alleles (79).

mRNA OF PLACENTAL ORIGIN IN MATERNAL PLASMA

The presence of fetal RNA in maternal plasma was first demonstrated in 2000 by Poon et al. (80) using Y-chromosome–specific zinc finger protein mRNA (ZFY). The detection rates of plasma fetal RNA in early and late pregnancies were 22% and 63%, respectively. This finding suggests that the concentration of fetal RNA in early pregnancy is lower than that in late pregnancy (80). Ng et al. took it further and studied mRNA of two placenta-expressed genes, human placental lactogen (hPL) and the βhCG in maternal plasma by quantitative RT-PCR. Placental hPL mRNA was detected in pregnant women at all gestational stages with concentration levels increasing with gestational age. βhCG mRNA was only detected in all women during the first trimester, decreasing in concentration toward term. Detection rates were 100%, 42%, and 7.7%, respectively, during first, second, and third trimesters. These results mirror the protein plasma levels of hPL and βhCG (30). A smaller study on βhCG mRNA in whole blood and serum of pregnant women also reported on concentrations in the first compared to the second trimester. In whole blood, data suggested a 30-fold higher concentration of βhCG mRNA in the early samples compared to the second trimester. No βhCG mRNA was detected in the corresponding sera (81).

Biology of Circulating RNA

Circulating mRNA During Pregnancy

The existence of RNA species in the circulation is a rather surprising finding, as free RNA is rapidly degraded in blood. After incubations with plasma for as short as 15 seconds, 99% of free added RNA can no longer be amplified. RNA in plasma of healthy volunteers obtained from uncentrifuged EDTA blood and stored in 4°C is surprisingly stable even after 24 hours. The stability of RNA in serum is less. To obtain stable RNA from serum, uncentrifuged clotted blood should be stored at 4°C and processed within 6 hours (82). Placental mRNA in maternal plasma has also been demonstrated to be very stable; hPL and the βhCG mRNA are stable for up to

24 hours at room temperature (32). An explanation can be found in the fact that plasma RNA is particle associated. Filtration studies have been performed to study this possibility. Plasma samples from pregnant women were filtered through 5-μm filter. No significant changes in maternal plasma hPL, βhCG, and GAPDH mRNA levels in pre- and postfiltration samples were observed. But if these plasma samples were passed through 0.45-μm filters, a clear reduction in mRNA levels was observed. This difference in levels after filtration through 5- or 0.45-μm filter was statistically significant (32). Filtration of plasma samples of healthy individuals and cancer patients was also studied. Unfiltered and filtered through 5-, 0.45-, and 0.22-μm pores, GAPDH mRNA and β-globin DNA concentrations were studied. GAPDH mRNA levels were not different between unfiltered and filtered through 5-μm pore samples. But filtered through smaller pores, 0.45 and 0.22 μm, levels reduce significantly. These results indicate that a significant proportion of GAPDH mRNA in plasma is particle associated. In contrast to these results, β-globin DNA concentrations did not differ between the filtered (all three pore sizes) and unfiltered samples, suggesting that most of the circulating β-globin DNA is nonparticle associated (83). It is likely that this particle association contributes to the stability of plasma RNA.

Circulating mRNA After Pregnancy

In blood of nonpregnant women who previously gave birth to at least one neonate, no βhCG mRNA could be detected (81). Clearance of hPL directly after delivery seems to be rapid (84). In predelivery plasma samples collected at a gestational age of 38–42 weeks, the median levels of hPL mRNA was 50.004 copies/mL. Twenty four hours after delivery, no hPL mRNA could be detected in any of these samples (32). The clearance of mRNA corticotropin-releasing hormone (CRH) was studied in uncomplicated pregnancies under controlled circumstances. Two hours post-cesarean section, no CRH mRNA was detectable anymore, indicating very rapid clearances under normal circumstances (85). These findings are comparable with the postpartum clearance of fetal DNA in maternal plasma. The mechanism of clearance is still unsolved.

Source and Mechanism of Release

The main source of the studied mRNA in maternal plasma is the placenta. Most studies concentrate on mRNA of genes uniquely expressed by the placenta, for example, hPL, βhCG (32), CRH (85), and glial cells missing-1 (GCM1) mRNA (86). It was expected that the placental mRNA demonstrated in maternal plasma would mainly originate from the extravillus trophoblasts, because of its close contact with the maternal circulation. But surprisingly this was not the outcome of these studies. hPL, βhCG, and GCM1 are synthesized by syncytiotrophoblast. There must be a regulation mechanism, yet unknown, releasing mRNA expressed by villus tropho-blast into the maternal circulation.

The possibility that fetal hematopoietic cells contribute to the pool of circulating cell-free fetal nucleic acids during pregnancy was studied by quantification of plasma γ-globin mRNA in the first trimester. GAPDH mRNA was used as house-keeping sequence. The concentration of γ-globin mRNA was significantly higher in pregnant women compared to nonpregnant individuals. In plasma taken 8–20 minutes after first-trimester termination of pregnancy, the concentrations were significantly lower than in the pretermination samples. GAPDH mRNA followed the same pattern. When termination of pregnancy was greater than nine weeks of gestation, the concentration of γ-globin mRNA was increased. The authors suggest that increased post-termination γ-globin mRNA concentration can be an indication that the source of this message is fetal hematopoietic cells. They propose further evaluation of γ-globin mRNA in maternal plasma after nine weeks in the perspective as being a marker for fetomaternal hemorrhage (87).

RNA from chromosome 21-encoded, placentally expressed gene, LOC 90625, was detected in first-trimester maternal plasma (88). It is very interesting that LOC 90625, also called 21 ORF 105, turned out to be a member of the human endogenous retrovirus (HERV)-F family (89). The RNA expression of various HERV families has recently been studied in an extensive range of cell types, tissues, and diseases. HERV-F is expressed in placental and fetal tissues (90,91). It became apparent that the placenta is unique in both the diverse range of HERV transcripts and their high level of expression (92). The transcriptional activity of HERVs has been studied. In the placenta three loci, syncytin, and syncytin2 were active. Three different patterns were observed: constant expression through gestation, gradually decrease as pregnancy proceeded, and a remarkable increase in term placentas (89). Products of the expression of certain HERV proteins in the placenta may have a variety of physiological roles: the envelope of HERV-W seems to be involved in cell fusion to form the syncytium and ERV3 Env is associated with cytotrophoblast differentiation.

POSSIBLE CLINICAL APPLICATIONS

The demonstration of placental mRNA in maternal plasma opens up the possibility of developing gender- and polymorphism-independent noninvasive prenatal diagnostic tools. Studies have been started on this challenging subject. In plasma collected in the third trimester from pregnant women with preeclampsia, the concentration of CRH mRNA was 10-fold higher compared to the uncomplicated pregnancies (85). A second study confirmed this finding, but a significant difference between mild and severe preeclampsia could not be demonstrated (93). RNA from a chromosome 21-encoded, placentally expressed gene, LOC 90625, was present in first-trimester maternal plasma and could be detected in 100% of samples when 1600 μL of plasma was used (88). This finding may allow development of plasma-RNA–based strategies for prenatal prediction of Down syndrome.

A more basic research field concerns the search for possible markers for clinical situations by systematic screening of placental mRNA in maternal plasma. Using RT-PCR, a large number of RNA targets ($n = 80$) known or expected to be present in extraembryonic tissues were screened in the first trimester of pregnancy in maternal plasma, plasma of nonpregnant women, and early placental tissue. With this strategy, eight genes were found positive in early placental tissue and plasma of pregnant women and tested negative in nonpregnant women. This approach not only permits rapid screening of potential new markers but also allows the detection of markers not accessible by conventional antibody-based assays (86). Using RT-PCR technique as a method of screening, the choice was made for a method with high sensitivity. Lower concentration levels of mRNA can be detected. The possibility of a high abundance screening method was also studied. Oligonucleotide microarray analysis has been applied as a systematic and high throughput strategy for the identification of new fetal RNA markers in maternal plasma. Gene expression profiles between placental tissues and corresponding peripheral blood from pregnant women in their first and third trimesters were compared. Six transcripts were selected for further evaluation by RT-PCR (84). Thus, genes expressed uniquely in placenta, which can be detected in maternal plasma (and not in plasma of nonpregnant women), can be seen as possible markers for clinical situations. The important advantage of this approach is that the markers are gender and polymorphism independent and hence are candidates for application in all pregnancies. These candidate markers will be further studied.

REFERENCES

1. van Wijk IJ, Van Vugt JM, Mulders MA, Konst AA, Weima SM, Oudejans CB. Enrichment of fetal trophoblast cells from the maternal peripheral blood followed by detection of fetal deoxyribonucleic acid with a nested X/Y polymerase chain reaction. Am J Obstet Gynecol 1996; 174(3):871–878.
2. van Wijk IJ, Griffioen S, Tjoa ML, et al. HLA-G expression in trophoblast cells circulating in maternal peripheral blood during early pregnancy. Am J Obstet Gynaecol 2001; 184(5):991–997.
3. Bianchi DW, Simpson JL, Jackson LG, et al. Fetal gender and aneuploidy detection using fetal cells in maternal blood: analysis of NIFTY I data. National Institute of Child Health and Development Fetal Cell Isolation Study. Prenat Diagn 2002; 22(7):609–615.
4. Lo YM, Corbetta N, Chamberlain PF, et al. Presence of fetal DNA in maternal plasma and serum. Lancet 1997; 350(9076):485–487.
5. Tungwiwat W, Fucharoen G, Ratanasiri T, Sanchaisuriya K, Fucharoen S. Non-invasive fetal sex determination using a conventional nested PCR analysis of fetal DNA in maternal plasma. Clin Chim Acta 2003; 334(1–2):173–177.
6. Honda H, Miharu N, Ohashi Y, Ohama K. Successful diagnosis of fetal gender using conventional PCR analysis of maternal serum. Clin Chem 2001; 47(1):41–46.
7. Sekizawa A, Kondo T, Iwasaki M, et al. Accuracy of fetal gender determination by analysis of DNA in maternal plasma. Clin Chem 2001; 47(10):1856–1858.
8. Lo YM, Tein MS, Lau TK, et al. Quantitative analysis of fetal DNA in maternal plasma and serum: implications for noninvasive prenatal diagnosis. Am J Hum Genet 1998; 62(4): 768–775.
9. Wataganara T, Chen AY, Leshane ES, et al. Cell-free fetal DNA levels in maternal plasma after elective first-trimester termination of pregnancy. Fertil Steril 2004; 81(3): 638–644.
10. Rijnders RJ, Van Der Luijt RB, Peters ED, et al. Earliest gestational age for fetal sexing in cell-free maternal plasma. Prenat Diagn 2003; 23(13):1042–1044.
11. Chan LY, Leung TN, Chan KC, et al. Serial analysis of fetal DNA concentrations in maternal plasma in late pregnancy. Clin Chem 2003; 49(4):678–680.
12. Zhong XY, Burk MR, Troeger C, Kang A, Holzgreve W, Hahn S. Fluctuation of maternal and fetal free extracellular circulatory DNA in maternal plasma. Obstet Gynecol 2000; 96(6):991–996.
13. Chan KC, Zhang J, Hui AB, et al. Size distributions of maternal and fetal DNA in maternal plasma. Clin Chem 2004; 50(1):88–92.
14. Li Y, Zimmermann B, Rusterholz C, Kang A, Holzgreve W, Hahn S. Size separation of circulatory DNA in maternal plasma permits ready detection of fetal DNA polymorphisms. Clin Chem 2004; 50(6):1002–1011.
15. Dhallan R, Au WC, Mattagajasingh S, et al. Methods to increase the percentage of free fetal DNA recovered from the maternal circulation. J Am Med Assoc 2004; 291(9): 1114–1119.
16. Lo YM, Zhang J, Leung TN, Lau TK, Chang AM, Hjelm NM. Rapid clearance of fetal DNA from maternal plasma. Am J Hum Genet 1999; 64(1):218–224.

17. Rijnders RJ, Christiaens GC, Soussan AA, van der Schoot CE. Cell-free fetal DNA is not present in plasma of nonpregnant mothers. Clin Chem 2004; 50(3):679–681.
18. Smid M, Galbiati S, Vassallo A, et al. No evidence of fetal DNA persistence in maternal plasma after pregnancy. Hum Genet 2003; 112(5–6):617–618.
19. Benachi A, Steffann J, Gautier E, et al. Fetal DNA in maternal serum: does it persist after pregnancy? Hum Genet 2003; 113(1):76–79.
20. Invernizzi P, Biondi ML, Battezzati PM, et al. Presence of fetal DNA in maternal plasma decades after pregnancy. Hum Genet 2002; 110(6):587–591.
21. Lambert NC, Lo YM, Erickson TD, et al. Male microchimerism in healthy women and women with scleroderma: cells or circulating DNA? A quantitative answer. Blood 2002; 100(8):2845–2851.
22. Bianchi DW, Zickwolf GK, Weil GJ, Sylvester S, DeMaria MA. Male fetal progenitor cells persist in maternal blood for as long as 27 years postpartum. Proc Natl Acad Sci USA 1996; 93(2):705–708.
23. Botezatu I, Serdyuk O, Potapova G, et al. Genetic analysis of DNA excreted in urine: a new approach for detecting specific genomic DNA sequences from cells dying in an organism. Clin Chem 2000; 46(8, Pt 1):1078–1084.
24. Al Yatama MK, Mustafa AS, Ali S, Abraham S, Khan Z, Khaja N. Detection of Y chromosome-specific DNA in the plasma and urine of pregnant women using nested polymerase chain reaction. Prenat Diagn 2001; 21(5):399–402.
25. Li Y, Zhong XY, Kang A, Troeger C, Holzgreve W, Hahn S. Inability to detect cell free fetal DNA in the urine of normal pregnant women nor in those affected by preeclampsia associated HELLP syndrome. J Soc Gynecol Investig 2003; 10(8):503–508.
26. Lau TW, Leung TN, Chan LY, et al. Fetal DNA clearance from maternal plasma is impaired in preeclampsia. Clin Chem 2002; 48(12):2141–2146.
27. Nelson M, Eagle C, Langshaw M, Popp H, Kronenberg H. Genotyping fetal DNA by non-invasive means: extraction from maternal plasma. Vox Sang 2001; 80(2):112–116.
28. Ariga H, Ohto H, Busch MP, et al. Kinetics of fetal cellular and cell-free DNA in the maternal circulation during and after pregnancy: implications for noninvasive prenatal diagnosis. Transfusion 2001; 41(12):1524–1530.
29. Jimbo M, Sekizawa A, Sugito Y, et al. Placenta increta: postpartum monitoring of plasma cell-free fetal DNA. Clin Chem 2003; 49(9):1540–1541.
30. Flori E, Doray B, Gautier E, et al. Circulating cell-free fetal DNA in maternal serum appears to originate from cyto- and syncytio-trophoblastic cells. Case report. Hum Reprod 2004; 19(3):723–724.
31. Guibert J, Benachi A, Grebille AG, Ernault P, Zorn JR, Costa JM. Kinetics of SRY gene appearance in maternal serum: detection by real time PCR in early pregnancy after assisted reproductive technique. Hum Reprod 2003; 18(8):1733–1736.
32. Ng EK, Tsui NB, Lau TK, et al. mRNA of placental origin is readily detectable in maternal plasma. Proc Natl Acad Sci USA 2003; 100(8):4748–4753.
33. Bianchi DW, Williams JM, Sullivan LM, Hanson FW, Klinger KW, Shuber AP. PCR quantitation of fetal cells in maternal blood in normal and aneuploid pregnancies. Am J Hum Genet 1997; 61(4):822–829.
34. Sekizawa A, Samura O, Zhen DK, Falco V, Farina A, Bianchi DW. Apoptosis in fetal nucleated erythrocytes circulating in maternal blood. Prenat Diagn 2000; 20(11):886–889.
35. Leung TN, Zhang J, Lau TK, Hjelm NM, Lo YM. Maternal plasma fetal DNA as a marker for preterm labour. Lancet 1998; 352(9144):1904–1905.
36. Hoesli I, Danek M, Lin D, Li Y, Hahn S, Holzgreve W. Circulating erythroblasts in maternal blood are not elevated before onset of preterm labor. Obstet Gynecol 2002; 100(5, Pt 1):992–996.
37. Costa JM, Benachi A, Gautier E. New strategy for prenatal diagnosis of X-linked disorders. N Engl J Med 2002; 346(19):1502.

38. Rijnders RJ, van der Schoot CE, Bossers B, de Vroede MA, Christiaens GC. Fetal sex determination from maternal plasma in pregnancies at risk for congenital adrenal hyperplasia. Obstet Gynecol 2001; 98(3):374–378.

39. Hromadnikova I, Houbova B, Hridelova D, et al. Replicate real-time PCR testing of DNA in maternal plasma increases the sensitivity of non-invasive fetal sex determination. Prenat Diagn 2003; 23(3):235–238.

40. Costa JM, Benachi A, Gautier E, Jouannic JM, Ernault P, Dumez Y. First-trimester fetal sex determination in maternal serum using real-time PCR. Prenat Diagn 2001; 21(12):1070–1074.

41. Lo YM, Leung TN, Tein MS, et al. Quantitative abnormalities of fetal DNA in maternal serum in preeclampsia. Clin Chem 1999; 45(2):184–188.

42. Zhong XY, Laivuori H, Livingston JC, et al. Elevation of both maternal and fetal extracellular circulating deoxyribonucleic acid concentrations in the plasma of pregnant women with preeclampsia. Am J Obstet Gynecol 2001; 184(3):414–419.

43. Swinkels DW, de Kok JB, Hendriks JC, Wiegerinck E, Zusterzeel PL, Steegers EA. Hemolysis, elevated liver enzymes, and low platelet count (HELLP) syndrome as a complication of preeclampsia in pregnant women increases the amount of cell-free fetal and maternal DNA in maternal plasma and serum. Clin Chem 2002; 48(4):650–653.

44. Cotter AM, Martin CM, O'Leary JJ, Daly SF. Increased fetal DNA in the maternal circulation in early pregnancy is associated with an increased risk of preeclampsia. Am J Obstet Gynecol 2004; 191(2):515–520.

45. Leung TN, Zhang J, Lau TK, Chan LY, Lo YM. Increased maternal plasma fetal DNA concentrations in women who eventually develop preeclampsia. Clin Chem 2001; 47(1):137–139.

46. Farina A, Sekizawa A, Sugito Y, et al. Fetal DNA in maternal plasma as a screening variable for preeclampsia. A preliminary nonparametric analysis of detection rate in low-risk nonsymptomatic patients. Prenat Diagn 2004; 24(2):83–86.

47. Zhong XY, Holzgreve W, Hahn S. The levels of circulatory cell free fetal DNA in maternal plasma are elevated prior to the onset of preeclampsia. Hypertens Pregnancy 2002; 21(1):77–83.

48. Levine RJ, Qian C, Leshane ES, et al. Two-stage elevation of cell-free fetal DNA in maternal sera before onset of preeclampsia. Am J Obstet Gynecol 2004; 190(3):707–713.

49. Lo YM, Lau TK, Zhang J, et al. Increased fetal DNA concentrations in the plasma of pregnant women carrying fetuses with trisomy 21. Clin Chem 1999; 45(10):1747–1751.

50. Zhong XY, Burk MR, Troeger C, Jackson LR, Holzgreve W, Hahn S. Fetal DNA in maternal plasma is elevated in pregnancies with aneuploid fetuses. Prenat Diagn 2000; 20(10):795–798.

51. Lee T, Leshane ES, Messerlian GM, et al. Down syndrome and cell-free fetal DNA in archived maternal serum. Am J Obstet Gynecol 2002; 187(5):1217–1221.

52. Farina A, LeShane ES, Lambert-Messerlian GM, et al. Evaluation of cell-free fetal DNA as a second-trimester maternal serum marker of Down syndrome pregnancy. Clin Chem 2003; 49(2):239–242.

53. Wald NJ, Rodeck C, Hackshaw AK, Walters J, Chitty L, Mackinson AM. First and second trimester antenatal screening for Down's syndrome: the results of the Serum, Urine and Ultrasound Screening Study (SURUSS). J Med Screen 2003; 10(2):56–104.

54. Hromadnikova I, Houbova B, Hridelova D, et al. Quantitative analysis of DNA levels in maternal plasma in normal and Down syndrome pregnancies. BMC Pregnancy Childbirth 2002; 2(1):4.

55. Ohashi Y, Miharu N, Honda H, Samura O, Ohama K. Quantitation of fetal DNA in maternal serum in normal and aneuploid pregnancies. Hum Genet 2001; 108(2):123–127.

56. Zhong XY, Holzgreve W, Li JC, Aydinli K, Hahn S. High levels of fetal erythroblasts and fetal extracellular DNA in the peripheral blood of a pregnant woman with idiopathic polyhydramnios: case report. Prenat Diagn 2000; 20(10):838–841.

57. Sekizawa A, Sugito Y, Iwasaki M, et al. Cell-free fetal DNA is increased in plasma of women with hyperemesis gravidarum. Clin Chem 2001; 47(12):2164–2165.

58. Sugito Y, Sekizawa A, Farina A, et al. Relationship between severity of hyperemesis gravidarum and fetal DNA concentration in maternal plasma. Clin Chem 2003; 49(10):1667–1669.

59. Sekizawa A, Jimbo M, Saito H, et al. Cell-free fetal DNA in the plasma of pregnant women with severe fetal growth restriction. Am J Obstet Gynecol 2003; 188(2):480–484.

60. Caramelli E, Rizzo N, Concu M, et al. Cell-free fetal DNA concentration in plasma of patients with abnormal uterine artery Doppler waveform and intrauterine growth restriction—a pilot study. Prenat Diagn 2003; 23(5):367–371.

61. Sekizawa A, Jimbo M, Saito H, et al. Increased cell-free fetal DNA in plasma of two women with invasive placenta. Clin Chem 2002; 48(2):353–354.

62. Lau TK, Lo KW, Chan LY, Leung TY, Lo YM. Cell-free fetal deoxyribonucleic acid in maternal circulation as a marker of fetal-maternal hemorrhage in patients undergoing external cephalic version near term. Am J Obstet Gynecol 2000; 183(3):712–716.

63. Smid M, Galbiati S, Vassallo A, et al. Fetal DNA in maternal plasma in twin pregnancies. Clin Chem 2003; 49(9):1526–1528.

64. Tang NL, Leung TN, Zhang J, Lau TK, Lo YM. Detection of fetal-derived paternally inherited X-chromosome polymorphisms in maternal plasma. Clin Chem 1999; 45(11): 2033–2035.

65. Tabor A, Bang J, Norgaard-Pedersen B. Feto-maternal haemorrhage associated with genetic amniocentesis: results of a randomized trial. Br J Obstet Gynaecol 1987; 94(6): 528–534.

66. Lo YM, Hjelm NM, Fidler C, et al. Prenatal diagnosis of fetal RhD status by molecular analysis of maternal plasma. N Engl J Med 1998; 339(24):1734–1738.

67. Rijnders RJ, Christiaens GC, Bossers B, van der Smagt JJ, van der Schoot CE, de Haas M. Clinical applications of cell-free fetal DNA from maternal plasma. Obstet Gynecol 2004; 103(1):157–164.

68. Faas BH, Beuling EA, Christiaens GC, dem Borne AE, van der Schoot CE. Detection of fetal RHD-specific sequences in maternal plasma. Lancet 1998; 352(9135):1196.

69. Finning KM, Martin PG, Soothill PW, Avent ND. Prediction of fetal D status from maternal plasma: introduction of a new noninvasive fetal RHD genotyping service. Transfusion 2002; 42(8):1079–1085.

70. Bianchi D, Avent N, Costa J, van der Schoot C. Current commentary. Non-invasive prenatal diagnosis of fetal Rhesus D: ready for prime(r) time. 2005. In Press.

71. Chen CP, Chern SR, Wang W. Fetal DNA in maternal plasma: the prenatal detection of a paternally inherited fetal aneuploidy. Prenat Diagn 2000; 20(4):355–357.

72. Chen CP, Chern SR, Wang W. Fetal DNA analyzed in plasma from a mother's three consecutive pregnancies to detect paternally inherited aneuploidy. Clin Chem 2001; 47(5): 937–939.

73. Gonzalez-Gonzalez MC, Garcia-Hoyos M, Trujillo MJ, et al. Prenatal detection of a cystic fibrosis mutation in fetal DNA from maternal plasma. Prenat Diagn 2002; 22(10): 946–948.

74. Nasis O, Thompson S, Hong T, et al. Improvement in sensitivity of allele-specific PCR facilitates reliable noninvasive prenatal detection of cystic fibrosis. Clin Chem 2004; 50(4):694–701.

75. Chiu RW, Lau TK, Leung TN, Chow KC, Chui DH, Lo YM. Prenatal exclusion of beta thalassaemia major by examination of maternal plasma. Lancet 2002; 360(9338): 998–1000.

76. Ding C, Chiu RW, Lau TK, et al. MS analysis of single-nucleotide differences in circulating nucleic acids: application to noninvasive prenatal diagnosis. Proc Natl Acad Sci USA 2004; 101(29):10762–10767.

77. Fucharoen S, Winichagoon P. Clinical and hematologic aspects of hemoglobin E beta-thalassemia. Curr Opin Hematol 2000; 7(2):106–112.

78. Amicucci P, Gennarelli M, Novelli G, Dallapiccola B. Prenatal diagnosis of myotonic dystrophy using fetal DNA obtained from maternal plasma. Clin Chem 2000; 46(2): 301–302.

79. Gonzalez-Gonzalez MC, Trujillo MJ, Rodriguez dA, et al. Huntington disease-unaffected fetus diagnosed from maternal plasma using QF-PCR. Prenat Diagn 2003; 23(3):232–234.

80. Poon LL, Leung TN, Lau TK, Lo YM. Presence of fetal RNA in maternal plasma. Clin Chem 2000; 46(11):1832–1834.

81. Costa JM, Benachi A, Olivi M, Dumez Y, Vidaud M, Gautier E. Fetal expressed gene analysis in maternal blood: a new tool for noninvasive study of the fetus. Clin Chem 2003; 49(6 Pt 1):981–983.

82. Tsui NB, Ng EK, Lo YM. Stability of endogenous and added RNA in blood specimens, serum, and plasma. Clin Chem 2002; 48(10):1647–1653.

83. Ng EK, Tsui NB, Lam NY, et al. Presence of filterable and nonfilterable mRNA in the plasma of cancer patients and healthy individuals. Clin Chem 2002; 48(8):1212–1217.

84. Tsui NB, Chim SS, Chiu RW, et al. Systematic micro-array based identification of placental mRNA in maternal plasma: towards non-invasive prenatal gene expression profiling. J Med Genet 2004; 41(6):461–467.

85. Ng EK, Leung TN, Tsui NB, et al. The concentration of circulating corticotropin-releasing hormone mRNA in maternal plasma is increased in preeclampsia. Clin Chem 2003; 49(5):727–731.

86. Go AT, Visser A, Mulders MA, Blankenstein MA, van Vugt JM, Oudejans CB. Detection of placental transcription factor mRNA in maternal plasma. Clin Chem 2004; 50(8): 1413–1414.

87. Wataganara T, Leshane ES, Chen AY, et al. Plasma gamma-globin gene expression suggests that fetal hematopoietic cells contribute to the pool of circulating cell-free fetal nucleic acids during pregnancy. Clin Chem 2004; 50(4):689–693.

88. Oudejans CB, Go AT, Visser A, et al. Detection of chromosome 21-encoded mRNA of placental origin in maternal plasma. Clin Chem 2003; 49(9):1445–1449.

89. Okahara G, Matsubara S, Oda T, Sugimoto J, Jinno Y, Kanaya F. Expression analyses of human endogenous retroviruses (HERVs): tissue-specific and developmental stage-dependent expression of HERVs. Genomics 2004; 84(6):982–990.

90. Kjellman C, Sjogren HO, Salford LG, Widegren B. HERV-F (XA34) is a full-length human endogenous retrovirus expressed in placental and fetal tissues. Gene 1999; 239(1): 99–107.

91. Yi JM, Kim HS. Expression analysis of endogenous retroviral elements belonging to the HERV-F family from human tissues and cancer cells. Cancer Lett 2004; 211(1):89–96.

92. Muir A, Lever A, Moffett A. Expression and functions of human endogenous retroviruses in the placenta: an update. Placenta 2004; 25(Suppl A):S16–S25.

93. Farina A, Chan CW, Chiu RW, et al. Circulating corticotropin-releasing hormone mRNA in maternal plasma: relationship with gestational age and severity of preeclampsia. Clin Chem 2004; 50(10):1851–1854.

10

Ethnic Population Screening

Lee P. Shulman
Department of Obstetrics and Gynecology, Division of Reproductive Genetics,
Feinberg School of Medicine, Northwestern University, Chicago, Illinois, U.S.A.

Genetic counseling in women's health care was initially applied, in large part, to the counseling of women and couples pregnant or considering pregnancy, and who either had a previous affected pregnancy or a personal or family history of a genetic condition. Genetic counseling was offered to assess the risk of recurrence (in the case of an affected previous pregnancy) or occurrence (in the case of a positive personal or family history) of that condition in the current or a subsequent pregnancy. This comprised the total information that such couples could obtain prior to the birth of their child.

The 1950s and 1960s witnessed profound changes in genetic medicine that entirely changed the counseling and evaluation of these women, couples, and families. The ability to identify heterozygote carriers of autosomal-recessive conditions such as Tay–Sachs disease (1) by the detection of aberrant levels of metabolites allowed for prenatal identification of carrier parents and affected children. In this way, genetic counseling went from a primarily mathematical risk-assessment exercise using Bayesian analysis to a clinical educational process that could provide specific information for some individuals at increased risk for a genetic disorder.

At this same time, the ability to detect genetic conditions in the fetus by amniocentesis (2) allowed for the aforementioned technological advances to identify fetuses with cytogenetic and certain mendelian disorders. This further altered and expanded the role of the genetic counselor for the woman or couple seeking information about their pregnancy. Subsequent progress in the delineation of genetic disease, in particular the increasing association of gene mutations with carrier (heterozygote) and affected (homozygote and compound heterozygote) states further expanded the scope and accuracy of genetic counseling and the capabilities of prenatal diagnosis to accurately detect an expanding number of fetal abnormalities.

Finally, the development of screening protocols for fetal neural tube defects, chromosome abnormalities, and some mendelian disorders provided the greatest expansion of the pool of potential patients for genetic counseling; now, women and couples with no personal or family history of disease could be offered highly effective screening that, if found positive, could identify individuals and pregnancies at increased risk for genetic conditions and allow for the appropriate offering of prenatal diagnostic procedures.

Technological developments such as complete genomic hybridization (CGH) and microarrays (3) will invariably further expand the application of molecular diagnostics for the identification of high-risk couples and pregnancies and facilitate the application of fetal diagnostic procedures to a potentially wider, but more accurately identifiable, cohort of women at increased risk for fetal genetic abnormalities. However, such changes will assuredly require the development of new approaches to genetic counseling (4), as clinicians will need to present the screening of numerous genetic disorders to the entire obstetrical population, review the screening protocols for their patients, and provide accurate explanations of those screening processes and potential outcomes. Using current practice guidelines, such a complicated and expansive screening process would be difficult, if not impossible, to properly implement.

PRENATAL SCREENING

Screening protocols are applied to populations to identify individuals who should be offered diagnostic tests; diagnostic testing is offered to individuals to determine a specific clinical outcome. Although the integration of molecular biological techniques has blurred this distinction with the ability of molecular screening protocols to provide exact information concerning the presence or absence of certain gene mutations, population screening for mendelian and non-mendelian conditions seeks to evaluate individuals who have a family history not characterized by a particular condition for that condition. The outcomes of screening tests are classically reported as "positive" or "negative" rather than "normal" or "abnormal"; reports of normal or abnormal outcomes should be reserved for diagnostic tests.

Optimal obstetrical care begins prior to pregnancy; a wide variety of issues concerning diet, medication use, and the preconception assessment for genetic and nongenetic conditions should be provided to women and couples seeking pregnancy. Accordingly, assessing the risk for genetic disease is best undertaken prior to pregnancy when the greatest selection of management options is available for that couple.

Fundamental to preconception genetic counseling is a detailed personal and family history. Such a history should identify the ages and racial and ethnic origin of both parents as well as the occurrence of any birth defects in any of the parents' family members. Indeed, the ACOG Committee on Gynecologic Practice, in its November 2003 Committee Opinion (5), states that for those women considering pregnancy, genetic counseling is warranted for those women >35 years at the time of delivery, for patient, partner, or family members with a history of genetic disorder or birth defect, exposure to teratogens, occurrence of consanguinity, or parental ancestry including one of the following:

- African,
- Acadian (Quebecois or Cajun),
- European Caucasian,
- Eastern European Jewish,
- Mediterranean, and
- Southeast Asian.

Once this information has been obtained, the offering of screening or diagnostic testing can be accomplished with counseling provided by the physician or by a genetic counselor or geneticist. Those women who are ≥35 years of age would be informed of their increased risk for fetal chromosome abnormalities; fathers who are ≥45–50 years should be informed of the increased likelihood of gene mutations leading to certain autosomal dominant and X-linked recessive disorders such as achondroplasia and X-linked hemophilia (6). For those individuals with a personal or family history of birth defects or genetic conditions, obtaining records to confirm the diagnosis and facilitate screening and diagnosis is critical, as an accurate diagnosis is essential to providing appropriate screening and diagnosis. If available, obtaining the results of molecular assays that confirmed the diagnosis of the genetic condition in an affected family member is of great value as this can permit a far more facile evaluation of the patient and a more precise assessment of the risk to the pregnancy.

For those individuals with ancestries that are associated with particular mendelian disorders, the disorders that are most commonly associated with particular ethnic and racial groups are autosomal-recessive conditions. Accordingly, the offering of screening to assess whether that individual (who is ostensibly unaffected and has no family history of the disorder) is a carrier of a gene that could place any offspring at an increased risk for inheriting the gene and, if the other parent is also a carrier, at an increased risk for being affected with the disorder, is an important part of preconception and prenatal screening (7).

Table 1 shows an outline of the genetic disorders associated with specific ethnic and racial groups; individuals who have at least one grandparent who is identified with one of these groups should be offered counseling and screening for these conditions, even if their spouse is not of the same ethnic and racial group. For example, the risk of an individual of Eastern European (Ashkenazi) Jewish ancestry of being a carrier for Tay–Sachs disease, a lethal autosomal-recessive condition, is 1 in 30. However, the carrier risk for Tay–Sachs among non-Jewish Caucasians is 1 in 300.

Table 1 Predisposition to Genetic Disorders in Various Ethnic and Racial Groups

Ethnic/racial group	Disorder	Screening test
Acadian/Quebecois	Tay–Sachs	DNA molecular analysis serum hexosaminidase-A
Non-White Africans	Sickle cell disease	Presence of sickle cell hemoglobin (sickledex); confirmatory hemoglobin electrophoresis
Ashkenazi Jews	Tay–Sachs	DNA molecular analysis serum hexosaminidase-A
	Canavan	DNA molecular analysis
	Familial dysautonomia	DNA molecular analysis
	Cystic fibrosis	DNA molecular analysis
Mediterranean people	β-Thalassemia	MCV <80% from CBC; confirmatory hemoglobin electrophoresis
Southeast Asian and Chinese ethnic groups	α-Thalassemia	MCV <80% from CBC; confirmatory hemoglobin electrophoresis
White Europeans and Ashkenazi Jews	Cystic fibrosis	DNA molecular analysis

Abbreviations: MCV, mean corpuscular volume; CBC, complete blood count.

Accordingly, a couple comprising an Ashkenazi Jewish individual who is a carrier for Tay–Sachs and a non-Jewish Caucasian individual would still be at risk ($1 \times 1/300 \times 1/4$ or $1/1200$) for having an affected child. Screening the non-Jewish partner would thus serve to either increase the risk to 1 in 4 (if found to be a carrier) or considerably reduce the a priori $1/1200$ risk, if found not to be a carrier. As no test is 100% accurate, finding the non-Jewish partner to be a noncarrier of Tay–Sachs does not absolutely guarantee that the couple would not have an affected child, but would considerably lower the risk and exclude the need for offering invasive testing.

In such cases where one partner has a mutation and the other partner does not, prenatal testing using molecular techniques cannot be used to diagnose the presence of an affected fetus as testing would only be able to demonstrate the presence or absence of one partner's detectable mutation. However, some mendelian conditions are amenable to accurate assessment by enzymatic assays as well as molecular analyses and thus may be used to assess the fetus in such situations. This may be particularly important for a couple who are both obligate carriers (e.g., have had a previous affected child) of a recessive condition amenable to molecular and enzymatic analyses (e.g., Tay–Sachs disease) but for whom molecular screening is not informative.

The list in Table 1 comprises the most common disorders in women seeking obstetrical care in the United States; however, other ethnic groups may have predispositions to other genetic disorders. For example, sickle cell disease (different mutation than the mutation causing sickle cell disease in people of African ancestry) is relatively common among Saudi Arabians (8) and β-thalassemia is relatively common (3.5% prevalence) in the West Bank Arab population (9). Practitioners should contact a geneticist or genetic center to determine whether a patient of a particular racial or ethnic group is at increased risk for genetic disease and whether screening is available or warranted for an individual with no family history of that disease.

The genetic disorders reviewed below occur most commonly in specific ethnic and racial groups but are by no means limited solely to these groups. Indeed, an overall decrease in endogamy in Europe and North America has already served to reduce the frequency of ethnic-based conditions in high-risk groups and increase mutation frequencies in individuals who may not self-identify as being in a high-risk group (10). Nonetheless, endogamous practices are still common in some communities at risk for certain single gene disorders, making counseling, screening, and diagnosis important for the preconception and prenatal care of individuals from these endogamous communities characterized by autosomal-recessive mendelian disorders (11). The conditions reviewed herein do not represent an exhaustive compilation of ethnic-associated genetic disease but rather provide insight into the role of ethnicity in genetic screening and obstetrical practice. Again, obstetrical care providers are urged to consult with geneticists and genetic counselors to determine whether individuals of particular racial or ethnic backgrounds may be at increased risk for detectable and screening conditions and thus may warrant the offering of such screening.

Cystic Fibrosis

A new model for genetic screening is found in the relatively recent incorporation of cystic fibrosis (CF) screening into obstetrical care. CF is an autosomal-recessive condition that results in thickened secretions of the exocrine glands leading to progressive organic dysfunction of the liver, pancreas, lung, and gastrointestinal system with an average life expectancy of 30 years for affected individuals. Although the past two decades have witnessed profound improvements in therapeutic approaches to the multiorgan failure resulting from the viscid mucus production and has led to increasing life expectancy and improving quality-of-life for affected individuals, many, if not most, children and adults with CF will face ongoing hospitalizations, medical and surgical interventions, and an overall adverse impact on quality-of-life and life expectancy (12).

CF results from mutations in the CF gene, mapped to chromosome 7, affecting the production and function of a transport protein called the cystic fibrosis transmembrane conductance regulator (CFTR). Abnormalities of CFTR lead to perturbations in the chloride channel that alter electrolyte movement across cell membranes and serve to thicken the mucus produced by these cells. Over 1200 mutations have been described, although 25 mutations comprise approximately 85% of mutations causing disease (13). Unfortunately, genotype–phenotype associations are highly variable, particularly in cases of compound heterozygosity when an individual is affected as a result of inheriting different mutations from each parent. The lack of firm genotype–phenotype associations makes for challenging counseling of women and couples at risk for having affected children, especially in situations resulting from different CF mutations.

CF most commonly occurs in Caucasian individuals of northern and central European and Ashkenazi Jewish ancestry. ΔF508 is the most common mutation observed in individuals with CF, and is the most common mutation in non-Jewish individuals of European ancestry, comprising almost three of four CF alleles in this group. However, this mutation accounts for a lower percentage of mutant alleles in other ethnic groups, although combining ΔF508 with certain ethnic-specific mutations has proven valuable for developing highly effective screening protocols in specific ethnic groups. For example, the ΔF508 and W1282X mutations together account for almost 90% of CF alleles in the Ashkenazi Jewish community (13).

In 1997, the National Institutes of Health issued a report of two conferences (1991 and 1997) that arrived at a consensus recommendation for CF screening. This report (14) recommended the offering of CF screening to:

- All couples with either partner having a personal or family history of CF, regardless of ethnicity or race.
- Couples planning a pregnancy who are at increased risk for CF.
- Couples seeking prenatal care who are at increased risk for CF.

Such population-based screening required time to be phased into practice, with clinical and educational counseling and laboratory standards and practices needing to be developed and distributed to all women's health care providers (15,16). In 2001, the American College of Obstetricians and Gynecologists introduced population-based CF screening as the standard-of-care (15) with the following practice guidelines:

- CF screening should be offered to all couples with a personal or family history of CF and all couples of European or Ashkenazi Jewish ancestry planning a pregnancy or seeking prenatal care. Information about CF screening should be made available to individuals of other racial and ethnic groups, with counseling and screening to be made available to individuals of lower-risk groups upon their request.

- Clinicians should identify women and couples who are at increased risk for CF, based on personal or family history or racial or ethnic background so as to offer them CF screening. Counseling and visual educational tools (e.g., pamphlets, videos, and internet) should be used to inform the woman and her partner, whenever possible. Clinicians can use simultaneous (screen both partners at the same time) or sequential (screen patient and then screen partner at a later time, especially if patient is positive) screening approaches.
- Obstetrical care providers should offer CF screening when possible and may choose to provide pretest counseling or refer the patient or couple for pretest counseling. Posttest counseling for couples with outcomes other than negative–negative may pose certain challenges for obstetrical care providers, and referral to genetic counselors or geneticists in such situations can be considered. In addition, referral to a geneticist or genetic counselor should be considered when there is a family or personal history of CF, when carriers are identified with mutations associated with congenital absence of the vas deferens (CAVD), or when an affected fetus is identified.

It should be recognized that negative screening results do not guarantee that an individual does not carry a CF mutation. Indeed, Table 2 shows the risk reduction, but not elimination, from negative screening outcomes in individuals of particular ethnic and racial groups. The degree of reduction of risk with a negative screening outcome will be dependent on the carrier-detection rate for each specific ethnic or racial group. For example, the carrier-detection rate for Ashkenazi Jews is approximately 97% so that a negative screening outcome results in a robust (1/29 to 1/930) reduction in risk. Conversely, the carrier-detection rate by screening for Hispanic-Americans is only 57%, so that a negative screening outcome for individuals of this group results in only a modest (1/46 to 1/105) reduction in risk for being a carrier (16,17).

However, the greatest challenges for obstetricians with CF screening are to obtain the requisite information from patients to properly assess risk, provide detailed and appropriate counseling to women and couples who are at risk for being carriers, and be able to interpret and communicate screening outcomes. All obstetrical care providers should be able to contact a geneticist, genetic counselor, or genetics center to assist in the management of specific screening and diagnostic outcomes, discussion of findings, or for referral in general.

Jewish Genetic Disease Screening

Specific autosomal-recessive conditions occur more frequently in certain racial and ethnic groups because of certain genetic mechanisms. The increased incidence

Table 2 Risk Reduction for Cystic Fibrosis Carrier State with Negative Screening Outcome in Specific Ethnic and Racial Groups

Ethnic/racial group	A priori carrier risk	After negative test
Non-Ashkenazi European Caucasian	1/29	~1/140
Ashkenazi Jewish	1/29	~1/930
African-American	1/65	~1/207
Hispanic-American	1/46	~1/105

Source: From Refs. 16, 17.

Table 3 Genetic Diseases Amenable to Screening in the Ashkenazi
Jewish Population

Disease[a]	Disease incidence	Carrier frequency	Screening detection rate
Tay–Sachs	1/3000	1/30	98% enzyme 94% DNA
Cystic fibrosis	1/3000	1/30	97%
Canavan disease	1/6400	1/40	98%
Familial dysautonomia	1/3600	1/32	99%
Gaucher's disease	1/900	1/15	95%
Bloom syndrome	1/40,000	1/100	96%
Mucolipidosis IV	1/62,500	1/127	95%
Niemann–Pick, type A	1/32,000	1/90	95%
Fanconi anemia, group C	1/32,000	1/89	99%

[a]Emboldened selections represent conditions for which screening is currently recommended
to be offered to individuals of Ashkenazi Jewish ancestry.
Source: Modified from ACOG 18.

of several autosomal-recessive conditions in the Eastern European, or Ashkenazi,
Jewish population (Table 3) is theorized to be the result of founder effect, resulting
from the social isolation of the Jewish community in Europe for the better part of the
first and second millennia (19). In the case of European Jewry, specific gene mutation
frequencies increased within a relatively small population isolated by social stigmatization perpetuated by the development of ghettos throughout Europe. Migration
of the Ashkenazi Jews from Europe began in earnest in the 19th and 20th centuries,
eventually resulting in a high frequency of specific gene mutations among individuals
of that community now living outside Europe, because of their ancestral origins from
those originally small and isolated communities. Founder effect also serves to
explain the high rate of Tay–Sachs disease within the French Quebecois and Acadian
communities, although the reason for the isolation of these communities was geographical separation rather than social stigmatization.

As most Jews in the United States are from Ashkenazi Jewish ancestry, most
individuals of Jewish ancestry are at increased risk for having offspring with one
of these conditions. Many of these conditions are lethal in nature or are associated
with considerable morbidity (19). As with CF screening, obstetrical care providers
may choose to refer individuals of Eastern European Jewish ancestry to a genetic
counselor or geneticist for formal genetic counseling to review the screening process,
disease-related issues, and family history.

Tay–Sachs disease was the first Jewish genetic disorder to be amenable to
carrier screening. As a result of extensive educational and out-reach programs
to the Jewish community, the incidence of Tay–Sachs among newborns has decreased by almost 90% since the inception of screening programs (20). Because of the
increased frequency of Tay–Sachs in the French Canadian and Acadian communities, Tay–Sachs screening is also recommended for individuals from these groups
as well. Initially, carrier screening and diagnosis was accomplished by measuring
levels of hexosaminidase A in serum, leukocytes, and for prenatal diagnostic procedures, amniotic fluid and chorionic villi. However, as advances in molecular technologies began to identify the actual genes responsible for Tay–Sachs and other Jewish

genetic disorders, molecular analysis became the primary approach for carrier screening and diagnostic testing for Tay–Sachs disease and other Jewish genetic disorders. Effective screening is possible using this more selective diagnostic approach because of the relatively few gene mutations responsible for each disease among Ashkenazi Jews, thus making gene analysis a highly sensitive approach to detecting disease carriers and affected fetuses and individuals within this community.

Current recommendations (18) call for the offering of carrier screening for Tay–Sachs disease, CF, Canavan disease, and familial dysautonomia (Riley–Day syndrome) to all individuals of Eastern European Jewish ancestry. However, extensive educational programs in the Jewish community have made individuals aware of other Jewish genetic disorders (Table 3). For those who inquire about screening for these conditions, educational materials should be provided so that an informed decision about screening can be made. When both partners are found to be carriers for a particular disorder, referral for genetic counseling and consideration of prenatal diagnosis is warranted.

Sickle Cell Disease

The term "sickle cell disease" derives from the effect of abnormal hemoglobin on the structure of the red blood cells, which become distorted into a variety of bizarre shapes that resemble a sickle. The basis for all sickle cell diseases is the abnormal hemoglobin, hemoglobin S (HbS), which replaces normal hemoglobin (HbA) when several gene mutations lead to the formation of an altered hemoglobin molecule. The most severe form of sickle cell disease is sickle cell anemia, or HbSS, and results from the homozygous state of two HbS alleles and the absence of HbA alleles. However, sickle cell disease encompasses a spectrum of hemoglobinopathies involving HbS and other abnormal hemoglobins. In general, these "compound heterozygote" conditions result in less severe disease than homozygous HbSS.

The sickled red blood cells lead to increased viscosity, hemolysis, and anemia. When sickling occurs in small blood vessels, the increased viscosity can lead to interruption of the blood supply to a variety of organs, a phenomenon known as vaso-occlusive crisis. These crises result in progressive interruption of normal perfusion and eventual organ failure, causing considerable pain and morbidity for affected individuals. Most individuals with HbSS will undergo splenectomy because of the progressive vaso-occlusive events in the spleen, reducing the ability of these individuals to fight off infection.

Sickle cell disease is an autosomal-recessive condition that occurs most commonly in people of sub-Saharan African origin. It is believed that the frequency of HbS is high among Africans because of heterozygosity advantage. For sickle cell disease, the advantage is the improved capability of the individual who is a sickle cell carrier to resist the adverse effects of malaria (21) and is thus a different mechanism than the one responsible (founder effect) for the high rate of heterozygosity of several other genetic disorders in the Ashkenazic Jewish community. Approximately 1 in 12 African-Americans is a carrier of sickle disease (HbAS and other heterozygotic states with HbS) and one in every 300 African-Americans has a form of sickle cell disease (22). Sickle mutations are also found in non-African populations, although the gene frequency in these populations is considerably less than that observed in the African population.

Sickle cell diseases are amenable to reliable diagnosis by hemoglobin electrophoresis. Solubility tests such as Sickledex are not capable of providing accurate diagnosis as they cannot differentiate heterozygous carrier individuals from homozygous affected individuals. However, such tests can serve as inexpensive screening tests to identify individuals who should be offered hemoglobin electrophoresis. Identifying individuals at risk for sickle cell disease is achieved by performing screening and diagnostic tests in high-risk (i.e., African-American) communities as well as evaluating family histories. For people with a family history of sickle cell disease, hemoglobin electrophoresis should be offered to detect carrier or disease states.

Screening for sickle cell disease is usually accomplished in the physician's office and does not require detailed counseling. As with CF, for those individuals who seek more in-depth discussion of sickle cell disease, referral for counseling should be provided. Individuals who are carriers of sickle cell disease and considering pregnancy should be offered counseling to review the genetics and heritability of sickle cell disease as well as available screening and diagnostic procedures. In order to provide prenatal testing, both partners should be screened to determine carrier status. In situations where both partners are carriers, discussion of sickle cell disease (based on the specific abnormal hemoglobin detected by electrophoresis) and available prenatal diagnostic testing should be provided; however, if only one individual is found to be a carrier, reassurance can be provided that their children will not be affected with sickle cell disease.

β- and α-Thalassemia

β-Thalassemia is an autosomal-recessive condition caused by a mutation in the β-globin gene that results in deficient or absent β-chain production. Such deficiency leads to abnormal or absent HbA. Individuals who are heterozygous for the mutation have a mild form of anemia known as β-thalassemia minor, whereas individuals who are homozygous for the mutation present with a severe anemia known as Cooley's anemia. Similar to sickle cell disease, individuals with β-thalassemia minor may be compound heterozygotes for other mutant hemoglobin genes that can exacerbate the relatively mild anemia associated with classic β-thalassemia minor. β-Thalassemia is commonly seen in individuals of Mediterranean, Asian, Middle Eastern, Hispanic, and West Indian descent (22).

Screening individuals at increased risk for β-thalassemia minor is accomplished by measuring red blood cell indices available from a complete blood count (CBC) test. Individuals with reduced mean corpuscular volumes (MCV) should be offered a serum ferritin test to determine whether iron deficiency is the cause of the low MCV as well as a hemoglobin electrophoresis to identify β-thalassemia and the presence of any other concomitant hemoglobinopathy. Counseling for β-thalassemia is similar to that of sickle cell disease, with couples who are both carriers being offered counseling and invasive prenatal testing in pregnancy situations.

α-Thalassemia results from a deletion of two or more of the four α-globin genes. α-Thalassemia is common among people of Southeast Asian, African, Mediterranean, and West Indian ancestry. Individuals who carry a single deletion are not identifiable by clinical presentation or laboratory values. Deletions of two genes result in a condition known as α-thalassemia minor that is characterized by a mild and usually asymptomatic anemia. The deletions can occur on the same chromosome (cis: αα/– –) or on different chromosomes (trans: α–α–); both genotypes are considered carrier states and increase the risk for severely affected offspring if two carriers conceive a child. Depending on the specific genotype of the carriers, children of carriers with deletions of either three or all four copies of the α-globin gene will have a clinically important anemia known as α-thalassemia major. Deletion of three α-globin chains results in a moderately severe anemia known as hemoglobin H disease, whereas the deletion of all four chains causes Hb Bart's, a condition associated with hydrops fetalis, intrauterine death, and preeclampsia (22). As with other genetic conditions found in several ethnic groups, specific mutations leading to α-globin chain deletions are unique to specific racial or ethnic groups.

As with other hemoglobinopathies, couples at risk for having an affected child may benefit from genetic counseling to review potential outcomes in offspring, the clinical course of α-thalassemia, their risk for affected offspring, and the availability of prenatal testing. However, identification of α-thalassemia carriers is not as straightforward as with sickle cell disease and β-thalassemia. Individuals of high-risk ethnic and racial groups should be initially offered a CBC to assess MCV. As many individuals with low MCV values are iron deficient, measuring serum ferritin levels will determine whether iron deficiency has caused the low MCV value. However, hemoglobin electrophoresis will not identify individuals with α-thalassemia trait. Accordingly, in individuals of high-risk groups with low MCV values, normal serum ferritin levels, and a normal hemoglobin electrophoresis, molecular genetic testing is needed to detect any α-globin gene deletions and thus determine risk for affected offspring (22).

Indeed, the aforementioned hemoglobinopathies are all amenable to highly accurate carrier determination and prenatal molecular genetic analysis; however, utilization of such testing in couples at risk for affected offspring is relatively low except for families with affected members (23). Nonetheless, individuals and couples at risk for hemoglobinopathies need to be identified and offered genetic counseling and prenatal diagnosis regardless of perceptions by the community or physicians concerning the expected or predicted choices of these individuals.

COUNSELING FOR SCREENING

Counseling of women identified to be at increased risk for mendelian disorders based on family history or positive screening outcomes encompasses all aspects of genetic counseling including obtaining a personal and family history, reviewing the specific aspects of the increased risk, as well as those factors that are not affected by the historical, screening, or ultrasound findings. All counseling should be done in a nondirective and culturally sensitive fashion, thus increasing the likelihood that the patient will make decisions based on the available information and her personal beliefs, rather than those of the physician or counselor. Counseling for such women is provided based on the understanding that such testing is chosen not solely for the purpose of pregnancy termination but rather to obtain information to help make informed decisions concerning pregnancy and newborn management. Indeed, each step of the screening and diagnostic processes is independent and does not require preordained decisions to be made in order to undergo that screening or diagnostic test.

Also critical in this process is emotional support, as learning that one is at increased risk for a genetic abnormality can be frightening and lead to adverse emotional responses by the woman, her partner, or her family. In the vast majority of cases, affirmation that neither partner did "something" to cause the increased risk can be valuable and reassuring information for the patient and her family. In addition, some patients may feel that they "have to" undergo or forego testing because of perceptions that it is the "right thing to do." Indeed, patients may feel that their physicians or certain family members or friends want them to undergo or forego the testing and that failure to do so would disappoint those people who are important to her. In this regard, counseling should empower women to make decisions based on their own convictions and to assure them that family members, close friends, and even their physician, despite wanting to have done what is "best" for the pregnancy and patient, do not likely have a complete view of the issues surrounding the high-risk pregnancy and, therefore, should not seek to coerce a particular decision from the patient.

An integral part of the counseling of these women is a discussion of the testing being considered. Gestational age plays a critical role in the decision, as chorionic villus sampling is usually performed in the latter portion of the first trimester, whereas amniocentesis should not be performed before 14 weeks' gestation (24,25). Indications for the two procedures are similar, except for several rare genetic conditions not amenable to diagnosis by analysis of chorionic villi (26). Risks, benefits, and limitations of the appropriate procedure for the patient should be discussed in detail and should include the risk of miscarriage, pregnancy- and maternal-related complications, and the possibility of not obtaining an accurate fetal assessment.

Regardless of the choice made by the patient, all women who undergo counseling should be sent a letter summarizing the counseling session and the decisions made by the patient. Follow-up counseling sessions should be made available to those women who wish further counseling; in some cases, counselors may wish to refer to other professionals including social workers, psychologists, psychiatrists, or other genetic counselors if information becomes available during the counseling that serves to indicate a need for further or different counseling.

Fetal Abnormalities

For women found to be carrying fetuses with mendelian abnormalities, counseling takes on a different perspective. In such cases, the counselor serves to communicate the extent and cause of the abnormality as well as the impact of the abnormality on the fetus and child. In many cases, referral to pediatric geneticists can provide invaluable information to women and couples considering difficult decisions concerning pregnancy management following the detection of fetal mendelian disorders. The need for further testing as well as the availability of pregnancy-management options is usually reviewed with the patient in cooperation with the referring physician. Although such counseling is difficult, it is usually greatly appreciated by patient and physician alike as it can facilitate communication of a spectrum of difficult, complex, and unpleasant information to a woman, couple, or family facing a life-altering decision concerning the pregnancy.

The counselor plays a vital role in helping the physician to provide complete and supportive care to the patient, responding to genetic, screening, diagnostic, and obstetrical issues as well as the need for emotional support during a time of great anxiety and fear for many patients. As anxiety and fear can obfuscate the communication of even simple facts, the counselor best serves the patient and physician by ensuring that important information is communicated in a clear and understandable manner, facilitating the decision-making process, and ensuring that a truly informed decision concerning prenatal screening, prenatal diagnosis, or pregnancy management following the detection of fetal mendelian disorders is made by the patient using the most accurate information and her own ethical and moral convictions (27).

REFERENCES

1. Volk BW, Aronson SM, Saifer SM. Fructose-1-phosphate aldolase deficiency in Tay–Sachs disease. Am J Med 1964; 36:481.
2. Nadler HL, Gerbie AB. Role of amniocentesis in the intrauterine detection of genetic disorders. N Engl J Med 1970; 282:596–599.
3. Pinkel D, Albertson DG. Comparative genomic hybridization. Annu Rev Genomics Hum Genet 2005; 6:331–354.
4. Elias S, Annas GJ. Generic consent for genetic screening. N Engl J Med 1994; 330:1611–1613.
5. ACOG. Committee on Gynecologic Practice Committee Opinion. Primary and Preventive Care: Periodic Assessments. Washington, DC: American College of Obstetricians and Gynecologists, 2003:292.
6. Crow JF. How much do we know about spontaneous human mutation rates? Environ Mol Mutagen 1993; 21:122–129.
7. Musci TJ. Screening for single gene genetic disease. Gynecol Obstet Invest 2005; 60:19–26.
8. Meshikhes AW, Mubarek MA, Abu-Alrahi AI, et al. The pattern of indications and complications of splenectomy in Eastern Saudi Arabia. Saudi Med J 2004; 25:1892–1895.
9. Darwish HM, El-Khatib FF, Ayesh S. Spectrum of beta-globin gene mutations among thalassemia patients in the West Bank region of Palestine. Hemoglobin 2005; 29:119–132.
10. Bittles AH. Endogamy, consanguinity and community genetics. J Genet 2002; 81:91–98.
11. Bittles AH. Endogamy, consanguinity and community disease profiles. Community Genet 2005; 8:17–20.
12. Gee L, Abbott J, Hart A, et al. Associations between clinical variables and quality of life in adults with cystic fibrosis. J Cyst Fibros 2005; 4:59–66.
13. Shulman LP. Cystic fibrosis screening. J Midwifery Womens Health 2005; 50:205–210.
14. NIH Consensus Development Report. No. 106. Genetic testing for cystic fibrosis. NIH Consens Statement 1997; 15:1–37.
15. ACOG and ACMG. Preconception and Prenatal Carrier Screening for Cystic Fibrosis. Washington, DC: American College of Obstetricians and Gynecologists, 2001.
16. Grody WW, Cutting GR, Klinger KW, et al. Laboratory standards and guidelines for population-based cystic fibrosis carrier screening. Genet Med 2001; 3:149–154.
17. Simpson JL, Elias S. Genetics in Obstetrics and Gynecology. 3rd ed. Philadelphia: Saunders, 2003:93–98.
18. ACOG. Committee on Genetics Committee Opinion. Prenatal and Preconceptional Carrier Screening for Genetic Diseases in Individuals of Eastern European Jewish Descent. Washington, DC: American College of Obstetricians and Gynecologists, 2004:298.
19. Charrow J. Ashkenazi Jewish genetic disorders. Fam Cancer 2004; 3:201–206.
20. Kaback M, Lim-Steele J, Dabholkar D, et al. Tay–Sachs disease—carrier screening, prenatal diagnosis and the molecular era. An international perspective, 1970 to 1993. The international TSD data collection network. J Am Med Assoc 1993; 270:2307–2315.
21. Richer J, Chudley AE. The hemoglobinopathies and malaria. Clin Genet 2005; 68:332–336.
22. ACOG. ACOG Practice Bulletin. Hemoglobinopathies in Pregnancy. Washington, DC: American College of Obstetricians and Gynecologists, 2005:64.
23. Bowman JE. Minority health issues and genetics. Community Genet 1998; 1:142–144.
24. Shulman LP, Elias S. Amniocentesis and chorionic villus sampling. West J Med 1993; 159:260–268.

25. CEMAT. Randomised trial to assess safety and fetal outcome of early and midtrimester amniocentesis. The Canadian Early and Mid-trimester Amniocentesis Trial (CEMAT) Group. Lancet 1998; 351:242–247.
26. ACOG. ACOG Practice Bulletin. Prenatal Diagnosis of Fetal Chromosomal Abnormalities. Washington, DC: American College of Obstetricians and Gynecologists, 2001:27.
27. Djurdjinovic L. Psychosocial counseling. In: Baker DL, Schuette JL, Uhlmann WR, eds. A Guide to Genetic Counseling. New York: Wiley-Liss, 1998:127–166.

11
Pathophysiology of Increased Nuchal Translucency

Monique C. Haak, Mireille N. Bekker, and John M. G. van Vugt
Department of Obstetrics and Gynecology, VU University Medical Center, Amsterdam, The Netherlands

INTRODUCTION

First trimester ultrasound offers the advantages of identifying and measuring small subcutaneous collections of fluid behind the fetal back and neck (1), later known as nuchal translucency (NT) (Fig. 1) (2–4). The size of NT increases with gestational age (GA) and fetal crown–rump length (CRL) (5–8). The translucent area disappears after 14 weeks' GA, when the subcutaneous tissue becomes more echogenic. NT is therefore a transient phenomenon (9). This translucent area in the fetal neck can be considerably enlarged (Fig. 2), which is defined as NT above the 95th percentile for the GA (5–7). An NT >95th percentile is strongly associated with fetal chromosomal abnormalities (2–4,10–24), although some centers report less significant results (25,26). Currently, it is possible to estimate the individual risk of chromosomal abnormalities in a fetus by combining maternal age with NT thickness (4).

In the presence of a normal karyotype in fetuses with enlarged NT, there is still an increased risk of isolated heart defects, intrauterine fetal demise, structural malformations, and rare genetic syndromes (18,20,27–43). Not explained are the cases in which a markedly increased NT resolves spontaneously around 14 weeks of gestation (7,44). The significance of this phenomenon is still uncertain. The frequent occurrence of a healthy outcome, as well as the variety of malformations and syndromes found in these fetuses, makes the understanding of the pathophysiology of increased NT difficult.

This chapter describes the different hypotheses on increased NT, aiming to give an overview and comparison of the theories on the pathophysiology of an increased NT. Knowledge of the etiology of nuchal edema provides the opportunity to understand the described association of enlarged NT with aneuploidy and a variety of syndromes and malformations. Furthermore, parental counseling could improve with more knowledge on the etiology of increased NT.

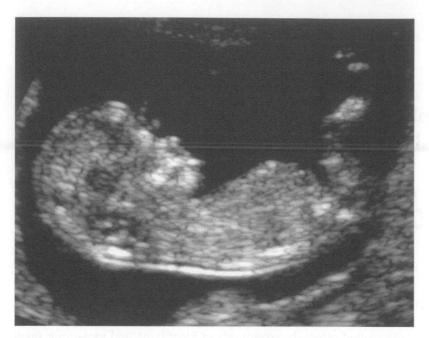

Figure 1 Ultrasound picture of a fetus at 12 + 4 weeks GA, with a normal NT (CRL 67 mm, NT 1.4 mm). *Abbreviations*: NT, nuchal translucency; CRL, crown–rump length; GA, gestational age.

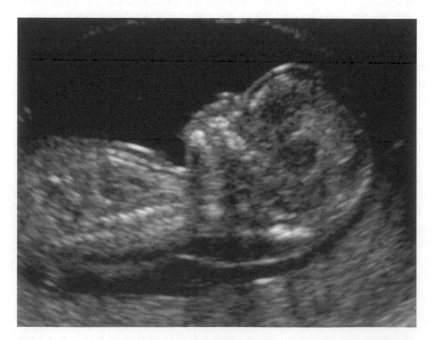

Figure 2 Ultrasound picture of a fetus at 12 + 5 weeks GA, with an increased NT (trisomy 21, CRL 70 mm, NT 4.2 mm). *Abbreviations*: NT, nuchal translucency; CRL, crown–rump length; GA, gestational age.

METHODS

Using a computerized database (PubMed), articles on the etiology of NT were retrieved. The search strategy consisted of the keywords "nuchal translucency" and "hygroma colli." Then, articles on NT as a screening method for chromosomal abnormalities and follow-up studies were excluded. Finally, the cited references in the studied articles were used to find additional articles.

CARDIAC MALFORMATIONS AND DYSFUNCTION

Studies on Cardiac Malformations

Hyett et al. examined fetal heart morphology in a group of 36 fetuses with increased NT and trisomy 21 (45). Twenty out of 35 (55%) had either a ventricular septal defect or an atrioventricular septal defect and the incidence of these defects was correlated with NT thickness (45). They concluded that the frequency of these defects is higher than in newborns with Down syndrome. This overrepresentation of heart defects in fetuses with increased NT was interpreted as a possible causal factor in the development of NT enlargement. In trisomy 18 fetuses, Hyett et al. demonstrated, however, the same frequency of cardiac defects compared to new-borns with trisomy 18 (46). The defects consisted of perimembranous ventricular septal defects and valvular abnormalities (46). In the same year this group published on aortic arch measurements in 34 trisomy 21 fetuses with increased NT (47). In these fetuses a narrowing of the aortic isthmus, which is the part of the aortic arch immediately before the entry of the ductus arteriosus, was demonstrated. There was a positive association between the size of the fetal NT and the extent of aortic isthmus narrowing of the examined fetuses, suggesting that a more severe narrowing produced a larger NT. In this publication, the development of an increased NT was explained as an overperfusion of the fetal head due to preferential blood flow to the head and neck because of the obstruction in the aortic arch. The overperfusion would result in subcutaneous edema in the fetal neck. The transient nature of NT was explained by subsequent differential growth of the aortic arch with advancing gestation, by which the hemodynamic consequences of the narrowing would be overcome. In this hypothesis, however, edema of the upper extremities should also be expected, as the offspring of the subclavian arteries lies before the aortic isthmus. Edema of the upper extremities is, however, seldom encountered in fetuses with increased NT. Furthermore, only 49% of the studied fetuses with increased NT actually had an aortic isthmus <5th percentile.

The same group of authors published reports on cardiac defects and aortic arch malformation in a larger group of fetuses, consisting of 60 trisomy 21 fetuses, 29 trisomy 18 fetuses, 17 trisomy 13 fetuses, 6 monosomy X fetuses, and 21 euploid fetuses (32). These fetuses were all included in the study because of an increased risk of chromosomal abnormalities, based on maternal age and NT measurement. Compared to newborns with the same type of aneuploidy, the prevalence of cardiac defects was higher in trisomy 21 fetuses, but the same in trisomy 13, trisomy 18, and monosomy X fetuses. Narrowing of the aortic isthmus in the trisomy 21, 18, 13, monosomy X, and chromosomally normal fetuses was present in, respectively, 55%, 36%, 77%, 100%, and 57% of the cases. In the trisomy 13 and monosomy X fetuses the aortic isthmus narrowing was, however, accompanied by a narrowing of the ascending aorta, immediately above the aortic valve. This is in contrast to the findings in the trisomy 21 and 18 fetuses, in which this part of the aorta was widened. Therefore, NT enlargement in trisomy 13 and monosomy X fetuses cannot be explained by overperfusion of the fetal head and neck, as the ascending aorta was relatively hypoplastic.

The aforementioned results prompted Martinez et al. (48) to study the flow velocity waveforms in the carotid artery and the jugular vein of first-trimester fetuses with increased NT, to examine the theory that overperfusion of the fetal head causes the fluid accumulation in the fetal neck. No differences were found between the data of normal fetuses compared to fetuses with increased NT. Furthermore, no correlation was found between the pulsatility index of the carotid artery and the jugular vein and the size of the NT. The authors conclude that overperfusion or venous congestion of the head does not appear to be a causative mechanism in increased NT.

Following the morphological reports, Hyett et al. found increased levels of mRNA of both atrial natriuretic peptide and brain natriuretic peptide in trisomic fetuses with increased NT (49). From these findings, they stated that analogous to induced heart failure in adult rats, human trisomic fetuses with increased NT suffer from cardiac failure due to an increase in afterload resulting from the narrowing of the aortic isthmus. In adults, cardiac failure can result in the development of edema, but the fact that in first trimester fetuses with increased NT the edema is restricted to the nuchal area is not explained with this finding. A second molecular biological study did not show any difference in the level of calcium ATPase in the cardiac tissue of normal and increased NT fetuses (50). Calcium ATPase is known to be downregulated in heart failure in adults. The authors state that with these results, cardiac failure has not proven to be absent because the total expression of calcium ATPase in fetal life is already low and therefore a further downregulation would be difficult to detect.

Studies on Cardiac Function

Besides the aforementioned morphological findings in the fetal hearts, several Doppler studies were performed to assess the hemodynamics in fetuses with increased NT. All these studies showed remarkable changes in the flow velocity waveforms of the ductus venosus of fetuses with increased NT and chromosomal abnormalities (51–55). The demonstrated low forward, or even absent or reversed, velocity during the atrial contraction of the fetal heart (a-wave) was attributed to cardiac failure, analogous to the observation in second- and third-trimester fetuses with overt cardiac failure (56,57). The underlying cardiac defects in aneuploid fetuses are suggested as the causal factor for the cardiac decompensation (51–55,58,59). It has been reported that abnormal ductus venosus flow velocities in euploid fetuses with increased NT identifies fetuses with an underlying major cardiac defect (60). This is also supported by the finding that abnormal ductus venosus flow velocities in fetuses with increased NT and a normal karyotype are associated with isolated heart defects or intrauterine fetal demise (55,60). Some authors have even hypothesized that the majority of spontaneously aborted fetuses may have a cardiac defect, suggesting that the same process that causes the excessive fluid accumulation in the nuchal region may also be responsible for their fetal demise (33).

The relationship of the ductus venosus flow velocities (as an indicator of the severity of the cardiac failure) and the thickness of the NT, however, remains unclear. In two studies there was found to be no correlation between NT thickness and the ductus venosus pulsatility index for veins (53,54), in contrast to another study that indeed did describe a correlation (55). In interpreting the results of the latter study, it has to be considered that there is a strong association between NT thickness and the frequency of aneuploidy. The results of this study may have been biased by the high frequency of aneuploidy in the group of fetuses studied, since in aneuploid fetuses abnormal ductus venosus flow velocity waveforms are more frequently encountered than in euploid fetuses (61).

Two publications described longitudinal follow-up of aneuploid fetuses with abnormal ductus venosus flow velocity waveforms with advancing gestation (52,62). In these three cases, both the NT enlargement and the abnormal ductus venosus velocities resolved. The authors concluded the cardiac failure to be temporary.

It is still unclear if the demonstrated hemodynamic changes in the fetuses of the described publications can solely be explained by cardiac failure. The fact that abnormal ductus venosus velocities are also found in trisomic fetuses with increased NT and a normal heart (63) is, for instance, still not explained by cardiac failure. The description of a trisomy 18 fetus with an abnormal heart and an abnormal flow velocity waveform in the ductus venosus, but with a normal NT (1.2 mm; GA, 13 weeks), also suggests that there is no direct causative link between altered hemodynamics and increased NT (64). Low or reversed velocities during the atrial contraction of the heart indicate that the pressure in the right atrium is higher than in the portal circulation. This does not necessarily mean that the fetal heart is "failing" (65).

More recent studies focus on the assessment of the cardiac function by intracardiac Doppler measurements across the AV valves (66–68). Rizzo et al. (67) found a decrease of the e-wave of both the mitral and the tricuspid valve. They ascribe their findings to reduced fetal myocardial relaxation. A major limitation of this study is that their data were collected between a GA of 20 and 23 weeks, with the inclusion of only euploid and structurally normal fetuses. In all but two of the studied fetuses, the fluid accumulation in the fetal neck had already disappeared at the time of the data collection and no relationship between the size of the NT and the e-wave values was found. Furthermore, their findings are not in accordance with the findings in the ductus venosus of first-trimester fetuses with increased NT, because then specifically changes in the a-wave should be expected and not in the e-wave only. Hata et al. (66) studied intracardiac flow velocities in normal fetuses between 11 and 13 weeks. They found a relationship between the size of the NT (<p95) and the values of the e- and a-waves across the mitral and tricuspid valve. They concluded that cardiac performance therefore influences NT size. However, NT is GA dependent, as are the e- and a-wave values (69). Hata, however, did not succeed in reproducing the latter relationship (66), probably due to the small number of fetuses studied. Increasing GA is most probably the explanation why the e- and a-waves are associated with NT size, within the normal limits.

Two other studies compared intracardiac flow velocity waveforms between normal fetuses and fetuses with increased NT, either euploid or aneuploid and with or without a heart defect (68,70). Huggon et al. performed these measurements in a large population of fetuses and found no differences in the cardiac Doppler parameters between normal fetuses and euploid fetuses with increased NT. The E/A ratio was slightly increased in trisomy 21 fetuses but not in the other groups of aneuploidies. Furthermore, the myocardial performance index was decreased in the trisomy 21 group, implying better cardiac performance, but again, this was not found in the other aneuploid fetuses. They concluded that the magnitude and/or the direction of the differences found does not support a major role for cardiac functional abnormality in the development of NT. Others performed a similar study, but in a smaller study population (70). Postmortem examination of the fetal heart was performed if the pregnancy was terminated, to ascertain the heart defects diagnosed by ultra-sound. No differences were found in the intracardiac flows between normal fetuses and fetuses with NT >p95. Within the group of fetuses with increased NT, those with aneuploidy showed decreased e- and a-waves compared to the euploid fetuses. This, however, could not be explained by the presence of cardiac defects, because there was no difference in the intracardiac flows between fetuses with and without a cardiac defect, within the group of fetuses with increased NT. Thus, neither study could prove cardiac dysfunction in fetuses with increased NT.

Another study (71) using intracardiac Doppler, showed regurgitation across the tricuspid valve in the 27% of fetuses with increased NT, of whom 83% were aneuploid. The regurgitation was found in fetuses with a heart defect as well as in fetuses with a normal heart, although less frequent in the latter group. The authors question the role of their findings in the development of increased NT, because the findings are not consistent in all types of aneuploidies which presented with increased NT. The findings were not explained as cardiac failure, because in a subgroup of fetuses without a heart defect, this finding was also present, especially in fetuses with trisomy 21. The authors speculate on subtle changes in pre- or afterload explaining this finding.

An increased heart rate in trisomy 21, trisomy 13, and monosomy X fetuses, is mentioned as a compensatory response to cardiac failure (72). In contrast, in trisomy 18 and triploid fetuses, the heart rate was lower than normal (72). No significant association between NT thickness and heart rate was found (72). No differences could be demonstrated in the pulsatility index of the umbilical artery of normal fetuses and fetuses with increased NT, irrespective of the karyotype (73). Cardiac failure is mentioned as the causal factor in the development of increased NT in a diversity of other syndromes and conditions, such as twin-to-twin transfusion syndrome (74); 22q11 deletion syndrome (75); umbilical cord encircling the fetal neck (76), present in about 8% of the screened fetuses (77); or congenital arthrogryposis (40).

Studies Opposed to Cardiac Dysfunction

Morphological studies and population based studies (30,38,78,79) demonstrate a clear association between abnormalities of the heart and great arteries and enlarged NT. This association was, however, less obvious in two large studies among an unselected population (11,80). The association between enlarged NT and heart defects does not, however, provide a uniform pathophysiological explanation for the development of enlarged NT in the different trisomies and in fetuses with normal outcome. Two recent publications in which the types of cardiac lesions were studied among fetuses with increased NT oppose the theory that increased NT is caused by cardiac failure (65,81). Simpson and Sharland demonstrated no difference in the types of heart malformations between fetuses with and without enlarged NT. Defects primarily characterized by left heart obstruction, right heart obstruction, and septal defects were equally represented in both the group with and the group without increased NT (65). They stated that if increased NT is due to abnormal fetal hemodynamics, it remains unknown why some fetuses with a particular cardiac lesion have an increased NT and others do not. In another study among a mixed population of euploid and aneuploid fetuses with increased NT, septal defects were the most commonly found defects (81). The authors state that this type of cardiac defect is not commonly associated with hemodynamic compromise during fetal life. The high pulmonary pressure minimizes shunting of blood across such defects and thus, changes in hemodynamics are not easily explained by the presence of these defects. Therefore the authors concluded that the increased NT in these fetuses could not be caused by cardiac failure (81).

ALTERATIONS IN THE EXTRACELLULAR MATRIX

The first studied extracellular matrix component in the skin of normal and trisomy 21 fetuses was collagen VI (82). In skin samples of trisomy 21 fetuses, collagen VI was found to form a dense, intensely staining, but randomly oriented network, reaching from the epidermal basal membrane to the subcutis (82,83). In normal fetuses, collagen VI was only sparsely present in the dermis (82,83). These changes were explained by the presence of a triplicate set of the genes encoding for collagen VI, as the genes of two of the three chains of collagen VI are located on chromosome 21 (COL6A1 and 2). The overexpression of genes was confirmed by a later study that demonstrated increased expression of mRNA of the α1 chain of collagen VI in the skin of trisomy 21 fetuses (84). Collagen VI is known to bind hyaluronan, a hydrophilic glycosaminoglycan. The distribution of hyaluronan precipitate was found abundantly in the skin of the trisomy 21 fetuses, in contrast to the small amount of hyaluronan found in the normal (82,83) and trisomy 13 and 18 fetuses (85). Lymphatic and blood vessels were neither dilated nor hyperplastic in these skin samples (82,83). With these findings, the authors explained NT as an interstitial edema, due to the presence of large amounts of hyaluronan, which binds interstitial fluid because of its negative charge (82,83). Furthermore, the authors hypothesized an additional effect of an overexpression of super-oxide-dismutase gene, also coded on chromosome 21, which stabilizes the hyaluronan molecule against free radicals. This would increase the amount of hyaluronan. All the demonstrated changes in the extracellular matrix components were, however, similar in samples of the nuchal skin and in samples of the skin of the fetal leg. The authors explained the edema to be restricted to the nuchal region due to a less close attachment of the skin to the underlying tissues in this area (82,83). A relationship between the severity of the extracellular matrix changes and the size of the NT thickness was not explored.

Following these findings, collagen VI, hyaluronan, and other extracellular matrix components were studied in normal and trisomy 21, 13, and 18 fetuses (83,85,86). Additionally, the skin of trisomy 16 mouse embryos (the animal model for human Down syndrome, which also demonstrates nuchal edema) and normal littermates were studied by light and electron microscopy (86). Although trisomy 21, 13, and 18 fetuses are all known to demonstrate an increased NT in the majority of cases (4,17), the extracellular matrix showed a characteristic composition for each trisomy (Fig. 3) (86). In trisomy 21, the findings were as described in the preceding text. Additionally, collagen I fiber bundles were found to be more widely spaced than in the skin of normal fetuses (86). In trisomy 18, intercellular cavities and dilated vessels were found (Fig. 3). The collagen fibers, predominantly collagen III (encoded by chromosome 2), were thinner and shorter (86). In trisomy 13, the collagen fiber bundles alternate between loosely arranged areas with little precipitate and "patchy," more dense areas with intense staining and excessive collagen type III and VI (Fig. 3) (86). In the trisomy 16 mouse embryos wide intercellular spaces were found that contained precipitate of glycosaminoglycans, resembling the pattern in human trisomy 21 fetuses (86). In the mouse embryos this cannot be the effect of

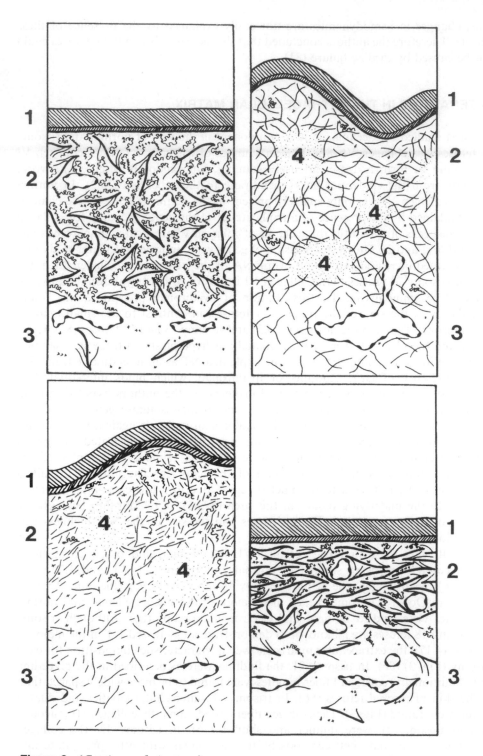

Figure 3   (*Caption on facing page*)

overexpression of collagen VI, because the genes encoding COL6A1 and COL6A2 are located on the mouse chromosome 10. The super-oxide-dismutase gene is, however, located on the mouse chromosome 16.

The authors conclude that the changes in the extracellular matrix components can only partially be explained by single dosage effects of genes on the extra chromosome 21, 18, or 13 (86). A similar study by the same group of investigators focused on the distribution of a number of other glycosaminoglycans (dermatan, heparan sulfate, keratan sulfate, chondroitin-6-sulfate, and chondroitin-4-sulfate proteoglycan) and biglycan (BGN, gene encoding for BGN is located on the X chromosome) in the extracellular matrix (87). Chondroitin-6-sulfate and chondroitin-4-sulfate proteoglycan were increased in Turner syndrome fetuses. BGN seemed to be underexpressed in these fetuses compared with controls. The other studied glycosaminoglycans showed a similar distribution in trisomies 21, 13, and 18 compared with normals (87).

The common phenotype of nuchal edema in all these aneuploidies remains difficult to explain solely by the altered extracellular matrix components. Furthermore, it does not explain the transient nature of the NT. The changed extracellular matrix could, however, contribute to an impairment of cell migration (83,87,88). Many organs receive cell contributions from the neural crest, like the fetal heart, aortic arch, face, and the enteric nervous system. This may lead to alterations in the development of these different organs (83,87,88). The specific pathophysiological relation to the nuchal edema is, however, not yet elucidated and remains to be investigated.

Alteration of the extracellular matrix is mentioned as the causal factor in the development of increased NT in a diversity of other syndromes, such as achondrogenesis type II, achondroplasia, thanatophoric dysplasia, and Zellweger syndrome (37).

STUDIES ON MORPHOLOGY OF THE FETAL NECK

Before the extensive use of first-trimester ultrasound, it was already known that spontaneously aborted fetuses could show cystic hygromas (89,90). The morphology of the lymphatic vessels in the nuchal skin and other organs were already being studied in the late seventies in second-trimester fetuses with cystic hygromas and assumed monosomy X (89) or proven monosomy X (90). Malformations of both the main lymphatic trunks and the peripheral lymphatic system were found (89). Van der Putte as well as Byrne speculated that the development of cystic hygromas

---

Figure 3 (*Figure on facing page*) Schematic drawing illustrating the main morphological characteristics of the nuchal skin of fetuses with trisomy 21 (*top left*), trisomy 18 (*top right*), and trisomy 13 (*bottom left*) and the nuchal skin of a normal control fetus (*bottom right*). In trisomy 21, there is a high number of collagen bundles in waveforms, irregularly arranged and densely packed; there are no cavities; the dermis is thickened; collagen type VI and glycosaminoglycans (hyaluronan) are abundant in the dermis; and collagen type I fiber bundles are more widely spaced than in the normal control. In trisomy 18, the dermis contains fluid-filled cavities and dilated vessels crossing from the subcutis to dermis; the collagen fibers are thinner and shorter, predominantly collagen type III. In trisomy 13, the collagen fibers alternate between loosely arranged areas with little precipitate and "patchy" more dense areas with intense staining and excess of collagen types III and VI. 1, epidermis; 2, dermis; 3, subcutis; 4, fluid-filled cavities; fibrillar bundles of collagen type I [◢], collagen type III [◿], collagen type VI [✗], hyaluronan [𝟛], blood and/or lymphatic vessels [𝟛], free interstitial fluid [∶∙∶∙∶]. *Source*: Courtesy of von Kaisenberg.

would be the result of impaired lymphatic drainage due to malformations of the jugular lymphatic sacs, which results in a lack of connection with the venous system in these monosomy X fetuses (89,90). Chervenak et al. described and defined cystic hygroma in monosomy X fetuses by ultrasound and agreed with the theory of impaired lymphatic drainage of the jugular lymphatic sacs (91). Others link the supposed enlargement of these lymphatic sacs to aortic arch malformations in monosomy X fetuses due to compression of the ascending aorta by these sacs (92). In the skin of the limbs, van der Putte found hypoplasia of the lymphatics or extremely dilated lymphatic vessels (89). Chitayat et al. studied the nuchal region and the lymphatic morphology in the skin of four monosomy X fetuses, two trisomy 21, one trisomy 13, and two euploid fetuses with nuchal edema (93). In this study all fetuses were karyotyped. The results were compared to five apparently normal fetuses. The walls of the cystic hygromas of monosomy X fetuses were lined by endothelial cells. In the trisomy 21, trisomy 13, and euploid fetuses with nuchal edema, the cavities were, however, lined by connective tissue. In the latter group, the cavities were smaller in size (93), which was confirmed by others (88). In the monosomy X fetuses, the peripherical lymphatic vessels were absent or hypoplastic, whereas in the trisomic and euploid fetuses with nuchal edema these vessels were numerous and dilated. Thus, the contradicting description of the lymphatic vessels in the skin of the limbs described in the study of van der Putte can be explained by the fact that karyotyping was not performed in these fetuses and the assumption that some of these fetuses had other kinds of aneuploidies than monosomy X (89). Chitayat et al. agreed with the hypothesis of van der Putte (89) that in monosomy X fetuses the cystic hygroma is the result of a delayed connection between the jugular lymphatic sac and the venous system (93). They explained the generalized cutaneous edema in monosomy X fetuses as the result of peripherical lymphatic hypoplasia (93). In the non-45 X fetuses Chitayat et al. hypothesized the cutaneous edema to be the result of abnormal proliferation of the lymphatic vessels; an explanation for the cystic hygroma was not given (93). The lymphatic hypoplasia in the monosomy X fetuses was confirmed by von Kaisenberg et al. with immunohistochemical staining methods (94). In this study, however, the distribution of lymphatic vessels in the nuchal skin of trisomy 21, 18, and 13 fetuses was similar to normal fetuses (94). Von Kaisenberg et al. attributed the abnormal lymphatic development to changes in the extracellular matrix (94).

When normal lymphatic development is studied in detail, jugular lymphatic sacs are found to derive from early veins, which thereafter become isolated and relatively large and subsequently reorganize into lymph nodes and reconnect to the jugular vein (95–97). This process is completed in human embryos of 10 weeks' GA. It is tempting to speculate that a delay or a maldevelopment of these structures could result in edema of the fetal neck, on the basis of the GA at which this process should be completed, which is the time NT starts to develop.

The development of these jugular lymphatic sacs was studied in normal and trisomy 16 mouse (the animal model for human Down syndrome, presenting with cardiac defects and nuchal edema) (98–100) embryos. Extremely enlarged lymphatic sacs were found in the trisomy 16 mouse embryos (101). The fact that the lymphatic distension presents at an earlier developmental stage than the occurrence of the nuchal edema suggests that it is less likely that the lymphatic distension is a secondary phenomenon to the increased NT (101). Using transvaginal ultrasound in first trimester fetuses with increased NT, the enlarged lymphatic sacs could be visualized in transverse sections through the fetal neck in the majority of cases (Fig. 4), in which

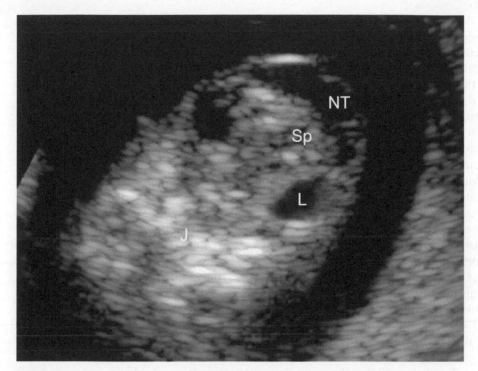

Figure 4 Transverse plane ultrasound picture through the neck of a human fetus at 12+6 weeks GA, with an increased NT (46 XX, CRL 66 mm, NT 3.4 mm). The enlarged bilateral jugular lymphatic sacs can be seen. *Abbreviations*: J, jaw; Sp, spine; L, jugular lymphatic sac; NT, nuchal translucency; CRL, crown–rump length; GA, gestational age.

trisomy 21, trisomy 18, as well as normal outcome fetuses were represented (101,102). The authors speculated that the enlargement of the jugular lymphatic sacs could be the result of a delay in reconnection with the venous system. Further morphological investigation of aneuploid human fetuses and trisomy 16 embryos with nuchal edema showed that the endothelial differentiation of the enlarged jugular sacs is disturbed and differs significantly from cases without nuchal edema (103). In this study, the enlarged jugular sacs occasionally contained blood cells, and the subendothelium of the enlarged lymphatic sac expressed smooth muscle actine, which is normally observed only in blood vessels or the large collecting lymph vessels (104). The endothelium of the enlarged jugular sacs showed an upregulation of vascular endothelial growth factor-A (VEGF-A), which is associated with edema, and a downregulation of podoplanin, which is described to cause lymphatic distension (105,106). Furthermore, the fetuses with increased NT showed an overexpression of neuropilin-1 (NP-1), a receptor for VEGF-A, which is also involved in neurogenesis (107). Interestingly, VEGF-A and NP-1 are also involved in cardiovascular development and could therefore be involved in the development of cardiac abnormalities seen in fetuses with increased NT (107,108). The overexpression of NP-1 is also in agreement with the impaired neurogenesis seen in the heart and neck and ductus venosus region of trisomy 16 mice embryos (109). The authors therefore speculate that a disturbed interaction between vasculogenesis and neurogenesis seems to be a common denominator that links different aspects of the spectrum of anomalies associated with increased NT.

With continued development, the lymphatic sacs are remodeled into lymph nodes and the excess fluid drains away, which explains the transient nature of the increased NT (101). The formation of lymph nodes was delayed but not morphologically altered in the fetus with increased NT (103). At a GA of 14 weeks, the changes in the placental circulation will result in a drop in peripheral resistance that will help to drain the excess fluid. The mechanism leading to the increased NT in Turner's syndrome could also be due to abnormal development of the jugular lymphatic sacs (101). In these cases, the enlarged lymphatic jugular sacs become only partly reorganized and do not find a proper reconnection into the jugular veins. This leads to the formation of a large amount of fluid in the posterior neck region, which is not transient and is called "hygroma colli." This hypothesis is supported by the study of Chitayat et al. (93), in which the walls of the cavities of a cystic hygroma of four fetuses with monosomy X were lined by endothelial cells. These posterior cavities are therefore most probably the enlarged lymphatic sacs that extend to the posterior neck region. It has been suggested that an unseptated enlarged NT may be more representative of a developmental delay whereas a septated or "notched" appearance may represent an abnormal lymphatic or cardiovascular development (110,111). Translucent cystic areas in the human fetal lateral neck were described earlier and were assumed to be the jugular lymphatic sacs (112). A relationship with increased NT could not, however, be established in this study, possibly due to the exclusion of fetuses with septated nuchal enlargement and the definition of increased NT as >4 mm.

To explore if the abnormal flow velocity patterns in the ductus venosus in fetuses with increased NT could be caused by local changes in morphology or development, this tiny fetal vessel was studied in trisomy 16 mouse embryos (109). The ductus venosus sphincter contains neural crest-derived adrenergic nerves, causing contraction and relaxation, which could influence the blood flow. Morphological data of trisomy 16 mice embryos show a thickening of the endothelium of the ductus venosus and an upregulation of neural cell adhesion molecule (NCAM), which is involved in vasculogenesis as well as neurogenesis and effects migration of neural crest cells. Interestingly, the NCAM upregulation was not linked to a specific cardiac morphology. The morphological alterations in the endothelium might explain the ductus venosus blood flow alterations in human fetuses with increased NT, which are also observed in fetuses without cardiac anomalies.

MISCELLANEOUS THEORIES

Venous Congestion

In fetuses with congenital diaphragmatic hernia and esophageal atresia, it has been proposed that mediastinal compression causes increased impedance to venous return and therefore causes venous congestion of the head and neck (31,36,39). In congenital diaphragmatic hernia, the increased intrathoracic pressure is caused by the intrathoracic herniation of abdominal viscera (39). In esophageal atresia, it is speculated that a distension of the blind ending of the esophagus causes compression of the great vessels of the head and neck (36).

In some skeletal dysplasias, increased intrathoracic pressure occurs due to impaired thoracic growth. In these cases, the association with increased NT can also be explained by venous congestion of the head and neck or impaired cardiac function due to the high intrathoracic pressure (113).

Fetal Infection

In a study of 426 chromosomally normal fetuses with first trimester increased NT, maternal serum infection screening was carried out (114). The incidence of fetal infection was similar to the general population. Therefore, the authors concluded that first trimester increased NT is not associated with fetal infection, in contrast to fetuses with second- or third-trimester hydrops, where an increased incidence of infections was found (114). They advised not to screen for maternal infections in chromosomally normal fetuses with increased NT, unless the translucency evolves into second- or third-trimester edema or generalized hydrops. In three cases with fetal hydrops at 12 weeks' GA, due to a parvovirus infection, it was suggested that the hydrops was the result of cardiac failure due to (a temporary) myocardial infection (115). In all three fetuses the hydrops resolved in the second trimester and healthy neonates were delivered.

COMMENT

A complete pathophysiologic explanation for increased NT, encompassing both normal outcome as well as the wide variety of malformations, has been lacking until now. Based on ultrasonographic and postmortem morphological studies in human fetuses as well as in trisomy 16 mouse embryos, it can be concluded that the findings in enlarged NT fetuses can be classified into three categories. First, there is an association between cardiac abnormalities (30,32,45,47,116), abnormal ductus venosus flow velocities (58), and increased NT. Second, various kind of abnormalities are found in the extracellular matrix of the nuchal skin of fetuses with increased NT (82–86). Third, abnormal lymphatic development is demonstrated in trisomy 16 mouse embryos and also in human fetuses (94,101–103).

A pathophysiological explanation for increased NT must, in our opinion, consider and preferably fit in, all aforementioned findings and associations. The link between all three categories of abnormal findings is, in our opinion, delayed or altered development.

The local accumulation of fluid in the nuchal region is best explained by the alterations in the jugular lymphatic sacs (101). It seems logical that a local disturbance of a system, which is responsible for the drainage of interstitial fluid, produces edema in that specific region. The jugular lymphatic system undergoes a finalization of its development at the time an increased NT normally occurs (95–97). A delay in this process explains the local accumulation of fluid in the nuchal region and not in other areas of the fetal body, as the drainage of interstitial fluid of the nuchal area is served by the jugular lymphatic sacs. Jugular sac distention was demonstrated in human fetuses with increased NT with different types of trisomies as well as fetuses with normal karyotypes. Furthermore, it gives an explanation for the time window in fetal development in which increased NT occurs. With advancing GA and the fetus increasing in size, a system that drains interstitial fluid back to the circulation is necessary. A delay in the development of such a system results in edema. It is hypothesized that there is a delay in remodeling of the endothelial system at the time the jugular lymphatic sacs differentiate from the early venous system (101). With continued development, the lymphatic sacs are remodeled into lymph nodes, reconnect to the venous system, and the excess fluid can drain away. This explains the transient nature of the increased NT. The disturbance of endothelial development and neurogenesis provides a link to the cardiac abnormalities found, including aortic arch malformations, as endothelial development and innervation fulfils an important role in cardiac (and aortic arch) development (117).

The interaction between endothelial development and the changes in the extracellular matrix is not yet elucidated. It is, however, not unlikely that an altered environment affects developmental processes that have to take place at that site. The variations in the extracellular matrix between the different types of trisomies could actually explain the fact that some trisomies have larger NT than others, by an unequal effect on local developmental processes, with effects differing in site or extent. An example of such interaction between developmental processes is the impaired migration of the neural crest cells in a changed extracellular matrix, which is a possible explanation of the link between cardiac defects and nuchal edema, first proposed by Miyabara et al. (88).

The abnormal ductus venosus velocities could be the result of abnormal endothelial development and innervation at that specific region (109). On the other hand, the absent or reversed a-wave of the ductus venosus can solely be explained as the result of delayed development. Only few data are available on ductus venosus flow velocity waveforms before a GA of 10 weeks (118). It is not known if reversed, absent, or low velocities during atrial contractions are physiological before 10 weeks' GA. Furthermore, the ductus venosus flow velocity waveforms could be secondary to the increased NT, as the amount of fluid that is accumulated in the nuchal region might have an effect on the blood viscosity and therefore might produce hemodynamic changes.

Despite the numerous publications on increased NT and the frequent use of this measurement to inform women about their specific risk of fetal aneuploidies, the exact etiology is still unknown. Many theories are based on associations and speculations. This study provides an overview of the different theories and an attempt to fit the different associations in one common abnormal developmental process. Further research, however, is needed to explore the etiology of increased NT, to be able to provide an answer to the parents' question why their fetus demonstrates nuchal edema, especially in cases with normal karyotypes.

REFERENCES

1. Szabo J, Gellen J. Nuchal fluid accumulation in trisomy-21 detected by vaginosonography in first trimester. Lancet 1990; 336:1133.
2. Pandya PP, Snijders RJM, Johnson SP, De Lourdes Brizot M, Nicolaides KH. Screening for fetal trisomies by maternal age and fetal nuchal translucency thickness at 10 to 14 weeks of gestation. Br J Obstet Gynaecol 1995; 102:957–962.
3. Nicolaides KH, Azar G, Byrne D, Mansur C, Marks K. Fetal nuchal translucency: ultrasound screening for chromosomal defects in first trimester of pregnancy. Br Med J 1992; 304:867–869.
4. Snijders RJ, Noble P, Sebire N, Souka A, Nicolaides KH. UK multicentre project on assessment of risk of trisomy 21 by maternal age and fetal nuchal-translucency thickness at 10–14 weeks of gestation. Lancet 1998; 352:343–346.
5. Pajkrt E, De Graaf IM, Mol BWJ, Van Lith JMM, Bleker OP, Bilardo CM. Weekly nuchal translucency measurements in normal fetuses. Obstet Gynecol 1998; 91:208–211.
6. Yagel S, Anteby EY, Rosen L, Yaffe E, Rabinowitz R, Tadmor O. Assessment of first-trimester nuchal translucency by daily reference intervals. Ultrasound Obstet Gynecol 1998; 11:262–265.

7. Pajkrt E, Bilardo CM, Van Lith JMM, Mol BWJ, Bleker OP. Nuchal translucency measurement in normal fetuses. Obstet Gynecol 1995; 86:994–997.

8. Braithwaite JM, Morris RW, Economides DL. Nuchal translucency measurements: frequency distribution and changes with gestation in a general population. Br J Obstet Gynaecol 1996; 103:1201–1204.

9. Roberts LJ, Bewley S, Mackinson AM, Rodeck CH. First trimester fetal nuchal translucency: problems with screening the general population. 1. Br J Obstet Gynaecol 1995; 102:381–385.

10. Sherod C, Sebire NJ, Soares W, Snijders RJM, Nicolaides KH. Prenatal diagnosis of trisomy 18 at the 10–14 weeks ultrasound scan. Ultrasound Obstet Gynecol 1997; 10: 387–390.

11. Schwarzler P, Carvalho JS, Senat MV, Masroor T, Campbell S, Ville Y. Screening for fetal aneuploidies and fetal cardiac abnormalities by nuchal translucency thickness measurement at 10–14 weeks of gestation as part of routine antenatal care in an unselected population. Br J Obstet Gynaecol 1999; 106:1029–1034.

12. Hafner E, Schuchter K, Liebhart E, Philipp K. Results of routine fetal nuchal translucency measurement at weeks 10–13 in 4233 unselected pregnant women. Prenat Diagn 1998; 18:29–34.

13. Economides DL, Whitlow BJ, Kadir R, Lazanakis M, Verdin SM. First trimester sonographic detection of chromosomal abnormalities in an unselected population. Br J Obstet Gynaecol 1998; 105:58–62.

14. Taipale P, Hiilesmaa V, Salonen R, Ylostalo P. Increased nuchal translucency as a marker for fetal chromosomal defects. N Engl J Med 1997; 337:1654–1658.

15. Jauniaux E, Brown R, Snijders RJM, Noble P, Nicolaides KH. Early prenatal diagnosis of triploidy. Am J Obstet Gynecol 1997; 176:550–554.

16. Pandya PP, Santiago C, Snijders RJM, Nicolaides KH. First trimester fetal nuchal translucency. Curr Opin Obstet Gynecol 1995; 7:95–102.

17. Pandya PP, Brizot ML, Kuhn P, Snijders RJM, Nicolaides KH. First-trimester fetal nuchal translucency thickness and risk for trisomies. Obstet Gynecol 1994; 84: 420–423.

18. Pandya PP, Kondylios A, Hilbert L, Snijders RJ, Nicolaides KH. Chromosomal defects and outcome in 1015 fetuses with increased nuchal translucency. Ultrasound Obstet Gynecol 1995; 5:15–19.

19. Van Vugt JMG, Zalen-Sprock RMv, Kostense PJ. First-trimester nuchal translucency: a risk analysis on fetal chromosome abnormality. Radiology 1996; 200:537–540.

20. Zalen-Sprock RMv, Van Vugt JMG, van Geijn HP. First-trimester diagnosis of cystic hygroma—course and outcome. Am J Obstet Gynecol 1992; 167:94–98.

21. Snijders RJ, Sundberg K, Holzgreve W, Henry G, Nicolaides KH. Maternal age- and gestation-specific risk for trisomy 21. Ultrasound Obstet Gynecol 1999; 13:167–170.

22. Snijders RJ, Sebire NJ, Nayar R, Souka A, Nicolaides KH. Increased nuchal translucency in trisomy 13 fetuses at 10–14 weeks of gestation. Am J Med Genet 1999; 86:205–207.

23. Snijders RJ, Sebire NJ, Nicolaides KH. Maternal age and gestational age-specific risk for chromosomal defects. Fetal Diagn Ther 1995; 10:356–367.

24. Sebire NJ, Snijders RJ, Brown R, Southall T, Nicolaides KH. Detection of sex chromosome abnormalities by nuchal translucency screening at 10–14 weeks. Prenat Diagn 1998; 18:581–584.

25. Kornman LH, Morssink LP, Beekhuis JR, de Wolf BT, Heringa MP, Mantingh A. Nuchal translucency cannot be used as a screening test for chromosomal abnormalities in the first trimester of pregnancy in a routine ultrasound practice. Prenat Diagn 1996; 16:797–805.

26. Brambati B, Cislaghi C, Tului L, et al. First-trimester Down's syndrome screening using nuchal translucency: a prospective study in patients undergoing chorionic villus sampling. Ultrasound Obstet Gynecol 1995; 5:9–14.

27. Brady AF, Pandya PP, Yuksel B, Greenough A, Patton MA, Nicolaides KH. Outcome of chromosomally normal livebirths with increased fetal nuchal translucency at 10–14 weeks' gestation. J Med Genet 1998; 35:222–224.
28. Bilardo CM, Pajkrt E, De Graaf IM, Mol BW, Bleker OP. Outcome of fetuses with enlarged nuchal translucency and normal karyotype. Ultrasound Obstet Gynecol 1998; 11:401–406.
29. Cha'Ban FK, van Splunder IP, Los FJ, Wladimiroff JW. Fetal outcome in nuchal translucency with emphasis on normal fetal karyotype. Prenat Diagn 1996; 16:537–541.
30. Hyett JA, Perdu M, Sharland GK, Snijders RSM, Nicolaides KH. Increased nuchal translucency at 10–14 weeks of gestation as a marker for major cardiac defects. Ultrasound Obstet Gynecol 1997; 10:242–246.
31. Souka AP, Snijders RJM, Novakov A, Soares W, Nicolaides KH. Defects and syndromes in chromosomally normal fetuses with increased nuchal translucency thickness at 10–14 weeks of gestation. Ultrasound Obstet Gynecol 1998; 11:391–400.
32. Hyett J, Moscoso G, Papapanagiotou G, Perdu M, Nicolaides KH. Abnormalities of the heart and great arteries in chromosomally normal fetuses with increased nuchal translucency thickness at 11–13 weeks of gestation. Ultrasound Obstet Gynecol 1996; 7:245–250.
33. Pajkrt E, Mol BW, Bleker OP, Bilardo CM. Pregnancy outcome and nuchal translucency measurements in fetuses with a normal karyotype. Prenat Diagn 1999; 19: 1104–1108.
34. Hyett J, Perdu M, Sharland G, Snijders R, Nicolaides KH. Using fetal nuchal translucency to screen for major congenital cardiac defects at 10–14 weeks of gestation: population based cohort study. Br Med J 1999; 318:81–85.
35. Michailidis GD, Economides DL. Nuchal translucency measurement and pregnancy outcome in karyotypically normal fetuses. Ultrasound Obstet Gynecol 2001; 17:102–105.
36. Brown RN, Nicolaides KH. Increased fetal nuchal translucency: possible association with esophageal atresia. Ultrasound Obstet Gynecol 2000; 15:531–532.
37. Nicolaides KH, Heath V, Cicero S. Increased fetal nuchal translucency at 11–14 weeks. Prenat Diagn 2002; 22:308–315.
38. Ghi T, Huggon IC, Zosmer N, Nicolaides KH. Incidence of major structural cardiac defects associated with increased nuchal translucency but normal karyotype. Ultrasound Obstet Gynecol 2001; 18:610–614.
39. Sebire NJ, Snijders RJ, Davenport M, Greenough A, Nicolaides KH. Fetal nuchal translucency thickness at 10–14 weeks' gestation and congenital diaphragmatic hernia. Obstet Gynecol 1997; 90:943–946.
40. Hyett J, Noble P, Sebire NJ, Snijders R, Nicolaides KH. Lethal congenital arthrogryposis presents with increased nuchal translucency at 10–14 weeks of gestation. Ultrasound Obstet Gynecol 1997; 9:310–313.
41. Van Vugt JMG, Tinnemans BW, Zalen-Sprock RMv. Outcome and early childhood follow-up of chromosomally normal fetuses with increased nuchal translucency at 10–14 weeks' gestation. Ultrasound Obstet Gynecol 1998; 11:407–409.
42. Maymon R, Jauniaux E, Cohen O, Dreazen E, Weinraub Z, Herman A. Pregnancy outcome and infant follow-up of fetuses with abnormally increased first trimester nuchal translucency. Hum Reprod 2000; 15:2023–2027.
43. Adekunle O, Gopee A, el Sayed M, Thilaganathan B. Increased first trimester nuchal translucency: pregnancy and infant outcomes after routine screening for Down's syndrome in an unselected antenatal population. Br J Radiol 1999; 72:457–460.
44. Fukada Y, Yasumizu T, Takizawa M, Amemiya A, Hoshi K. The prognosis of fetuses with transient nuchal translucency in the first and early second trimester. Acta Obstet Gynecol Scand 1997; 76:913–916.
45. Hyett JA, Moscoso G, Nicolaides KH. First-trimester nuchal translucency and cardiac septal defects in fetuses with trisomy 21. Am J Obstet Gynecol 1995; 172:1411–1413.

46. Hyett JA, Moscoso G, Nicolaides KH. Cardiac defects in 1st-trimester fetuses with trisomy 18. Fetal Diagn Ther 1995; 10:381–386.

47. Hyett J, Moscoso G, Nicolaides K. Increased nuchal translucency in trisomy 21 fetuses: relationship to narrowing of the aortic isthmus. Hum Reprod 1995; 10:3049–3051.

48. Martinez JM, Echevarria M, Gomez O, et al. Jugular vein and carotid artery blood flow in fetuses with increased nuchal translucency at 10–14 weeks' gestation. Ultrasound Obstet Gynecol 2003; 22:464–469.

49. Hyett JA, Brizot ML, von Kaisenberg CS, McKie AT, Farzaneh F, Nicolaides KH. Cardiac gene expression of atrial natriuretic peptide and brain natriuretic peptide in trisomic fetuses. Obstet Gynecol 1996; 87:506–510.

50. Kaisenberg CS, Huggon I, Hyett JA, Farzaneh F, Nicolaides KH. Cardiac expression of sarcoplasmic reticulum calcium ATPase in fetuses with trisomy 21 and trisomy 18 presenting with nuchal translucency. Fetal Diagn Ther 1997; 12:270–273.

51. Matias A, Montenegro N, Areias JC, Brandao O. Anomalous fetal venous return associated with major chromosomopathies in the late first trimester of pregnancy. Ultrasound Obstet Gynecol 1998; 11:209–213.

52. Matias A, Gomes C, Flack N, Montenegro N, Nicolaides KH. Screening for chromosomal abnormalities at 10–14 weeks: the role of ductus venosus blood flow. Ultrasound Obstet Gynecol 1998; 12:380–384.

53. Borrell A, Antolin E, Costa D, Farre MT, Martinez JM, Fortuny A. Abnormal ductus venosus blood flow in trisomy 21 fetuses during early pregnancy. Am J Obstet Gynecol 1998; 179:1612–1617.

54. Antolin E, Comas C, Torrents M, et al. The role of ductus venosus blood flow assessment in screening for chromosomal abnormalities at 10–16 weeks of gestation. Ultrasound Obstet Gynecol 2001; 17:295–300.

55. Bilardo CM, Muller MA, Zikulnig L, Schipper M, Hecher K. Ductus venosus studies in fetuses at high risk for chromosomal or heart abnormalities: relationship with nuchal translucency measurement and fetal outcome. Ultrasound Obstet Gynecol 2001; 17:288–294.

56. Kiserud T, Eik-Nes SH, Blaas HG, Hellevik LR, Simensen B. Ductus venosus blood velocity and the umbilical circulation in the seriously growth-retarded fetus. Ultrasound Obstet Gynecol 1994; 4:109–114.

57. Kiserud T, Eik-Nes SH, Hellevik LR, Blaas HG. Ductus venosus blood velocity changes in fetal cardiac diseases. J Matern Fetal Invest 1993; 3:15–20.

58. Montenegro N, Matias A, Areias JC, Castedo S, Barros H. Increased fetal nuchal translucency: possible involvement of early cardiac failure. Ultrasound Obstet Gynecol 1997; 10:265–268.

59. Mol BW. Down's syndrome, cardiac anomalies, and nuchal translucency. Br Med J 1999; 318:70–71.

60. Matias A, Huggon I, Areias JC, Montenegro N, Nicolaides KH. Cardiac defects in chromosomally normal fetuses with abnormal ductus venosus blood flow at 10–14 weeks. Ultrasound Obstet Gynecol 1999; 14:307–310.

61. Zoppi MA, Putzolu M, Ibba RM, Floris M, Monni G. First-trimester ductus venosus velocimetry in relation to nuchal translucency thickness and fetal karyotype. Fetal Diagn Ther 2002; 17:52–57.

62. Huisman TWA, Bilardo CM. Transient increase in nuchal translucency thickness and reversed end-diastolic ductus venosus flow in a fetus with trisomy 18. Ultrasound Obstet Gynecol 1997; 10:397–399.

63. Haak MC, Twisk JWR, Bartelings MM, Gittenberger-de Groot AC, Van Vugt JMG. Ductus venosus flow velocities in relation to the cardiac defects in first-trimester fetuses with enlarged nuchal translucency. Am J Obstet Gynecol 2003; 188:727–733.

64. Martinez Crespo JM, Del Rio M, Gomez O, et al. Prenatal diagnosis of hypoplastic left heart syndrome and trisomy 18 in a fetus with normal nuchal translucency and

abnormal ductus venosus blood flow at 13 weeks of gestation. Ultrasound Obstet Gynecol 2003; 21:490–493.

65. Simpson JM, Sharland GK. Nuchal translucency and congenital heart defects: heart failure or not? Ultrasound Obstet Gynecol 2000; 16:30–36.

66. Hata T, Inubashiri E, Kanenishi K, et al. Nuchal translucency thickness and fetal cardiac flow velocity in normal fetuses at 11–13 weeks of gestation. Gynecol Obstet Invest 2002; 53:209–213.

67. Rizzo G, Muscatello A, Angelini E, Capponi A. Abnormal cardiac function in fetuses with increased nuchal translucency. Ultrasound Obstet Gynecol 2003; 21:539–542.

68. Huggon IC, Turan O, Allan LD. Doppler assessment of cardiac function at 11–14 weeks' gestation in fetuses with normal and increased nuchal translucency. Ultrasound Obstet Gynecol 2004; 24:390–398.

69. van Splunder IP, Stijnen T, Wladimiroff JW. Fetal atrioventricular flow-velocity waveforms and their relation to arterial and venous flow-velocity waveforms at 8 to 20 weeks of gestation. Circulation 1996; 94:1372–1378.

70. Haak MC, Twisk JWR, Bartelings MM, Gittenberger-de Groot A, Van Vugt JMG. First-trimester fetuses with enlarged nuchal translucency do not show changed intracardiac flow velocities. Ultrasound Obstet Gynecol 2005; 25(3):246–252.

71. Huggon IC, DeFigueiredo DB, Allan LD. Tricuspid regurgitation in the diagnosis of chromosomal anomalies in the fetus at 11–14 weeks of gestation. Heart 2003; 89:1071–1073.

72. Hyett JA, Noble PL, Snijders RJ, Montenegro N, Nicolaides KH. Fetal heart rate in trisomy 21 and other chromosomal abnormalities at 10–14 weeks of gestation. Ultrasound Obstet Gynecol 1996; 7:239–244.

73. Zoppi MA, Ibba RM, Putzolu M, Floris M, Monni G. First trimester umbilical artery pulsatility index in fetuses presenting enlarged nuchal translucency. Prenat Diagn 2000; 20:701–704.

74. Sebire NJ, D'Ercole C, Hughes K, Carvalho M, Nicolaides KH. Increased nuchal translucency thickness at 10–14 weeks of gestation as a predictor of severe twin-to-twin transfusion syndrome. Ultrasound Obstet Gynecol 1997; 10(2):86–89.

75. Lazanakis MS, Rodgers K, Economides DL. Increased nuchal translucency and CATCH 22. Prenat Diagn 1998; 18:507–510.

76. Maymon R, Herman A, Dreazen E, Tovbin Y, Bukovsky I, Weinraub Z. Can nuchal cord cause transient increased nuchal translucency thickness? Hum Reprod 1999; 14:556–559.

77. Schaefer M, Laurichesse-Delmas H, Ville Y. The effect of nuchal cord on nuchal translucency measurement at 10–14 weeks. Ultrasound Obstet Gynecol 1998; 11:271–273.

78. Zosmer N, Souter VL, Chan CS, Huggon IC, Nicolaides KH. Early diagnosis of major cardiac defects in chromosomally normal fetuses with increased nuchal translucency. Br J Obstet Gynaecol 1999; 106:829–833.

79. Moselhi M, Thilaganathan B. Nuchal translucency: a marker for the antenatal diagnosis of aortic coarctation. Br J Obstet Gynaecol 1996; 103:1044–1045.

80. Mavrides E, Cobian-Sanchez F, Tekay A, et al. Limitations of using first-trimester nuchal translucency measurement in routine screening for major congenital heart defects. Ultrasound Obstet Gynecol 2001; 17:106–110.

81. Haak MC, Bartelings MM, Gittenberger-de Groot AC, Van Vugt JMG. Cardiac malformations in first trimester fetuses with increased nuchal translucency: ultrasound diagnosis and postmortem morphology. Ultrasound Obstet Gynecol 2002; 20:14–21.

82. Brand-Saberi B, Floel H, Christ B, Schulte-Vallentin M, Schindler H. Alterations of the fetal extracellular matrix in the nuchal oedema of Down's syndrome. Ann Anat 1994; 176:539–547.

83. Brand-Saberi B, Epperlein HH, Romanos GE, Christ B. Distribution of extracellular matrix components in nuchal skin from fetuses carrying trisomy 18 and trisomy 21. Cell Tissue Res 1994; 227:465–475.

84. von Kaisenberg CS, Brand-Saberi B, Christ B, Vallian S, Farzaneh F, Nicolaides KH. Collagen type VI gene expression in the skin of trisomy 21 fetuses. Obstet Gynecol 1998; 91:319–323.

85. Bohlandt S, von Kaisenberg CS, Wewetzer K, Christ B, Nicolaides KH, Brand-Saberi B. Hyaluronan in the nuchal skin of chromosomally abnormal fetuses. Hum Reprod 2000; 15:1155–1158.

86. von Kaisenberg CS, Krenn V, Ludwig M, Nicolaides KH, Brand-Saberi B. Morphological classification of nuchal skin in human fetuses with trisomy 21, 18, and 13 at 12–18 weeks and in a trisomy 16 mouse. Anat Embryol 1998; 197:105–124.

87. von Kaisenberg CS, Prols F, Nicolaides KH, Maas N, Meinhold-Heerlein I, Brand-Saberi B. Glycosaminoglycans and proteoglycans in the skin of aneuploid fetuses with increased nuchal translucency. Hum Reprod 2003; 18:2544–2561.

88. Miyabara S, Sugihara H, Maehara N, et al. Significance of cardiovascular malformations in cystic hygroma: a new interpretation of the pathogenesis. Am J Med Genet 1989; 34:489–501.

89. Van der Putte SC. Lymphatic malformation in human fetuses. A study of fetuses with Turner's syndrome or status Bonnevie-Ullrich. Virchows Arch A Pathol Anat Histol 1977; 376:233–246.

90. Byrne J, Blanc WA, Warburton D, Wigger J. The significance of cystic hygroma in fetuses. Hum Pathol 1984; 15:61–67.

91. Chervenak FA, Isaacson G, Blakemore KJ, et al. Fetal cystic hygroma. Cause and natural history. N Engl J Med 1983; 309:822–825.

92. Clark EB. Neck web and congenital heart defects: a pathogenic association in 45 X- O Turner syndrome? Teratology 1984; 29:355–361.

93. Chitayat D, Kalousek DK, Bamforth JS. Lymphatic abnormalities in fetuses with posterior cervical cystic hygroma. Am J Med Genet 1989; 33:352–356.

94. von Kaisenberg CS, Nicolaides KH, Brand-Saberi B. Lymphatic vessel hypoplasia in fetuses with Turner syndrome. Hum Reprod 1999; 14:823–826.

95. Sabin FR. The lymphatic system in human embryos, with a consideration of the morphology of the system as a whole. Am J Anat 1909; 9:43–91.

96. Van der Putte SC. The development of the lymphatic system in man. Adv Anat Embryol Cell Biol 1975; 51:3–60.

97. Van der Putte SC, van Limborgh J. The embryonic development of the main lymphatics in man. Acta Morphol Neerl Scand 1980; 18:323–335.

98. Reeves RH, Irving NG, Moran TH, et al. A mouse model for Down's syndrome exhibits learning and behaviour deficits. Nat Genet 1995; 11:177–184.

99. Miyabara S, Gropp A, Winking H. Trisomy 16 in the mouse fetus associated with generalized edema and cardiovascular and urinary tract anomalies. Teratology 1982; 25:369–380.

100. Holtzman DM, Bayney RM, Li Y, et al. Dysregulation of gene expression in mouse trisomy 16, an animal model of Down's syndrome. EMBO J 1992; 11:619–627.

101. Haak MC, Bartelings MM, Jackson DG, Webb S, Van Vugt JMG, Gittenberger-de Groot AC. Increased nuchal translucency is associated with jugular lymphatic distension. Hum Reprod 2002; 17:1086–1092.

102. Bekker MN, Haak MC, Rekoert-Hollander M, Twisk JWR, Van Vugt JMG. Increased nuchal translucency and distended jugular lymphatic sacs by first-trimester ultrasound. Ultrasound Obstet Gynecol. 2005; 25:239–245.

103. Bekker MN, van den Akker NMS, Bartelings MM, et al. Gittenberger-de Groot Nuchal edema and venous-lymphatic phenotype disturbance in human fetuses and mouse embryos with aneuploidy. J Soc Gynecol Invest 2006; 13.

104. Petrova TV, Karpanen T, Norrmen C, et al. Defective valves and abnormal mural cell recruitment underlie lymphatic vascular failure in lymphedema distichiasis. Nat Med 2004; 10:974–981.

105. Nagy JA, Vasile E, Feng D, et al. Vascular permeability factor/vascular endothelial growth factor induces lymphangiogenesis as well as angiogenesis. J Exp Med 2002; 196:1497–1506.
106. Schacht V, Ramirez MI, Hong YK, et al. T1alpha/podoplanin deficiency disrupts normal lymphatic vasculature formation and causes lymphedema. EMBO J 2003; 22: 3546–3556.
107. Kawasaki T, Kitsukawa T, Bekku Y, et al. A requirement for neuropilin-1 in embryonic vessel formation. Development 1999; 126:4895–4902.
108. Carmeliet P, Ferreira V, Breier G, et al. Abnormal blood vessel development and lethality in embryos lacking a single VEGF allele. Nature 1996; 380:435–439.
109. Bekker MN, Arkesteijn JB, Van Den Akker NM, et al. Increased NCAM expression and vascular development in trisomy 16 mouse embryos: relationship with nuchal translucency. Dev Dyn. Pediatr Res 2005; 58:1222–1227.
110. Landwehr JB Jr, Johnson MP, Hume RF, Yaron Y, Sokol RJ, Evans MI. Abnormal nuchal findings on screening ultrasonography: aneuploidy stratification on the basis of ultrasonographic anomaly and gestational age at detection. Am J Obstet Gynecol 1996; 175:995–999.
111. Maymon R, Dreazen E, Buckovsky I, Weinraub Z, Herman A. Does a 'notched' nuchal translucency indicate Down's syndrome fetuses or other adverse pregnancy outcome? Prenat Diagn 2001; 21:403–408.
112. Achiron R, Yagel S, Weissman A, Lipitz S, Mashiach S, Goldman B. Fetal lateral neck cysts: early second-trimester transvaginal diagnosis, natural history and clinical significance. Ultrasound Obstet Gynecol 1995; 6:396–399.
113. Ben Ami M, Perlitz Y, Haddad S, Matilsky M. Increased nuchal translucency is associated with asphyxiating thoracic dysplasia. Ultrasound Obstet Gynecol 1997; 10: 297–298.
114. Sebire NJ, Bianco D, Snijders RJ, Zuckerman M, Nicolaides KH. Increased fetal nuchal translucency thickness at 10–14 weeks: is screening for maternal–fetal infection necessary? Br J Obstet Gynaecol 1997; 104:212–215.
115. Petrikovsky BM, Baker D, Schneider E. Fetal hydrops secondary to human parvovirus infection in early pregnancy. Prenat Diagn 1996; 16:342–344.
116. Hyett J, Moscoso G, Nicolaides K. Abnormalities of the heart and great arteries in first trimester chromosomally abnormal fetuses. Am J Med Genet 1997; 69:207–216.
117. Carmeliet P. Blood vessels and nerves: common signals, pathways and diseases. Nat Rev Genet 2003; 4:710–720.
118. van Splunder IP, Huisman TWA, de Ridder MAJ, Wladimiroff JW. Fetal venous and arterial flow velocity waveforms between 8 and 20 weeks of gestation. Pediatr Res 1996; 40:158–162.

12

Invasive Prenatal Diagnostic Techniques

James D. Goldberg and Thomas J. Musci
San Francisco Perinatal Associates, San Francisco, California, U.S.A.

The ability to obtain fetal tissue has been a major advance in the field of prenatal diagnosis. While most invasive prenatal diagnostic procedures obtain either amniocytes or chorionic villi, certain diagnoses require sampling of other fetal tissues. This chapter will review currently available invasive prenatal diagnostic techniques, emphasizing the technical aspects of the sampling procedures and the associated risks.

AMNIOCENTESIS

Jacobson and Barter reported the first prenatal diagnosis of a chromosomal abnormality from cultured cells, obtained from amniocentesis, in 1967 (1). The following year, the prenatal diagnosis of Down syndrome was reported (2,3). Since that time, mid-trimester amniocentesis has become the most commonly performed invasive prenatal diagnostic procedure. In 1997, the International Genetic Laboratory Directory indicated that as many as 190,000 genetic amniocenteses were performed in the United States (4). Amniocentesis has become the "gold standard" against which all other prenatal diagnostic procedures are compared.

The procedure is most commonly performed between 15 and 18 weeks of gestation. Following ultrasound evaluation of the fetus, an insertion site chosen to avoid the fetus is marked on the abdomen. While many practitioners attempt to avoid traversing the placenta, there does not appear to be an increased risk of pregnancy loss if this is necessary (5). The abdomen is then prepped with povidone–iodine and/or alcohol. A local anesthetic may be used, although this probably does not significantly reduce the discomfort associated with the procedure (6). Under direct, real-time ultrasound guidance, a 22-gauge spinal needle is inserted into the amniotic space and 20–30 mL of amniotic fluid is aspirated. The use of concurrent ultrasound guidance has been shown to reduce the number of needle insertions and to reduce the incidence of bloody taps (7). In addition, patient anxiety appears to be reduced by the use of ultrasound guidance. If bloody fluid is aspirated, a small amount of heparin should be added to reduce clumping of the amniocytes in clotted blood. The first 1–2 mL of amniotic fluid should be discarded to reduce the incidence of maternal cell contamination (8).

Risk

Surprisingly, given the large number of amniocenteses performed over the last 30 years, the risk of the procedure is still uncertain. The most commonly quoted risk for the procedure is 0.25–0.5% (9). The origin of this risk figure is somewhat unclear.

Several studies in the 1970s looked at the safety of mid-trimester amniocentesis. A National Institutes of Health (NIH)-sponsored, prospective, nonrandomized, collaborative study found an overall loss rate of 3.5% between the time of the procedure and delivery compared to a loss rate of 3.2% in matched controls (10). A Canadian prospective study, which did not include a control group, found a similar overall loss rate of 3.2% following mid-trimester amniocentesis (11). A British collaborative study, however, found a higher loss rate following amniocentesis compared to controls (2.6% vs. 1%) (12). The British study included many patients whose indication for amniocentesis was an elevated maternal serum α-fetoprotein (AFP), which in subsequent studies has been shown to be associated with adverse perinatal outcome. The only prospective randomized trial looking at the risk of amniocentesis was a Danish study published in 1986 (13). The study group consisted of 4606 women aged 25–34 years of age who had no known risk factors to increase their risk of pregnancy loss. There was a statistically significant difference in the loss rate between the two groups with the amniocentesis group at 1.7% compared to 0.7% in controls. The procedures in this study were performed with an 18-gauge needle (as compared with a 22-gauge needle in most of the other studies), which many thought might be a factor in the increased loss rate compared to other studies. However, the authors subsequently reported that most procedures were performed with a 20-gauge needle (14).

In an attempt to accurately assess the risk of amniocentesis, Seeds examined the literature reporting all series of amniocenteses that had both greater than 1000 cases and sufficient detail for analysis (15). He found 29 studies (published between 1976 and 2002), which included 68,119 procedures. Of these, 33,975 used preamniocentesis ultrasound only and 34,144 used concurrent ultrasound. Unfortunately, only 10 reports had control groups and of these only four had matched controls. The Danish study noted above was the only prospective randomized study. Looking at more recent studies, all of which used concurrent ultrasound, the excess risk of pregnancy loss compared to controls was 0.33% (95% CI, 0.09, 0.56). Among only the controlled studies, the excess loss rate was 0.6% (95% CI, 0.32, 0.90). The reviewed studies also showed no increase in fetal loss following placental puncture.

A recent report by Eddleman et al. described a procedure-related loss rate of 0.15% in 1605 women undergoing mid-trimester amniocentesis compared with 26,187 controls (16). These patients were a subset of the NICHD's (National Institute of Child Health and Human Development) first- and second-trimester evaluation of risk for aneuploidy (FASTER) trial.

Thus, it appears that the procedure-related risk attributable to mid-trimester amniocentesis is less than the commonly quoted figure of 0.5%, although the exact magnitude is still unclear. Given the fact that there is unlikely to be a new, large, prospective randomized study in the future, this will remain the best data we have to present to patients.

There has been concern that certain conditions may lead to an increased loss rate following amniocentesis. One of these has been the presence of leiomyomata. Salvador et al. in a retrospective study, found no increased loss rate as compared with women with leiomyomata who had not undergone amniocentesis (17). The loss rate, however, was significantly higher than controls without leiomyomas (6.3% vs. 0.8%) suggesting that women with leiomyomata are at increased risk of fetal loss. Another concern has been a history of bleeding and/or of a subchorionic hematoma noted on ultrasound. Papantoniou et al. found a 2.4 times greater risk of fetal loss in women who had a history of bleeding in the index pregnancy (18). There are no studies in the literature looking at the risk of amniocentesis following the finding of a subchorionic hematoma by ultrasound. Several indirect pieces of evidence suggest the possibility of increased risk. These include the increased baseline risk of loss with a subchorionic hematoma (19). Also, several investigators have reported an increased loss rate following the aspiration of discolored amniotic fluid (10,20–23). This fluid has been shown to most commonly contain breakdown hemoglobin products suggesting that past bleeding had taken place (24). The precise level of this potential risk is unknown.

There have been a number of case reports suggesting direct fetal injury following amniocentesis (25–42). Almost all of these reports offer no direct evidence that the amniocentesis actually caused the injury. The true incidence of fetal trauma during amniocentesis is unknown but appears to be very low. It is likely that with the use of concurrent ultrasound, the incidence of fetal injury will further diminish.

Leakage of amniotic fluid following amniocentesis is seen in a small percentage of women. Unlike oligohydramnios caused by other conditions, there is frequently a reaccumulation of fluid (43,44). Expectant management is indicated in these cases.

The Society of Obstetricians and Gynecologists of Canada recently reviewed the literature from 1966 to 2002 regarding the infectious risks of mid-trimester amniocentesis in women with hepatitis B, hepatitis C, and human immunodeficiency virus (HIV) (45). Of 115 hepatitis B surface antigen positive women reported in the literature who underwent mid-trimester amniocentesis, the rate of postnatal seroconversion in their infants was no different than in women who did not have an amniocentesis. All of the infants received hepatitis B vaccination and immunoprophylaxis beginning at birth. There is only one series of 22 hepatitis C positive women reported in the literature who underwent mid-trimester amniocentesis. No infants in this series were found to be hepatitis C RNA positive on postnatal testing. This included one woman with hepatitis C RNA positive amniotic fluid.

Amniocentesis in women who are HIV positive does appear to increase the vertical transmission rate, although the number of exposed fetuses in the literature is very small. There is no data available on the vertical transmission risk of women who are on antenatal retroviral therapy.

Giorlandino et al. has shown that following amniocentesis, the amniotic fluid is commonly contaminated with maternal blood (46). They also reported that the amount of contamination was significantly increased when an anterior placenta was present. This suggests that in women with hepatitis or HIV, transversing the placenta during amniocentesis should be avoided.

Thus, while the literature has shown no increase in the risk of vertical transmission of hepatitis B and C, the number of exposed cases in the literature is extremely small. In women with HIV, the risk of transmission does appear to be increased, although the effect of antiretroviral therapy is unknown. It seems prudent to discuss noninvasive screening options in these women.

EARLY AMNIOCENTESIS

Because of the gestational age at which amniocentesis has traditionally been performed and the need for long-term culture of the amniocytes, there has   been significant interest in developing procedures that could be performed earlier in gestation. Historically, the reason that amniocentesis was not performed earlier in pregnancy had been the difficulty in obtaining amniotic fluid. This was most likely due to the poor quality of ultrasound that was then available. With modern ultrasound equipment this is not an issue, and several investigators have reported their experience with amniocentesis as early as 10 weeks of gestation (47,48). Until recently, however, there had been no large prospective trials looking at the safety of this approach.

Results of a Canadian prospective, randomized trial of early amniocentesis [(between 11(+0) and 12(+6) gestational weeks (days)] versus mid-trimester amniocentesis [between 15(+0) and 16(+6) gestational weeks (days)] revealed a significantly increased loss rate in the early amniocentesis group (7.6% vs. 5.9%) (49). In addition, there was a significantly increased incidence of talipes equinovarus in the early amniocentesis group (1.3% vs. 0.1%). The increased incidence of talipes has been confirmed in other studies (50–52).

Twins

The amniocentesis procedure in twins is very similar to the procedure for singletons. Following ultrasound survey of the fetuses and evaluation of chorionicity, the sampling sites for the amniocentesis are chosen. Most commonly, two separate needle insertions are performed for each fetus. A single puncture technique, which punctures the dividing membrane has been described (53–55). There is concern that this may lead to mixing of the aspirated fluid and/or dissection of the punctured dividing membrane leading to cord strangulation. If the complete course of the fetal membrane cannot be seen, indigo carmine dye can be injected into the first sac following aspiration of amniotic fluid. If clear fluid is aspirated from the second sac it assures that the other fetus has been sampled. In the past, methylene blue was used for this purpose. Studies have shown an increased incidence of small intestine atresia and fetal death following its use (56).

There is a paucity of risk data concerning twins in the literature. Anderson et al. in 1991, reported on amniocentesis in 330 twins and 9 triplets (57). The loss rate to 28 weeks in this series was 3.57%. There was no twin control group in this series. Ten years later, Yukobowich et al. reported on a series of 476 twins, 489 singletons, and 477 twins' not undergoing amniocentesis (58). The loss rates were 2.7%, 0.6%, and 0.6%, respectively. Unfortunately, this series was not matched for maternal age and adjusted for indication for amniocentesis.

CHORIONIC VILLUS SAMPLING

The use of chorionic villus sampling (CVS) for prenatal diagnosis was first reported by the Chinese in 1975 (59). The procedure was performed by passing a small catheter next to the gestational sac and aspirating chorionic villi without ultrasound guidance. The villi were analyzed by sex chromatin evaluation without full karyotyping being performed. Since that report, the procedure has evolved into a sonographically guided procedure performed either transcervically or transabdominally (60). The type of procedure is dictated by the location of the implantation site and the position of the uterus. Typically with an anterior placental implantation site and an anteflexed uterus, the procedure is most easily performed transabdominally. With a posterior implantation or a retroflexed uterus, the transcervical approach is usually easiest. While many centers today offer only a transabdominal approach, there are situations when sampling can only be performed transcervically. Because of this, centers should ideally have the capability of performing both types of procedures.

The procedure is most commonly performed between 10 and 12 gestational weeks. Procedures performed earlier in gestation have been shown to be associated with an increased incidence of adverse outcomes (see later). Later procedures can be safely performed transabdominally (61–64). This is especially useful in situations of oligohydramnios where karyotype analysis is needed. Prior to performing either a transcervical or transabdominal CVS, an ultrasound examination is performed to assess fetal anatomy, heart rate, and to identify the implantation site. The presence of an empty gestational sac, in addition to the normal gestational sac, should also be ascertained. A CVS performed in the presence of an unrecognized empty sac could lead to the erroneous sampling of that placental tissue and result in an inaccurate diagnosis (65). Frequently, by having the patient fill or empty her bladder, the position of the uterus can be optimized for the sampling procedure. At our center, patients are counseled that the practitioner will suggest the preferable approach at the time of the ultrasound.

If a transcervical procedure is to be performed, the patient is put in lithotomy position. A sterile speculum is inserted and the cervix visualized. The cervix and vagina are prepped with a povidone–iodine solution. In most cases, a tenaculum is not necessary but may be helpful in some cases to rotate the uterus or apply traction. A thin (approximately 16-gauge) polyethylene catheter with a malleable stainless steel obturator is then guided to the area of the trophoblast under direct ultrasound vision. The catheter can be curved to facilitate placement. Care is taken to avoid inserting the catheter close to the fetal membranes or maternal decidua. A small amount of cramping may be felt by the patient as the catheter passes through the internal os. No anesthesia is necessary. Communication between the sonologist and the person inserting the catheter is critical for successful placement of the catheter. A 20 mL syringe is then attached to the catheter after removing the obturator, negative pressure is applied, and the catheter is slowly withdrawn. The sample is then aspirated into transport media and immediately examined under a low-power dissecting microscope to determine its adequacy.

Transabdominal CVS is performed in a similar manner to amniocentesis. The insertion site is marked on the maternal abdomen and the site prepped with povidone–iodine and alcohol. A local anesthetic is injected to anesthetize the skin and subcutaneous layers. Under ultrasound guidance, a 20-gauge spinal needle is inserted into the long axis of the trophoblast. Some practitioners utilize a two-needle technique where an 18-gauge needle is inserted into the myometrium and a smaller needle inserted through this needle to obtain a sample. The advantage of this technique is that a second needle insertion is not needed if the sample is inadequate. However, in over 90% of cases, in most centers, a second insertion is not necessary and thus most centers use the single needle approach. A 20 mL syringe is attached, negative pressure applied, and the needle is moved up and down several times within the placenta to obtain a sample. The sample is then aspirated into transport media and examined for adequacy as above.

Risk

The procedure-related risk of pregnancy loss following CVS appears to be the same as mid-trimester amniocentesis when performed in experienced centers. The Canadian collaborative experience, published in 1989, showed no significant increase in fetal loss following CVS when compared to mid-trimester amniocentesis (66). Shortly thereafter, data from the American collaborative series was reported that also showed no significant difference in loss between CVS and amniocentesis (67). In contrast to this, a collaborative European trial [Medical Research Council (MRC) Working Party on the Evaluation of CVS] reported a 4.6% increased loss rate following CVS as compared to mid-trimester amniocentesis (68). Examining the studies, it appears that the MRC study was performed at a greater number of centers and with more practitioners than the other studies. In addition, each practitioner performed fewer procedures than in the North American trials. Thus, it has been suggested that the relative lack of experience might have contributed to the increased loss rate in the MRC study.

There has been much discussion in the literature regarding the association of CVS and fetal limb reduction defects following the report by Firth in 1991 of five infants born with limb reduction defects following CVS in a series of 539 women (69). Four of the infants had the oromandibular-limb hypogenesis syndrome and one had a terminal transverse limb reduction defect. All of the CVS procedures in the affected infants were between 55 and 66 days of gestation and were done by transabdominal sampling. Several other small series have also reported an increased incidence of limb reduction defects following CVS (70–72). The most common association seems to be with procedures performed early (prior to 70 days of gestation), although not all reports have found this. In an effort to further study this association, over 140,000 cases submitted to the World Health Organization (WHO) registry were analyzed with no increase in limb reduction defects over baseline being found (73). Thus, it appears that procedures performed after 10 weeks of gestation in experienced centers carry no increased risk of limb reduction defects.

Twins

Several series have been reported in the literature describing CVS in twins (74–77). There are two issues of concern regarding the use of CVS in twins. These are the risk of fetal loss and the accuracy of the diagnosis. The above studies suggest that the fetal loss rated following twin CVS is not significantly increased. Several studies have reported that there is an increased incidence of inaccurate diagnoses and/or mixed results, which contain cells from both fetuses (75–77). The exact incidence of an inaccurate diagnosis is unclear but appears to be low. This finding will require further studies to establish a precise risk figure.

Technically the CVS sampling procedure is straightforward when two separate placental sites are present. A combination of transabdominal and transcervical sampling can be used to obtain a sample from each site. It is important not to traverse the placental site of one fetus to reach the other. If the placentas are fused, sampling becomes more difficult. Brambati has suggested that by directing the sampling needle close to the umbilical cord insertion site, an accurate diagnosis may be obtained (74).

Rh Isoimmunization

It has become standard practice to administer Rh(D) immunoglobulin (RhIG) to Rh-negative women after amniocentesis and CVS despite conflicting data in the literature on the risk of sensitization. The American College of Obstetricians and Gynecologists currently recommends a 300 µg dose of RhIG after second-trimester amniocentesis or first-trimester CVS (78). Due to the possibility of enhancement, where very low circulating antibody levels may enhance antibody production to an antigen challenge, a repeat dose of RhIG should be given every 12 weeks until delivery (79).

PERCUTANEOUS UMBILICAL BLOOD SAMPLING

The early motivation to sample fetal blood was first for the diagnosis of hemoglobinopathies, which at the time was not possible using fetal DNA. While there are many more genetic diagnoses that can be made using fetal DNA obtained either through CVS or amniocentesis, there remains a place, albeit reduced, for direct sampling of fetal blood to resolve prenatal diagnostic dilemmas.

Fetal blood sampling was first introduced in the early 1970s using fetoscopy to sample fetal vessels on the surface of the placenta under direct visualization (80,81). The risk of fetal loss associated with the procedure was not insignificant (4 5%) (82) as there were difficulties in obtaining an adequate sample free of maternal blood admixture or amniotic fluid (83).

Along with the technical improvements in ultrasound came the first reports of a sonographically guided percutaneous technique to sample fetal blood from the umbilical cord in 1983 (84,85). The report of Daffos et al. described 66 cases that were all accomplished without maternal blood contamination and without dilution in all but two cases. The majority of cases were done for the prenatal diagnosis of infectious or genetic disease. The work by Daffos and colleagues established some important principles of the technique which are utilized today, such as the rapid analysis of the blood sample on an automated analyzer to measure mean corpuscular volume (MCV), thereby, assuring that fetal blood has been sampled. This paper was followed shortly by a report from Hobbins et al. in 1985 demonstrating the usefulness of cordocentesis in the diagnosis of hematologic disease, for clarification of chromosomal disorders, and in the management of other diagnostic problems in the second and third trimester of pregnancy (86). It also established important principles of the technique and demonstrated success in using a 25-gauge needle for sampling in contrast to the 20-gauge needle technique of Daffos. In either case, the facility of an ultrasound-guided percutaneous approach as opposed to a fetoscopic technique was a major advance. The ability to obtain fetal blood samples, with an apparent decreased fetal and maternal risk, opened up many new diagnostic possibilities. For example, fetal blood was suddenly being used to diagnose hemoglobinopathies and fetal infection, for obtaining rapid chromosome analysis, to evaluate fetal hydrops and fetal acid–base status in growth restriction and for the diagnosis and management of isoimmunization (87,88). The technique today is performed in a similar manner as originally described; however, the list of indications for prenatal diagnosis and the overall necessity to perform percutaneous umbilical blood sampling (PUBS) has diminished.

Indications

As the risk of percutaneous umbilical blood sampling (PUBS) is greater than for other prenatal diagnostic procedures (discussed later), fetal blood sampling is reserved for those pregnancies in which the information required about the fetus cannot be obtained by other diagnostic procedures either accurately or in sufficient time. For example, when rapid knowledge of fetal blood type, fetal hematocrit, chromosomes, or infectious disease status is essential for appropriate pregnancy management, direct fetal blood sampling may be indicated. However, in recent years there have been major advances in cytogenetic, molecular, and ultrasound techniques that have diminished the need for fetal blood-based diagnosis. The use of fetal blood for rapid chromosome analysis for trisomies 13, 18, and 21 has been largely replaced by fluorescence in situ hybridization. This technique applied to amniocytes can typically provide chromosome results within 1–2 days. Polymerase chain reaction–based assays for the diagnosis of certain fetal viral exposures can now be made on amniotic fluid specimens. Lastly, increased use of ultrasound for fetal surveillance (biophysical profile and Doppler studies) has reduced the need for direct fetal blood assessment of fetal acid–base status.

Nonetheless, it is clear that fetal blood sampling has played a major role in prenatal diagnosis. It remains the method of choice for diagnosis and therapeutic intervention for erythroblastosis fetalis. In many perinatal centers, fetal platelet count is assessed by PUBS in cases of alloimmune thrombocytopenia and in idiopathic thrombocytopenia purpura. In certain cases of fetal chromosome mosaicism detected in cultured amniocytes or chorionic villi, it remains useful for direct cytogenetic analysis of uncultured fetal nucleated blood cells or short-term fetal lymphocytes (89,90). This can be particularly useful when fetal structural abnormalities are detected late in the second trimester of pregnancy and knowledge of fetal karyotype would have implications for parental decision making or in late third trimester for decisions regarding delivery.

Technique

Although the procedure is similar to an amniocentesis, it requires a high-level of physician's expertise and a support team facile with the handling and analysis of fetal blood. PUBS is generally performed beginning in the mid-second–trimester and beyond. There have been reports of first-trimester percutaneous blood sampling but the number of cases are relatively few to obtain clear data with regard to safety and efficacy (91).

An initial ultrasound examination is performed to visualize the cord, its fetal and placental insertion sites, and precise location of the placenta. The skin of the abdomen is then prepped with povidone–iodine solution and draped in a sterile manner consistent with amniocentesis. The skin insertion site is typically infiltrated with approximately 5 mL of 1% lidocaine or a mixture of lidocaine and sodium bicarbonate. The basic approach taken by most practitioners is to insert a spinal needle (the largest being a 22-gauge, and most often 25-gauge) under direct ultrasound visualization into the umbilical vein, most often where it inserts into the placenta and is least mobile. Once entry into the umbilical vein is established, the obturator of the spinal needle is removed and a small amount of blood is aspirated using a small volume syringe (3 or 5 mL). An automated blood cell analyzer can be used to rapidly assess blood cell volume of the sample for the presence of fetal erythrocytes. In order to confirm that the sample is fetal in origin, the MCV of the sample is determined and should be >100 mL. After this initial sample is drawn, a new syringe is placed on the needle and the diagnostic sample is aspirated. Once an adequate sample is obtained, the needle is withdrawn and the fetal status is directly observed by ultrasound. While fetal blood has been aspirated from the umbilical artery, the umbilical vein is preferred because it is larger and is less likely to constrict and cause a fetal bradycardia when punctured.

A brief period of fetal monitoring is usually performed. For pregnancies in the early third trimester and beyond, a longer period of fetal surveillance is recommended. This should be done in a location near the delivery suite where severe fetal heart rate abnormalities can be dealt with either by external resuscitation methods (maternal oxygen, intravenous fluids, and position change) or by expedient delivery. It should be remembered that transient fetal bradycardia is a common finding during and immediately after cordocentesis.

Risks

Although there have been no data to demonstrate that the risk of fetal loss from PUBS is definitely related to the number of prior procedures a given operator has performed, there appears to be general agreement based on suggestive evidence that an important factor related to the overall safety of the procedure is operator experience (92). To date, there have been no studies done directly comparing loss rates in patients undergoing PUBS to an appropriate control group. However, in the first large series published, the reported loss rate based on 606 consecutive cases was 2%, which included a 0.8% spontaneous abortion rate (fetal loss before 28 weeks gestation) and a 1.1% in utero death rate (93).Other series have reported higher rates, especially those with a smaller overall number of procedures (94). However, fetuses with ultrasound structural abnormalities, metabolic disease, or karyotypic abnormalities appear to fair worse overall (95). The only comprehensive review of the complications of fetal blood sampling was reported in 1993, by Ghidini et al. (92). In this review, the authors compiled all reports from the English language literature up until 1992 and tabulated loss rates for low-risk patients from series reporting >100 cases. Data from six reports between 1985 and 1991 were combined resulting in a "total fetal loss" rate of 2.7%, with equal numbers before and after 28 weeks. In more recently published guidelines, the procedure-related loss rate, taking into account all indications, is reported to be <2% (96).

The list of complications that have been reported to be associated with PUBS include fetal death, chorioamnionitis, fetal bradycardia (either transient or persistent), bleeding from the puncture site in the umbilical cord, umbilical cord hematomas, fetomaternal hemorrhage, and abruptio placenta. Bleeding from the cord puncture site is the most common complication and is usually self-limited. Factors postulated to affect the duration of bleeding after cord puncture are needle size, fetal platelet count, and whether the artery or vein was punctured (97). Some reports have found significant correlation between fetal platelet count and incidence and duration of postpuncture bleeding (97,98), while others have found none (99). Paidas et al. reported on a number of cases of fetal exsanguination following cordocentesis for alloimmune thrombocytopenia (98). These fetuses had significantly reduced platelet counts compared to surviving control cases.

A reduction in the incidence of bleeding has been reported with the use of a 25-gauge needle rather than a 20-gauge needle, which was the way the technique was originally described (84,100). Bleeding from the puncture site is typically short-lived and the majority of cases last <60 seconds; published reports have documented bleeding nearly twice that long (97). The duration of bleeding has been demonstrated to be longer following umbilical artery puncture compared with sampling the umbilical vein (99). Nevertheless, exsanguinations have been responsible for fetal losses in a number of reports and must be regarded as a potential complication and given appropriate attention in postprocedure surveillance (93). Most reports of persistent bleeding describe fetal bradycardia as the primary clinical sign (98,99); however, persistent fetal tachycardia after funipuncture, without a preceding fetal bradycardia, has been reported (101).

FETAL TISSUE BIOPSY

Muscle Biopsy

Percutaneous fetal muscle biopsy is a rare procedure reserved for the definitive diagnosis of genetic myopathies that are not amenable to diagnosis by direct DNA analysis (102). Since the cloning and characterization of the dystrophin gene in 1987 (103), prenatal diagnosis of Duchenne muscular dystrophy for high-risk families has been in large part successful using deletion analysis or linkage analysis on DNA isolated from either amniocytes or chorionic villi (104,105). However, in rare cases molecular methods fail to provide a definitive diagnosis, or a rare myopathy may require direct mitochondrial analysis (102,106). In these cases, fetal muscle biopsy may serve as a useful diagnostic option. The technique involves ultrasound-guided percutaneous placement of a suitable biopsy needle. The biopsy needle is most commonly directed into the fetal gluteal muscle. This requires an experienced operator, support team, and pathologist with particular interest in this procedure (102,107,108).

Fetal Skin Biopsy

As with umbilical blood sampling, fetoscopy was initially used to obtain fetal skin to diagnose hereditary skin disorders (109). These disorders, often called genodermatoses, are not always amenable to diagnosis using fetal DNA derived from amniocytes or chorionic villi. The fetal skin biopsy technique has been described in detail by Elias et al. and essentially involves a similar approach as is done with PUBS (110).

Indications

The number of genetic skin disorders that can be diagnosed by direct fetal DNA analysis has increased over recent years. With advances in molecular technology, informatics, and progress with the human genome project, the molecular basis of over 60% of genodermatoses have been elucidated (111). The prototypic disease, epidermolysis bullosa, is a clinically and genetically diverse group of heritable mechanobullous disorders. This disorder, in its severe form, most often results in early prenatal demise and until the early 1990s could only be characterized by microscopy (111,112). Congenital ichthyosis, a severe, generally lethal disorder, can be definitively diagnosed prenatally in high-risk families only by fetal skin biopsy. However, even in this disorder, imaging of the associated facial dysmorphic features using three-dimensional ultrasound has been reported to be diagnostic and may obviate the need for an invasive procedure in some cases (113). Clearly, the indications for the procedure have diminished considerably in recent years and there are few reports in the literature since 1994.

Other Tissues

Biopsy of the fetal liver has been used to diagnose suspected cases of inborn metabolic disorders for which direct analysis of fetal DNA was not diagnostic. In these cases, enzymatic analysis has been performed on fetal liver cells (114). However, as the mutations and deletions in genes responsible for these disorders have been elucidated, the need for direct liver analysis has diminished greatly.

In certain suspected fetal conditions, there is no genetic lesion but simply a histologic abnormality that requires microscopic diagnosis. As an example, congenital nephrosis is one disorder that has been reported to be accurately diagnosed in utero by histologic analysis of a fetal kidney biopsy (115). In the reported case, the combination of an elevated amniotic fluid AFP, negative acetylcholinesterase, and a negative ultrasound examination was investigated by direct fetal kidney biopsy resulting in a definitive diagnosis. These interventions, biopsy of fetal liver or kidney, hold a small place in the diagnostic armamentarium of the prenatal geneticist. However, in rare cases, they may help to resolve diagnostic dilemmas for high-risk families with a history of a previous affected child. These procedures should only be performed by centers with special expertise in invasive fetal biopsy techniques.

REFERENCES

1. Jacobson CB, Barter RH. Intrauterine diagnosis and management of genetic defects. Am J Obstet Gynecol 1967; 99(6):796–807.
2. Nadler HL. Antenatal detection of hereditary disorders. Pediatrics 1968; 42(6):912–918.
3. Valenti C, Schutta EJ, Kehaty T. Prenatal diagnosis of Down's syndrome. Lancet 1968; 2(7561):220.
4. Association of Genetic Technologists. International Genetic Laboratory Directory. Lenexa, KS: Association of Genetic Technologists, 1998.
5. Bombard AT, Powers JF, Carter S, Schwartz A, Nitowsky HM. Procedure-related fetal losses in transplacental versus nontransplacental genetic amniocentesis. Am J Obstet Gynecol 1995; 172(3):868–872.
6. Van Schoubroeck D, Verhaeghe J. Does local anesthesia at mid-trimester amniocentesis decrease pain experience? A randomized trial in 220 patients. Ultrasound Obstet Gynecol 2000; 16(6):536–538.
7. Romero R, Jeanty P, Reece EA, et al. Sonographically monitored amniocentesis to decrease intraoperative complications. Obstet Gynecol 1985; 65(3):426–430.
8. ACMG. Standards and Guidelines for Clinical Genetics Laboratories. 3rd ed. Bethesda, MD: American College of Medical Genetics, 2002.
9. Olney RS, Moore CA, Khoury MJ, et al. Chroionic villus sampling and amniocentesis: recommendations for prenatal counseling. MMWR Morb Mortal Wkly Rep 1995; 44(RR-9):1–12.
10. Midtrimester amniocentesis for prenatal diagnosis. Safety and accuracy. J Am Med Assoc 1976; 236(13):1471–1476.
11. Simpson NE, Dallaire L, Miller JR, et al. Prenatal diagnosis of genetic disease in Canada: report of a collaborative study. Can Med Assoc J 1976; 115(8):739–748.
12. An assessment of the hazards of amniocentesis. Report to the Medical Research Council by their Working Party on Amniocentesis. Br J Obstet Gynaecol 1978; 85(Suppl 2):1–41.
13. Tabor A, Philip J, Madsen M, Bang J, Obel EB, Norgaard-Pedersen B. Randomised controlled trial of genetic amniocentesis in 4606 low-risk women. Lancet 1986; 1(8493):1287–1293.
14. Tabor A, Philip J, Bang J, Madsen M, Obel EB, Norgaard-Pedersen B. Needle size and risk of miscarriage after amniocentesis. Lancet 1988; 1(8578):183–184.
15. Seeds JW. Diagnostic mid trimester amniocentesis: how safe? Am J Obstet Gynecol 2004; 191(2):607–615.
16. Eddleman K, Berkowitz R, Kharbutli Y, et al. Pregnancy loss rates after midtrimester amniocentesis: the faster trial. Am J Obstet Gynecol 2003; 189:S111.
17. Salvador E, Bienstock J, Blakemore KJ, Pressman E. Leiomyomata uteri, genetic amniocentesis, and the risk of second-trimester spontaneous abortion. Am J Obstet Gynecol 2002; 186(5):913–915.

18. Papantoniou NE, Daskalakis GJ, Tziotis JG, Kitmirides SJ, Mesogitis SA, Antsaklis AJ. Risk factors predisposing to fetal loss following a second trimester amniocentesis. Br J Obstet Gynecol 2001; 108(10):1053–1056.

19. Borlum KG, Thomsen A, Clausen I, Eriksen G. Long-term prognosis of pregnancies in women with intrauterine hematomas. Obstet Gynecol 1989; 74(2):231–233.

20. Golbus MS, Loughman WD, Epstein CJ, Halbasch G, Stephens JD, Hall BD. Prenatal genetic diagnosis in 3000 amniocenteses. N Engl J Med 1979; 300(4):157–163.

21. Dacus JV, Wilroy RS, Summitt RL, et al. Genetic amniocentesis: a twelve years' experience. Am J Med Genet 1985; 20(3):443–452.

22. Karp LE, Schiller HS. Meconium staining of amniotic fluid at midtrimester amniocentesis. Obstet Gynecol 1977; 50(1 Suppl):47S–49S.

23. Zorn EM, Hanson FW, Greve LC, Phelps-Sandall B, Tennant FR. Analysis of the significance of discolored amniotic fluid detected at midtrimester amniocentesis. Am J Obstet Gynecol 1986; 154(6):1234–1240.

24. Hankins GD, Rowe J, Quirk JG Jr, Trubey R, Strickland DM. Significance of brown and/or green amniotic fluid at the time of second trimester genetic amniocentesis. Obstet Gynecol 1984; 64(3):353–358.

25. Young PE, Matson MR, Jones OW. Fetal exsanguination and other vascular injuries from midtrimester genetic amniocentesis. Am J Obstet Gynecol 1977; 129(1):21–24.

26. Broome DL, Wilson MG, Weiss B, Kellogg B. Needle puncture of fetus: a complication of second-trimester amniocentesis. Am J Obstet Gynecol 1976; 126(2):247–252.

27. Karp LE, Hayden PW. Fetal puncture during midtrimester amniocentesis. Obstet Gynecol 1977; 49(1):115–117.

28. Gillberg C, Rasmussen P, Wahlstrom J. Long-term follow-up of children born to women who had amniocentesis. Lancet 1979; 1(8130):1341.

29. Epley SL, Hanson JW, Cruikshank DP. Fetal injury with midtrimester diagnostic amniocentesis. Obstet Gynecol 1979; 53(1):77–80.

30. Swift PG, Driscoll IB, Vowles KD. Neonatal small-bowel obstruction associated with amniocentesis. Br Med J 1979; 1(6165):720.

31. Merin S, Beyth Y. Uniocular congenital blindness as a complication of midtrimester amniocentesis. Am J Ophthalmol 1980; 89(2):299–301.

32. Youroukos S, Papadelis F, Matsaniotis N. Porencephalic cysts after amniocentesis. Arch Dis Child 1980; 55(10):814 815.

33. Therkelsen AJ, Rehder H. Intestinal atresia caused by second trimester amniocentesis. Case report. Br J Obstet Gynaecol 1981; 88(5):559–562.

34. Stock RJ. Fetal death secondary to needle laceration during 2nd trimester amniocentesis: a case report. Prenat Diagn 1982; 2(2):133–137.

35. Bruce S, Duffy JO, Wolf JE Jr. Skin dimpling associated with midtrimester amniocentesis. Pediatr Dermatol 1984; 2(2):140–142.

36. Raimer SS, Raimer BG. Needle puncture scars from midtrimester amniocentesis. Arch Dermatol 1984; 120(10):1360–1362.

37. Finegan JA, Quarrington BJ, Hughes HE, et al. Infant outcome following mid-trimester amniocentesis: development and physical status at age six months. Br J Obstet Gynaecol 1985; 92(10):1015–1023.

38. Admoni MM, BenEzra D. Ocular trauma following amniocentesis as the cause of leukocoria. J Pediatr Ophthalmol Strabismus 1988; 25(4):196–197.

39. BenEzra D, Sela M, Peer J. Bilateral anophthalmia and unilateral microphthalmia in two siblings. Ophthalmologica 1989; 198(3):140–144.

40. Chong SK, Levitt GA, Lawson J, Lloyd U, Newman CG. Subarachnoid cyst with hydrocephalus—a complication of mid-trimester amniocentesis. Prenat Diagn 1989; 9(9):677–679.

41. Eller KM, Kuller JA. Porencephaly secondary to fetal trauma during amniocentesis. Obstet Gynecol 1995; 85(5, Pt 2):865–867.

42. Raymond GV. Rare neurologic injury from amniocentesis. Birth Defects Res A Clin Mol Teratol 2003; 67(3):205–206.

43. Simpson JL, Socol ML, Aladjem S, Elias S. Normal fetal growth despite persistent amniotic fluid leakage after genetic amniocentesis. Prenat Diagn 1981; 1(4):277–279.

44. Crane JP, Rohland BM. Clinical significance of persistent amniotic fluid leakage after genetic amniocentesis. Prenat Diagn 1986; 6(1):25–31.

45. Davies G, Wilson RD, Desilets V, et al. Amniocentesis and women with hepatitis B, hepatitis C, or human immunodeficiency virus. J Obstet Gynaecol Can 2003; 25(2):145–148 (see also 149–152).

46. Giorlandino C, Gambuzza G, D'Alessio P, Santoro ML, Gentili P, Vizzone A. Blood contamination of amniotic fluid after amniocentesis in relation to placental location. Prenat Diagn 1996; 16(2):180–182.

47. Diaz Vega M, De La Cueva P, Leal C, Aisa F. Early amniocentesis at 10–12 weeks' gestation. Prenat Diagn 1996; 16(4):307–312.

48. Hanson FW, Tennant F, Hune S, Brookhyser K. Early amniocentesis: outcome, risks, and technical problems at less than or equal to 12.8 weeks. Am J Obstet Gynecol 1992; 166(6, Pt 1):1707–1711.

49. Randomised trial to assess safety and fetal outcome of early and midtrimester amniocentesis. The Canadian Early and Mid-trimester Amniocentesis Trial (CEMAT) Group. Lancet 1998; 351(9098):242–247.

50. Nicolaides K, Brizot Mde L, Patel F, Snijders R. Comparison of chorionic villus sampling and amniocentesis for fetal karyotyping at 10–13 weeks' gestation. Lancet 1994; 344(8920):435–439.

51. Philip J, Silver RK, Wilson RD, et al. Late first-trimester invasive prenatal diagnosis: results of an international randomized trial. Obstet Gynecol 2004; 103(6):1164–1173.

52. Sundberg K, Bang J, Smidt-Jensen S, et al. Randomised study of risk of fetal loss related to early amniocentesis versus chorionic villus sampling. Lancet 1997; 350(9079):697–703.

53. Buscaglia M, Ghisoni L, Bellotti M, et al. Genetic amniocentesis in biamniotic twin pregnancies by a single transabdominal insertion of the needle. Prenat Diagn 1995; 15(1):17–19.

54. Jeanty P, Shah D, Roussis P. Single-needle insertion in twin amniocentesis. J Ultrasound Med 1990; 9(9):511–517.

55. van Vugt JM, Nieuwint A, van Geijn HP. Single-needle insertion: an alternative technique for early second-trimester genetic twin amniocentesis. Fetal Diagn Ther 1995; 10(3):178–181.

56. Kidd SA, Lancaster PA, Anderson JC, et al. Fetal death after exposure to methylene blue dye during mid-trimester amniocentesis in twin pregnancy. Prenat Diagn 1996; 16(1):39–47.

57. Anderson RL, Goldberg JD, Golbus MS. Prenatal diagnosis in multiple gestation: 20 years' experience with amniocentesis. Prenat Diagn 1991; 11(4):263–270.

58. Yukobowich E, Anteby EY, Cohen SM, Lavy Y, Granat M, Yagel S. Risk of fetal loss in twin pregnancies undergoing second trimester amniocentesis (1). Obstet Gynecol 2001; 98(2):231–234.

59. Fetal sex pridiction by sex chromatin of chorionic villi cells during early pregnancy. Chin Med J (Engl) 1975; 1(2):117–126.

60. Wapner RJ. Chorionic villus sampling. Obstet Gynecol Clin North Am 1997; 24(1):83–110.

61. Cameron AD, Mathers AM, Wisdom S, et al. Second-trimester placental biopsy for rapid fetal karyotyping. Am J Obstet Gynecol 1990; 163(3):931–934.

62. Holzgreve W, Miny P, Gerlach B, Westendorp A, Ahlert D, Horst J. Benefits of placental biopsies for rapid karyotyping in the second and third trimesters (late chorionic villus sampling) in high-risk pregnancies. Am J Obstet Gynecol 1990; 162(5):1188–1192.

63. Pijpers L, Jahoda MG, Reuss A, Wladimiroff JW, Sachs ES. Transabdominal chorionic villus biopsy in second and third trimesters of pregnancy to determine fetal karyotype. Br Med J 1988; 297(6652):822–823.

64. Podobnik M, Ciglar S, Singer Z, Podobnik-Sarkanji S, Duic Z, Skalak D. Transabdominal chorionic villus sampling in the second and third trimesters of high-risk pregnancies. Prenat Diagn 1997; 17(2):125–133.

65. Tharapel AT, Elias S, Shulman LP, Seely L, Emerson DS, Simpson JL. Resorbed cotwin as an explanation for discrepant chorionic villus results: non-mosaic 47,XX,+16 in villi (direct and culture) with normal (46,XX) amniotic fluid and neonatal blood. Prenat Diagn 1989; 9(7):467–472.

66. Multicentre randomised clinical trial of chorion villus sampling and amniocentesis. first report. Canadian Collaborative CVS-Amniocentesis Clinical Trial Group. Lancet 1989; 1(8628):1–6.

67. Rhoads GG, Jackson LG, Schlesselman SE, et al. The safety and efficacy of chorionic villus sampling for early prenatal diagnosis of cytogenetic abnormalities. N Engl J Med 1989; 320(10):609–617.

68. Medical Research Council European trial of chorion villus sampling. MRC working party on the evaluation of chorion villus sampling. Lancet 1991; 337(8756):1491–1499.

69. Firth HV, Boyd PA, Chamberlain P, MacKenzie IZ, Lindenbaum RH, Huson SM. Severe limb abnormalities after chorion villus sampling at 56–66 days' gestation. Lancet 1991; 337(8744):762–763.

70. Brambati B, Simoni G, Travi M, et al. Genetic diagnosis by chorionic villus sampling before 8 gestational weeks: efficiency, reliability, and risks on 317 completed pregnancies. Prenat Diagn 1992; 12(10):789–799.

71. Hsieh FJ, Shyu MK, Sheu BC, Lin SP, Chen CP, Huang FY. Limb defects after chorionic villus sampling. Obstet Gynecol 1995; 85(1):84–88.

72. Mastroiacovo P, Tozzi AE, Agosti S, et al. Transverse limb reduction defects after chorion villus sampling: a retrospective cohort study. GIDEF—Gruppo Italiano Diagnosi Embrio-Fetali. Prenat Diagn 1993; 13(11):1051–1056.

73. Froster UG, Jackson L. Limb defects and chorionic villus sampling: results from an international registry, 1992–94. Lancet 1996; 347(9000):489–494.

74. Brambati B, Tului L, Guercilena S, Alberti E. Outcome of first-trimester chorionic villus sampling for genetic investigation in multiple pregnancy. Ultrasound Obstet Gynecol 2001; 17(3):209–216.

75. De Catte L, Liebaers I, Foulon W. Outcome of twin gestations after first trimester chorionic villus sampling. Obstet Gynecol 2000; 96(5, Pt 1):714–720.

76. van den Berg C, Braat AP, Van Opstal D, et al. Amniocentesis or chorionic villus sampling in multiple gestations? Experience with 500 cases. Prenat Diagn 1999; 19(3):234–244.

77. Wapner RJ. Genetic diagnosis in multiple pregnancies. Semin Perinatol 1995; 19(5):351–362.

78. ACOG. Prevention of Rh D Alloimmunization. ACOG Practice Bulletin. Washington, DC: American College of Obstetricians and Gynecologists, 1999:4.

79. Bowman JM. Hemolytic disease. In: Creasy RK, Resnik R, eds. Maternal–Fetal Medicine. Saunders: Philadephia: W.B. Saunders, 1999:736–767.

80. Valenti C. Antenatal detection of hemoglobinopathies. A preliminary report. Am J Obstet Gynecol 1973; 115(6):851–853.

81. Hobbins JC, Mahoney MJ, Goldstein LA. New method of intrauterine evaluation by the combined use of fetoscopy and ultrasound. Am J Obstet Gynecol 1974; 118(8):1069–1072.

82. The status of fetoscopy and fetal tissue sampling. The results of the first meeting of the International Fetoscopy Group. Prenat Diagn 1984; 4(1):79–81.

83. Cao A, Furbetta M, Angius A, et al. Haematological and obstetric aspects of antenatal diagnosis of beta-thalassaemia: experience with 200 cases. J Med Genet 1982; 19(2):81–87.

84. Daffos F, Capella-Pavlovsky M, Forestier F. A new procedure for fetal blood sampling in utero: preliminary results of fifty-three cases. Am J Obstet Gynecol 1983; 146(8):985–987.

85. Daffos F, Capella-Pavlovsky M, Forestier F. Fetal blood sampling via the umbilical cord using a needle guided by ultrasound. Report of 66 cases. Prenat Diagn 1983; 3(4):271–277.

86. Hobbins JC, Grannum PA, Romero R, Reece EA, Mahoney MJ. Percutaneous umbilical blood sampling. Am J Obstet Gynecol 1985; 152(1):1–6.

87. Copel JA, Scioscia A, Grannum PA, Romero R, Reece EA, Hobbins JC. Percutaneous umbilical blood sampling in the management of Kell isoimmunization. Obstet Gynecol 1986; 67(2):288–290.

88. Ludomirski A, Nemiroff R, Johnson A, Ashmead GG, Weiner S, Bolognese RJ. Percutaneous umbilical blood sampling. A new technique for prenatal diagnosis. J Reprod Med 1987; 32(4):276–279.

89. Tharapel AT, Moretti ML, Meyers CM, et al. Diagnosis of trisomy 18 using spontaneously dividing cells from fetal umbilical cord blood: a novel approach for rapid late second and third trimester prenatal diagnosis. Am J Perinatol 1990; 7(3):211–213.

90. Tipton RE, Tharapel AT, Chang HH, Simpson JL, Elias S. Rapid chromosome analysis with the use of spontaneously dividing cells derived from umbilical cord blood (fetal and neonatal). Am J Obstet Gynecol 1989; 161(6, Pt 1):1546–1548.

91. Orlandi F, Jakil C, Damiani G, et al. First trimester fetal blood sampling. Acta Eur Fertil 1988; 19(1):23–24.

92. Ghidini A, Sepulveda W, Lockwood CJ, Romero R. Complications of fetal blood sampling. Am J Obstet Gynecol 1993; 168(5):1339–1344.

93. Daffos F, Capella-Pavlovsky M, Forestier F. Fetal blood sampling during pregnancy with use of a needle guided by ultrasound: a study of 606 consecutive cases. Am J Obstet Gynecol 1985; 153(6):655–660.

94. Hogge WA, Thiagarajah S, Brenbridge AN, Harbert GM. Fetal evaluation by percutaneous blood sampling. Am J Obstet Gynecol 1988; 158(1):132–136.

95. Maxwell DJ, Johnson P, Hurley P, Neales K, Allan L, Knott P. Fetal blood sampling and pregnancy loss in relation to indication. Br J Obstet Gynaecol 1991; 98(9):892–897.

96. ACOG. Prenatal diagnosis of fetal chromosomal abnormalities (practice bulletin). Washington, DC: American College of Obstetricians and Gynecologists, 2001.

97. Segal M, Manning FA, Harman CR, Menticoglou S. Bleeding after intravascular transfusion: experimental and clinical observations. Am J Obstet Gynecol 1991; 165(5, Pt 1):1414–1418.

98. Paidas MJ, Berkowitz RL, Lynch L, et al. Alloimmune thrombocytopenia: fetal and neonatal losses related to cordocentesis. Am J Obstet Gynecol 1995; 172(2, Pt 1):475–479.

99. Weiner CP, Wenstrom KD, Sipes SL, Williamson RA. Risk factors for cordocentesis and fetal intravascular transfusion. Am J Obstet Gynecol 1991; 165(4, Pt 1):1020–1025.

100. Bovicelli L, Orsini LF, Grannum PA, Pittalis MC, Toffoli C, Dolcini B. A new funipuncture technique: two-needle ultrasound and needle biopsy-guided procedure. Obstet Gynecol 1989; 73(3, Pt 1):428–431.

101. Seligman SP, Young BK. Tachycardia as the sole fetal heart rate abnormality after funipuncture. Obstet Gynecol 1996; 87(5, Pt 2):833–834.

102. Evans MI, Hoffman EP, Cadrin C, Johnson MP, Quintero RA, Golbus MS. Fetal muscle biopsy: collaborative experience with varied indications. Obstet Gynecol 1994; 84(6):913–917.

103. Koenig M, Hoffman EP, Bertelson CJ, Monaco AP, Feener C, Kunkel LM. Complete cloning of the Duchenne muscular dystrophy (DMD) cDNA and preliminary genomic organization of the DMD gene in normal and affected individuals. Cell 1987; 50(3):509–517.

104. Darras BT, Koenig M, Kunkel LM, Francke U. Direct method for prenatal diagnosis and carrier detection in Duchenne/Becker muscular dystrophy using the entire dystrophin cDNA. Am J Med Genet 1988; 29(3):713–726.

105. Forrest SM, Smith TJ, Cross GS, et al. Effective strategy for prenatal prediction of Duchenne and Becker muscular dystrophy. Lancet 1987; 2(8571):1294–1297.

106. Heckel S, Favre R, Flori J, et al. In utero fetal muscle biopsy: a precious aid for the prenatal diagnosis of Duchenne muscular dystrophy. Fetal Diagn Ther 1999; 14(3):127–132.

107. Nevo Y, Shomrat R, Yaron Y, Orr-Urtreger A, Harel S, Legum C. Fetal muscle biopsy as a diagnostic tool in Duchenne muscular dystrophy. Prenat Diagn 1999; 19(10):921–926.

108. Overton TG, Smith RP, Sewry CA, Holder SE, Fisk NM. Maternal contamination at fetal muscle biopsy. Fetal Diagn Ther 2000; 15(2):118–121.

109. Elias S, Esterly NB. Prenatal diagnosis of hereditary skin disorders. Clin Obstet Gynecol 1981; 24(4):1069–1087.

110. Elias S, Emerson DS, Simpson JL, Shulman LP, Holbrook KA. Ultrasound-guided fetal skin sampling for prenatal diagnosis of genodermatoses. Obstet Gynecol 1994; 83(3):337–341.

111. Uitto J, Richard G. Progress in epidermolysis bullosa: from eponyms to molecular genetic classification. Clin Dermatol 2005; 23(1):33–40.

112. Pfendner EG, Nakano A, Pulkkinen L, Christiano AM, Uitto J. Prenatal diagnosis for epidermolysis bullosa: a study of 144 consecutive pregnancies at risk. Prenat Diagn 2003; 23(6):447–456.

113. Bongain A, Benoit B, Ejnes L, Lambert JC, Gillet JY. Harlequin fetus: three-dimensional sonographic findings and new diagnostic approach. Ultrasound Obstet Gynecol 2002; 20(1):82–85.

114. Golbus MS, Simpson TJ, Koresawa M, Appelman Z, Alpers CE. The prenatal determination of glucose-6-phosphatase activity by fetal liver biopsy. Prenat Diagn 1988; 8(6):401–404.

115. Wapner RJ, Jenkins TM, Silverman N, Kaufmann M, Hannau C, McCue P. Prenatal diagnosis of congenital nephrosis by in utero kidney biopsy. Prenat Diagn 2001; 21(4):256–261.

13

Prenatal Diagnosis of Multifetal Pregnancies

Lee P. Shulman and Leeber Cohen
Department of Obstetrics and Gynecology, Division of Reproductive Genetics,
Feinberg School of Medicine, Northwestern University, Chicago, Illinois, U.S.A.

INTRODUCTION

Advances in assisted reproductive technologies and delay in childbearing have led to a considerable increase in the frequency of multiple gestations (1,2). The latter finding is due to the fact that twinning and multiple gestations increase with maternal age in spontaneous pregnancies. Many of these women are at increased risk for fetal chromosome abnormalities because of maternal age. Increased screening for a wide variety of Mendelian disorders has also led to more counseling and consideration of invasive prenatal diagnosis for women carrying singleton and multiple gestations.

The obstetrical management of multiple gestations is fraught with considerable challenges for the obstetrician including prematurity, growth disparity, fetal abnormalities, and delivery management among other maternal and fetal clinical issues (3). The prenatal detection of fetal abnormalities in multifetal pregnancies is no less challenging, with substantial challenges placed on well-accepted screening and diagnostic protocols and procedures (4). These challenges can be related to the presence of more than one fetus or can be the result of the zygosity and chorionicity of the pregnancy. Current approaches to the prenatal screening and diagnosis of multiple pregnancies will be reviewed in this chapter.

MULTIFETAL PREGNANCIES

The risk of twinning and multiple gestation increases with maternal age among women carrying spontaneous pregnancies. Utilization of assisted reproductive technologies further increases that risk so that approximately 2% of all pregnancies are now twins or higher-order pregnancies (5).

Approximately 80% of twin pregnancies are dizygotic and are the result of the fertilization of two distinct eggs (Fig. 1) (1). Race, age, and use of ovulation stimulating agents play an important role in the rate of dizygotic twins (and higher order multifetal gestations) (6). As dizygotic twins account for approximately 80% of all

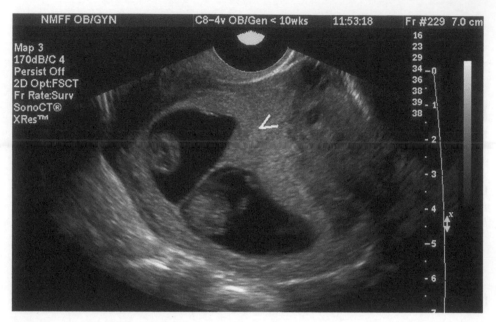

Figure 1 Dichorionic, diamniotic twin gestation in the first trimester. Note relatively thick membrane separating the two gestations emanating from separate placentas. *Arrowhead* points to lambda sign.

multifetal gestations, these factors play an important role in the overall rate of multiple gestations. In dizygotic twins, there are two separate placentas and the membrane that separates the gestations appears to be thick because of the juxtaposition of two separate amnionic and chorionic membranes. In the first trimester, the junction of the membranes with the placenta gives an ultrasonographic appearance of the Greek letter "lambda" (Fig. 2) and is used to identify di- or multiple zygotic twin and higher-order pregnancies.

The remaining 20% of twin pregnancies are monozygotic gestations and arise from a single cell that splits at some time during the first 2 weeks after fertilization into two (or more) distinct cell masses that then proceed to differentiate into separate gestations. The rate of monozygotic twins appears to be relatively constant in all populations at 3–4 per 1000 births and is independent of race, age, or the use of ovulation stimulating regimens, in contradistinction of dizygotic twins. Ultrasonographic evaluation of such pregnancies shows either a thin separating membrane with no lambda sign (diamniotic–monochorionic) (Fig. 3) or no membrane at all (monoamniotic–monochorionic) (Fig. 4). In some monozygotic cases, cell mass splitting occurs in the first 3 days after fertilization and leads to separate placentas with the lambda sign. If cell splitting occurs after 3 days, the common blood vessels join the two placentas and result in de facto monozygosity even if the placentas are visually separate by ultrasound. The degree of separateness of placentas and gestations in monozygotic gestations, as well as the presence of certain fetal anomalies such as acardiac twins and conjoined twins is based on the timing of the cell splitting.

Determination of zygosity and chorionicity is a critical and central part of the overall management of twin and higher-order pregnancies (3,4). Sebire and colleagues (7,8) have shown that such ultrasound evaluations not only can determine chorionicity and zygosity but also provide essential information concerning the

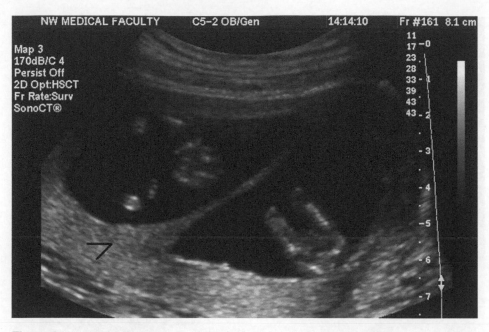

Figure 2 *Arrowhead* points to lambda sign, characteristic of a diamniotic twin gestation.

management of such pregnancies and the counseling of women carrying these pregnancies. Ultrasonographic equipment and expertise now make it possible to evaluate fetuses in the first trimester for some abnormalities (e.g., nuchal translucency, structural abnormalities) (9) and to accurately assess fetal placentation in

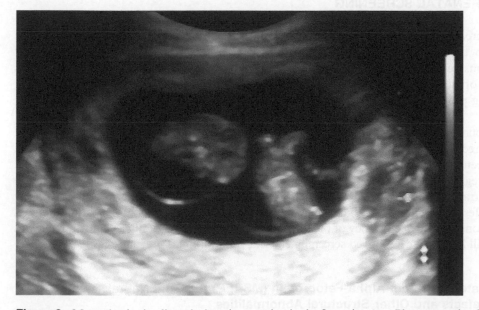

Figure 3 Monochorionic, diamniotic twin gestation in the first trimester. Please note the thin separating membrane between the two gestations as compared to the separating membrane in Figures 1 and 2. In addition, no lambda sign is present.

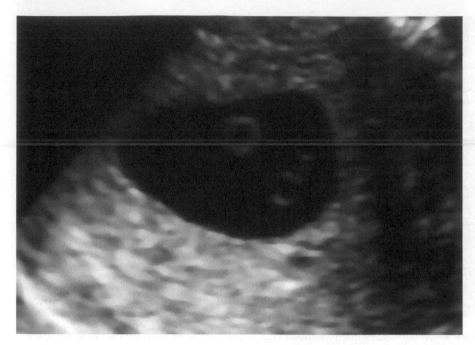

Figure 4 Monochorionic, monoamniotic twin gestation in the early first trimester.

the first trimester with the lambda sign, with such determination being central to prenatal screening and diagnosis of multifetal pregnancies (3,4).

PRENATAL SCREENING

Screening protocols for determining risk for fetal abnormalities are primarily based on the assessment of singleton pregnancies at the time of screening. Only after considerable information concerning detection rates for "screen positive" outcomes is obtained from large trials is consideration given for the application of the screening protocol for multifetal pregnancies.

The ability of first and second trimester screening protocols to assess risk for fetal abnormalities in twin and higher-order multiple gestations is based on the mode of screening. In general, screening protocols based on maternal serum analytes alone have been consistently shown to have considerably reduced screening efficiency in multifetal pregnancies compared to singleton pregnancies (10). For those protocols that utilize ultrasonographic measurements, it appears that risk assessment may not be as adversely affected by multiple gestations as those protocols that use maternal serum analytes alone, although efficiency of protocols using a combination of ultrasound and analytes will likely have a reduced screening efficiency in multifetal pregnancies (10).

Maternal Serum Alpha-Fetoprotein (MSAFP) for Fetal Neural Tube Defects and Other Structural Abnormalities

Detecting women at increased risk for carrying fetuses with structural abnormalities such as neural tube defects, gastroschisis, and omphalocele is frequently accomplished by setting an upper-limit concentration of maternal serum alpha-feto-protein (MSAFP; usually 2.0–2.5 MoM) (MoM = multiples of the median) above which ultrasound evaluation, genetic counseling, and invasive testing should be offered.

As one would expect, the concentration of MSAFP is proportional to the number of fetuses in the pregnancy. Early studies showed that MSAFP levels in twin pregnancies were, on average, twice the concentration as found in singleton pregnancies and that higher-order pregnancies were similarly likely to have increased MSAFP levels commensurate with the number of fetuses present at the time of evaluation (11,12). Interestingly, Wald and colleagues (11) showed that MSAFP levels in monozygotic twin gestations tended to be higher than found in dizygotic twins, with such differences potentially affecting the ability of such screening to accurately assess the risk of all the fetuses in a multiple gestation. Accordingly, the assessment for zygosity in the multifetal pregnancies is a vital part of the screening process for open neural tube defects.

As 2.5 MoM is typically used as the upper-limit cutoff for MSAFP screening of singleton pregnancies for open fetal defects, a value of 5.0 MoM is typically used as the upper-limit value for twin pregnancies. Ghosh et al. (12) found that in cases of twin pregnancies where the MSAFP concentration was greater than 5.0 MoM, 59% of these cases resulted in fetal demise, stillbirth, or demise of one of the gestations. With regard to fetal structural abnormalities, Cuckle et al. (13) evaluated 46 twin pregnancies in which one fetus was found to have an open neural tube defect. They found that using a cutoff of 5.0 MoM resulted in a detection rate of 83% for fetal anencephaly and 39% for open spinal defects. The ability of MSAFP screening to detect open spinal defects in multifetal pregnancies is clearly less efficient than MSAFP screening in singleton pregnancies utilizing a 2.5 MoM cutoff, although such screening will apparently detect many pregnancies with at least one affected fetus.

A finding of an MSAFP level of 5.0 MoM or greater should thus precipitate a targeted ultrasound; if twins are detected, a thorough assessment for neural tube defects and other open defects should be performed. If no abnormalities are detected by ultrasound, consideration of invasive testing to assess amniotic fluid AFP and acetylcholinesterase levels, along with fetal chromosomes, is warranted and strongly suggested.

Maternal Serum Screening for Fetal Down Syndrome and Other Chromosome Abnormalities

The incorporation of multiple serum markers into first- and second-trimester screening protocols has increased the ability to detect fetuses with Down syndrome and other specific chromosome abnormalities such as trisomy 18. However, the use of multimarker protocols with multifetal pregnancies requires data to determine whether such protocols can be applied to the detection of those fetal abnormalities in twin and multifetal pregnancies. In a study by Cuckle in 1998 (14), a meta-analysis showed that values for AFP, free β-hCG, hCG, and unconjugated estriol (uE3) were approximately 2 MoM in twin pregnancies. Watt and colleagues (15) reported that the median level of inhibin A in unaffected twin pregnancies was 1.99 MoM. With regard to first-trimester PAPP-A, Spencer (16) and Spencer and Nicolaides (17) showed the median level of PAPP-A in unaffected pregnancies to also be approximately 2 MoM.

Despite the aforementioned data that demonstrates that each fetus in a twin pregnancy appears to be responsible for a similar impact on serum analytes used for Down syndrome and trisomy 18 risk assessment as is observed with singleton pregnancies, the calculation of a fetal-specific risk using maternal serum analytes alone is not possible in a multifetal pregnancy because the fetal-specific contributions to each serum analyte measurement cannot be determined. A pregnancy-related risk can be calculated based on estimates for the contribution of each fetus and evaluating the total concentration of each analyte. However, Meyers and colleagues (18) have shown that the screening efficiency for twin pregnancies at all ages is considerably lowered compared to singleton pregnancies. Again, as with MSAFP screening for open neural tube defects, physicians and patients need to be aware of the reduced efficiency of biochemical screening protocols for twin pregnancies but recognize that such protocols do provide some information for pregnancy management, even if that information is not as robust as that obtained in singleton pregnancies. Indeed, consideration of screening for twins should reinforce some fundamental issues regarding prenatal screening; namely, that the detection and false positive rates for all prenatal biochemical screening protocols preclude its use as a substitute or alternative for prenatal diagnostic procedures that are highly accurate. In addition, utilization of screening modalities that use only biochemical markers should not be applied for assessment of triplet or higher-order pregnancies as there are little data concerning these protocols in such pregnancies and the existing information shows that such protocols have considerably reduced detection rates (19).

Maternal Screening Protocols Using Nuchal Translucency Measurement

Sebire and colleagues (20) showed that nuchal translucency (NT) measurement alone (with maternal age) was equally effective in identifying Down syndrome fetuses in twin pregnancies as in singleton pregnancies. Determination of chorionicity is again a central issue in the use of NT to assess risk for fetal Down syndrome. Increased NT measurements have been associated with an increased risk for fetal Down syndrome and other chromosome abnormalities as well as fetal cardiac malformations, skeletal dysplasias, and some genetic syndromes (Fig. 5). Increased NT measurements in twin pregnancies have also been associated with a higher frequency of twin-to-twin transfusion in monochorionic multiple gestations (21).

When NT is used alone (without serum analytes but with maternal age) to assess risk for fetal Down syndrome in a dichorionic gestation, NT is measured in each fetus and separate and distinct risks are calculated for each fetus. If the risk for chromosome abnormality is found to be increased for any fetus, chorionic villus sampling (CVS) or amniocentesis (at a later date) can be offered to assess the specific fetal chromosome complement. In cases of monochorionic multifetal gestations, the calculation of risk is based on the greatest NT measurement among the fetuses (5). If CVS or amniocentesis is chosen, only a single sample of placenta or amniotic fluid is required.

With screening protocols that use NT and biochemical markers, either a risk for each individual fetus is calculated or an overall pregnancy-related risk is determined. However, the limitations mentioned earlier concerning the inability to determine fetal-specific contributions to overall biochemical marker measurements still have an adverse impact on the efficiency of screening protocols that utilize both NT measurements and biochemical assays (10). Accordingly, many programs, including our own, use a pregnancy-related, rather than a fetal-specific, calculation

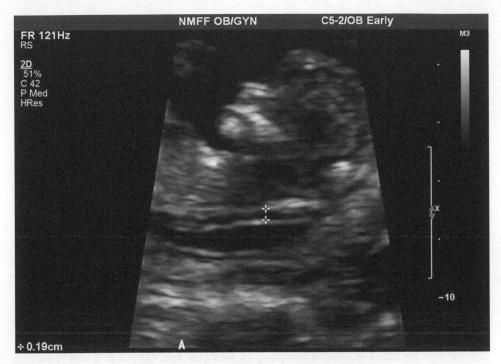

Figure 5 Nuchal translucency measurement in a twin gestation.

providing a risk assessment that at least one fetus (of a twin gestation) has Down syndrome. As with protocols using NT alone, chorionicity must be determined prior to calculation and is incorporated in a similar fashion with combination protocols as with NT-alone protocols.

PRENATAL DIAGNOSIS

Chorionic Villus Sampling

The use of CVS for detecting abnormalities in multiple gestations is now recognized to be an acceptable, safe, and reliable approach for prenatal diagnosis. The potential benefits of CVS in multiple gestations are similar to those in singleton pregnancies, that is, to provide safe and reliable prenatal diagnosis of detectable fetal abnormalities. However, CVS in multifetal gestations also provides unique benefits as well as challenges. Specifically, the ability to perform prenatal diagnosis in a multifetal pregnancy allows for early detection of fetal abnormalities that may lead to the consideration of fetal reduction. Diagnosing such problems in the first trimester allows for first trimester fetal reduction, a procedure that is likely safer and less emotionally taxing than a second trimester reduction (22). Conversely, CVS in multifetal gestations is usually challenging and requires experience with all approaches to CVS: transcervical, transabdominal, and transvaginal (23). Indeed, a unique and daunting challenge with CVS in multifetal pregnancies is not just to perform a safe procedure but to do so while obtaining a specimen or specimens that are correctly associated with specific fetuses.

Early reports of the benefits and risks of CVS in multiple gestations showed that it could be successfully accomplished, although there were cases characterized by admixture of cell lines, either representing the results of more than one fetus or maternal cell contamination (23–25). All reports showed that some patients (42% of subjects in Ref. 23) would require a discordant approach to secure appropriate specimens from all fetuses. Brambati et al. (22) and De Catte et al. (26) later reported on the use of CVS as a tool for facilitating first trimester fetal reduction. De Catte et al. (26) presented information showing no fetal losses among 32 multifetal pregnancies undergoing CVS prior to consideration of multifetal pregnancy. Loss rates from these early studies range from 0% to 6% and were similar, in comparative studies, to twin pregnancies not undergoing invasive testing or amniocentesis. Similar findings were later reported by Appelman et al. (27), De Catte et al. (28), and Brambati et al. (29). Appelman et al. (27) reported no spontaneous losses or incorrect cytogenetic outcomes among 28 twin and 14 triplet fetuses undergoing CVS. De Catte et al. (28) reported a total fetal loss rate of 5.5% (including selective terminations) among 262 consecutive women carrying twin gestations undergoing CVS. Uncertain cytogenetic results complicated the management of only 3 of the 262 cases. Brambati et al. (29) reported on the outcomes of 198 sets of twins and nine sets of triplets undergoing CVS and compared outcomes with 63 dichorionc twin pregnancies undergoing no invasive testing. Unlike the De Catte et al. (23) experience, all but one case was performed transabdominally. Brambati and colleagues found no difference in fetal or perinatal loss rate; interestingly, they reported a higher rate of delivery before 37 weeks' gestation and of low birth weight babies in the control group. In addition, the authors reported successful sampling in all cases and only four cases requiring more than one pass (1.0%).

In contradistinction to the experience reported by Brambati and coworkers (29), Casals and colleagues (30) reported on the use of a biopsy forceps for the transcervical sampling of placentas; however, loss rates and the need for follow-up amniocentesis were somewhat higher in this series compared to the experience of other centers. Accordingly, our center, in concordance with the paper by De Catte et al. (23), chooses to forego a transcervical approach for more than one fetus. Brambati and colleagues (29) have also reported on the successful use of a double coaxial needle system that can be used, when two placentas are fused, to reliably sample both placentas in a transabdominal manner. One first samples the most accessible placenta in a conventional manner. In order to sample the other placenta, a double coaxial needle is then passed through the already sampled placenta and guided to the unsampled placenta. The sampling needle is then introduced through the outer needle shaft (which has already traversed the sampled placenta) and into the heretofore unsampled placenta. Aspiration of villi is then achieved without an increased risk for contamination from the previously sampled placenta. Brambati and colleagues (29) have found this double coaxial approach to be highly successful with regard to safety (no losses) and accuracy (no inaccurate diagnoses).

As with multifetal screening protocols using NT, determination of chorionicity is an important and required initial step before CVS is performed. If multichorionic gestations with distinct placentas are observed, each placenta is approached as with a singleton gestation (Fig. 6A and B), except that needles or catheters must not traverse one placenta to access another for fear of specimen contamination [unless a coaxial needle system as described by Brambati et al. (29) is used]. In cases of monochorionic gestations, a single specimen can be obtained to assess all fetuses.

In cases characterized by fused placentas, ultrasonography may not be able to accurately determine chorionicity. In such cases, sampling placental areas that are most likely to be associated with specific fetuses should be considered. Such sampling

(A)

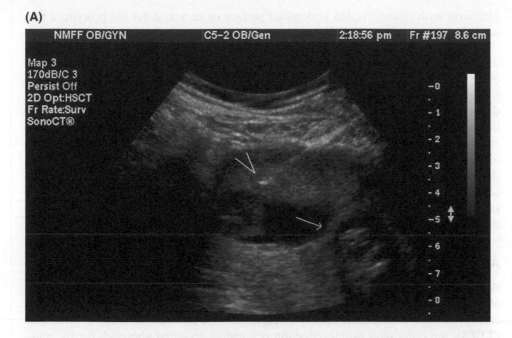

(B)

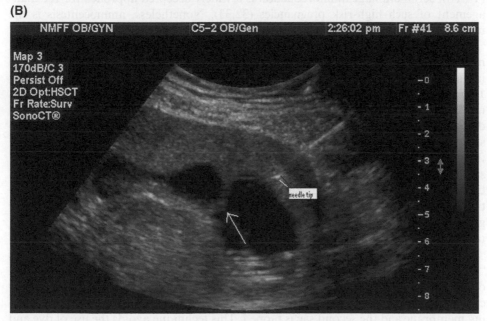

Figure 6 (A) Chorionic villus sampling (CVS) in a dichorionic twin gestation. *Arrowhead* points to needle tip whereas the *arrow* points to the thick separating membrane. (B) CVS of twin B. The *arrow* points to the separating membrane and the needle tip is labeled.

areas could be close to each individual umbilical insertion site or at the edges of the placenta far from the fusion of the placentas. At our center, we utilize sites determined from the latter approach; if we are unable to identify and access such placenta sampling sites, we alter bladder volume to change the relative positions of the placentas with relation to the abdominal surface or cervix, defer the procedure to a later date, or consider second-trimester amniocentesis.

If there is concern about diagnostic accuracy regarding same-sex findings from distinct samples in a di- or multichorionic gestation, DNA polymorphisms can be evaluated to identify differences between the samples. If such studies cannot be performed or are inconclusive, consideration of second-trimester ultrasonographic studies and amniocenteses is warranted. Patients must be made aware of the possible limitations of multifetal CVS and the potential need for further (i.e., second trimester) procedures to obtain accurate prenatal diagnoses. Finally, physicians must recognize the technical challenges in performing multifetal CVS and be willing to defer procedures to a later date or for amniocentesis. However, we and others (28,29,31) strongly believe that CVS in multifetal pregnancies is a safe and effective prenatal diagnostic procedure for well-counseled women when performed by skilled operators in experienced centers.

Amniocentesis

Amniocentesis is readily performed in multiple gestations if sufficient fluid is available and an unimpeded access to the sac is available. Unlike CVS, amniocentesis also can serve as a therapeutic option in cases of twin-to-twin transfusion syndrome (TTTS); serial drainage amnioreduction is a widely accepted approach for the management of such high-risk pregnancies (32,33). Nonetheless, amniocentesis is the most widely used method for prenatal diagnosis in multifetal pregnancies.

At our center, we perform amniocentesis in multifetal pregnancies utilizing a needle puncture for each amniotic sac (34). Following aspiration of fluid from the initial sac, $10 \, cm^3$ of a dilute indigo carmine solution ($1 \, cm^3$ indigo carmine: $10 \, cm^3$ normal saline) is injected into the sac before removing the needle. A second needle is then inserted into the second sac for the second gestation, and so forth depending on the number of fetuses (Fig. 7). The initial $2–3 \, cm^3$ aspirate of each subsequent aspiration is evaluated for a greenish-blue tint that would indicate whether the needle was in a previously tapped sac or leakage between two distinct gestational sacs had occurred; aspiration of clear fluid confirms that a previously tapped amniotic sac had not been reentered. Before early amniocentesis (before 14 weeks' gestation) had been shown to be less safe than conventional amniocentesis or CVS, our group (35) had shown that this technique could be successfully applied to the prenatal diagnosis of twin pregnancies before 14 weeks' gestation.

Another approach to amniocentesis of multifetal gestations is by the so-called "single-needle" technique (36–38). As opposed to the aforementioned approach, only a single needle puncture is performed. After amniocentesis of the initial sac is completed, the needle is redirected under ultrasound guidance to traverse the dividing membrane and the second sac is tapped. This technique avoids the use of dye and multiple needle punctures of the uterus.

Evaluation of both techniques shows a relatively low rate of pregnancy loss following amniocentesis and a high rate of diagnostic accuracy, although the number of documented cases with both techniques is relatively small. The single-needle technique requires an operator and ultrasonographer who are highly experienced with invasive procedures; not all multiple gestations, especially triplets and those that are higher order, are amenable to such sampling. In addition, there is a potential for diagnostic inaccuracy due to amniotic fluid admixture in traversing one sac to another. Finally, some have opined that the manipulation needed to direct the needle

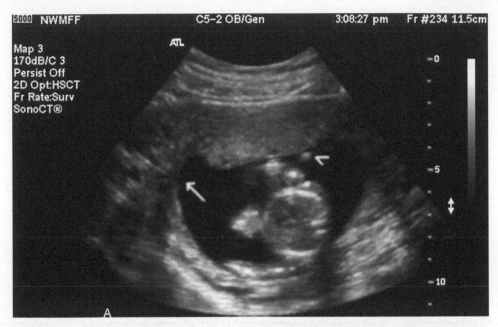

Figure 7 Amniocentesis of a dichorionic, diamniotic twin gestation. The *arrow* points to separating membrane and *arrowhead* to the needle tip within the amniotic cavity of twin A.

into the second sac could result in higher rates of fetal morbidity and mortality resulting from membrane shearing, amniotic band syndrome, and fetal injury. Although the multiple needle insertion technique precludes the need for such needle manipulation, that technique does require multiple needle punctures of the uterus that could also lead to an increased risk of bleeding, infection and fetal loss. Suffice it to say that both techniques are reasonably safe and reliably, although successful use of the single-needle technique likely requires a more experienced operator and center.

Loss rates with amniocentesis in multiple pregnancies appear to be low and, possibly, similar to loss rates observed with singleton pregnancies. Anderson and colleagues (39) reported a loss rate (up to 28 weeks) of 3.6% compared to a 0.6% spontaneous loss rate observed among singleton pregnancies not undergoing invasive testing. The authors reported that the increased loss rate was likely representative of the expected loss rate observed in multifetal pregnancies and was likely not related to the amniocentesis. Conversely, Yukobowich and colleagues (40) compared 476 women carrying twins and undergoing amniocentesis to 489 women carrying a singleton pregnancy and undergoing amniocentesis and 477 women with twins undergoing no invasive procedure in a retrospective review. The authors found a miscarriage rate (up to 4 weeks following the procedure) in the twins/amnio group of 2.73% compared to 0.63% in the twins/no amnio group and 0.6% in the singleton/amnio group). Although maternal age and other factors that could have impacted clinical outcomes were not controlled in this study, it does suggest that the risk of loss may be somewhat higher than others have reported. These studies do not indicate a considerably increased risk of loss with twin amniocentesis compared with singleton amniocentesis; however, a formal comparative study of twin amniocentesis is needed to best determine the specific risks of the procedure.

CONCLUSIONS

An increasing number of women choosing to have children later in life and the expanding use of assisted reproductive technologies have markedly increased the rate of multifetal gestations over the past two decades. As many of these women are at increased risk for detectable fetal abnormalities, the use of invasive prenatal procedures has been more frequently applied to women carrying multifetal pregnancies. In addition, many women, even at recognized increased risk for detectable fetal abnormalities, are requesting information about and choosing to undergo prenatal screening protocols that do not expose the fetus to an increased risk of loss or injury, but also do not provide diagnostic information as do invasive procedures.

In general, the information concerning screening efficiencies of first- and second-trimester screening protocols and the safety and efficacy of first- and second-trimester invasive prenatal diagnostic procedures is considerably less for multifetal pregnancies than what is available concerning singleton pregnancies. Regardless, there are certain basic tents of multifetal screening and diagnosis that have emerged. First, ultrasound plays a vital role in screening and diagnostic protocols in determining chorionicity and zygosity of the pregnancy and detecting fetal structural abnormalities. Second, all screening protocols using biochemical markers are profoundly less efficient in multifetal pregnancies than singleton pregnancies. Third, all invasive procedures involving multifetal gestations tend to be more complicated to perform and are more likely to result in an incorrect result or with no result at all compared to invasive testing in singleton pregnancies. However, the overall safety of CVS and amniocentesis in twin pregnancies does not appear to be considerably inferior than that observed in singleton pregnancies.

This chapter primarily presents information on twin gestations. There is little to no meaningful information on triplet and higher-order multiple gestations, save for occasional case reports and very small series (41). The management of such pregnancies should thus be individualized with regard to screening or diagnosis with several considerations. Ultrasound will likely play the most important role in screening these pregnancies for fetal chromosome abnormalities as biochemical protocols should not be used in the evaluation of triplet or higher-order multifetal pregnancies. Although CVS and amniocentesis can be used to diagnose fetal abnormalities in such pregnancies, performing these procedures will likely be technically challenging and may not result in obtaining fetal information in all cases.

The obstetrical management of twins and higher-order pregnancies is challenging and involves increased risk to mother and fetuses alike. Prenatal screening and diagnosis can provide important information concerning fetal outcomes, but patients and physicians must recognize the considerable limitations of screening protocols and invasive procedures in such pregnancies.

REFERENCES

1. Hirtenlehner-Ferber K, Krampl E, Strohmer H, et al. Multiple pregnancy (German). Ther Umsch 2002; 59:683–688.
2. Rochon M, Stone J. Invasive procedures in multiple gestations. Curr Opin Obstet Gynecol 2003; 15:167–175.
3. Sperling L, Tabor A. Twin pregnancy: the role of ultrasound in management. Acta Obstet Gynecol Scand 2001; 80:287–299.

4. Picone O, Dommergues M. Strategies of antenatal diagnosis and management of pathologies related to multiple pregnancies (French). Gynecol Obstet Fertil 2004; 32: 153–159.

5. Ville YG, Nicolaides KH, Campbell S. Prenatal diagnosis of fetal malformations by ultrasound. In: Milunsky A, ed. Genetic Disorders and the Fetus: Diagnosis, Prevention and Treatment. 5th ed. Baltimore, MD: The Johns Hopkins University Press, 2004: 836–900.

6. MacGillivary I, Nylander POS, Corney G, et al. Human Multiple Reproduction. London: WB Saunders, 1975.

7. Sebire NJ, Snijders RJ, Hughes K, et al. The hidden mortality of monochorionic twin pregnancies. Br J Obstet Gynaecol 1997a; 104:1203–1207.

8. Sebire NJ, Thornton S, Hughes K, et al. The prevalence and consequences of missed abortion in twin pregnancies at 10 to 14 weeks of gestation. Br J Obstet Gynaecol 1997b; 104:847–848.

9. Timor-Tritsch IE, Bashiri A, Monteagudo A, et al. Qualified and trained sonographers in the US can perform early fetal anatomy scans between 11 and 14 weeks. Am J Obstet Gynecol 2004; 191:1247–1252.

10. Cuckle HS, Arbuzova S. Multimarker maternal serum screening for chromosomal abnormalities. In: Milunsky A, ed. Genetic Disorders and the Fetus: Diagnosis, Prevention and Treatment. 5th ed. Baltimore, MD: The Johns Hopkins University Press, 2004:795–835.

11. Wald NJ, Cuckle HS, Peck S, et al. Maternal serum alpha-fetoprotein in relation to zygosity. Br Med J 1979; 1(6161):455.

12. Ghosh A, Woo JSK, Rawlinson HA, et al. Prognostic significance of raised serum alpha-fetoprotein levls in twin pregnancies. Br J Obstet Gynaecol 1982; 89:817–820.

13. Cuckle HS, Wald NJ, Stevenson JD, et al. Maternal serum alpha-fetoprotein screening for open neural tube defects in twin pregnancies. Prenat Diagn 1990; 10:71–77.

14. Cuckle H. Down's syndrome screening in twins. J Med Screen 1998; 5:3–4.

15. Watt HC, Wald NJ, George L. Maternal serum inhibin-A levels in twin pregnancies: implications for screening for Down's syndrome. Prenat Diagn 1996; 16:927–929.

16. Spencer K. Screening for trisomy 21 in twin pregnancies in the first trimester using free beta-hCG and PAPP-A, combined with fetal nuchal translucency thickness. Prenat Diagn 2000; 20:91–95.

17. Spencer K, Nicolaides KH. Screening for trisomy 21 in twins using first trimester ultrasound and maternal serum biochemistry in a one-stop clinic: a review of three years experience. Br J Obstet Gynaecol 2003; 110:276–280.

18. Meyers C, Adam R, Dungan J, et al. Aneuploidy in twin pregnancies: when is maternal age advanced? Obstet Gynecol 1997; 89:248–251.

19. Spencer K, Salonen R, Muller F. Down's syndrome screening in multiple pregnancies using alpha-fetoprotein and free beta hCG. Prenat Diagn 1994; 14:537–542.

20. Sebire NJ, Snijders RJ, Hughes K, et al. Screening for trisomy 21 in twin pregnancies by maternal age and fetal nuchal translucency thickness at 10–14 weeks of gestation. Br J Obstet Gynaecol 1996; 103:999–1003.

21. Borruto F, Comparetto C, Acanfora L, et al. Role of ultrasound evaluation of nuchal translucency in prenatal diagnosis. Clin Exp Obstet Gynecol 2002; 29:235–241.

22. Brambati B, Tului L, Alberti E. Prenatal diagnosis by chorionic villus sampling. Eur J Obstet Gynecol Reprod Biol 1996; 65:11–16.

23. De Catte L, Liebaers I, Foulon W, et al. First trimester chorionic villus sampling in twin gestations. Am J Perinatol 1996; 13:413–417.

24. Pergament E, Schulman JD, Copeland K, et al. The risk and efficacy of chorionic villus sampling in multiple gestations. Prenat Diagn 1992; 12:377–384.

25. Wapner RJ, Johnson A, Davis G, et al. Prenatal diagnosis in twin gestations: a comparison between second-trimester amniocentesis and first-trimester chorionic villus sampling. Obstet Gynecol 1993; 82:49–56.

26. De Catte L, Camus M, Bonduelle M, et al. Prenatal diagnosis by chorionic villus sampling in multiple pregnancies prior to fetal reduction. Am J Perinatol 1998; 15:339–343.
27. Appelman Z, Vinkler C, Caspi B. Chorionic villus sampling in multiple pregnancies. Eur J Obstet Gynecol Reprod Biol 1999; 85:97–99.
28. De Catte L, Liebaers I, Foulon W, et al. Outocme of twin gestations after first trimester chorionic villus sampling. Obstet Gynecol 2000; 96:714–720.
29. Brambati B, Tului L, Guercilena S, et al. Outcome of first-trimester chorionic villus sampling for genetic investigation in multiple pregnancy. Ultrasound Obstet Gynecol 2001; 17:209–216.
30. Casals G, Borrell A, Martinez JM, et al. Transcervical chorionic villus sampling in multiple pregnancies using a biopsy forceps. Prenat Diagn 2002; 22:260–265.
31. Appelman Z, Furman B. Invasive genetic diagnosis in multiple pregnancies. Obstet Gynecol Clin North Am 2005; 32:97–103.
32. Fieni S, Gramellini D, Piantelli G, et al. Twin-twin transfusion syndrome: a review of treatment option. Acta Biomed Ateneo Parmense 2004; 75(Suppl 1):34–39.
33. Johnsen SL, Albrechtsen S, Pirhonen J. Twin-twin transfusion syndrome treated with serial amniocenteses. Acta Obstet Gynecol Scand 2004; 83:326–329.
34. Elias S, Gerbie AB, Simpson JL, et al. Genetic amniocentesis in twin gestations. Am J Obstet Gynecol 1980; 138:169–174.
35. Shulman LP, Elias S, Phillips OP, et al. Early twin amniocetesis prior to 14 weeks' gestation. Prenat Diagn 1992; 12:625–626.
36. Jeanty P, Shah D, Roussis P. Single-needle insertion in twin amniocentesis. J Ultrasound Med 1990; 9:511–517.
37. Buscaglia M, Ghisoni L, Bellotti M, et al. Genetic amniocentesis in biamniotic twin pregnancies by a single transabdominal insertion of the needle. Prenat Diagn 1995; 15:17–19.
38. van Vugt JM, Nieuwint A, van Geijn HP. Single-needle insertion: an alternative technique for early second-trimester genetic twin amniocentesis. Fetal Diagn Ther 1995; 10:178–181.
39. Anderson RL, Goldberg JD, Golbus MS. Prenatal diagnosis in multiple gestations: 20 years experience with amniocentesis. Prenat Diagn 1991; 11:263–270.
40. Yukobowich E, Anteby EY, Cohen SM, et al. Risk of fetal loss in twin pregnancies undergoing second trimester amniocentesis. Obstet Gynecol 2001; 98:231–234.
41. Wald NJ, Cuckle HS, Peck S, et al. Maternal serum alpha-fetoprotein levels in triplet and quadruplet pregnancies. Br J Obstet Gynaecol 1978; 85:124–126.

14

Embryoscopy in the First Trimester of Pregnancy

T. Philipp

Department of Obstetrics and Gynecology, Danube Hospital, Vienna, Austria

EMBRYOSCOPY

Embryoscopy is an invasive technology that allows direct visualization of the embryo. In ongoing pregnancies, an endoscope is introduced at 10 to 11 weeks' gestation into the *exocoelomic space*, by either transcervical or transabdominal route. At about 12 weeks of gestation, chorion and amnion fuse and, therefore, make the procedure impossible (1).

Fetoscopy is the examination of the fetus at a later gestational age. The scope is entered directly into the amniotic cavity.

Embryoscopy is rarely used today in *ongoing pregnancies*, because of complications such as rupture of the amnion and embryonic death. As a result of the improvements in ultrasound technology and the relatively high risk of spontaneous abortion associated with the technique, embryoscopy finds only a limited number of indications in *ongoing pregnancies*:

- very early in pregnancy (9–10 gestational weeks) in families affected by recurrent genetic conditions in pregnancy diagnosable by characteristic external features;
- to confirm or rule out suspected fetal anomalies in the early ultrasound examination (10–14 gestational weeks).

There is a tendency to abandon the transcervical approach of embryoscopy because of the higher risk of spontaneous abortion associated with the technique.

In *failed first-trimester pregnancies*, scheduled for instrumental evacuation of the uterus, transcervical embryoscopy is the method to be favored in examination of the dead conceptus (2). Most of the losses occur when the conceptus is still very small and the resolution of ultrasound does not allow for a precise visualization. Embryoscopy in early spontaneous abortions spots subtle morphologic abnormalities

(A)   (B)

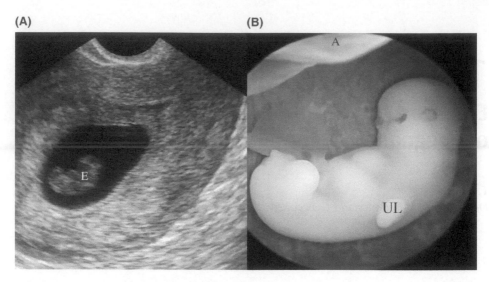

Figure 1 (**A**) Endovaginal sonography before embryoscopy showing no heart action of the embryo (E) measuring 15 mm in CRL. Embryoscopic examination of the same embryo from a lateral view (**B**) showed a microcephalic embryo with a dysplastic face. UL are paddle-shaped, indicating retarded development relative to CRL. Remnants of the amnion are labeled A. Chromosome analysis revealed a normal (46,XY) karyotype. *Abbreviations*: CRL, crown–rump length; UL, upper limbs. (*B*: *See color insert*.)

undetectable by ultrasound (Fig. 1A,B). The technique used prior to dilatation and curettage in cases of early failed pregnancies enables investigators to visualize the embryo in utero, unaffected by the damage resulting from instrumental evacuation or spontaneous passage.

TECHNIQUE OF TRANSCERVICAL EMBRYOSCOPY IN CASES OF EARLY SPONTANEOUS ABORTIONS (MISSED ABORTIONS)

Morphological Evaluation

Embryoscopy and subsequent curettage of early spontaneous abortion is performed under intravenous general anesthesia. After careful dilatation of the cervix, and *before curettage* is performed, a rigid hysteroscope (12° angle of view with both the biopsy and the irrigation working channel, Circon Ch 25-8 mm) is passed transcervically into the uterine cavity. A continuous normal saline flow should be used throughout the procedure (pressure, 40–120 mmHg) to help distend, clean, and thus provide a clear view. After inspection of the uterine cavity, the gestational sac has to be localized. The chorion is opened with microscissors (CH 7-2 mm) and the embryo first viewed through the amnion. Since amniotic rupture need not be avoided in cases of failed pregnancies, the hysteroscope is then passed into the amniotic cavity after opening this membrane with microscissors. Usually, the amnion obscures vision by reflecting the light. Documentation of delicate embryonic details can be better achieved inside the amniotic cavity. All procedures may be viewed on a TV monitor by connecting a video camera (Circon Microdigital III, a 3-CCD color camera) to the eyepiece of the endoscope, and can be recorded for later analysis. A complete examination of the conceptus includes visualization of the head, face, dorsal and ventral walls, limbs, and umbilical cord.

Technique of Tissue Sampling

Karyotyping should be attempted in all cases and evaluated morphologically (see section on Developmental Defects with Chromosomal Aberrations). In missed abortions, chorionic villi can be obtained either by curettage, or direct chorion biopsies can be taken embryoscopically at the end of the morphologic examination (3,4). In our studies, direct chorionic villus sampling was performed under visual monitoring using a microforceps (CH 7-2 mm). At the end of the procedure, chorionic villi should be placed in normal saline and carefully dissected. Samples from the curettage material have to be freed from decidual cells and blood, and washed in normal saline several times. The chorionic villi should be placed in culture medium and immediately forwarded to the cytogenetic laboratory for further processing. In our studies, the tissue was subsequently cultured and analyzed cytogenetically, using standard G-banding cytogenetic techniques.

Special Features of the Technique

For the operator to become proficient, a number of cases are required during the initial learning curve. The success rate for a complete embryoscopic examination is above 85%. However, a tight amniotic sac, or a short umbilical cord closely attaching the embryo to the chorionic plate can make the complete embryoscopic examination of the conceptus impossible (5).

The small size, the usually long intrauterine retention time, and particularly the high rate of chromosomal anomalies among malformed embryos (see section on Developmental Defects with Chromosomal Aberrations) are certain characteristics that mark *early* spontaneous abortion specimens.

The size of the embryo makes high demands on image resolution. At the end of the eighth week it measures 30 mm but already possesses several thousand named structures. The development of the human embryo is a particularly dynamic process with a constantly changing anatomical appearance of the conceptus. Therefore, it is important to get as close as possible to the target with the embryoscope to document minute developing structures like the developing limbs (Fig. 2A,B).

It is important for the investigator to develop the ability to evaluate the developmental age (DA) of embryos accurately, as the diagnosis of an embryonic defect is dependent on precise staging (6). Without a basic knowledge of the developing anatomy of the human embryo, early diagnosis of developmental defects by embryoscopy is not possible (Fig. 3). The term *gestational age*, used in clinical terminology and ultrasound, should not be used in this study of missed abortions, as most of these specimens are usually retained in utero. The actual DA can be derived from the crown–rump length (CRL), measured by ultrasonography, and from the developmental stage assessed by embryoscopy (7).

The incidence of developmental defects (see section on Common Morphologic Defects in Early Abortion Specimens Diagnosed Embryoscopically) and the rate of chromosomal anomalies (see section on Developmental Defects with Chromosomal Aberrations) among early abortion specimens are particularly high. Therefore, the difference between an embryo and a fetus is more than a matter of terminology and the specific definitions should be used in studies of abortions.

(A)

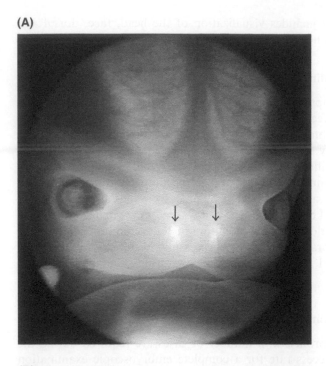

(B)

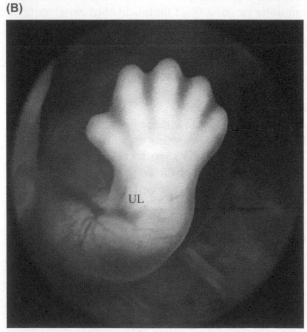

Figure 2   Close view of the face (**A**) and the right hand (**B**) of an embryo measuring 22 mm in CRL. The nostrils (*arrows*) and upper lip formation are depicted on front view (**A**). The fingers are distinct but still webbed (**B**).The elbow region can be recognized on the UL. *Abbreviations*: CRL, crown–rump length; UL, upper limb.

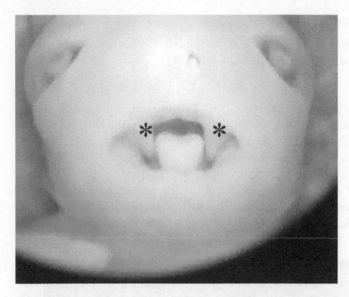

Figure 3 Close-up anterior view of the face of an embryo measuring 22 mm CRL (eighth week of development). Physiological cleft of soft palate (*) is visible. Cleft palate can only be diagnosed in the fetal period, since fusion is completed after the 10th week of development (see section on Facial Clefts). *Abbreviation*: CRL, crown–rump length.

DEFINITIONS USED IN THE STUDY OF ABORTIONS

Abortion is defined as the premature expulsion or removal of the conceptus from the uterus before it is able to sustain life on its own. *Early spontaneous abortion* occurs in the embryonic period, up to the end of the eighth developmental week (8). The *DA* or *conceptional age* of an embryo or fetus extends from the day of fertilization to the day of intrauterine death or expulsion. In contrast, in abortion specimens, *gestational* or *menstrual age* extends from the first day of the last menstrual period to the expulsion or removal of the conceptus.

The developing human is considered to be an *embryo* from conception until the end of the eighth week. From the beginning of the ninth week until birth, the developing human is called a *fetus*.

COMMON MORPHOLOGICAL DEFECTS IN EARLY ABORTION SPECIMENS DIAGNOSED EMBRYOSCOPICALLY

Though the incidence of developmental defects in specimens of early spontaneous abortions is high (5,9), a detailed morphological examination of the embryo is rarely performed for practical reasons. Most early abortion specimens are difficult to evaluate morphologically because they are either incomplete or damaged, mainly during instrumental evacuation of the uterus (10).

Embryoscopy in early spontaneous abortions spots subtle morphologic abnormalities undetectable by ultrasound and the diagnostic potential of transcervical embryoscopy in missed abortions is just beginning to unfold. The following section is an overview of developmental defects that we were able to diagnose with this technique.

Embryonic Growth Disorganization

Based on the degree of abnormal embryonic development, four categories of growth
disorganization (GD 1–GD 4), can be distinguished (11).

Growth Disorganization 1

GD 1 represents an empty sac or an embryonic sac. The amnion, if present, is usually
closely applied to the chorion (Fig. 4A) (fusion of the amnion to the chorion prior to
10 weeks of gestation is abnormal).

Growth Disorganization 2

GD 2 conceptuses show embryonic tissue 3–5 mm with no recognizable external
embryonic landmarks and no retinal pigment (Fig. 4B). It is not possible to differentiate
a caudal and a cephalic pole. Often the embryo is directly attached to the chorionic plate.

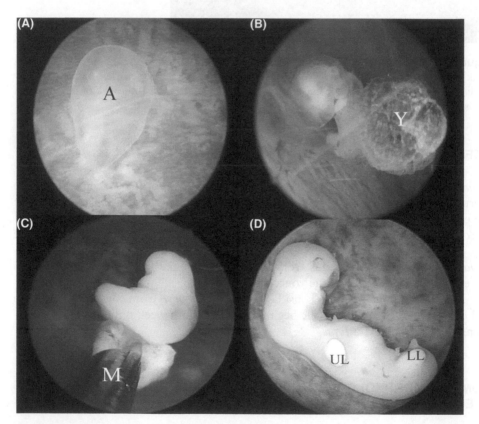

Figure 4 The amnion (A) is fused to the chorion. Note the absence of an embryo and yolk
sac. The 45,X GD 1 embryo resulted from IVF (**A**). A trisomy 16 (47,XY,+16) embryo 6 mm
in length. The yolk sac (Y) is clearly discernible. The GD 2 embryo showed no recognizable
external structures after the amnion was opened (**B**). Lateral view of a GD 3 embryo with a
CRL of 7 mm. An apparently normal karyotype (46,XY) was diagnosed cytogenetically.
"M" marks the microscissor (**C**). Lateral view of a trisomy 15 (47,XX,+15) embryo, 15 mm
in length. Based on the CRL the head of the macerated GD 4 embryo is too small, the face
is highly abnormal and the UL and LL buds are profoundly retarded in development (**D**).
Abbreviations: GD, growth disorganization; IVF, in vitro fertilization; CRL, crown–rump
length; UL, upper limb; LL, lower limb. (*See color insert.*)

Growth Disorganization 3

GD 3 embryos are up to 10-mm long. They lacked limb buds but retinal pigment is often present. A cephalic and caudal pole could be differentiated (Fig. 4C).

Growth Disorganization 4

The GD 4 embryos have a CRL of over 10 mm with a discernible head, trunk, and limb buds. The limb buds show marked retardation in development and the development of the facial structures is highly abnormal (Fig. 4D).

In our experience, growth-disorganized embryos show a high frequency (92%) of autosomal trisomies, trisomy 16 being the most common, accounting for the majority (46%) of abnormal karyotypes (12).

Localized Defects

Localized defects can be isolated or combined. Morphologically, they are similar to developmental defects seen in fetuses.

Neural Tube Defects

Previous pathological investigations demonstrated that the incidence of neural tube defects (NTDs) differs between early and late pregnancy loss. Studies examining both embryos and fetuses in spontaneous abortion revealed an incidence of 3.6% to 4.1% (13,14). Studies confined to embryonic specimens registered NTDs in about 7% of the intact embryos (15).

Morphology. There is a difference in the phenotype of NTDs at early DAs. *Spina bifida* previously described in embryos (16) and frequently observed embryoscopically includes a plaque-like protrusion of neural tissue over the caudal spine (Fig. 5A). It is not fully understood whether these defects are of a different cause or whether they are precursor lesions of spina bifida observed in fetuses.

Encephaloceles present themselves on embryoscopy as a bulge in the cranium, often covered by adherent discolored skin (Fig. 5B). Contrary to fetuses where the defect usually occurs in the occipital area, encephalocele may be observed embryoscopically in embryos in the frontal and parietal region. Their sizes range from small encephaloceles to large defects involving most of the cranium of the embryo.

In *anencephalic embryos*, the brain tissue may still be present and this condition is called exencephaly. The developing cerebral structures subsequently undergo varying degrees of destruction, leaving a mass of vascular structure and degenerated neural tissue (Fig. 5C,D).

NTDs can be multifactorial in origin, caused by a lethal gene defect or nongenetic mechanism like amniotic bands, amnion rupture sequence (ARS). Chromosomal anomalies are the most common cause of *embryonic* NTDs (13–15,17,18). The most common chromosome abnormalities are triploidy (*spina bifida*), 45,X (encephalocele), and trisomies 9 and 14 (19).

Facial Clefts

Lateral cleft lip and/or palate is present in about one in 700 live births. Median cleft lip accounts for only 0.2% to 0.7% of cases of cleft lip. The incidence of median cleft lip in embryos from early spontaneous abortions seems to be higher.

Morphology. *Cleft Lip.* Lateral and median cleft lip can be distinguished embryoscopically. Lateral clefts may be unilateral or bilateral. Cleft lip occurs when the maxillary prominence and the united medial nasal prominence fail to fuse.

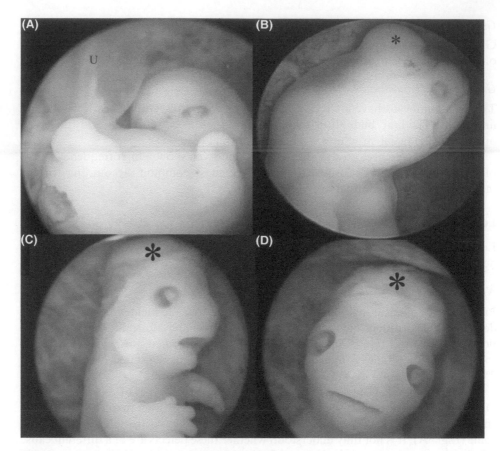

Figure 5 Posterior overview of a triploid (69,XXY) embryo. The 15-mm-long embryo had a large open neural tube defect of the lower lumbar and sacral spine. "U"marks the umbilical cord (**A**). Close-up lateral view of the upper portion of a 45,X embryo with a parietal encephalocele (∗). The brownish pigmentations of the 14-mm-long embryo are indicative of degeneration. Based on the CRL, the head is too small and the limb buds (*not seen in these pictures*) were retarded in their development (**B**). Close-up lateral (**C**) and anterior (**D**) view of an embryo with exencephaly, 22 mm in length. The brain tissue (∗) is still present. A normal karyotype was diagnosed cytogenetically (46,XX). *Abbreviation*: CRL, crown–rump length. (*See color insert.*)

The midline cleft lip represents a fusion defect of the median nasal swelling. In the embryo, cleft lip cannot be diagnosed until after seven weeks of development, since fusion does not occur until that time.

Cleft lip may be part of malformation syndromes. Irregular clefting may be caused by amniotic bands. In embryos, clefting defects occur commonly with chromosomal errors, especially trisomy 13.

Cleft Palate.   Cleft palate occurs if the primary anterior palate, lateral palatine processes, and nasal septum fail to unite. Cleft palate can only be diagnosed in the fetal period, since fusion is completed after the 10th week of development.

Hand Malformations

Polydactyly.   Polydactyly is one of the most common limb abnormalities in the embryo. Polydactyly may be on the radial (preaxial) (Fig. 6) or ulnar (postaxial)

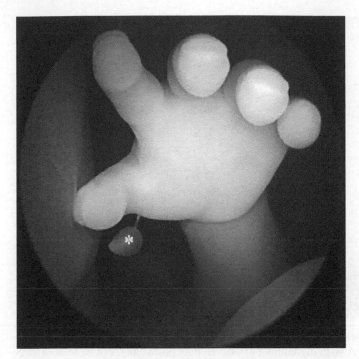

Figure 6 The early fetus measured 58-mm CRL. On the right side a sixth digit (*), developing preaxially, can be seen. *Abbreviation*: CRL, crown–rump length.

(Fig. 7) site. Polydactyly may occur as an isolated malformation or may be part of malformation syndromes. *Postaxial* polydactyly is common in trisomy 13 (20).

    Syndactyly. In syndactyly two or more of the fingers or toes are joined together. This joining can involve the bones or just the skin between the digits. At the end of the eighth developmental week, fingers become free and syndactyly can be diagnosed embryoscopically.

    Syndactyly may be part of malformation syndromes. Syndactyly of *digits III and IV* is common in triploidy (20,21).

    Split-Hand Malformation. Split-hand malformation means a malformation of the limbs with syndactyly, median clefts of the hands and feet, and aplasia and/or hypoplasia of the phalanges, the metacarpals, and the metatarsals. The split-hand/split-foot malformation involves ectrodactyly. The hand is divided into two parts, which are opposed like a lobster claw. In the second anatomical type, the radial rays are absent with only the fifth digit remaining (Fig. 8A,B) (22). Split hand can be part of numerous syndromes. In embryos with split-hand malformation, chromosomal abnormality (trisomy 15) can also be found.

    Transverse Limb Reduction Defect. In transverse limb reduction defect, distal structures of the limb are absent with proximal parts being more or less normal (Fig. 9). These limb defects are regarded as a disruption sequence, which is presumed to be a result by peripheral ischemia (23). The recurrence risk in future pregnancies is minimal (20).

Duplication Anomalies

    Chorangiopagus Parasiticus (CAPP) or Acardius. *Morphology.* The most severe defect in the acardiac conceptus is usually seen in the cranial pole. The parasitic

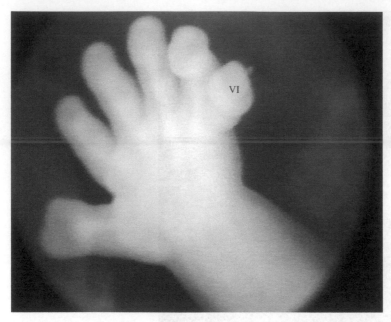

Figure 7　Fingers of well-preserved embryo with trisomy 13 (47,XX,+13) measuring 30-mm CRL were fully separated. A sixth digital ray (VI), developing postaxially, can be seen. *Abbreviation*: CRL, crown–rump length.

twin usually is a markedly edematous mass. The upper portion of the conceptus has missing or highly abnormal facial structures and only remnants of the upper extremities. Usually, well-developed lower limbs can be found. The pump twin is usually developmentally abnormal (24). The circulation is through the normal pump twin by a return reversed flow through direct artery to artery, or vein to vein, anastomoses of the cord or chorionic surface vessels. The observed anomalies of the parasitic twin are presumed to be caused by a combination of a primary developmental defect and decreased oxygenation of the recipient twin with disruption of organogenesis.

Conjoined Twins.　Conjoined twinning is the result of late and incomplete twin formation at the latest possible moment when the embryonic axis is being laid down (embryonic division between 13 and 15 days postconception). Most classifications are descriptive and based on the anatomical zones of coalescence. Fusion of the thorax (thoracopagus) is most commonly (70%) reported (Fig. 10). It is extremely important to identify these rare duplication anomalies (25). Parents can be reassured of the fact that the anomalies are an accidental sequel of twinning, with no additional risk of recurrence in future pregnancies (21).

Amnion Rupture Sequence

The pathogenesis of amniotic bands is still debated and a variety of different theories have been proposed in the past (26). The theory of early amnion rupture, as proposed by Torpin (27), with subsequent formation of amniotic bands interfering with normal embryonic development to cause malformations or disruptions has gained most acceptance and is designated as the ARS (28). Although uncommon among liveborn infants, its frequency may be as high as 1 in 56 in previable fetuses.

(A)

(B)

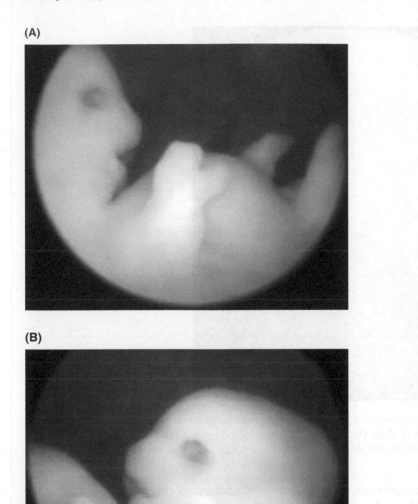

Figure 8 The specific limb defect of this macerated, microcephalic embryo, 21-mm CRL, presented as split right hand (**A**). The finding of rudimentary development of the left limb (UL) (**B**) was consistent with monodactyly, the second anatomical type of split hand. Cytogentic investigation revealed an abnormal (47,XX,+15) karyotype. *Abbreviations*: CRL, crown–rump length; UL, upper limb.

Bands that constrict the umbilical cord are recognized as the main cause of death (29). ARS may cause abnormalities that are detectable by embryoscopy, such as encephaloceles, cleft lip, and amputations. When aberrant sheets or bands of tissue attached to the conceptus with characteristic deformities in a nonembryologic distribution are visualized on embryoscopy, a diagnosis of amniotic band syndrome or ARS can be made (30).

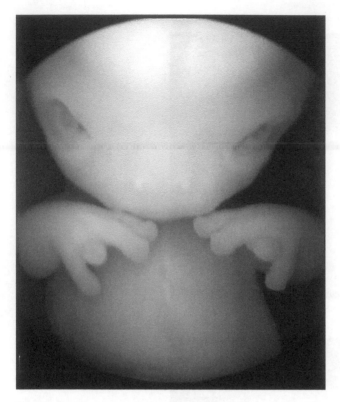

Figure 9 Close-up anterior view of the upper portion of an embryo with a distal symmetric transverse defect of digit IV. The embryo measured 24-mm CRL. A normal karyotype was diagnosed cytogenetically (46,XY). *Abbreviation*: CRL, crown–rump length.

Amniotic bands can occur as a result of abdominal trauma (31), chorionic villus sampling (32), and connective tissue abnormalities (33). In most cases of ARS no such cause can be identified. Therefore, most authors consider ARS a sporadic event with a negligible risk of recurrence.

ETIOLOGY OF DEVELOPMENTAL DEFECTS IN EARLY MISSED ABORTIONS

Developmental Defects with Chromosomal Aberrations

A total of 6% stillbirths (34) and about 0.5% of liveborns (35) have chromosomal aberrations. During the previable fetal period, the reported prevalence of chromosomal abnormality is between 4% and 7% (36). The most common trisomies observed among fetuses are those that involve chromosomes 13, 18, or 21.

Contrary to this comparably "low frequency" of chromosomal abnormality, 60% to 70% of *early spontaneous abortions* have chromosomal abnormalities (37,38). The main classes of chromosomal abnormalities being autosomal trisomies, sex chromosome monosomy, and polyploidy. About 2% to 5% of abnormal karyotypes that occur in early spontaneous abortions are structural chromosomal anomalies. Trisomies for *all* chromosomes with the exception of chromosome 1 are described in *early* spontaneous abortions (37). The majority of the chromosomal

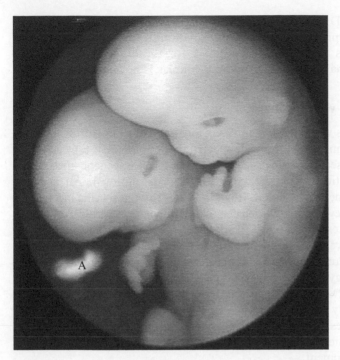

Figure 10 Fetoscopic examination of twins with a CRL of 32 mm from an anterolateral view showed thoracophagus conjoined twins with a fused thorax and upper abdomen, and separate heads. "A"marks the remnants of the amnion. A normal karyotype (46,XX) was diagnosed cytogenetically. *Abbreviation*: CRL, crown–rump length.

abnormalities observed among early spontaneous abortions are incompatible with survival to term; these include tetraploids and all trisomies except trisomies 8, 9, 13, 18, 21, and 22. The estimated prenatal survival of these chromosomal abnormalities ranges between 1% (trisomies 8, 9, and 22 and monosomy X), 3% (trisomy 13), and 5% (trisomy 18). The probability of abortion for trisomy 21 is about 74%.

Correlation of embryonic morphology and karyotype in early abortion specimens shows that a high rate of chromosomal anomalies can be found in *phenotypically abnormal embryos*. The highest rate of chromosomal anomalies (86%) can be found in the category of embryos with combined developmental defects (5,10). Among grossly disorganized embryos, about 70% are cytogenetically abnormal and a comparably "low frequency" of chromosomal abnormality is registered in phenotypically normal embryos (48%).

In summary, aneuploidy/polyploidy is the major factor affecting normal embryonic development in early intrauterine deaths. This might secure as an explanation that though the incidence of developmental defects in specimens of early spontaneous abortions is high, spontaneous abortion is usually a sporadic event in a patient's reproductive history. Most (95%) of the observed chromosomal mutations are not hereditary and carry no increased risk for future pregnancies. They originate de novo either in parental gametes (trisomy and monosomy) or are the result of failure of normal fertilization (triploidy and tetraploidy) and cleavage (tetraploidy).

Therefore, it is necessary to *supplement all embryoscopic findings by the results of cytogenetic analysis* to distinguish between nonchromosomal and chromosomal causes of malformation. Detected aneuploidy/polyploidy in cases of a phenotypically abnormal embryo provides a causal explanation for these developmental defects and also indicates that the recurrence risk for the observed developmental defect and chromosomal abnormality in these couples is not increased (39).

Developmental Defects with Normal Karyotype

Embryonic malformations with an apparently normal karyotype might be heterogenous in their origin. They might cover a wide spectrum of etiologies as they can be of multifactorial origin, caused by a single gene defect, or a non-genetic–mechanism (amniotic bands, duplication anomalies, and vascular disruptions). An accurate description of these specimens is essential. It helps to identify the specific mechanism leading to the observed developmental defects. This information would be completely lost if morphological examination of the demised embryo had not been carried out and the particular developmental defects remained undetected.

The probability of recurrence of these defects in future pregnancies differs depending on their etiology.

If the observed defects are multifactorial in origin, the risk of recurrence of the observed defect is generally around 2% to 5%. It may be much higher for autosomal dominant or recessive genes or not significantly increased if non-genetic–mechanisms (amniotic bands, duplication anomalies, and vascular disruptions) interfered with normal embryonic development.

Multiple developmental defects *without* a chromosomal anomaly are an indicator of a single gene defect, and a high risk of recurrence in future pregnancies cannot be excluded. A specific syndrome diagnosis is usually not possible at these early stages.

In the light of this increased risk, examination of early intrauterine deaths is extremely important, as the information obtained from such an examination may identify patients who can be offered genetic counseling. First-trimester ultrasonographic examination has already become invaluable for women at increased risk of hereditary conditions (40). It is extremely important to obtain an accurate description of specific development, as such information may support early prenatal ultrasonographic examination for the exclusion of recurrence in subsequent pregnancies.

If we are correct in hypothesizing that single gene defects exist in chromosomally normal abortions with developmental defects, the finding might serve as an explanation why detection of a normal karyotype in early abortion specimens is usually interpreted as a poor prognostic sign (41,42).

CLINICAL SIGNIFICANCE OF A DETAILED MORPHOLOGICAL AND CYTOGENETIC EVALUATION OF EARLY SPONTANEOUS ABORTION

Whether embryoscopy and cytogenetic studies should be offered to all women with missed abortion is debatable. This policy has the advantage of providing comprehensive etiological data, but has the disadvantage of requiring an invasive procedure and of inducing extra costs for the management of a condition with a low risk of recurrence.

However, a detailed embryoscopic examination of the dead embryo is likely to be useful in couples who have experienced recurrent abortion or have reproductive loss after IVF (4). In such cases, chromosome analysis is generally recommended (43).

The value of karyotyping early abortion specimens is limited by frequent false-negative results caused by maternal contamination and the finding of a 46,XX karyotype *in the curettage material* is not a reliable result (44). Transcervical embryoscopy in missed abortions allows selective reliable sampling of chorionic tissues with a minimal potential for maternal contamination (3). Apart from this evident benefit, *abnormal embryonic development* documented by embryoscopy in cases *with normal chromosomes* will confront investigators with factors usually *not* considered to be etiologically related to early pregnancy loss and will assist gynecologists in answering specific questions from parents concerning the probable cause of death and the risk of recurrence in a subsequent pregnancy.

ACKNOWLEDGMENT

To a wonderful embryopathologist and teacher, who introduced me to embryopathology, Prof. Dr. D. K. Kalousek.

REFERENCES

1. Cullen MT, Reece A, Wetham J, Hobbins JC. Embryoscopy: description and utility of a technique. Am J Obstet Gynecol 1990; 162:82–86.
2. Philipp T, Kalousek DK. Transcervical embryoscopy in missed abortion. J Assist Reprod Genet 2001; 18:285–290.
3. Ferro J, Martinez MC, Lara C, Pellicer A, Remohi J, Serra V. Improved accuracy of hysteroembryoscopic biopsies for karyotyping early missed abortions. Fertil Steril 2003; 80:1260–1264.
4. Philipp T, Feichtinger W, Van Allen M, Separovic ER, Rainer A, Kalousek DK. Abnormal embryonic development diagnosed embryoscopically in early intrauterine deaths after in vitro fertilization (IVF): a preliminary report of 23 cases. Fertil Steril 2004; 82:1337–1342.
5. Philipp T, Philipp K, Reiner A, Beer F, Kalousek DK. Embryoscopic and cytogenetic analysis of 233 missed abortions: factors involved in the pathogenesis of developmental defects of early failed pregnancies. Hum Reprod 2003; 18:1724–1732.
6. Philipp T. Atlas der Embryologie. In: Embryoskopische Aufnahmen der normalen und abnormen Embryonalentwicklung. Wien: Facultas Verlag, 2004.
7. Moore KL. The Developing Human—Clinically Orientated Embryology. 5th ed. Philadelphia: W.B. Saunders, 1993.
8. Kalousek DK, Fitch N, Paradice BA. Pathology of the Human Embryo and Previable Fetus. New York: Springer Verlag, 1990.
9. Shiota K. Development and intrauterine fate of normal and abnormal human conceptuses. Congenit Anom 1991; 31:67–80.
10. Kalousek DK, Pantzar T, Tsai M, Paradice B. Early spontaneous abortion: morphologic and karyotypic findings in 3912 cases. Birth Defects 1993; 29:53–61.
11. Poland BJ, Miller JR, Harris M, Livingston J. Spontaneous abortion: a study of 1961 women and their conceptuses. Acta Obstet Gynecol Scand 1981; 102(suppl):5–32.
12. Philipp T, Kalousek DK. Generalized abnormal embryonic development in missed abortion: embryoscopic and cytogenetic findings. Am J Med Genet 2002; 111:41–47.
13. Creasy MR, Alberman ED. Congenital malformations of the central nervous system in spontaneous abortions. J Med Genet 1976; 13:9–16.
14. Bell JE, Gosden CM. Central nervous system abnormalities-contrasting patterns in early and late pregnancy. Clin Genet 1978; 13:387–396.

15. Mc Fadden DE, Kalousek DK. Survey of neural tube defects in spontaneously aborted embryos. Am J Med Genet 1989; 32:356–358.
16. Patten BM. Overgrowth of the neural tube in young human embryos. Anat Rec 1952; 113:381–393.
17. Coerdt W, Miller K, Holzgreve W, Rauskolb R, Schwinger E, Rehder H. Neural tube defects in chromosomally normal and abnormal human embryos. Ultrasound Obstet Gynecol 1997; 10:410–415.
18. Philipp T, Kalousek DK. Neural tube defects in missed abortions—embryoscopic and cytogenetic findings. Am J Med Genet 2002; 107:52–57.
19. Philipp T, Grillenberger K, Separovic ER, Philipp K, Kalousek DK. Effects of triploidy on early human development. Prenat Diagn 2004; 242:276–281.
20. Ramsing M, Duda V, Mehrain Y, et al. Hand malformations in the aborted embryo: an informative source of genetic information. Birth Defects 1996; 30:79–94.
21. Dimmick JE, Kalousek DK. Developmental Pathology of the Embryo and Fetus. Philadelphia: J.B. Lippincott Company, 1992.
22. Birch-Jensen A. Congenital Deformities of Upper Extremities. Copenhagen: Enjar Munksgaard, 1949.
23. Golden CM, Ryan LM, Holmes LB. Choronic villus sampling: a distinctive teratogenic effects on fingers? Birth Defects Res 2003; 67:557–562.
24. Napolitani FD, Schreiber I. The acardiac monster. A review of the world literature and presentation of two cases. Am J Obstet Gynecol 1960; 82:708–711.
25. Philipp T, Separovic ER, Philipp K, Reiner A, Kalousek DK. Trancervical fetoscopic diagnosis of structural defects in four first trimester monochorionic twin intrauterine deaths. Prenat Diagn 2003; 12:964–969.
26. Evans MI. Amniotic bands. Ultrasound Obstet Gynecol 1997; 10:307–308.
27. Torpin R. Amniochorionic mesoblastic fibrous strings and amniotic bands. Associated constricting fetal anomalies or fetal death. Am J Obstet Gynecol 1965; 91:65–75.
28. Kalousek DK, Bamforth S. Amnion rupture sequence in previable fetuses. Am J Med Genet 1988; 3:63–73.
29. Hong CY, Simon MA. Amniotic bands knotted about umbilical cord. A rare cause of fetal death. Obstet Gynecol 1963; 222:667–670.
30. Philipp T, Kalousek DK. Amnion rupture sequence in a first trimester missed abortion. Prenat Diagn 2001; 21:835–838.
31. Ossipoff V, Hall BD. Etiologic factors in the amniotic band syndrome. A study of 24 patients. Birth Defects 1977; 13:117–132.
32. Firth HV, Boyd PA, Chamberlain P, Mackenzie IZ, Lindenbaum RH, Huson SM. Severe limb abnormalities after chorion villus sampling at 56–66 days gestation. Lancet 1991; 337:762–763.
33. Young ID, Lindenbaum RH, Thompsen EM, Pemburg ME. Amniotic bands in connective tissue disorders. Arch Dis Child 1985; 60:1061–1063.
34. Jacobs PA, Hassold TJ. Chromosome abnormalities origin and ethiology in abortions and stillbirths. In: Vogel F, Sperling K, eds. Human Genetics. New York: Springer Verlag, 1987.
35. Sperling K. Chromosomen-anomalien beim menschen: häufigkeit und entstehung. Biol I Unserer Ziet 1983; 13:144–156.
36. Craver RD, Kalousek DK. Cytogenetic abnormalities among spontaneously aborted previable fetuses. Am J Med Gen 1987; 3(suppl):113–120.
37. Eiben B, Bartels I, Bähr–Porsch S, et al. Cytogenetic analysis of 750 spontaneous abortions with the direct-preparation method of chorionic villi and its implicationsfor studying genetic causes of pregnancy wastage. Am J Hum Genet 1990; 47:656–663.
38. Tariverdian G, Paul M. Genetische Diagnostik in Geburtshilfe und Gynäkologie. In: Ein Leitfaden für Klinik und Praxis. Heidelberg: Springer Verlag, 1999.
39. Warburton D, Kline J, Stein Z, Hutzler M, Chin A, Hassold T. Does the karyotype of a spontaneous abortion predict the karyotype of a subsequent abortion?—Evidence

from 273 women with two karyotyped spontaneous abortions. Am J Hum Genet 1987; 41:465–483.

40. Blaas HG. The examination of the embryo and early fetus: how and by whom? Ultrasound Obstet Gynecol 1999; 14:153–158.

41. Osagawara M, Aoki K, Okada S, Suzumori K. Embryonic karyotype of abortuses in relation to the number of previous miscarriages. Fertil Steril 2000; 73:300–304.

42. Stephenson M, Awartani KA, Robinson WP. Cytogenetic analysis of miscarriages from couples with recurrent miscarriage: a case–control study. Hum Reprod 2002; 17:446–451.

43. Wolf GC, Horger EO. Indication for examination of spontaneous abortion specimens: a reassessment. Am J Obstet Gynecol 1995; 5:1364–1367.

44. Bell KA, Van Deerlin PG, Haddad BR, Feinberg RF. Cytogenetic diagnosis of "normal 46,XX" karyotypes in spontaneous abortions frequently may be misleading. Fertil Steril 1999; 71:334–341.

45. Jauniaux E, Barnea E, Edwards R. Embryonic Medicine and Therapy. New York: Oxford University Press, 1997.

15

Prenatal Diagnosis of Chromosome Abnormalities

Kamlesh Madan
Department of Clinical Genetics, VU University Medical Center,
Amsterdam, The Netherlands

INTRODUCTION

The correct human chromosome number was determined to be 46 in 1956 (1,2). In the following 10 years, most of the common chromosomal disorders such as Down syndrome, Turner syndrome, Edwards syndrome, Klinefelter syndrome, and Patau syndrome were identified.

Cells taken from amniotic fluid were first used to determine the sex of the fetus nearly 50 years ago (3). However, it was a decade later, in 1966, that cells from amniotic fluid taken in the second trimester of pregnancy were first cultured for karyotyping of cells of the fetus (4). Since then there have been developments on several fronts. Increase in experience and improvement in sampling methods on the one hand and in culture techniques on the other, have led to improvement in the quality of prenatal diagnosis of chromosome abnormalities. With the development of chromosome banding techniques in the seventies and molecular cytogenetic methods in the nineties there has been an increase in the number of structural abnormalities that can be identified, including imbalance of very small and even submicroscopic chromosome segments.

In the 1980s the introduction of chorionic villus sampling (5) opened up the possibility for early prenatal diagnosis in the first trimester. The possibility of sampling cord blood for prenatal diagnosis in the second trimester of pregnancy (6) increased the scope of prenatal diagnosis in fetuses found to have abnormalities detected by ultrasound later in pregnancy.

In this chapter, I shall attempt to give an overview of prenatal diagnosis (PD) of chromosomal disorders. For technical details of methodology I shall refer the reader to text books and review articles. This chapter will focus on chromosome abnormalities in general, the indications for PD, the type of chromosome abnormalities that can be expected in the various indication groups, and the difficulties and pitfalls in the interpretation of some of the findings.

NORMAL CHROMOSOMES AND VARIANTS

A normal human cell has two sex chromosomes, or gonosomes, and 22 pairs of autosomes. A woman has two identical sex chromosomes called X, and a man has an X and a Y. The karyotypes are 46,XX and 46,XY, respectively (Fig. 1). Chromosomes are visible during cell division and are normally examined in the metaphase stage of cell division. At this stage, the chromosomes appear double as the chromatids are still held together at the centromere and have not yet separated into the two daughter cells. The two arms of the chromosome on either side of the centromere are conventionally designated the letters *p* (for the short arm) and *q* (for the long arm). The chromosomes are usually examined using G-banding or, less frequently, R-banding (7). These banding techniques produce bands along the length of the chromosome so that each chromosome has a unique banding pattern (Fig. 1). The identification of each chromosome and each chromosome band (by p or q and the number of the band) has been standardized and is described in the International System for Cytogenetic Nomenclature which is regularly updated, the last update having taken place in 2005 (7).

Also described in this publication are the so-called normal polymorphic *variants*. Certain chromosome segments that are usually composed of genetically inactive, darkly staining (with C-banding) heterochromatin may vary in size without being associated with any phenotypic effect (7). The short arms of the acrocentric chromosomes (i.e., chromosomes with very short arms: 13, 14, 15, 21, and 22) may vary in size or may have so-called satellites (e.g., the left chromosome 13 in Fig. 1). The heterochromatic segments next to the centromeres of most chromosomes may also vary in size. In some cases the centromeric heterochromatin may be shifted from the long arm to the short arm due to a pericentric inversion (see following text). Inversion of chromosome 9 with breakpoints in bands p11 and q13, i.e., inv(9)(p11q13), is the most common example and is found in about 2% of the population. The heterochromatic portion in the distal arm of the long arm of the Y chromosome can also vary considerably in size.

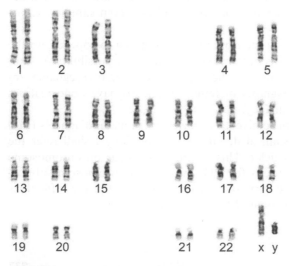

Figure 1 Normal male karyotype 46,XY.

A number of families have been described in which the short arm of an acrocentric chromosome (most commonly chromosome 22) has a very large heterochromatic segment originating from the long arm of the Y chromosome. Both male and female carriers in these families are phenotypically normal. In fact such a variant is no different from other variants except that the heterochromatin is from the Y. In cases of unusual or exceptionally large variants it is necessary to examine the chromosomes of the parents or other relatives to establish that one is dealing with a variant.

In addition to the G-banding, other staining techniques are used to identify specific chromosome regions (7). The fluorescence in situ hybridization (FISH) technique, which is discussed in Chapter 16, is regularly used to investigate chromosome abnormalities in a routine cytogenetics laboratory. FISH can be used with probes that are specific for centromeric regions, telomeric regions (ends of chromosomes) or specific disease loci on individual chromosomes or for specific whole chromosomes (using whole chromosome paints). Spectral karyotyping (SKY) and multicolor FISH methods whereby each chromosome gets a specific color, are extra tools for identifying chromosome abnormalities.

CHROMOSOME ABNORMALITIES

Chromosome abnormalities can be described as numerical or structural.

Numerical Chromosome Abnormalities

Aneuploidy

The most common numerical abnormality is either the presence of an extra chromosome or the absence of a chromosome (aneuploidy). Aneuploidy arises when a pair of chromosomes fails to separate (nondisjunction, ND) during cell division, leading to an extra chromosome (trisomy) or a missing chromosome (monosomy) in one of the daughter cells. This can occur during one of the two stages of meiosis (the cell division in the gonads that leads to the formation of spermatozoa or ova) or during mitosis (the cell division in somatic cells) (Fig. 2). Aneuploid cells as well as normal cells may be present in the same individual. Such a chromosome constitution in which two or more cell lines are present is described as a mosaic. Mosaicism arises by ND in a mitotic cell division in the zygote. If one of the normal cells with 46 chromosomes in the early zygote undergoes ND, for example, chromosome 21, one of the daughter cells would have 47 chromosomes with an extra 21 and the other 45 chromosomes in which the 21 is absent. The latter cell line would not be viable. The resulting individual would be a mosaic with two cell lines, one with 46 and the other with 47 chromosomes (Fig. 3A). In a zygote that is trisomic to begin with, the extra chromosome may be lost (trisomy rescue) during one of the cell divisions by a process called anaphase lag. In one of the cells the extra chromosome is left behind and does not get included in either of the two daughter cells (Fig. 3B). This would also lead to a mosaic karyotype with 46 and 47 chromosomes.

The best-known example of aneuploidy is the presence of an extra chromosome 21 (trisomy 21), described as 47,XX or XY,+21, in individuals with Down syndrome. Trisomy 21, trisomy 13 (Patau syndrome), and trisomy 18 (Edwards

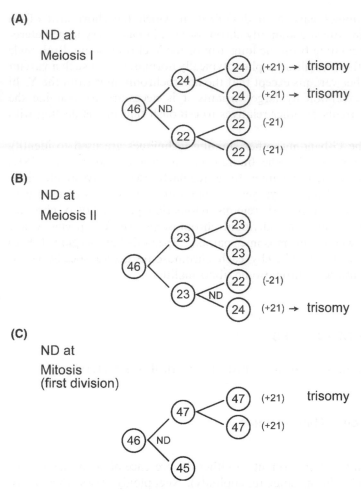

Figure 2 Origin of aneuploidy by nondisjunction (ND) during: **(A)** the first meiotic division, **(B)** the second meiotic division, or **(C)** the first mitotic division of the zygote. The gametes with the extra chromosomes in (A) and (B) would give rise to trisomy after fertilization. The cell with 45 chromosomes in **(C)** would not be viable.

syndrome) (Fig. 4) are the only autosomal trisomies that are compatible with live birth. These chromosome abnormalities may also be found in a mosaic form. Mosaic trisomy 9 and mosaic trisomy 8 are known to be compatible with live birth. Mosaic trisomies for other chromosomes are usually lost spontaneously early in pregnancy. A few survive longer and have been found in phenotypically abnormal liveborn children (see following text under mosaicism at amniocentesis). Autosomal monosomy is not normally viable. Sex chromosome aneuploidies, such as 47,XXX, 47,XXY (Klinefelter syndrome), and 47,XYY, are compatible with live birth. All these aneuploidies may occur as mosaics. The only monosomy that can survive to birth is monosomy X (45,X), which is associated with Turner syndrome. The 45,X cell line may occur together with different cell lines including those with structural abnormalities of the X or the Y chromosome, with variable phenotype (8). For phenotypes associated with the abnormal karyotypes described previously, the reader is referred to the textbook by Gardner and Sutherland (9).

(A)

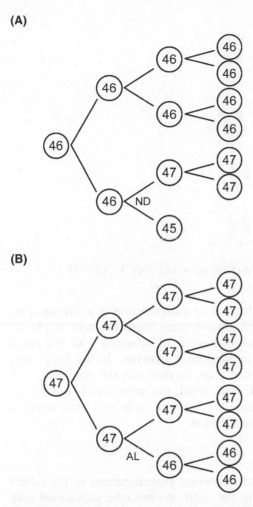

(B)

Figure 3 Origin of mosaicism with two cell lines with 46 and 47 chromosomes: **(A)** due to nondisjunction (ND) in an embryo with a normal karyotype (the cell with 45 chromosomes would not be viable) and **(B)** due to anaphase lag (AL) in a trisomic embryo.

Triploidy

In a triploid individual there is a whole extra set of chromosomes (Fig. 5). Triploidy occurs in 1% of all conceptions and originates from the fertilization of an ovum by two spermatozoa or by fusion of a fertilized ovum with a polar body (see following text). Most fetuses with triploidy 69,XXX or 69,XXY, abort spontaneously but sometimes they are stillborn or die shortly after birth. Ultrasonographic abnormalities have been described in triploids (10) as well as in diploid/triploid mosaics (11).

Chromosome Structural Abnormalities

When segments of chromosomes are rearranged without loss of genetic information, the rearrangement can be described as a balanced rearrangement. Such a rearrangement is usually found in one of the partners of a couple referred for postnatal chromosome analysis following two or more spontaneous abortions, or in one of

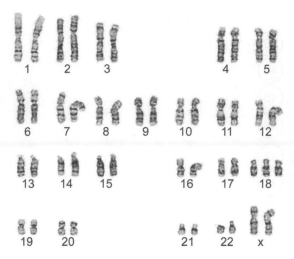

Figure 4   Karyotype of a girl with trisomy 18 (Edwards syndrome): 47,XX,+18.

the parents of an abnormal child with a deletion or a duplication of a chromosome segment. Carrier of a balanced structural chromosome rearrangement is phenotypically normal but has an increased risk of having an offspring with too much or too little chromosome material, an unbalanced karyotype. If the karyotypic imbalance is too big the conceptus will not grow further and the pregnancy will end in a spontaneous abortion. If, on the other hand, the imbalance is not so big, it may be compatible with life. In that case the liveborn child will have multiple congenital abnormalities and/or mental retardation.

Meiosis

In order to understand how a balanced chromosome rearrangement in the parent can give rise to chromosome imbalance in the child one must be acquainted with the process of gametogenesis, and particularly with the process of meiosis. Meiosis is the cell division that takes place in the testes and the ovaries in the parents whereby the number of chromosomes is reduced from 46 (a diploid number) to 23 (a haploid number) in the ovum or the spermatozoon (Fig. 6). After fertilization, the zygote

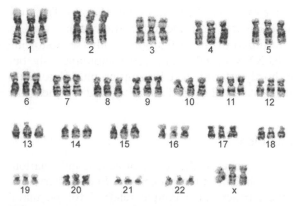

Figure 5   Karyotype of a triploid fetus showing 69 chromosomes: 69,XXX.

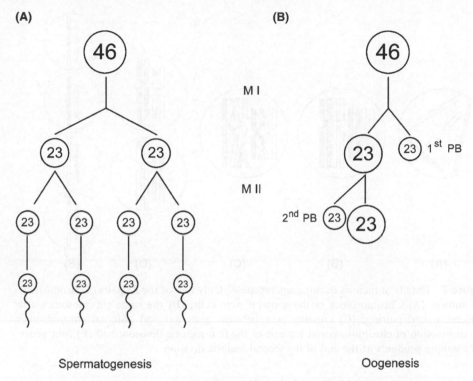

Spermatogenesis

Oogenesis

Figure 6 Stages of (**A**) spermatogenesis and (**B**) oogenesis from a gonadal stem cell with 46 chromosomes through first (M I) and second (M II) meiotic divisions to gametes with 23 chromosomes. Each spermatogonium gives rise to four spermatozoa. During oogensis, the cytoplasm divides unequally in both meiotic divisions as a result of which there is only one mature ovum and two polar bodies (PBs). The first PB sometimes also divides during the second meiotic division.

gets 46 chromosomes. An important step in the process is recombination during which the homologous chromosomes of maternal and paternal origin in the individual come together to pair, to exchange material and then separate. As a result, although each individual passes on one chromosome of a pair to the offspring, this chromosome contains material from both, the mother and father, i.e., the child receives genetic information from all four grandparents. At the end of meiosis four genetically unique products are formed, each with 23 chromosomes (Fig. 7).

Reciprocal Translocations

A reciprocal translocation results from breaks in two nonhomologous chromosomes followed by an exchange of the chromosome segments. In carriers of structural rearrangements the process of separating of chromatids following the pairing and the recombination during meiosis is disturbed. The pairing and segregation of chromosomes involved in a reciprocal translocation can take place in various ways (7). The chromosomes involved in the translocation can segregate in such a way that the gametes that are formed give rise to a balanced karyotype in the zygote. This happens with a so-called 2:2 alternate segregation. In the example of a translocation t(8;15) shown in Figure 8, gamete (A) gets both the normal chromosomes, i.e., chromosomes

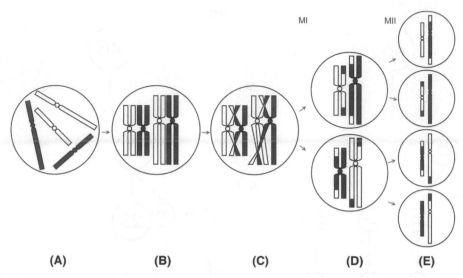

Figure 7 Details of meiosis during gametogenesis. Only two of the 23 pairs of chromosomes are shown. (**A**) Chromosomes in the gonadal stem cells; (**B**) the same chromosomes after replication and pairing; (**C**) crossing over between maternal and paternal chromosomes; (**D**) disjunction of chromosomes at the end of the first meiotic division; and (**E**) four genetically unique products at the end of the second meiotic division.

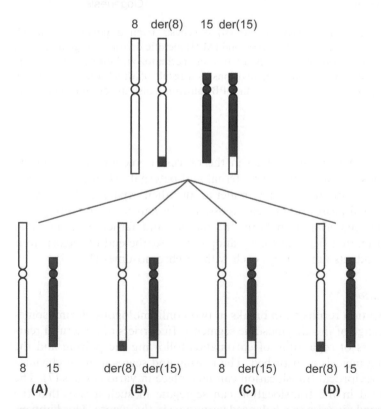

Figure 8 Segregation in a carrier of a translocation t(8;15) between the long arms of chromosomes 8 and 15 (see text). The first two gametes (A and B) are the result of an alternate segregation and would result in balanced karyotypes after fertilization. The last two (C and D) are a result of a 2:2 adjacent 1 segregation and would give rise to zygotes with unbalanced karyotypes.

8 and 15 and the other, gamete (B) both the derived chromosomes involved in the translocation, i.e., der(8) and der(15). After fertilization by a normal gamete both of these would result in a phenotypically normal child, one with normal chromosomes and the other with the balanced translocation like the parent. This type of segregation takes place in carriers of all reciprocal translocations (Fig. 9A).

Unbalanced karyotypes can arise by other 2:2 segregations (so called adjacent 1 or adjacent 2 segregations, see below) or by a 3:1 segregation whereby one gamete receives three and the other only one chromosome. The various types of segregations are illustrated in Figure 9.

A 2:2 adjacent 1-segregation is also shown in the example in Figure 8. The normal 8 segregates together with the der(15) [gamete (C)] and the der(8) with the normal 15 [gamete (D)]. Both of these would give rise to unbalanced gametes. The first would have too much material from chromosome 8 and too little from chromosome 15. The second would have too little material from chromosome 8 and too much from chromosome 15. The zygotes resulting from these gametes would either end up in an early abortion or in a phenotypically abnormal child. This is the most common segregation by which karyotypic imbalance can arise. It occurs mostly when the size of the exchanged segments is relatively small (Figs 9B and 10A).

Also in the 2:2 adjacent 2 type of segregation, each gamete gets the correct number of chromosomes, i.e., two. However, instead of one chromosome of each pair separating into different gametes, both centromeres of one pair end up in the same gamete resulting in both gametes being chromosomally unbalanced (Figs 9C and 10B). This type of segregation is more likely to occur when the breakpoints of the translocation are close to the centromere and relatively long chromosome segments have been exchanged. In a 3:1 segregation (Fig. 9D and E), one gamete receives three chromosomes and results in a zygote with 47 chromosomes (Fig. 10C and D). The other corresponding gamete gets only one and results in a zygote with 45 chromosomes (Fig 10E). A 3:1 segregation is likely to take place if the sizes of the exchanged segments are very unequal and if one of the chromosomes involved is small, an acrocentric chromosome (13, 14, 15, 21, or 22) or chromosome 9 with a break in the heterochromatic segment.

Most reciprocal translocations can be identified using standard G-banded preparations. In some cases, however, the size of the exchanged segments is so small that the translocation can be identified only by means of molecular cytogenetic techniques using subtelomere probes, as described in Chapter 16.

The risk of a carrier of a reciprocal translocation having a liveborn child with an unbalanced karyotype depends on several factors. These are: the chromosomes involved, the position of the breakpoints and the size of the segments exchanged, whether the segments contain genetically active (euchromatin) or inactive (heterochromatin) material, and the extent of the imbalance in the unbalanced product, i.e., whether it is compatible with life or not.

For the calculation of the risk of a liveborn child with a chromosome imbalance, one needs to estimate the most likely mode of segregation as described earlier and illustrated in Figure 9. The potential imbalance (which segment would be duplicated and which will be deleted) can then be worked out. In general, extra chromosome material is tolerated better by the developing embryo than is the loss of chromosome material. Based on other published cases and/or on possible unbalanced cases in the family, one can work out the chance of the particular imbalance being compatible with live birth. In the absence of sufficient information, a very rough estimate of the risk of a child with an unbalanced karyotype can be made by considering the mode of ascertainment. If the translocation was

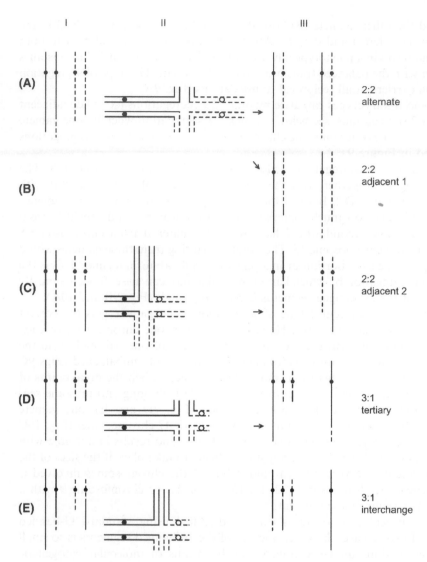

Figure 9 Types of segregation in reciprocal translocations. Column I: the translocation in the parent. Column II: pairing of the chromosomes after duplication of chromatids during meiosis. Column III: the distribution of the chromosomes in the gametes. The different types of segregation are: (**A**) *Alternate* segregation in which both types of gametes would result in a zygote with a balanced karyotype after fertilization. This segregation can take place in all four translocations shown. (**B–E**) Types of segregations that produce unbalanced gametes. (**B**) Unbalanced gametes (see text) resulting from a *2:2 adjacent 1*-segregation. This usually occurs when the size of the translocated segments is relatively small. (**C**) Unbalanced gametes resulting from a *2:2 adjacent 2* type of segregation. This occurs when the translocated segments are relatively long and the centric segments are short. (**D**) Gametes resulting from a *3:1* segregation that after fertilization would give rise to zygotes with tertiary trisomy and monosomy. (**E**) Gametes resulting from a *3:1* segregation that would give rise to zygotes with interchange trisomy and monosomy. The 3:1 segregations described in (**D**) and (**E**) occur usually when there is an asymmetrical exchange and where one of the chromosomes involved is very small (an acrocentric or the short arm of chromosome 9).

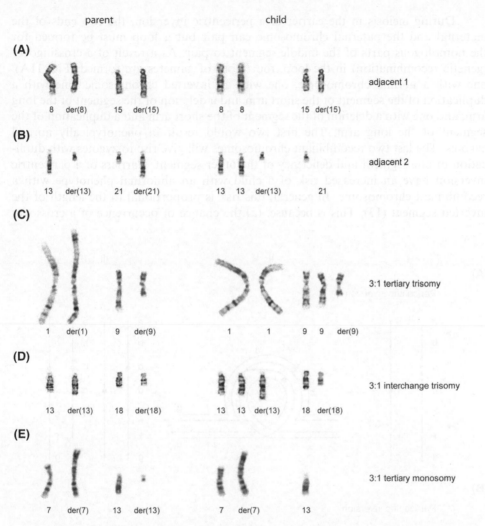

Figure 10 Partial karyotypes showing a reciprocal translocation in a phenotypically normal parent (*left*) and the resulting unbalanced karyotype in the child (*right*) with congenital abnormalities due to different modes of segregation (see text).

ascertained through spontaneous abortion or was an accidental finding, the risk is 1.5–5% (lower risk associated with a paternal carrier). If the ascertainment was through a previous child with an unbalanced karyotype the risk increases to about 20% (12).

Inversions

A chromosomal inversion is a result of two breaks followed by reinsertion of the segment between the two breaks after it has been rotated by 180°. If one of the breaks is in the short arm and the other in the long arm of the chromosome, it is called a *pericentric inversion*. If both the breaks are in the same arm of the chromosome, it is called a *paracentric inversion*. Carriers of such inversions are phenotypically normal. The reproductive consequence is different for the two types of inversions.

During meiosis in the carrier of a pericentric inversion, the two ends of the maternal and the paternal chromosome can pair but a loop must be formed for the homologous parts of the middle segment to pair. As a result of a crossingover (genetic recombination) in the loop, four types of gametes are formed (Fig. 11A): one with a normal chromosome; one with an inverted chromosome; one with a duplication of the segment of the short arm and a deletion of the segment of the long arm; and one with a deletion of the segment of the short arm and a duplication of the segment of the long arm. The first two would result in phenotypically normal zygotes. The last two recombinant chromosomes will give rise to zygotes with duplication of one segment and deficiency of the other segment. Carriers of a pericentric inversion have an increased risk of a child with an abnormal phenotype with a recombinant chromosome. In general, this risk is proportional to the length of the inverted segment (13). This is because: (a) the chance of occurrence of a crossover

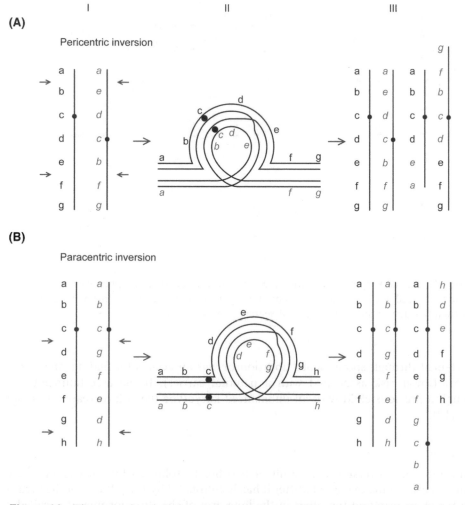

Figure 11 The normal and the inverted chromosome of the parent (column I), the inversion loop showing a crossover during meiosis (column II), and the normal, the inverted and two recombinant chromosomes in the four gametes (column III) resulting from **(A)** a pericentric inversion and **(B)** a paracentric inversion (see text).

and the formation of recombinants is greater if the inverted segment is long; (b) recombinant chromosomes arising from a long inversion have short segments that have been duplicated and deleted; and (c) zygotes with imbalance of relatively short segments have a higher chance of survival. Figure 12A shows a pericentric inversion in chromosome 6.

Also for a paracentric inversion, a loop has to be formed for the homologous segments to pair (Fig. 11B). In this case, however, the two resulting recombinants will be either an acentric fragment (segment without a centromere) or a dicentric chromosome (with two centromeres). Neither of the zygotes from these gametes will be viable. The risk of an abnormal child for a carrier of a paracentric inversion is extremely low (14). There are very few exceptions. Two cases of chromosome 14 (15,16), one of chromosome 15 (17), and one of chromosome 9 (18), have been published, where a dicentric chromosome has stabilized itself by inactivation of one of the two centromeres. In all these cases there was a live-born child with phenotypic abnormalities. A word of caution is warranted here. In rare cases some inverted intrachromosomal insertions (see following text), can be indistinguishable from a paracentric inversion (19). Many previously reported recombinants thought

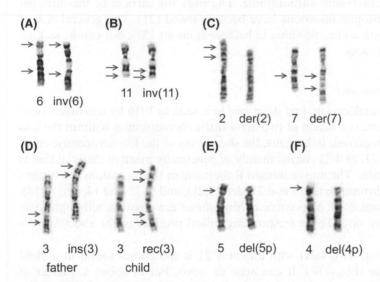

Figure 12 Partial karyograms. (**A**) A normal chromosome 6 and a 6 with a pericentric inversion, inv(6)(p25q21), found in a woman referred for recurrent abortions. (**B**) A normal chromosome 11 and an 11 with a paracentric inversion, inv(11)(q21q23), found in a normal woman referred for prenatal diagnosis for maternal age. The same inversion was found in the amniotic fluid cells. (**C**) Interchromosomal insertion, ins(7;2)(q22;p23p13), in which a segment from the short arm of chromosome 2, (2p13 → p23), is inverted and inserted into the long arm of chromosome 7 in band 7q22. This insertion was found in a man referred for infertility. (**D**) Intrachromosomal insertion of a segment from the long arm of chromosome 3, (3q13.2 → q25), into band p25.3 in the short arm of the same chromosome. The *left* pair of chromosomes is from the phenotypically normal father (karyotype: 46, XY, ins(3)(p25.3q13.2q25)). The *right* pair is from the child with congenital abnormalities. The recombinant chromosome in the child (right one of the pair) has a duplication of the inserted segment. (**E**) Deletion of a part of the short arm of chromosome 5 in a child with Cri-du-Chat syndrome. (**F**) Deletion of a part of the short arm of chromosome 4 in a child with Wolf–Hirshhorn syndrome.

to have arisen from a paracentric inversion have later been reinterpreted to have arisen from insertions (19). It is important to distinguish between the two, as paracentric inversions are found relatively commonly and are associated with a very low risk of abnormal offspring, and insertions on the other hand are very rare and are associated with a high risk. Figure 12B shows a paracentric inversion of chromosome 11.

Insertions

There are two kinds of insertions: *interchromosomal* and *intrachromosomal*. In an interchromosomal insertion an interstitial segment from one chromosome is inserted interstitially into another nonhomologous chromosome (Fig. 12C). The risk of a liveborn abnormal child with a deletion or a duplication of the inserted segment for carriers of these insertions is high, about 35% (12,20).

In an intrachromosomal insertion a chromosomal segment is moved from its original position to another position in the same chromosome, either in the same arm or in the other arm of the chromosome (Fig. 12D). Pairing of homologous segments during meiosis is complicated and crossing over can lead to an unbalanced karyotype with a recombinant chromosome. The risks for carriers of the different types of intrachromosomal insertions have been reviewed (21). The general risk of an abnormal child with a chromosomal imbalance is about 15%, but can be as high as 50% in individual cases.

Robertsonian Translocations

In a Robertsonian translocation, first described in insects in 1916 by a cytogeneticist called Robertson, there is a fusion of two acrocentric chromosomes without the loss of genetically active material. In humans, the short arms of the five acrocentric chromosomes 13, 14, 15, 21, and 22 consist mainly of genetically inactive material that is usually heterochromatic. The most common Robertsonian translocations are fusions of the long arms of chromosomes 14 and 21, der(14;21), and of 13 and 14, der(13;14). However, combinations of all acrocentric chromosomes are possible, although some of them are extremely rare. The corresponding fusion product of the short arms is usually lost.

The translocation der(14;21) with an extra 21 is sometimes found in a child with Down syndrome (Fig. 13B). It can arise de novo, but in about a quarter of the cases one of the parents is a carrier of the balanced translocation, der(14;21). A carrier of a balanced Robertsonian translocation has 45 chromosomes with one 14, one 21, and a der(14;21) (Fig. 13A). The carrier is phenotypically normal but has an increased risk of having a child with Down syndrome. The segregation of the chromosomes into the gametes is shown in Figure 14. The risk of a child with Down syndrome is 1% for a male carrier and about 10% for a female carrier (9). Carriers of a der(13;14) have a risk of having a child with Patau syndrome with an extra chromosome 13, but this risk is very low, 0.5–0.7% (9). In general, female carriers are identified following the birth of a child with Patau syndrome, whereas male carriers are often identified because of infertility (22,23).

The risk of abnormalities due to uniparental disomy (UPD), particularly if chromosomes 14 and 15 are involved, is increased for children of carriers (24).

Uniparental Disomy. UPD is a rare phenomenon in which a person receives both chromosomes of a pair from only one parent instead of one from each

(A)

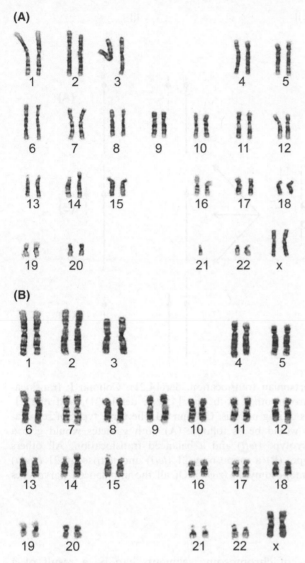

Figure 13 Karyograms from **(A)**, a phenotypically normal woman with a Robertsonian translocation between chromosomes 14 and 21, karyotype 45,XX,der(14;21), and **(B)** her child with Down syndrome and karyotype 46,XY,der(14,21), +21.

parent. In some cases this can give rise to an abnormal phenotype. For more insight into UPD, the reader is referred to review articles and a textbook (25–28). UPD of chromosome 15 is the best-known example. Maternal UPD of 15 causes Prader–Willi syndrome whereas paternal UPD of chromosome 15 causes Angelman syndrome. In rare situations, in an initially trisomic zygote, the aneuploidy may be "corrected" by loss of one of the three chromosomes (a process described as "trisomy rescue," see preceding text). In about one-third of the cases the trisomy rescue will lead to both remaining chromosomes being from the same parent, i.e., UPD. UPD of certain chromosomes is associated with congenital abnormalities (see following text).

I   II   III

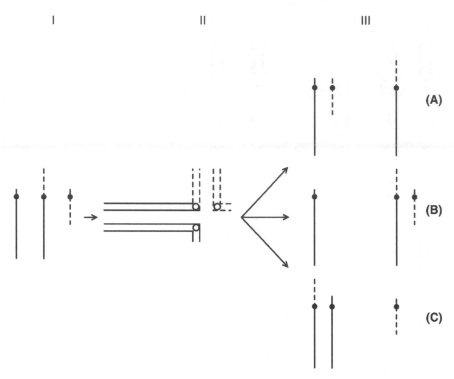

Figure 14 Segregation of a Robertsonian translocation, der(14;21). Column I: translocation in the parent who has 45 chromosomes, with one 14, one der(14;21), and one 21. Column II: pairing of chromosomes during meiosis. Column III: the three types of segregation. After fertilization the results would be as follows: (**A**) both gametes would give a balanced karyotype, a normal karyotype (*left*) and a balanced translocation. All others would give an unbalanced karyotype: (**B**) a monosomy 21 (*left*) and a trisomy 21 (*right*) and (**C**) a trisomy 14 (*left*) and a monosomy 14 (*right*). Of all the unbalanced karyotypes only trisomy 21 is viable.

Deletions and Duplications

Both deletions and duplications of chromosome segments can be a result of a balanced rearrangement in one of the parents. Therefore, when a deletion or a duplication is found in a child referred for congenital abnormalities, it is essential to investigate the parents in order to exclude a translocation. However, a de novo deletion or duplication can occur in any chromosome. A deletion may involve a terminal or an interstitial chromosomal segment. For a full review of deletions, the reader is referred to the textbook by Gardner and Sutherland (9). A few relatively common deletions are associated with certain syndromes. Cri-du-Chat syndrome is associated with a terminal deletion of the short arm of chromosome 5, del(5p) (Fig. 12E) and patients with Wolf–Hirshhorn syndrome have a deletion of the short arm of chromosome 4, del(4p) (Fig. 12F). A submicroscopic interstitial deletion in band q11.2 in chromosome 7, del(7)(q11.2), is found in patients with Williams syndrome. In patients with Miller–Dieker syndrome there is an interstitial deletion in chromosome 17, del(17)(p13.3). The last two, like many so-called microdeletion syndromes, can be identified only with the aid of molecular cytogenetic techniques as discussed in Chapter 16.

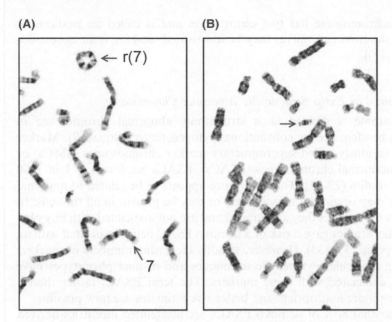

Figure 15 Partial metaphases showing (**A**), a ring derived from chromosome 7 found in a child with congenital abnormalities and (**B**) a marker chromosome, i(22p), derived from chromosome 22 in which the short arm with the satellite is duplicated (see text). This de novo marker was found in all cells in the amniotic fluid of a woman referred for maternal age. A normal child was born.

Ring Chromosomes

A ring chromosome may replace one of the chromosomes. It is formed by a deletion of a segment of the short arm and a deletion of the long arm followed by fusion of the two ends (Fig. 15A). Ring chromosomes are very unstable during the mitotic cell division. As a result, an individual with a ring chromosome has cells with a ring or a double-sized ring or cells in which the ring has been lost. The associated phenotype may be due to del(p), del(q), trisomy and monosomy of the chromosome involved.

Very small ring chromosomes in which most of the short arm as well as the long arm is missing are sometimes found as an extra chromosome. These are discussed in a subsequent section on "marker" chromosomes.

Isochromosomes

Isochromosomes are "mirror image" chromosomes with two identical arms on either side of the centromere. Isochromosomes of the long arm of the X chromosome are sometimes found in patients with Turner syndrome, usually in a mosaic form with a monosomy X cell line, karyotype: 45,X/46,X,i(Xq). Isochromosomes may involve one arm or one arm and a part of the other arm of a chromosome, in which case it is a dicentric chromosome in which one of the centromeres is inactivated (pseudodicentric) in order to stabilize the dicentric during cell division. Isochromosomes of chromosome 15 are some of the most frequently found marker chromosomes (see marker chromosomes in the next section). If only the short arm of chromosome 15 is involved, it is an isochromosome of the short arm [i(15p)]. If also the long arm is involved the isochromosome has two centromeres and is called an isodicentric [idic (15)]. One of the two centromeres may be inactivated, making it an isopseudo-dicentric [ipsu dic (15)].

Marker Chromosomes, or Extra Structurally Abnormal Chromosomes

A marker chromosome is defined as a structurally abnormal chromosome in which no part can be identified by conventional cytogenetic techniques (7). Marker chromosomes are variously called supernumerary marker chromosomes (SMCs) or extra structurally abnormal chromosomes (ESACs). ESACs are found in 1 in 1000 fetuses in prenatal studies (29–31). The occurrence appears to be related to maternal age (32). A marker may occur in a mosaic form or may be present in all the cells. In approximately 40% of the cases they are familial and are not associated with any phenotypic effect. Earlier studies gave a risk of a de novo ESAC being associated with an abnormal phenotype as 13% (33). However, steadily increasing numbers of markers are identified using molecular cytogenetic techniques and distinct phenotypes have been found to be associated with these markers. The term ESAC, rather than a marker, is becoming more appropriate and better risk estimates are now possible.

It is now clear that 80% of de novo ESACs are bisatellited dicentrics derived from acrocentric chromosomes. Half of these are from chromosome 15 and some are from chromosome 22 (30,34–36). The remaining 20% are either isochromosomes, mostly i(8p), i(9p), i(12p), or small ring chromosomes derived from the centromeric region of any of the other chromosomes. The risk of an ESAC being associated with an abnormal phenotype is directly related to its size and whether or not it contains any genetically active euchromatic material.

ESACs derived from the acrocentric chromosomes are usually harmless if they are small and contain only the short arm and centromere regions. A large ESAC derived from chromosome 15 containing a duplication of a euchromatic part of the long arm, 15q11–13 (which includes the Prader–Willi locus and which can be identified using FISH) is associated with an abnormal phenotype (37–39). The presence of euchromatic material from the long arm in i(22) is associated with the Cat-eye syndrome (40,41). Figure 15B shows a dicentric marker chromosome with a duplication of the short arm and the centromere of chromosome 22. Distinct abnormal phenotypes are known to be associated with isochromosomes of the short arms i(9p) (42), i(12p) (Pallister Killian syndrome) (43) and i(18p) (44). For a full overview of other rare ESACs that have been found in PD, the reader is referred to the textbook by Gardner and Sutherland (9). Crolla (45) has reviewed the risk of an abnormal phenotype being associated with a marker chromosome that cannot be identified. For those derived from an acrocentric chromosome (excluding 15) it is approximately 7% as compared to approximately 28% for one derived from a nonacrocentric chromosome.

TISSUE SAMPLES

Amniotic Fluid

Typically, 15–18 mL of amniotic fluid (AF) is taken from a woman in the 15th to 18th week of pregnancy by amniocentesis (Chapter 12). The sample is processed according to established protocols (46). The principle is as follows. Amniotic fluid contains epithelial cells from the fetus and the amniotic membrane. These cells are separated by centrifugation and are cultured at 37°C in a CO_2 incubator. The culture medium is regularly refreshed and the cultures are maintained until there is a sufficient number of dividing cells. This process takes between 7 and 10 days. The cultures are then harvested and preparations are made on microscope slides. The slides are treated and stained so as to produce banding patterns on the chromosomes and analyzed using a light microscope. The maximum time limit for producing the result in most laboratories is 21 days. This is in good time for the parents to be informed so that they can make decisions concerning possible termination of pregnancy, should an abnormality be found. The legal limit for termination of a pregnancy for medical indications varies from 22 to 24 weeks in most Western countries.

This method produces chromosomes of rather good quality and it is very reliable. As mentioned earlier, amniotic fluid contains cells of the fetus, so that the result obtained is fairly representative of the cells of the fetus (47,48). The increase in experience and improvement in sampling methods and laboratory procedures has considerably reduced the risk of maternal cell contamination (see following text) in the last 15 years. The risk of miscarriage following amniocentesis is in most centers < 0.5%.

In the late 1980s, there were a number of reports on results obtained from early amniocentesis in the 10th to the 13th weeks of pregnancy. However, the procedure did not become popular mainly because of higher procedure-related fetal losses, higher culture failure rate because of insufficient cells and because of concerns about the adverse effect on the fetus (49–52). Early amniocentesis has now been largely abandoned.

Chorionic Villi

A sample of about 10–20 mg of chorionic villi (CV), taken either transvaginally or transabdominally, in the 11th to the 13th week of pregnancy, is received by the laboratory. The CV are carefully cleaned by removing maternal tissue. Two types of cultures can be set up: short-term (ST) cultures, which take between a few hours to 24 hours, and long-term (LT) cultures, which take about 7–10 days. The chorionic villus sampling (CVS) technique is described in Chapter 12.

The cytotrophoblast (extra-embryonic ectoderm) layer of CV consists of actively dividing cells that are examined in the ST-CV culture. The cells of the inner mesodermal core (extra-embryonic mesoderm) are not actively dividing and require LT-CV culture to produce dividing cells. The cultures are harvested and the microscope preparations are stained and examined as in the case of amniotic fluid (46). The results of the ST culture are ready in about 2–7 days and the results of the LT are known in 7–14 days.

The biggest advantage of this method is that the result particularly of the ST culture is available early. Should termination of pregnancy be necessary this can be done by the vacuum suction-curettage method before the 14th week of pregnancy. When the CVS method was first introduced in the eighties, it was carried out as early as the 8th week. In 1991, Firth et al. (53) first reported limb deformities associated with the sampling procedure. This was followed by a number of other similar reports. Subsequent investigations suggested a correlation with the timing of the procedure (54–56) and led to the consensus that CVS before the 11th week was not advisable. Later, no significant difference in limb reduction defects was found between babies born following CVS and those in the normal population (57,58).

Nevertheless, the popularity of CVS, which was used in some European countries in nearly 50% of the cases in the late 1980s and early 1990s, has decreased considerably. This is partly because of concerns regarding limb defects (59). There are some disadvantages of CVS. Chromosomes from CV are less suitable for the detection of subtle structural abnormalities. There is also the problem of confined placental mosaicism (see following text). Both the trophoblast cells and the mesodermal cells of the CV are extra-embryonic in origin and are further removed from the fetus than the amniocytes; they are therefore less representative of the fetus (47,48). The risk of a miscarriage following CVS is 0.5–1% (60,61). However, CVS remains a very useful procedure. Many women still prefer it for quick results. It is particularly recommended when there is a high risk of a chromosome abnormality that is easily recognizable. CVS is also suitable for DNA studies.

Cord Blood

The procedure of sampling fetal blood from the umbilical cord of the fetus, cordocentesis, was first introduced in the early 1970s for prenatal diagnosis of hemoglobinopathies (62). It was later applied for a variety of indications for PD (6). Cordocentesis is generally carried out from about the 18th week of pregnancy. Before the blood sample is sent to the laboratory, it is checked to be sure that it is of fetal origin. As standard blood cultures take 48–72 hours, this method can give quick results when fetal abnormality is discovered by ultrasound later in pregnancy. It is also helpful for confirming chromosome abnormalities, including mosaicism, found in amniocytes or CV (63). The results are reliable (except for certain cases such as mosaicism involving trisomy 20 or i(12p) found in Pallister–Killian syndrome, see following text) and the quality of the chromosomes is good. The sampling method, however, carries a higher risk of miscarriage than other procedures, about 5% (64) and is therefore rarely used except in certain very high-risk situations.

In recent years, however, FISH analysis of nondividing (interphase) cells from amniotic fluid has largely replaced cord blood analyses in late pregnancy, as described in Chapter 16.

CHROMOSOME FINDINGS IN THE VARIOUS INDICATION GROUPS

Advanced Maternal Age

The risk of a child with an extra chromosome 13, 18, 21, or X is related to maternal age and increases sharply after the age of 35. The general frequency of a child with trisomy 21 is 1 in 700 births. It is 1 in 1400 births at 20 years, 1 in 380 births at 35 years, and 1 in 28 births at the age of 45 years (65). Detailed estimates for the different maternal ages and gestational weeks are available for trisomies 21, 13, and 18 and for sex chromosome aneuploidy (66,67). In spite of nearly 50 years of research, which is still being actively pursued, the exact reason for the association of increased aneuploidy with advanced maternal age is not clear. Hassold and Hunt (68) have reviewed the developments in this field. In most European countries and in the United States, advanced maternal age, starting from 35 to 38 years, is one of the most common reasons for referral for PD. This indication group represents more than 77% of the 12,624 of women referred for PD to our laboratory during a period of 10 years. However, a chromosome abnormality is found in only about 3% of the cases (see Table 1).

With the steady increase in the number of women undergoing screening tests (such as serum screening of maternal blood to look for biochemical markers and nuchal translucency measurements using ultrasound) described in Chapters 1–3 and 6, the number of women referred for maternal age has been declining during the last 2 years. The most frequent finding in PD in this group of women is trisomy 21 followed by trisomy 18 (Table 2). Trisomy 13 and sex chromosome aneuploidy are also found in this referral group. Other occasional findings are triploidy (69,XXX or 69,XXY). Balanced or unbalanced structural abnormalities may also be found in these women.

Ultrasound Abnormalities

Women are referred for PD following a finding of structural abnormalities in the fetus (Chapter 7). Developments in the technical quality of ultrasonographic equipment have led to an increasing number of physical abnormalities that can be detected by ultrasound. Autosomal trisomies, triploidy, and monosomy X can be often predicted by ultrasound. Although this group represents less than 10% of the total referrals, chromosome abnormalities are found in about 27% of the cases (Table 1). The most frequent findings in this group are the three trisomies, 21, 18, and 13, monosomy X, and triploidy (Table 2). One specific parameter of ultrasonographic scanning, namely the separation of the skin in the back of the neck from the underlying tissue by fluid, the so-called nuchal translucency (NT), which is assessed in the period between 11 and 14 weeks of pregnancy is important (Chapter 3). An NT measurement of 3 mm or more appears to be associated an autosomal trisomy and is also a good indicator of monosomy X. Intrauterine growth retardation (IUGR) detected by ultrasonography is an indicator of chromosome abnormalities such as trisomy 18 and triploidy, 69,XXX or 69,XXY.

Duplications or deletions of chromosomes may be identified in a considerable proportion of cases in this group (Table 2). These may be de novo changes or may represent unbalanced products of a parental rearrangement. For that reason the parents' karyotype must be determined after finding an unbalanced karyotype.

Table 1 Abnormalities Found in the Various Indication Groups in a Total of 12,637 Prenatal Diagnosis at the VU University in Amsterdam (1994–2003)

Reason for referral	Number of investigations	Number of abnormalities	Percentage abnormalities
Advanced maternal age	9,790	289	3.0
Ultrasound abnormalities	1,164	308	26.5
Parent carrier of chromosome rearrangement	127	75	59.1
Previous child with chromosome abnormality	436	14	3.2
Increased risk by first or second trimester serum test	408	28	6.9
Anxiety	465	15	3.4
Other	247	2	0.8
Total	12,637	731	5.8

Table 2 Number of Different Types of Chromosome Abnormalities Found in the Various Indication Groups

Abnormality	Advanced maternal age	Ultrasound	Parent carrier	Previous child with abnormality	Serum tests	Anxiety	Other	Total
Trisomy 21	91	93		5	19	5	1	214
Trisomy 18	39	81			1	1		121
Trisomy 13	13	28	1		1	1		43
47,XXX	12				1			13
47,XXY	18	5	1	2	1	1		28
47,XYY	4			1				5
48,XXXY or 49,XXXXY	2	1				1		4
45,X	10	39						49
69,XXX or 69,XXY	4	18						22
Tetraploidy	4	2						6
Trisomies 8 (mosaic), and 9	4	1			1			6
Other (mosaic) aneuploidy	19	1		1	1			22
Unbalanced karyotypes	16	30	13		2	2	1	64
ESACs	9	2						11
Balanced rearrangements	44	7	60	5	2	5		123
Total	289	308	75	14	28	15	2	731

Carriers of Balanced Chromosomal Rearrangements

In this category one is looking for an unbalanced product of the parental balanced chromosome rearrangement. As mentioned earlier, a carrier of such a rearrangement is phenotypically normal but has a risk of having a child with an unbalanced karyotype. This group represents only one percent of the total referrals but the chance of finding a chromosome abnormality is considerably higher than in any of the other groups. In 127 prenatal diagnoses, an abnormal karyotype was identified in 75 cases, an abnormality rate of nearly 60% (Table 1). It should be pointed out, however, that in 60 out of the 75 cases the karyotypic abnormality of the fetus was the same balanced rearrangement found in the parent, which is not expected to result in any phenotypical abnormality in the fetus (Table 2). In only 13 cases the karyotype showed a structural imbalance. Two cases showed aneuploidy. So the real rate of chromosome abnormality associated with an abnormal phenotype in the fetus in this group was about 12%.

When one partner is a carrier of an insertion (19), or a complex translocation (69), it is advisable to characterize the chromosome rearrangement fully, if necessary using FISH, before prenatal diagnosis. Also, in extremely rare situations where both partners are carriers of a different translocation, it is important to work out all the possible expected karyotypes in the fetus before embarking upon PD. This allows quick and accurate interpretation of the results of PD.

Previous Child with a Chromosome Abnormality

It has been estimated that following the birth of a child with chromosome aneuploidy the risk for the next pregnancy is about 1–2% (70). The risk following two previous pregnancies with trisomy 21 rises to 10–20% (9). In our series of 436 women referred in this category, we found 14 abnormal karyotypes (3.2%) (Table 1). One of the reasons for the higher rate in our series is that we included cases where the previous child was suspected of having a chromosomal syndrome but where chromosome analysis had not actually been carried out. Five of the 14 abnormal karyotypes in this group were in fact familial rearrangements (Table 2).

Serum Tests

The noninvasive tests such as screening of maternal blood serum for biochemical markers in the first or second trimester of pregnancy have been described in Chapters 1 and 2.

If the result of such a test indicates a risk of a chromosome abnormality equal to or greater than 1 in 250, there is an indication for PD. About 7% of cases referred in this category had a chromosome abnormality, mostly trisomy 21 (Tables 1 and 2).

Anxiety

In this group, I have included cases where women asked for a test, even if there was no official indication for a PD, often because someone in their circle of family or friends had a child with a chromosomal abnormality. Abnormalities were found in only three out of 290 cases, 1% (Table 1). However, this is an important group of women who need reassurance.

Other

Chromosome analysis is carried out for various reasons other than those mentioned previously. For example, if a prenatal sample is taken for carrying out a DNA or biochemical test, chromosome analysis is also performed on a part of the sample. It takes very little extra effort to exclude a chromosome abnormality, once the invasive procedure of amniocentesis or CVS has already been carried out.

For X-linked disorders that can be detected prenatally by biochemical tests, such as hemophilia or Duchenne muscular dystrophy, it is important to identify the sex of the fetus. This is often done on a part of the CV sample and is reported within 24 hours. Should the fetus turn out to be female, the DNA test need not be performed.

PROBLEMS OF INTERPRETATION OF RESULTS AND OTHER DILEMMAS

Unbalanced Karyotypes

If the results of PD show that the fetus has a deletion or a duplication of a chromosome segment, examination of the chromosomes of the parents is essential. A deletion or duplication in the fetus may be a result of a balanced rearrangement in one of the parents. Identification of the extra or the missing segment in the fetus may help to predict the phenotype of the child and may help in the decision-making process for the parents. Also, finding an extra unidentified chromosome in the fetus may be a result of a 3:1 segregation of a parental translocation (see the following section on marker chromosomes). Furthermore, finding a balanced rearrangement in one of the parents has implications for future pregnancies of the couple. Even if an apparently balanced chromosome rearrangement is found in the fetus, it is important to investigate the parents. Whereas for a familial rearrangement there is no risk, an apparently balanced rearrangement that has a risen de novo carries a risk of an abnormal phenotype (33). For de novo Robertsonian translocations this risk is less than 1%, including the risk of UPD (24). For other two-break rearrangements the risk varies from 6% to 10%. For complex de novo rearrangements the risk is likely to be higher and proportional to the number of breakpoints (69).

Variants

As mentioned previously, certain genetically inactive and usually heterochromatic regions of chromosomes can vary in size without producing any phenotypic effect. The acrocentric short arms can occasionally be considerably enlarged, increasing the length of the short arm by about 200% or more. The laboratory is usually able to confirm cases of variants by using staining techniques such as C-banding or Q-banding, which stain the heterochromatic regions. However, occasionally the laboratory may request blood samples from the parents to check if the parent is carrying the same variant and thus to exclude the possibility that the so-called variant is in fact an unbalanced product of a parental translocation. Therefore, even if the variant has been identified in the fetus as well as the parent, it is essential to carefully examine all the other chromosomes in the parent.

Marker Chromosomes or ESACs in PD

Finding a marker or an ESAC in a prenatal sample, which happens once in about 1000 samples, can cause a dilemma for both the cytogeneticist as well as the genetic counselor. This is because the marker may or may not be associated with an adverse phenotypic effect (see preceding text) and the origin of the ESAC needs to be determined urgently. The first step is to examine the chromosomes of the parents. If the same ESAC is present in one of the parents who is phenotypically normal, it is likely to be harmless. Another possibility is that the ESAC is actually a result of a 3:1 segregation of a translocation in one of the parents. In that case one can expect an abnormal phenotype. If both parents have a normal karyotype, the ESAC must be identified as far as possible by different staining methods. Hastings et al. (36) have suggested a management protocol for markers found in prenatal samples. Use of the so-called DA-DAPI staining method can identify an ESAC derived from chromosome 15. FISH using probes for all the acrocentric chromosomes (13, 14, 15, 21, and 22) and the X and the Y is another useful tool for identifying an ESAC derived from these chromosomes. FISH with band-specific probes or whole chromosome paints can be used for the identification of isochromosomes derived from 9, 12, or 18. Use of the C-banding method helps to distinguish between ESACs with only heterochromatin and those with euchromatin as well as heterochromatin. If the ESAC is derived from chromosome 15 or 22, further FISH studies are required to determine if euchromatic material from the long arm is present, in which case an abnormal phenotype can be expected. If all of the aforementioned origins of ESACs have been excluded, multicolor FISH or microdissection techniques may be used to identify the ESAC. However, in practice it is difficult to carry out all these procedures because of lack of facilities, time or patient material. If the marker is not identifiable and contains genetically active euchromatin there is a risk that the fetus will be phenotypically abnormal (45). This risk is about 7% if the marker is derived from an acrocentric chromosome and about 28% for markers of other origins. For chromosome 15 derived ESACs (even if inherited) there may be an added small risk of UPD which should be excluded by DNA studies (71).

Sex Chromosome Abnormalities

The finding of common sex chromosome aneuploidies, 47,XXX, 47,XXY, 47,XYY, and 45,X, whether in nonmosaic or mosaic form, can pose a dilemma for genetic counseling. Whereas infertility is nearly certain for 47,XXY and for 45,X is very likely, intellectual and psychological functioning for all these cases is less predictable. There is now a large body of data available on the long-term outcome in children with sex chromosome aneuploidy (72–74). There is also more information on the prognosis and genetic counseling of prenatally diagnosed cases (75–77). As more information has become available, there is a trend in higher rate of pregnancy continuation in these cases (78).

The finding of a 45,X karyotype in a ST-CV culture is not reliable and should always be confirmed if possible in CV-LT cultures or in amniotic fluid cultures (see the following section on false positive and false negative results). Also, one should always bear in mind the possibility that Y chromosome material may be present in cases of 45, X (8,79). It is important to examine a sufficient number of cells to exclude mosaicism involving the Y and to be aware of the possibility that a male child can be born. A woman with Turner syndrome and Y chromosome material has an increased risk for gonadoblastoma (80).

Other polysomies such as 48,XXXX, 48,XXXY, 48,XXYY, 49,XXXXX, and 49,XXXXY are usually associated with intellectual impairment (81). For other rare structural abnormalities of the sex chromosomes, the reader is referred to the textbook of Gardner and Sutherland (9). It should be pointed out that in the male, who has only one X chromosome, even a balanced structural abnormality such as an X-autosome translocation or an inversion, results in infertility (82).

Mosaicism at Amniocentesis

When normal as well as abnormal cells are found in the same specimen, it is difficult to distinguish between true mosaicism and pseudomosaicism. In amniotic fluid the abnormal cell line may be limited to a single cell or to cells from only one culture, or it may be found in all the cultures. In the first two cases the mosaicism is nearly always a result of a cultural artifact or of abnormal cells from extraembryonic tissue (psuedomosaicism), whereas in the last case the mosaic karyotype may well be representative of the karyotype of the fetus (true mosaicism). The rate of true mosaicism in amniotic samples from four surveys in Europe, Canada, and the United States is about 0.2% and that of (multiple cell) pseudomosaicism about 0.9% (83–86). The chromosome involved in the aneuploid cell line is an important consideration. Mosaic aneuploidy of chromosomes 8, 9, 13, 18, 21, X, and Y is known to be compatible with live birth and is associated with congenital abnormalities. The situation concerning mosaic trisomies of chromosomes 12 and 20 is not so clear. For both chromosomes there are reports of cases with no phenotypic effect as well as cases with an abnormal outcome (87,88). Trisomy of chromosome 7 or of 16 is a relatively common finding in CVS that is rarely confirmed at amniocentesis (89). However, both have been associated with an abnormal phenotype when detected at amniocentesis (90–93). Congenital abnormalities have also been found to be associated with mosaic trisomy 17 (94,95). Other rare mosaic trisomies have been reported by Hsu et al. (92) and have been reviewed by Gardner and Sutherland (9). There are guidelines which may help in distinguishing between pseudomosaicism, which is clinically not significant, and true mosaicism (86,96,97).

When mosaicism involving a common aneuploidy or a rare aneuploidy known to be associated with live birth and an abnormal phenotype is found, it is advisable to check the pregnancy with ultrasonography for signs of physical abnormalities in the fetus. Also, chromosome analysis should be repeated on a second tissue: amniotic fluid or cord blood. It should be noted, however, that blood is not a suitable tissue for confirming certain abnormalities. Isochromosome of 12p (Pallister–Killian syndrome) is found in amniocytes and skin cells but not in blood cells (43). The same is true for trisomy 20 (88).

Mosaics for balanced structural abnormalities are extremely rare (98). Mosaicism for an unbalanced structural abnormality usually turns out to be pseudomosaicism. However, when true mosaicism is suspected confirmation on another sample is recommended. Also, ultrasonography to look for phenotypic abnormalities is essential (99). Mosaicism with marker chromosomes has been discussed in the preceding sections.

Confined Placental Mosaicism

When mosaicism is detected in CV samples one must consider the question whether the abnormal cells are present also in the fetus or whether they are confined to the placenta (100). Whereas true mosaicism in the fetus is found in about 0.15% of the cases (101), mosaicism that is confined to the placenta is present in about

1–2% of the CV samples. In order to interpret mosaicism and confined placental mosaicism (CPM) one needs to understand something of the process of early embrogenesis and the origin of the embryonic and the extra-embryonic tissues (47,48). In short, the trophoblast (of the CV-ST culture) arises from the wall of the blastocyst and is separated at an early stage from the inner cell mass. Only three cells of the inner cell mass give rise to the entire embryo (47,102). The rest of the inner cell mass contributes to the formation of the inner cell wall of the amnion and the yolk sac. The yolk sac gives rise to the chorionic mesoderm (of the CV-LT cultures) and also contributes to the amniotic mesoderm. The question of the origin of the fetal blood is not quite resolved. It is thought to arise from fetal mesoderm as well as from the yolk sac. According to this model of Bianchi et al. (47), amniocentesis samples cells that more closely reflect the constitution of the fetus than CVS. CVS samples trophoblast cells (CV-ST cells) that separated early on from the cells that form the fetus, and cells from the chorionic mesoderm (CV-LT cells) that reflect a more-recently separated cell lineage. This model can explain all the discrepancies between the feto-placental tissues that have been described and are shown in Table 3. It also explains why amniocytes are more representative of the fetus than fetal blood cells.

Depending on when and where mosaicism originates one can expect varying degrees of mosaicism in the fetus and/or the placenta. In the great majority of pregnancies, there is complete concordance between the karyotypes of the CV and the fetal tissue (FT). In only about 1% there is discordance. The different types of placental-fetal discordance at CVS from two studies are shown in Table 3 (89,103). In 94% of the cases the mosaicism was confined to the placenta (Table 3 a, b, and c). In 55% of these it was confined to the cells of the CV-ST culture (Table 3, a), in 27% to the cells of the CV-LT culture, and in the remaining 18% to cells from both the CV-ST and the CV-LT cultures.

For mosaic trisomies associated with viable phenotypically abnormal fetuses that are found in CV-ST and/or CV-LT, ultrasound examination is recommended.

Table 3 Cytogenetic Discrepancies in 240 Cases of CVS, Combined Data from U.S. (61 Cases)[a] and European Studies (179 Cases)[b]

Group	CV-ST	CV-LT	FT/AF	No. of cases	Comment
a	Abnormal or mosaic	Normal	Normal	123	False positive ST (25/123 nonmosaic abnormal)
b	Normal	Abnormal or mosaic	Normal	62	False positive LT (3/62 nonmosaic abnormal)
c	Abnormal or mosaic	Abnormal or mosaic	Normal	40	False positive ST and LT
d	Normal	Abnormal or mosaic	Abnormal or mosaic	15	False negative ST
e	Abnormal or mosaic	Normal	Abnormal or mosaic	0	False negative LT
f	Normal	Normal	Abnormal or mosaic	0	False negative ST and LT
Total				240	

[a]From Ref. 103.
[b]From Ref. 89.

Mosaic results at CV-ST should be confirmed by CV-LT or by amniocentesis. Also, discrepancies between the results of ST-CV and LT-CV cultures should be resolved by amniocentesis. Again, a word of caution is warranted for the choice of second tissue for confirmation of chromosome results. As mentioned earlier, cord blood is not suitable for confirming i(12p) or trisomy 20. The opposite seems to be true for i(9p) which is missed on amniocentesis but is present in blood (104–106). Trisomy 8 and trisomy 9 mosaics may show tissue-specific variation (107–110).

If the conclusion of CPM has been reached, one can assume in general that the fetus will be normal but CPM itself can have some clinical consequences. Although CPM for aneuploidy of most autosomes appears to have no adverse effect on the pregnancy outcome (111), CPM for certain chromosomes, particularly chromosome 16, has been associated with intrauterine growth retardation (IUGR) (112–114). IUGR appears to be present in cases where the aneuploidy arose during maternal meiosis I as opposed to postzygotic mitosis (115). The high frequency of trisomic cells in the placenta in these cases is thought to cause placental insufficiency resulting in IUGR (116,117). This certainly applies to trisomy 16, which is the most common trisomy (1% of all clinically recognized pregnancies) and is often related to poor pregnancy outcome (93,113). It is maternal age-dependent and arises at maternal meiosis I (118). In addition, UPD in the fetus due to trisomy rescue, which occurs in these cases, has been implicated in IUGR (114). It is also possible, that low level and tissue specific mosaicism of trisomy 16 in the fetus itself may be responsible for the abnormalities (113).

If mosaic trisomy 15 has been identified at CVS but has not been confirmed at amniocentesis, the karyotype of the fetus is most likely to be normal. However, DNA analysis on the remaining amniotic fluid cultures is recommended to exclude UPD 15, because of a small risk of Prader–Willi syndrome (111).

False Positive and False Negative Results

If a sufficient number of cells are examined, the risk of false positive and false negative results at amniocentesis is extremely small. I shall discuss the role of maternal cell contamination (MCC) in the next section.

In CVS, however, it is possible in very rare situations that all the cells in the particular CV sample are normal while the cells in the fetus are abnormal, giving a false negative result (Table 3). On the other hand, the CV result may be abnormal whereas the fetus is normal, which is a false positive result. The reasons for these discrepancies have been explained under the section on CPM. False positive results are reported to occur in 0.15% (1 in 700) cases and false negative in 0.03% (1 in 3000) cases (89,119). In Table 3 the results from the fetal tissue are concordant with CV-LT in nearly 58% of the cases (Table 3, a and d) and with CV-ST in 25% of the cases (Table 3, b). It has been suggested that for the highest rate of accuracy both ST and LT cultures should be analyzed as neither the ST nor the LT culture is totally reliable by itself (103,120,121). Whereas false positive results have been found in both types of cultures (Table 3, c), there is only one case on record in which both ST and LT cultures gave a false negative result (122). So, combined results from both types of cultures should considerably reduce the rates of false positive and false negative results. However, analyzing both ST-CV and LT-CV cultures is labor intensive and some of the advantage of an early result is lost by having to wait for the result of the LT culture. In any case, both ST and LT cultures should be set up for high-risk groups, for example patients referred for ultrasound abnormalities (123,124).

The abnormal results at CVS should be checked by ultrasonography and by amniocentesis, thus reducing the chance of a false positive result. The risk of false negative results, though small, is always there.

Maternal Cell Contamination

There is a chance that cells of maternal origin may be present in amniotic fluid cultures or LT-CV cultures. Combined results from three large surveys show that male as well as female cells, ascribed to maternal cell contamination (MCC), in the same sample were detected in 0.17% of amniotic fluid samples (84,85,125). The frequency of MCC, allowing also for female fetuses, is therefore 0.34%. MCC in amniotic fluids appears to be associated with the sampling technique (126). In 1983, Benn and Hsu (125) made recommendations for improving both sampling techniques and laboratory procedures to reduce the problems of MCC. The current rate of MCC is probably much reduced. At present MCC is not usually a source of misinterpretation of results as it is only extremely rarely that only maternal cells are present. However, wrong assignment of sex due to MCC remains a possibility, especially if an amniotic fluid sample is contaminated with blood. One should also bear in mind the extremely remote possibility of finding an XX/XY chimera, where cells from genetically two individuals are present in one person (127,128). In 1992, Hsu (88) found only one case in 26,000 amniotic fluids where only 46,XX cells were found and a normal boy was born. The chance of finding only maternal cells and missing the fetal cells altogether in this series was $1/26,000 \times 2 = 1/13,000$ or 0.008%. So, if the risk for trisomy 21 for a pregnancy is 1 in 300, the chance of missing the trisomy altogether due to MCC would be $1/13,000 \times 1/300 = 1/3,900,000$. If the risk of trisomy for the pregnancy is 1 in 40, the risk of missing it is $1/520,000$.

The chance of MCC in LT-CV cultures is much higher, close to 1%. However, careful removal of all maternal tissue from the CV before setting up the culture can minimize the risk of MCC.

Tetraploid/Diploid Mosaicism

Tetraploid cells (with 92 instead of 46 chromosomes) are commonly seen in amniotic fluid samples and are usually considered a result of an in vitro cultural artifact. Although the presence of both tetraploid and diploid cells is nearly always an innocuous finding, caution is indicated as tetraploidy and tetraploid/diploid mosaicism have been reported in phenotypically abnormal individuals (129–131). Nonmosaic tetraploids can survive from a few hours to several months (129) whereas tetraploid/diploid mosaics can survive to adulthood with severe mental retardation (130). Although phenotypic abnormalities may be detectable by ultrasound only later in pregnancy, IUGR and placental abnormalities have been noted in the 19th week of gestation in one case of a tetraploid/diploid mosaic (131). In case of doubt, ultrasonography and, if necessary, cordocentesis is recommended.

Laboratory Errors

In 1986 the risk of laboratory errors, based on amniocentesis, varied from 0.1% to 0.6% in different surveys (88). These figures include errors due to MCC as well as laboratory or administrative errors. Laboratory errors due to misinterpretation of results, overlooking subtle unexpected structural abnormalities, mix up of specimens, and administrative errors always remain a possibility. The stringent requirements of the laboratory accreditation schemes in the recent years should contribute to reducing laboratory errors.

Monozygotic Twins

Although concordant karyotypes are expected in the case of monozygotic twins, there are numerous reports of discordance for Turner syndrome/female phenotype or Turner syndrome/male phenotype. A few of these have been diagnosed prenatally (132–134). There are also a few reports of discordance for Down syndrome (132,135). When one of the fetuses in a monochorionic diamniotic twin pregnancy shows ultrasound abnormatiles, neither fetal blood nor chorionic villi are suitable tissues for prenatal diagnosis. The blood sample is unreliable because of placental vascular anastomoses (132–134). Mosaicism can spread throughout the single placenta and there is no clear correlation between the karyotype of the CV sample, even if taken from a site close to the insertion of the umbilical cord, and the karyotype of the fetus (132). Amniocentesis from both amniotic sacs is the most reliable method of PD in these cases.

ACKNOWLEDGMENTS

I thank Aggie Nieuwint and John Wolstenholme for their comments. I am grateful to Aggie Nieuwint also for her help with the karyograms and to Madelon Paulis for the references. Professor A. Bansil kindly provided the facilities for writing this chapter at Northeastern University, Boston.

REFERENCES

1. Tjio JH, Levan A. The chromosome number in man. Hereditas 1956; 42:1–6.
2. Ford CE, Hamerton JL. The chromosomes of man. Nature 1956; 178:1020–1023.
3. Fuchs F, Riis P. Antenatal sex determination. Nature 1956; 177:330.
4. Steele MW, Breg WR Jr. Chromosome analysis of human amniotic-fluid cells. Lancet 1966; 1(7434):383–385.
5. Niazi M, Coleman DV, Loeffler FE. Trophoblast sampling in early pregnancy. Culture of rapidly dividing cells from immature placental villi. Br J Obstet Gynecol 1981; 88:1081–1085.
6. Daffos F, Capella-Pavlovsky M, Forestier F. Fetal blood sampling during pregnancy with use of a needle guided by ultrasound: a study of 606 consecutive cases. Am J Obstet Gynecol 1985; 153:655–660.
7. Shaffer LG, Tommerup N, eds. ISCN: An International System for Human Cytogenetic Nomenclature. Basel: S. Karger, 2005.
8. Jacobs P, Dalton P, James R, et al. Turner syndrome: a cytogenetic and molecular study. Ann Hum Genet 1997; 61:471–483.
9. Gardner RJM, Sutherland GR. Chromosome Abnormalities and Genetic Counseling. 3rd ed. Oxford: Oxford University Press, 2004.
10. Jauniaux E, Brown R, Rodeck C, Nicolaides KH. Prenatal diagnosis of triploidy during the second trimester of pregnancy. Obstet Gynecol 1996; 88:983–989.
11. Van de Laar I, Rabelink G, Hochstenbach R, Tuerlings J, Hoogeboom J, Giltay J. Diploid/triploid mosaicism in dysmorphic patients. Clin Genet 2002; 62:376–382.

12. Daniel A, Hook EB, Wulf G. Risks of unbalanced progeny at amniocentesis to carriers of chromosome rearrangements: data from United States and Canadian Laboratories. Am J Med Genet 1989; 31:14–53.

13. Kaiser P. Pericentric inversions. Problems and significance for clinical genetics. Hum Genet 1984; 68:1–47.

14. Madan K. Paracentric inversions: a review. Hum Genet 1995; 96:503–515.

15. Mules EH, Stamberg J. Reproductive outcomes of paracentric inversion carriers: report of liveborn dicentric recombinant and literature review. Hum Genet 1984; 67:126–131.

16. Whiteford ML, Baird C, Kinmond S, Donaldson B, Davidson HR. A child with bisatellited, dicentric chromosome 15 arising from a maternal paracentric inversion of chromosome 15q. J Med Genet 2000; 37(8):E11.

17. Lefort G, Blanchet P, Belgrade N, et al. Stable dicentric duplication-deficiency chromosome 14 resulting from crossing-over within a maternal paracentric inversion. Am J Med Genet 2002; 113:333–338.

18. Worsham MJ, Miller DA, Devries JM, et al. A dicentric recombinant 9 derived from a paracentric inversion: phenotype, cytogenetics, and molecular analysis of centromeres. Am J Hum Genet 1989; 44:115–123.

19. Madan K, Nieuwint AWM. Reproductive risks for paracentric inversion heterozygotes: inversion or insertion? That is the question [letter]. Am J Med Genet 2002; 107:340–343.

20. Van Hemel JO, Eussen HJ. Interchromosomal insertions. Identification of five cases and a review. Hum Genet 2000; 107:415–432.

21. Madan K, Menko FH. Intrachromosomal insertions: a case report and a review. Hum Genet 1992; 89:1–9.

22. De Braekeleer M, Dao T-N. Cytogenetic studies in male infertility: a review. Hum Reprod 1991; 6:245–250.

23. Tuerlings JHAM, de France HF, Hamers A, et al. Chromosome studies in 1792 males prior to intra-cytoplasmic sperm injection: the Dutch experience. Eur J Hum Genet 1998; 6:194–200.

24. Silverstein S, Lerer I, Sagi M, Frumkin A, Ben-Neriah Z, Abeliovich D. Uniparental disomy in fetuses diagnosed with balanced Robertsonian translocations: risk estimate. Prenat Diagn 2002; 22:649–651.

25. Engel E. Uniparental disomy revisited: the first twelve years. Am J Med Genet 1993; 46:670–674.

26. Engel E. Uniparental disomies in unselected populations. Am J Hum Genet 1998; 63:962–966.

27. Kotzot D. Complex and segmental uniparental disomy (UPD): review and lessons from rare chromosomal complements. J Med Genet 2001; 38:497–507.

28. Engel E, Antonaraki SE. Genomic Imprinting and Uniparental Disomy in Medicine: Clinical and Molecular Aspects. New York: Wiley-Liss, 2002.

29. Benn PA, Hsu LYF. Incidence and significance of supernumerary marker chromosomes in prenatal diagnosis. Am J Hum Genet 1984; 36:1092–1102.

30. Blennow E, Bui T-H, Kristoffersson U, et al. Swedish survey on extra structurally abnormal chromosomes in 39,105 consecutive prenatal diagnoses: prevalence and characterization by fluorescence in situ hybridization. Prenat Diagn 1994; 14:1019–1028.

31. Li MM, Howard-Peebles PN, Killos LD, Fallon L, Listgarten E, Stanley WS. Characterization and clinical implications of marker chromosomes identified at prenatal diagnosis. Prenat Diagn 2000; 20:138–143.

32. Hook EB, Schreinemachers DM, Willey AM, Cross PK. Rates of mutant structural chromosome rearrangements in human fetuses: data from prenatal cytogenetic studies and associations with maternal age and parental mutagen exposure. Am J Hum Genet 1983; 35:96–109.

33. Warburton D. De novo balanced chromosome rearrangements and extra marker chromosomes identified at prenatal diagnosis: clinical significance and distribution of breakpoints. Am J Hum Genet 1991; 49:995–1013.

34. Crolla JA, Howard P, Mitchell C, Long FL, Dennis NR. A molecular and FISH approach to determining karyotype and phenotype correlations in six patients with supernumerary marker (22) chromosomes. Am J Med Genet 1997; 72:440–447.

35. Crolla JA, Long F, Rivera H, Dennis NR. FISH and molecular study of autosomal supernumerary marker chromosomes excluding those derived from chromosomes 15 and 22: I. Results of 26 new cases. Am J Med Genet 1998; 75:355–366.

36. Hastings RJ, Nisbet DL, Waters K, Spencer T, Chitty LS. Prenatal detection of extra structurally abnormal chromosomes (ESACs): new cases and a review of the literature. Prenat Diagn 1999; 19:436–445.

37. Rineer S, Finucane B, Simon EW. Autistic symptoms among children and young adults with isodicentric chromosome 15. Am J Med Genet 1998; 81:428–433.

38. Wolpert CM, Menold MM, Bass MP, et al. Three probands with autistic disorder and isodicentric chromosome 15. Am J Med Genet 2000; 96:365–372.

39. Torrisi L, Sangiorgi E, Russo L, Gurrieri F. Rearrangements of chromosome 15 in epilepsy. Am J Med Genet 2001; 106:125–128.

40. Mears AJ, Duncan AMV, Budarf ML, Emanuel BS, Sellinger B, Siegel-Bartelt J. Molecular characterization of the marker chromosome associated with cat eye syndrome. Am J Hum Genet 1994; 55:134–142.

41. Mears AJ, El-Shanti H, Murray JC, McDermid HE, Patil SR. Minute supernumerary ring chromosome 22 associated with cat eye syndrome: further delineation of the critical region. Am J Hum Genet 1995; 57:667–673.

42. Dhandha S, Hogge WA, Surti U, McPherson E. Three cases of tetrasomy 9p. Am J Med Genet 2002; 113:375–380.

43. Horn D, Majewski F, Hildebrandt B, Körner H. Pallister-Killian syndrome: normal karyotype in prenatal chorionic villi, in postnatal lymphocytes, and in slowly growing epidermal cells, but mosaic tetrasomy 12p in skin fibroblasts. J Med Genet 1995; 32:68–71.

44. Kotzot D, Bundscherer G, Bernasconi F, et al. Isochromosome 18p results from maternal meiosis II nondisjunction. Eur J Hum Genet 1996; 4:168–174.

45. Crolla JA. FISH and molecular studies of autosomal supernumerary marker chromosomes excluding those derived from chromosome 15: II. Review of the literature. Am J Med Genet 1998; 75:367–381.

46. Rooney DE, ed. Human Cytogenetics: A Practical Approach. Constitutional Analysis. 3rd ed. Oxford: IRL Press, 2001; Vol. 1.

47. Bianchi DW, Wilkins-Haug LE, Enders AC, Hay ED. Origin of extraembryonic mesoderm in experimental animals: relevance to chorionic mosaicism in humans. Am J Med Genet 1993; 46:542–550.

48. Robinson WP, McFadden DE, Barrett IJ, et al. Origin of amnion and implications for evaluation of the fetal genotype in cases of mosaicism. Prenat Diagn 2002; 22: 1076–1085.

49. Nicolaides K, de Lourdes Brizot M, Patel F, Snijders R. Comparison of chorionic villus sampling and amniocentesis for fetal karyotyping at 10–13 weeks' gestation. Lancet 1994; 344:435–439.

50. Daniel A, Ng A, Kuah KB, Reiha S, Malafiej P. A study of early amniocentesis for prenatal cytogenetic diagnosis. Prenat Diagn 1998; 18:21–28.

51. The Canadian Early and Mid-trimester Amniocentesis Trial (CEMAT) Group. Randomised trial to assess safety and fetal outcome of early and midtrimester amniocentesis. Lancet 1998; 351:242–247.

52. Whittle MJ. Early amniocentesis: time for a rethink [commentary]. Lancet 1998; 351:226–227.

53. Firth H, Boyd PA, Chamberlain P, MacKenzie IZ, Huson SM. Limb defects and chorionic villus sampling [letter]. Lancet 1996; 347:1406.

54. Jahoda MGJ, Brandenburg H, Cohen-Overbeek T, Los FJ, Sachs ES, Wladimiroff JW. Terminal transverse limb defects and early chorionic villus sampling: evaluation of 4,300 cases with completed follow-up. Am J Med Genet 1993; 46:483–485.

55. Hsieh F-J, Shyu M-K, Sheu B-C, Lin S-P, Chen C-P, Huang F-Y. Limb defects after chorionic villus sampling. Obstet Gynecol 1995; 85:84–88.
56. Saura R, Longy M, Horovitz J, et al. Risks of transabdominal chorionic villus sampling before the 12th week of amenorrhea. Prenat Diagn 1990; 10:461–467.
57. Froster UG, Jackson L. Limb defects and chorionic villus sampling: results from an international registry, 1992–94. Lancet 1996; 347:489–494.
58. WHO/PAHO consultation on CVS. Evaluation of chorionic villus sampling safety. Prenat Diag 1999; 19:97–99.
59. Cutillo DM, Hammond EA, Reeser SL, et al. Chorionic villus sampling utilization following reports of a possible association with fetal limb defects. Prenat Diagn 1994; 14:327–332.
60. Brambati B, Tului L, Camurri L, Guercilena S. Early second trimester (13 to 20 weeks) transabdominal chorionic villus sampling (TA-CVS): a safe and alternative method for both high and low risk populations. Prenat Diagn 2002; 22:907–913.
61. Brun J-L, Mangione R, Gangbo F, et al. Feasibility, accuracy and safety of chorionic villus sampling: a report of 10,741 cases. Prenat Diagn 2003; 23:295–301.
62. Valenti C. Antenatal detection of hemoglobinopathies. Am J Obstet Gynecol 1973; 115:851–853.
63. Shalev E, Zalel Y, Weiner E, Cohen H, Shneur Y. The role of cordocentesis in assessment of mosaicism found in amniotic fluid cell culture. Acta Obstet Gynecol Scand 1994; 73:119–122.
64. Watson MS, Breg WR, Hobbins JC, Mahoney MJ. Cytogenetic diagnosis using midtrimester fetal blood samples: application to suspected mosaicism and other diagnostic problems. Am J Med Genet 1984; 19:805–813.
65. Connor JM, Ferguson-Smith MA. Essential Medical Genetics. 4th ed. Oxford: Blackwell Scientific Publications, 1993.
66. Snijders RJM, Sebire NJ, Nicolaides KH. Maternal age and gestational age-specific risk for chromosomal defects. Fetal Diagn Ther 1995; 10:356–367.
67. Snijders RJM, Sundberg K, Holzgreve W, Henry G, Nicolaides KH. Maternal age- and gestation-specific risk for trisomy 21. Ultrasound Obstet Gynecol 1999; 13:167–170.
68. Hassold T, Hunt P. To err (meiotically) is human: the genesis of human aneuploidy. Nat Rev Genet 2001; 2:280–291.
69. Madan K, Nieuwint AWM, van Bever Y. Recombination in a balanced complex translocation of a mother leading to a balanced reciprocal translocation in the child. Review of 60 cases of balanced complex translocations. Hum Genet 1997; 99:806–815.
70. Stene J, Stene E, Mikkelsen M. Risk for chromosome abnormality at amniocentesis following a child with a non-inherited chromosome aberration. Prenat Diag 1984; 4:81–95.
71. Kotzot D. Supernumerary marker chromosomes (SMC) and uniparental disomy (UPD): coincidence or consequence? J Med Genet 2002; 39:775–778.
72. Bender BG, Harmon RJ, Linden MG, Bucher-Bartelson B, Robinson A. Psychosocial competence of unselected young adults with sex chromosome abnormalities. Am J Med Genet 1999; 88:200–206.
73. Bender BG, Linden MG, Harmon RJ. Neuropsychological and functional cognitive skills of 35 unselected adults with sex chromosome abnormalities. Am J Med Genet 2001; 102:309–313.
74. Linden MG, Bender BG. Fifty-one prenatally diagnosed children and adolescents with sex chromosome abnormalities. Am J Med Genet 2002; 110:11–18.
75. Linden MG, Bender BG, Robinson A. Intrauterine diagnosis of sex chromosome aneuploidy. Obstet Gynecol 1996; 87:468–475.
76. Linden MG, Bender BG, Robinson A. Genetic counseling for sex chromosome abnormalities. Am J Med Genet 2002; 110:3–10.
77. Brun J-L, Gangbo F, Wen ZQ, et al. Prenatal diagnosis and management of sex chromosome aneuploidy: a report on 98 cases. Prenat Diagn 2004; 24:213–218.

78. Christian SM, Koehn D, MacDougall A, Wilson RD. Parental decisions following prenatal diagnosis of sex chromosome aneuploidy: a trend over time. Prenat Diagn 2000; 20:37–40.

79. Huang B, Thangavelu M, Bhatt S, Sandlin CL, Wang S. Prenatal diagnosis of 45,X and 45,X mosaicism: the need for thorough cytogenetic and clinical evaluations. Prenat Diagn 2002; 22:105–110.

80. Mendes JRT, Strufaldi MWL, Delcelo R, et al. Y-chromosome identification by PCR and gonadal histopathology in Turner's syndrome without overt Y-mosaicism. Clin Endocrinol 1999; 50:19–26.

81. Linden MG, Bender BG, Robinson A. Sex chromosome tetrasomy and pentasomy. Pediatrics 1995; 96:672–682.

82. Madan K. Balanced structural changes involving the human X: effect on sexual phenotype. Hum Genet 1983; 63:216–221.

83. Hsu LYF, Perlis TE. United States survey on chromosome mosaicism and pseudomosaicism in prenatal diagnosis. Prenat Diagn 1984; 4:97–130.

84. Worton RG, Stern R. A Canadian collaborative study of mosaicism in amniotic fluid cell cultures. Prenat Diagn 1984; 4:131–144.

85. Bui T-H, Iselius L, Lindsten J. European collaborative study on prenatal diagnosis: mosaicism, pseudomosaicism and single abnormal cells in amniotic fluid cell cultures. Prenat Diagn 1984; 4:145–162.

86. Hsu LYF, Kaffe S, Jenkins EC, et al. Proposed guidelines for diagnosis of chromosome mosaicism in amniocytes based on data derived from chromosome mosaicism and pseudomosaicism studies. Prenat Diagn 1992; 12:555–573.

87. Brosens JJ, Overton C, Lavery SA, Thornton S. Trisomy 12 mosaicism diagnosed by amniocentesis. Acta Obstet Gynecol Scand 1996; 75:79–81.

88. Hsu LYF. Prenatal diagnosis of chromosomal abnormalities through amniocentesis. In: Milunski A, ed. Genetic Disorders and the Fetus: Diagnosis, Prevention and Treatment. 3rd ed. Baltimore, MD: The Johns Hopkins University Press, 1992.

89. Hahnemann JM, Vejerslev LO. European collaborative research on mosaicism in CVS (EUCROMIC)—fetal and extrafetal cell lineages in 192 gestations with CVS mosaicism involving single autosomal trisomy. Am J Med Genet 1997; 70:179–187.

90. Kivirikko S, Salonen R, Salo A, von Koskull H. Prenatally detected trisomy 7 mosaicism in a dysmorphic child. Prenat Diagn 2002; 22:541–544.

91. Warburton D. Trisomy 7 mosaicism: prognosis after prenatal diagnosis [letter]. Prenat Diagn 2002; 22:1239–1240.

92. Hsu LYF, Yu M-T, Neu RL, et al. Rare trisomy mosaicism diagnosed in amniocytes, involving an autosome other than chromosomes 13, 18, 20 and 21: karyotype/phenotype correlations. Prenat Diagn 1997; 17:201–242.

93. Hsu W-T, Shchepin DA, Mao R, et al. Mosaic trisomy 16 ascertained through amniocentesis: evaluation of 11 new cases. Am J Med Genet 1998; 80:473–480.

94. Collado FK, Fisher AJ, Bombard AT. Counseling patients with trisomy 17 mosaicism found at genetic amniocentesis [letter]. Prenat Diagn 2003; 23:948–950.

95. Terhal P, Sakkers R, Hochstenbach R, et al. Cerebellar hypoplasia, zonular cataract and peripheral neuropathy in trisomy 17 mosaicism. Am J Med Genet 2004; 130A:410–414.

96. Sikkema-Raddatz B, Castedo S, te Meerman GJ. Probability tables for exclusion of mosaicism in prenatal diagnosis. Prenat Diagn 1997; 17:115–118.

97. Hsu LYF, Benn PA. Revised guidelines for the diagnosis of mosaicism in amniocytes [letter]. Prenat Diagn 1999; 19:1081–1090.

98. Opheim KE, Brittingham A, Chapman D, Norwood TH. Balanced reciprocal translocation mosaicism: how frequent? Am J Med Genet 1995; 57:601–604.

99. Pipiras E, Dupont C, Chantot-Bastaraud S, et al. Structural chromosomal mosaicism and prenatal diagnosis. Prenat Diagn 2004; 24:101–103.

100. Kalousek DK, Dill FJ. Chromosomal mosaicism confined to the placenta in human conceptions. Science 1983; 221:665–667.

101. Hahnemann JM, Vejerslev LO. Accuracy of cytogenetic findings on chorionic villus sampling (CVS)- diagnostic consequences of CVS mosaicism and non-mosaic discrepancy in centres contributing to EUCROMIC 1986–1992. Prenat Diagn 1997; 17:801–820.

102. Markert CL, Petters RM. Manufactured hexaparental mice show that adults are derived from three embryonic cells. Science 1978; 202:56–58.

103. Ledbetter DH, Zachary JM, Simpson JL, et al. Cytogenetic results from the U.S. collaborative study on CVS. Prenat Diagn. 1992; 12:317–345.

104. Grass FS, Parke JC Jr, Kirkman HN, et al. Tetrasomy 9p: tissue-limited idic(9p) in a child with mild manifestations and a normal CVS result. Report and review. Am J Med Genet 1993; 47:812–816.

105. Eggerman T, Rossier E, Theurer-Mainka U, et al. New case of mosaic tetrasomy 9p with additional neurometabolic findings. Am J Med Genet 1998; 75:530–533.

106. Lloveras E, Pérez C, Solé F, et al. Two cases of tetrasomy 9p syndrome with tissue limited mosaicism. Am J Med Genet 2004; 124A:402–406.

107. Kaffe S, Benn PA, Hsu LYF. Fetal blood sampling investigation of chromosome mosaicism in amniotic fluid cell culture. Lancet 1988; 332:284.

108. Schwartz S, Ashai S, Meijboom EJ, Schwartz MF, Sun CC-J, Cohen MM. Prenatal detection of trisomy 9 mosaicism. Prenat Diagn 1989; 9:549–554.

109. Klein J, Graham JM Jr, Platt LD, Schreck R. Trisomy 8 mosaicism in chorionic villus sampling: case report and counselling issues. Prenat Diagn 1994; 14:451–454.

110. Chen C-P, Chern S-R, Town D-D, Wang W, Liao Y-W. Fetoplacental and fetoamniotic chromosomal discrepancies in prenatally detected mosaic trisomy 9 [letter]. Prenat Diagn 2003; 23:1019–1021.

111. Wolstenholme J, Rooney DE, Davison EV. Confined placental mosaicism, IUGR, and adverse pregnancy outcome: a controlled retrospective U.K. collaborative survey. Prenat Diagn 1994; 14:345–361.

112. Kalousek DK, Howard-Peebles PN, Olson SB, et al. Confirmation of CVS mosaicism in term placentae and high frequency of intrauterine growth retardation association with confined placental mosaicism. Prenat Diagn 1991; 11:743–750.

113. Benn P. Trisomy 16 and trisomy 16 mosaicism: a review. Am J Med Genet 1998; 79:121–133.

114. Robinson WP, Barrett IJ, Bernard L, et al. Meiotic origin of trisomy in confined placental mosaicism is correlated with presence of fetal uniparental disomy, high levels of trisomy in trophoblast, and increased risk of fetal intrauterine growth restriction. Am J Hum Genet 1997; 60:917–927.

115. Kalousek DK. Pathogenesis of chromosomal mosaicism and its effect on early human development. Am J Med Genet 2000; 91:39–45.

116. Wolstenholme J. An audit of trisomy 16 in man. Prenat Diagn 1995; 15:109–121.

117. Yong PJ, Barrett IJ, Kalousek DK, Robinson WP. Clinical aspects, prenatal diagnosis, and pathogenenis of trisomy 16 mosaicism. J Med Genet 2003; 40:175–182.

118. Hassold T, Merrill M, Adkins K, Freeman S, Sherman S. Recombination and maternal age-dependent nondisjunction: molecular studies of trisomy 16. Am J Hum Genet 1995; 57:867–874.

119. Saura R, Roux D, Maugey-Laulon B, et al. False-negative results of trisomy 21 on direct analysis on chorionic villus sampling [letter]. Prenat Diagn 1998; 18:862–869.

120. Wang BT, Peng W, Cheng K-T, et al. Chorionic villi sampling: laboratory experience with 4,000 consecutive cases. Am J Med Genet 1994; 53:307–316.

121. Smith K, Lowther G, Maher E, Hourihan T, Wilkinson T, Wolstenholme J. On behalf of the Association of Clinical Cytogeneticists Prenatal Working Party. The predictive value of findings of the common aneuploidies, trisomies 13, 18 and 21, and numerical

sex chromosome abnormalities at CVS: experience from the ACC U.K. collaborative study. Prenat Diagn 1999; 19:817–826.

122. Pindar L, Whitehouse M, Ocraft K. A rare case of a false-negative finding in both direct and culture of a chorionic villus sample. Prenat Diagn 1992; 12:525–527.

123. Caspari D, Bartels I, Rauskolb R, Prange G, Osmers R, Eiben B. Discrepant karyo-types after second- and third-trimester combined placentacentesis/amniocentesis. .Prenat Diagn 1994; 14:569–576.

124. Los FJ, van de Berg C, van Opstal D, et al. Abnormal karyotypes in semi-direct chor-ionic villus preparations of women with different cytogenetic risks. Prenat Diagn 1998; 18:1023–1040.

125. Benn PA, Hsu LYF. Maternal cell contamination of amniotic fluid cell cultures: results of a U.S. nationwide survey. Am J Med Genet 1983; 15:297–305.

126. Nuss S, Brebaum D, Grond-Ginsbach C. Maternal cell contamination in amniotic fluid samples as a consequence of the sampling technique. Hum Genet 1994; 93:121–124.

127. Freiberg AS, Blumberg B, Lawce H, Mann J. XX/XY chimerism encountered during prenatal diagnosis. Prenat Diagn 1988; 8:423–426.

128. Amor D, Delatycki MB, Susman M, et al. 46,XX/46,XY at amniocentesis in a fetus with true hermaphroditism [letter]. J Med Genet 1999; 36:866–869.

129. Teyssier M, Gaucherand P, Buenerd A. Prenatal diagnosis of a tetraploid fetus. Prenat Diagn 1997; 17:474–478.

130. Edwards MJ, Park JP, Wurster-Hill DH, Graham JM Jr. Mixoploidy in humans: two surviving cases of diploid-tetraploid mixoploidy and comparison with diploid-triploid mixoploidy. Am J Med Genet 1994; 52:324–330.

131. Meiner A, Holland H, Reichenbach H, Horn L-Ch, Faber R, Froster UG. Tetraploidy in an growth-retarded fetus with a thick placenta. Prenat Diagn 1998; 18:864–865.

132. Nieuwint A, van Zalen-Sprock R, Hummel P, et al. 'Identical' twins with discordant karyotypes. Prenat Diagn 1999; 19:72–76.

133. Schmid O, Trautmann U, Ashour H, Ulmer R, Pfeiffer RA, Beinder E. Prenatal diag-nosis of heterokaryotypic mosaic twins discordant for fetal sex. Prenat Diagn 2000; 20:999–1003.

134. Gilbert B, Yardin C, Briault S, et al. Prenatal diagnosis of female monozygotic twins discordant for Turner syndrome: implications for prenatal genetic counseling. Prenat Diagn 2002; 22:697–702.

135. Rogers JG, Voullaire L, Gold H. Monozygotic twins discordant for trisomy 21. Am J Med Genet 1982; 11:143–146.

16

Prenatal DNA Testing

Eugene Pergament
*Department of Obstetrics and Gynecology, Northwestern University,
Chicago, Illinois, U.S.A.*

INTRODUCTION

This chapter is concerned with the application of molecular (DNA) testing for the prenatal diagnosis of genetic disorders. From a population perspective, prenatal DNA testing is applied to a relatively limited number of families when compared to the prenatal diagnosis of chromosome aberrations for women of advanced maternal age. From the perspective of individual reproductive risk, however, for prenatal DNA testing of single gene disorders, this risk characteristically ranges from 25% to 50% versus a 0.5% to 5% risk of a chromosome aberration in the case of women 35 to 45 years of age at the time of delivery. From a diagnostic perspective, prenatal DNA testing represents a greater challenge due to the rapidly expanding number of disease entities identified through molecular technologies versus the limited number of laboratories experienced and qualified to provide such testing. In almost all cases of prenatal DNA testing, therefore, the obstetrician–gynecologist as well as the reproductive geneticist serves as counselor and coordinator between the at-risk couple and the laboratory performing the genetic analysis. It is the aim of this chapter to provide practical guidance to obstetricians, recognizing that detailed descriptions of laboratory techniques concerning DNA analyses are beyond the scope of this chapter.

SOURCES OF PATIENTS

There are two primary sources of patients undergoing prenatal DNA testing: (i) couples identified through carrier detection programs, e.g., screening of Caucasians for cystic fibrosis (CF), of the Ashkenazim for Tay–Sachs, and of African-Americans for sickle cell disease and (ii) couples determined to be at risk because of the birth of a child with an established diagnosis of a single gene mutation either for an autosomal recessive, autosomal dominant, or X-linked disorder. Thus, in each of these clinical situations presenting to the obstetrician–gynecologist, the molecular basis of the specific disease entity under consideration for prenatal DNA testing has already been fully defined and, thereby, in many but not all instances also identifies the laboratory capable of performing the prenatal genetic analysis.

THE FIRST STEP: CONFIRMING THE DIAGNOSIS

A critical and essential first step in providing prenatal genetic diagnosis is obtaining laboratory documentation to confirm the specific mutation(s) involved, either the carrier status of both parents or that of the affected relative. Laboratories serving as referral sources characteristically require that documentation of the diagnosis accompany the specimen being sent for prenatal diagnosis, unless they had performed the original DNA studies. There will be cases whereby a laboratory will repeat the DNA analyses on the prospective parents, to confirm the diagnosis as well as to rule out maternal contamination in the prenatal sample either of chorionic villi or amniotic fluid cells.

THE SECOND STEP: LEARNING MORE ABOUT THE DISEASE AND DETERMINING WHETHER PRENATAL DIAGNOSIS IS POSSIBLE

Following confirmation of the genetic diagnosis and the accurate assessment of the reproductive risk, the next step is to determine whether prenatal DNA testing is in fact possible and if so, the specific laboratories which are experienced and are able to conduct such testing. An extremely valuable resource toward this end is Gene Tests™, a comprehensive database of genetic laboratories funded by the Maternal and Child Health Bureau and the National Institutes of Health Library of Medicine. The URL is www.genetests.org and access is available to any health professional who registers as a user so as to gain access to information concerning specific genetic disease entities. Gene Tests lists over 700 genetic diseases as well as more than 450 laboratories which provide DNA testing. Within the description of each genetic disease will be included the names of those laboratories performing DNA testing throughout the Western world and whether such testing is on a research basis only or is available for clinical and/or prenatal diagnosis. And, of immeasurable value, the descriptions will contain the name of a contact person for each laboratory. This in turn makes it possible for the referring physician to discuss a specific case before obtaining and properly preparing the sample prior to sending it for prenatal DNA testing. Gene Tests actually allows one to perform "comparative shopping" by listing cost and turn-around time between different laboratories.

Although the need to document the diagnosis leading to prenatal testing may seem obvious, there have been times when prenatal DNA testing was applied incorrectly either because of incorrect diagnosis, lack of medical/laboratory documentation, or failure to be aware that there are still many recognized single gene disorders for which prenatal diagnosis is currently unavailable. And, since the field of molecular biology is rapidly evolving, families previously counseled that the underlying molecular basis of a particular gene is unknown must also be encouraged to maintain contact if they are considering a pregnancy to determine if any advances have occurred in the case of their genetic disorder.

THE THIRD STEP: WHEN AND HOW OF PRENATAL DNA TESTING

There are several practical considerations that must be arranged for each genetic condition and each couple undergoing prenatal DNA testing. These include special arrangements with the laboratory performing the DNA analysis; clear understanding of the nature and source of payment, either by the couple themselves or by preauthorization from the insurance company as a covered benefit; the preparation, handling, and shipping of the sample; and, most important, the completion of any special consent forms required by the referral laboratory.

Having established that prenatal DNA testing is available, the at-risk couple must select either first-trimester chorionic villus sampling (CVS) or second-trimester amniocentesis. One of the obvious advantages of CVS is that it can be performed earlier than amniocentesis, usually between 10 and 13 weeks' gestation, thereby, providing results weeks earlier. Most laboratories will require up to 14 days for completion of a prenatal DNA analysis. As such couples are considered to be at a very high risk of recurrence, there are very significant obstetrical benefits identifying couples with affected pregnancies as early as possible. Therefore, it is not surprising that CVS has basically replaced amniocentesis in the case of the prenatal diagnosis of diseases for which DNA testing is available. After more than two decades, the technical expertise associated with the performance of CVS in the hands of experienced samplers has reached a level whereby it is claimed that the risk of fetal loss with CVS as a direct consequence of the procedure is now regarded as the same risk as amniocentesis.

THE FOURTH STEP: AN OVERVIEW OF DNA ANALYSIS

The number of genetic disorders that can be diagnosed as well as the precision and efficiency of DNA analyses are increasing rapidly as new approaches are developed, new mutations are characterized, and additional genetic diseases are mapped and sequenced. Prenatal diagnosis of genetic disorders by DNA analysis can be performed either by means of closely linked markers or by direct detection of the mutation. Direct detection of mutations is performed in the case of point mutations; larger DNA segments, e.g., deletions, insertions, inversions, and rearrangements such as translocations; and, expansion of trinucleotide repeats. In each case, there are a variety of methods (Table 1) and any technique used for direct mutation screening can be applied to prenatal diagnosis, a reflection in part of the nature of the mutations undergoing DNA analysis as well as the experience and expertise of the referral laboratory. Basic to the development and application of these methods are three fundamental tools of molecular genetics that underlie all forms of DNA testing; they are: (i) Southern blotting, (ii) polymerase chain reaction (PCR) amplification; and (iii) DNA sequencing (1).

Southern blotting uses restriction endonucleases and probes (2). Restriction endonucleases are used to produce genomic fragments of DNA of suitable size for analysis. Since these endonucleases cleave DNA at specific nucleotide sequences, termed "restriction sites," the resulting DNA fragments are of reproducible size and composition. In order to perform a Southern blot, aliquots of genomic DNA are incubated with a restriction endonuclease and the resulting DNA fragments are subjected to gel electrophoresis to separate them by size (described in the following section on PCR). After separation, the DNA fragments are denatured in order to make them single-stranded; these fragments are then transferred and attached to a solid membrane. The membrane is then incubated or hybridized in a solution containing labeled DNA segments termed "probes." After hybridization and removal of excess probe, the membrane is exposed to film, and genomic DNA fragments containing sequences complementary to the probe appears as bands. The sizes and

Table 1 Overview of Recombinant DNA Techniques Used for Prenatal Testing of
Genetic Mutations

Method	Gene deletion	Gene duplication	Indirect linkage	Direct point mutation
Southern blot	+	+		
Restriction fragment length polymorphism			+	
Variable number tandem repeat			+	
Polymerase chain reaction	+	+	+	+
DNA sequencing				+
Mismatch cleavage				+
Oligonucleotide specific hybridization				+
Denaturing gradient gel electrophoresis				+
Single-stranded conformational polymorphism				+
Protein truncation test				+

number of bands are determined by the number and locations of restriction endonuclease sites in the segment undergoing analysis. Although Southern blotting can
identify chromosome fragments, deletions, and rearrangements and is particularly
useful in determining the size of trinucleotide repeats, e.g., CGG repeats in the case
of the fragile X syndrome, PCR is now the method of choice for routine diagnostic
testing.

PCR is a primer-directed enzymatic amplification of specific DNA sequences
(3). Assuming that a specific set of mutations have already been identified in the case
of prospective parents seeking prenatal DNA testing, the application of the polymerase chain reaction is the most common method currently used for primary mutation
analysis. Specificity of PCR amplification results from the selection of unique primers
flanking the DNA segment to be amplified. The primers are allowed to anneal to
opposite genomic strands by lowering the denaturing temperature of 95°C to the
annealing temperature specific for the primer pair being used, usually around 37°C.
Following annealing, Taq polymerase, or a polymerase with similar properties,
directs DNA synthesis during incubation at 72°C. And, following this primer directed
synthesis, the genomic segments and copies are denatured again at 95°C for another
round of amplification.

With each amplification cycle, the number of copies synthesized doubles; after
30 such cycles, the number of copies will be in the order of 10^6 to 10^7. Thus, PCR can
easily increase the number of target copies by 100 million-fold in a matter of
2 to 3 hours in a test tube. Starting from 100 ng of hugely complex human genomic
DNA, for example, a large amount, >1 μg, of a homogenous 300 base-pair target
sequence can be produced. This sequence is in fact a copy of the corresponding
target region from the total genomic DNA and in turn can be analyzed for the presence or absence of any genetic mutation present in the sample undergoing prenatal
testing (Table 1). To increase the sensitivity and/or specificity of PCR, "nested"
primers, i.e., two sets of juxtaposed primers can be used in two complete rounds
of PCR amplification.

Separation and accurate size estimation of the DNA derived from the PCR is the final step in the prenatal diagnosis for single gene disorders. A change in the DNA sequence for a particular gene causes changes either in the size, charge, or folded structure of the DNA, which in turn alters its mobility on a nondenaturing gel. Under the influence of an electric current, therefore, DNA molecules migrate toward the positive electrode at a differential rate depending on size, charge, or number of folds, in a sequence-specific manner. After electrophoresis, the DNA is usually visualized by staining the gel with fluorescent dye, ethidium bromide, which binds to DNA.

The accuracy of the diagnosis approaches 100% when direct detection of a mutation is possible. However, prenatal diagnosis by DNA analysis is not predictive of the exact clinical presentation in the case of an affected pregnancy. Most couples undertaking prenatal DNA testing have already finalized their course of action if the pregnancy proves to be genetically abnormal. It must also be emphasized, however, that in most cases, there is a 50% to 75% chance that the pregnancy is unaffected and, therefore, the results of prenatal DNA testing permit prospective parents to continue their pregnancy free of the fear of delivering a child whose life will be significantly compromised qualitatively and, in many instances, quantitatively as well.

DNA sequencing is usually performed by the Sanger or dideoxy method (4). In principle, the dideoxy method makes use of a single-stranded phage (bacterial virus) called M13. Once the DNA fragment to be sequenced has been subcloned into M13, the DNA polymerase is used to synthesize a complementary radioactive copy of the insert. During the DNA polymerase reaction, $2',3'$-dideoxynucleotides of adenine, cytosine, guanine, or thymidine are added to four separate reactions containing one of the deoxyribonucleotides radiolabeled with 32P or 35S. When one of the dideoxynucleotides is incorporated, the $3'$-end of the reaction is no longer a substrate for chain elongation, and the growing DNA chain is terminated. Thus, in each of these four separate reactions there is a population of DNA molecules that is radioactive with a common $5'$-end, but of varying length because of the incorporation of a specific $3'$-end. Next, each of the four reaction products are subjected to electrophoresis, and autoradiograph and sequence deduction are performed. Comparison of mutant and standard sequences enables deduction of the mutation. Sequencing not only identifies the mutation but can enable derivation of short oligonucleotide sequences. These sequences can be used as probes in Southern blots or as allele-specific primers for PCR amplification to detect the presence of a specific mutation in the genomic DNA of samples obtained in the course of prenatal diagnosis. Recent modifications of this methodology employ automation and the use of dideoxynucleotides that have been chemically modified to fluoresce under ultraviolet light, i.e., each nucleotide has its own unique color, producing bands of alternating colors reflecting the sequence of the nucleotides comprising the DNA fragment of interest.

PRENATAL DNA DIAGNOSIS: THREE EXAMPLES

The prenatal DNA diagnoses of three disorders have been selected to illustrate some of the common but significant clinical and laboratory issues that must be considered in the course of providing such a service; these are CF, autosomal recessive polycystic kidney disease (ARPKD), and myotonic dystrophy (DM).

Illustrative Study Case 1: Cystic Fibrosis

Prenatal diagnosis of CF is of considerable interest because of the high frequency of carriers, approaching 3% in the Caucasian population, and consequently it is the most common lethal genetic disease in this ethnic group. This autosomal recessive disorder is caused by as many as 1000 different mutations in a gene termed the "cystic fibrosis transmembrane conductance regulator," with the type and frequency of mutations significantly varying between different ethnic populations (5–7). The first and most common mutation, F508del, accounts for 70% of the CF mutations among Northern Europeans. Common mutations present in other ethnic populations only occur in frequencies of 1% to 2%, although specific mutations in a given ethnic group may be higher. For most ethnic populations, DNA analyses for F508del and these common mutations will identify approximately 85% of all mutations in the CF gene; however, the detection rate can vary from less than 50% to as high as 97%, depending on the type and number of mutations analyzed for any one ethnic group.

Given the fact that mutations in the CF gene occur in Caucasians at a considerable frequency, it is likely that one of the most frequent uses for prenatal DNA testing will be for CF. This is as a direct consequence of the widespread adoption in the United States and Europe of carrier screening for all such couples at reproductive risk, fostered in the United States, for example, by recommendations of the National Institutes of Health as well as by publications by the American College of Obstetrics and Gynecology and guidelines established by the American College of Medical Genetics (http://acmg.net).

When both parents are carriers of the F508del mutation, prenatal DNA testing is rather straightforward and the clinical outcome predictable. Conducting prenatal DNA testing for CF may be complicated when at-risk parents have different mutations within the CF gene. In such a case, when each prospective parent passes on a mutation, forming what is termed, "a compound heterozygote," the phenotype may not be easily predictable in terms of organ system involvement, e.g., respiratory, digestive, etc., and in terms of clinical severity. There may be other complications in relating genotype to phenotype, as the CF gene is also involved in other disorders such as congenital bilateral absence of the vas deferens (8), disseminated bronchiectasis (9), and chronic pancreatitis (10). The results of prenatal DNA testing with regard to these disease entities presents many prospective parents with enormous dilemmas in decision-making concerning their pregnancy.

Perhaps the most confusing element in screening and prenatal diagnosis of CF concerns the 5T polymorphism at the Tn locus in intron 8 of the CF gene (11). 5T by itself is considered a polymorphism (a mutation occurring in >1% of a population) without clinical significance. If a mutation designated R117H is found, the results at the Tn locus become significant, since R117H can be either present in combination with a 5T or T7 allele. R117H-5T is only found in CF patients, whereas, R117H-T7 is found both in CF patients and patients with congenital bilateral absence of the vas deferens. Confusion arises when one parent carries the 5T polymorphism and the other parent carries a defined mutation in the CF gene: the R117H mutation must be on the same chromosome as the 5T polymorphism in order for there to be the potential for an affected offspring.

Prenatal DNA testing for CF can be conducted either on chorionic villus cells or amniocytes. Most laboratories will require cultured cells, as direct preparations are very likely to fail and have a negative impact by reducing the sample size for culture, thereby, affecting turnaround time, and disappointing parental expectations. It also cannot be emphasized too often that CF testing, like other genetic analyses, is complex and prone to errors, as demonstrated in quality assurance programs concerned with carrier screening for CF (12), and therefore, the laboratory performing prenatal DNA testing for CF should document their history and experience in this regard.

Illustrative Study Case 2: Autosomal Recessive Polycystic Kidney Disease

Autosomal recessive polycystic kidney disease (ARPKD) involves fusiform dilation of the renal collecting ducts and congenital hepatic fibrosis with hyperplastic bile ducts and portal fibrosis. The prognosis in the perinatal cases is usually extremely poor with neonatal death occurring in a considerable number of affected individuals. For those that survive the neonatal period, about 15% will develop end stage renal failure in childhood; in juveniles, there may be severe complications with rupture of esophageal varices; and, in most cases, the treatment involves kidney–liver transplantation (13). Due to the poor renal- and liver-related morbidity and mortality, there is a strong demand for prenatal diagnosis (14). Ultrasound evaluation often fails to detect kidney enlargement and increased echogenicity, as well as oliogohydramnios, well into the second trimester of pregnancy. Early and reliable prenatal diagnosis for families with a history of ARPKD is not possible on the basis of fetal ultrasonography.

The gene for polycystic kidney and hepatic disease 1 (PKHD1), has been mapped to chromosome 6p21-cen, i.e., on the short arm of chromosome 6, somewhere between band 21 and the centromere. This makes possible indirect molecular analysis for the prenatal diagnosis of ARPKD with the use of several closely linked markers. This approach is both robust and reliable in the majority of ARPKD cases. Nevertheless, there are significant limitations of prenatal diagnosis based on genetic linkage. First, DNA linkage testing is a procedure that requires analysis of families and cannot be applied to isolated individuals or to apparently sporadic cases of the disease. The unavailability of key family members, essential for interpretation of linkage data, may prevent the application of the indirect method of molecular analysis. The linkage analysis will be totally inaccurate if there is undisclosed non-paternity. Second, linkage analysis cannot be used to confirm a doubtful diagnosis, for unlike direct mutation analysis, the actual mutation causing the disease is never observed. Therefore, the diagnosis of ARPKD must be secure on other grounds if linkage is to be used for prenatal diagnosis. And, third, there is the possibility of genetic recombination, a normal event, but one that reduces the accuracy of the DNA analysis relative to the distance between the disease gene such as PKHD1 and the marker(s).

The PKHD1 gene has been identified (15,16). The gene encodes a protein (fibrocystin/polyductin) whose function, while presently unknown, is hypothesized to be involved in cellular adhesion, repulsion, and proliferation as well as intercellular signaling and ciliary function. The identification of the PKHD1 gene offers the option of prenatal diagnostic testing for families at risk for ARPKD without anatomically proven diagnosis in an index case or in the presence of diagnostic doubts, as well as for those families without available sources of DNA from the index case.

The mutation detection rate of the PKHD1 mutation has been reported to be >75%, involving both severely as well as moderately affected ARPKD (17). In a recent study of ARPKD patients, at least one mutation in the PKHD1 gene was identified in 96% and no mutation in only 4% (17). The diagnosis is definitely established only if two mutations are detected in the proband but ARPKD is also assumed if only one mutation is identified. Therefore, it may be expected that a small set of families with a history of ARPKD may present for prenatal diagnosis with the following genetic information: an anatomically documented case wherein only one PKHD1 mutation is identified in the proband and in one but not the other parent. Nevertheless, in such instances, a combination of direct and indirect mutation analysis can be offered as long as the relationship of the markers to the PKHD1 gene has been established through family analysis in the parent whose mutation in the PKHD1 gene has not been identified.

The possibility of a misinterpretation has to be addressed in prenatal genetic counseling for ARPKD. Approximately two-thirds of the mutations were predicted to truncate the protein of the PKHD1 gene as a result of missense changes, point mutations resulting in a change in an amino-acid–specifying codon (17). This makes the interpretation especially difficult in cases with only one identified base pair exchange, as a polymorphism without clinical significance may be misinterpreted as a disease-related mutation. Therefore, a comparison with known PKHD1 mutations in the PKHD1 mutation database is essential (http://ww.humgen.rwth-aachen.de). The presence of a second defined mutation makes the risk of misinterpretation less likely.

Illustrative Study Case 3: Myotonic Dystrophy

DM is an autosomal dominant disorder which presents with myotonia, muscle atrophy, and cataracts. Pregnancies of women with DM can be complicated by polyhydramnios, decreased fetal movement, breech presentation, and prematurity, signifying the likelihood of a more severe, congenital form of DM, which is characterized by hypotonia, respiratory and feeding difficulties, delayed motor development, and mental retardation (18). The gene responsible for DM, myotonin protein kinase, has been mapped to chromosome 19q13.2 (the long arm of chromosome 19, within band 13.2). This gene contains an unstable DNA sequence identified as a CTG trinucleotide repeat within the 3'-untranslated region. This CTG repeat is highly polymorphic: present from 5 to 30 times in the general population, it is amplified up to several thousand repeats in DM patients. It has been observed that expanded CTG repeats are basically unstable, altering their lengths from generation to generation and tending to expand when transmitted from affected mother to child. In the case of congenital DM, the repeat size is unusually large, consistent with the hypothesis of "anticipation," the manifestation of the disease with increasing severity in successive generations.

Prenatal diagnosis of DM is possible by using direct mutation analysis and detection of the CTG repeat expansion within the MPK gene. In most cases of congenital DM, the CTG repeat expansion in the fetus is larger than that of the affected mother. However, there is at least one case of a fetus affected with congenital DM in which prenatal diagnosis performed on amniocytes demonstrated that the size of the repeats (580) was less than that of the mother's (980), whereas the repeat size in blood cells of the infant were higher (1384) (19). Such a result based on amniocytes would predict DM but not the congenital form. This case may illustrate that in the case of disorders caused by trinucleotide expansion, e.g., fragile X syndrome, there is likely to be somatic instability resulting in different sizes of trinucleotide expansion in different tissues of the same individual (and likely, somatic mosaicism within a single tissue type). Studies have demonstrated that CTG expansion is greater in brain, skeletal muscle, cardiac muscle, testes, thyroid, and liver when compared to leukocytes (20).

Genetic counseling of pregnant patients affected with DM can be challenging due to a number of factors associated with the clinical expression of the disorder. Such counseling must clearly describe the clinical findings of DM and congenital DM as well as an explanation of the risks associated with intergenerational expansion of the CTG repeat during maternal transmission resulting in offspring with congenital DM. Intergenerational contraction, that is, reduced CTG repeat size in fetal chorionic villi or amniocytes compared to maternal blood, can occur but is still likely to result in either DM or congenital DM.

A FINAL NOTE OF CAUTION

As the base of knowledge of the human genome has increased, it has become evident that clinical and genetic heterogeneity is standard in almost all human diseases. The basis of any prenatal DNA testing, therefore, demands that the diagnosis of the disorder under investigation be rigorous, definitive, and definable. In the last example DM is simply too broad a term, for at least four clinical forms are recognized: DM type 1, DM type 2, proximal myotonic myopathy, and proximal DM. And, there have been cases of DM reported with no trinucleotide repeat expansion (21). Written documentation of the clinical diagnosis as well as results of laboratory analyses is paramount before undertaking prenatal DNA testing.

REFERENCES

1. Taylor CF, Taylor GR. Current and emerging techniques for diagnostic mutation detection: an overview of Methods for Mutation Detection. In: Elles R, Mountford R, eds. Molecular Diagnosis of Genetic Diseases. Clifton, U.K.: Humana Press, 2004:9–44.
2. Southern EM. Blotting at 25. Trends Biochem Sci 2000; 25(12):585–588.
3. Mullis K. Specific enzymatic amplification of DNA in vitro: the polymerase chain reaction. Cold Spring Harbor Symposium. Quant Biol 1975; 51:263–273.
4. Sanger F, Nicklen S, Coulson AR. DNA sequencing with chain-terminating inhibitors. Proc Natl Acad Sci USA 1977; 74:5463–5467.
5. Riordan JR, Rommens JM, Kerem BS, et al. Identification of the cystic fibrosis gene: cloning and characterization of complementary DNA. Science 1989; 245:1066–1073.
6. Zielenski J, Rozmahel R, Bozon D, et al. Genomic DNA sequence of the cystic fibrosis transmembrane conductance regulator (CFTR) gene. Genomics 1991; 10:214–228.
7. The Cystic Fibrosis Genetic Analysis Consortium. Cystic Fibrosis Mutation Database. (November 21, 2005 at http://www.genet.sickkids.on.ca/cftr/).
8. Chillon M, Casals T, Mercier B, et al. Mutations in the cystic fibrosis gene in patients with congenital absence of the vas deferens. N Engl J Med 1995; 332:1475–1480.
9. Pignatti PF, Bombieri C, Margio C, et al. Increased incidence of cystic fibrosis gene mutations in adults with disseminated bronchiectasis. Hum Mol Genet 1995; 4:635–639.
10. Scharer N, Schwarz M, Malone G, et al. Mutations of the cystic fibrosis gene in patients with chronic pancreatitis. N Engl J Med 1998; 339:645–652.
11. Cuppens H, Lin W, Jaspers M, et al. Polyvariant mutant cystic fibrosis transmembrane conductance regulator genes—the polymorphic (TG)m locus explains the partial penetrance of the T5 polymorphism as a disease mutation. J Clin Investig 1998; 101:487–496.

12. Dequeker E, Cassiman JJ. Genetic testing and quality control in diagnostic laboratories. Nat Genet 2000; 25:259–260.
13. Bergmann C, Senderek J, Windelen E, et al. Clinical consequences of PKHD1 mutations in 164 patients with autosomal-recessive polycystic kidney disease (ARPKD). Kidney Int 2005; 67:829–848.
14. Zerres K, Senderek J, Rudnik-Schoneborn S, et al. New options for prenatal diagnosis in autosomal recessive polycystic kidney disease by mutation analysis of the PKHD1 gene. Clin Genet 2004; 66(1):53–57.
15. Harris PC, Rossetti S. Molecular genetics of autosomal recessive polycystic kidney disease. Mol Genet Metab 2004; 81(2):75–85.
16. Rossetti S, Torra R, Coto E, et al. A complete mutation screen of PKHD1 in autosomal-recessive polycystic kidney disease (ARPKD) pedigrees. Kidney Int 2003; 64(2):391–403.
17. Bergmann C, Senderek J, Schneider F, et al. PKHD1 mutations in families requesting prenatal diagnosis for autosomal recessive polycystic kidney disease (ARPKD). Hum Mutat 2004: 23(5):487–495.
18. Upadhyay K, Thomson A, Luckas MJ. Congenital myotonic dystrophy. Fetal Diagn Ther 2005; 20(6):512–514.
19. Geifman-Holtzman O, Fay K. Prenatal diagnosis of congenital myotonic dystrophy and counseling of the pregnant mother: case report and literature review. Am J Med Genet 1998; 78:250–253.
20. Thornton CA, Johnson K, Moxley RT. Myotonic dystrophy patients have larger CTG expansions in skeletal muscle than in leukocytes. Ann Neurol 2004; 35:104–107.
21. Thornton CA, Griggs RC, Moxley R. Myotonic dystrophy with no trinucleotide repeat expansion. Ann Neurol 2004; 35:269–272.

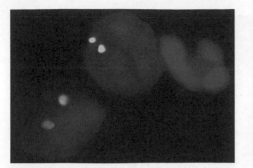

Figure 8.1 (*See p. 123*)

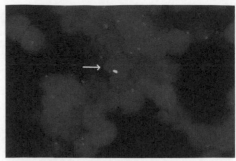

Figure 8.2A (*See p. 129*)

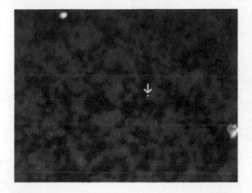

Figure 8.2B (*See p. 129*)

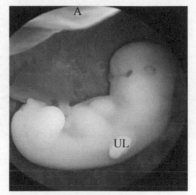

Figure 14.1B (*See p. 220*)

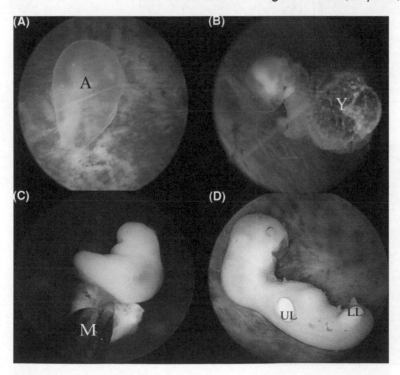

Figure 14.4 (*See p. 224*)

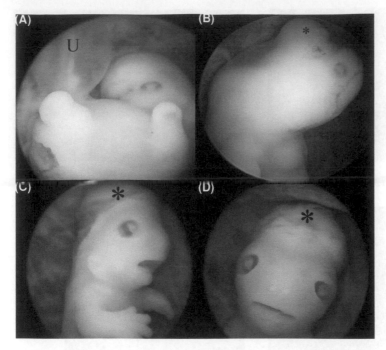

Figure 14.5 (*See p. 226*)

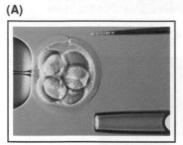 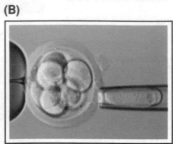

Figure 17.1 (*See p. 288*)

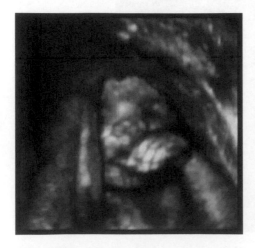 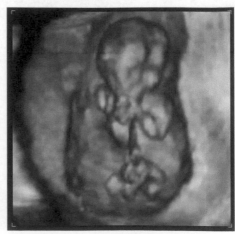

Figure 19.1 (*See p. 354*)   **Figure 19.7** (*See p. 358*)

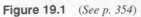

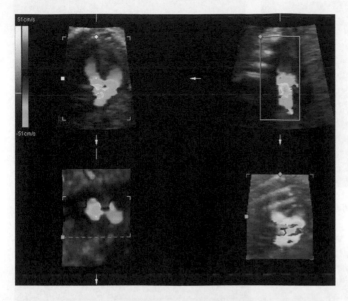

Figure 19.11 (*See p. 362*)

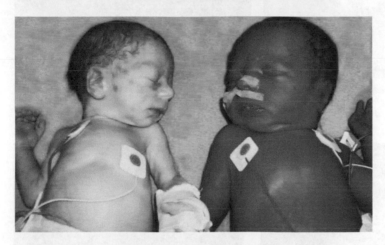

Figure 25.4 (*See p. 450*)

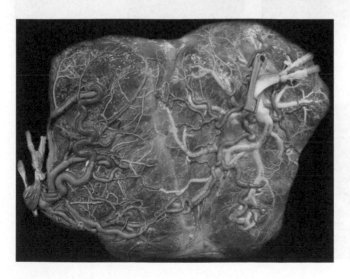

Figure 25.5 (*See p. 451*)

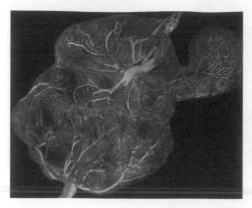

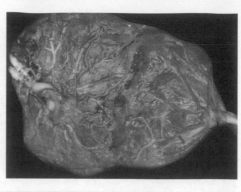

Figure 25.16B-1 (*See p. 464*)

Figure 25.16A-1 (*See p. 464*)

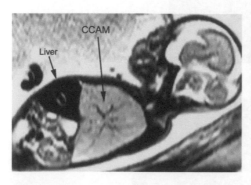

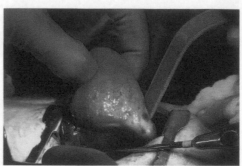

Figure 27.1 (*See p. 498*)

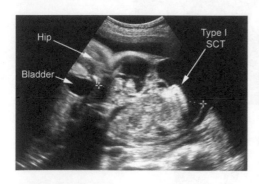

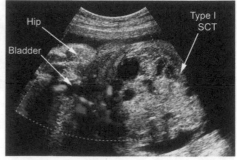

Figure 27.3 (*See p. 501*)

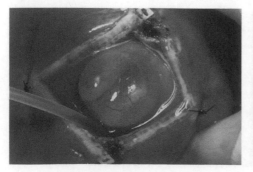

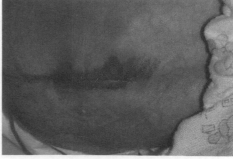

Figure 27.4 (*See p. 503*)

17

Preimplantation Genetic Diagnosis

Norman Ginsberg
Feinberg School of Medicine, Northwestern University,
Chicago, Illinois, U.S.A.

INTRODUCTION

The incidence of severe congenital and genetic disorders that cause early death or lifelong chronic disease ranges from 15 to 45 per 1000 live births. The main goal in the management of genetic disorders, like other diseases, is prevention when possible and treatment when not. Until recently, many of these conditions were not detected until birth, because there was no safe or reliable way to detect them.

To reduce the number of liveborn children with genetic handicaps, screening was introduced. Carrier detection before and during pregnancy is now widely used for such common diseases as sickle cell anemia, thalassemia, Tay–Sach's disease, and cystic fibrosis. In the United States, Tay–Sach's screening programs have been highly effective, leading to a decrease in the incidence of the disease by over 90% (1). This disease is the classic example of the power of effective screening. Thalassemia is a common disorder in populations of Mediterranean origin. Thalassemia major may affect 0.18 per 1000 liveborn children in this area of the world. Screening for this disease is simple and effective. Carriers have a characteristic microcytic mild anemia. A simple hemoglobin electrophoresis of hemoglobin A2 is diagnostic. Screening for cystic fibrosis is more complex since there are over 600 mutations and the disease impact of some of these mutations is not well understood. While screening may be effective for some common diseases, the majority of genetic disorders do not have a readily available biochemical marker or clear molecular marker.

It is important to be aware that not all genetic disorders are incurable. Individuals with phenylketonuria can lead normal lives if they strictly adhere to certain dietary restrictions. Effective cures are possible for certain vitamin-responsive inborn errors of metabolism. Better therapies for pulmonary infections and other innovations have extended the lifespan for children afflicted with cystic fibrosis that they may live beyond 25–30 years.

Nevertheless, numerous genetic diseases are not compatible with survival or a satisfactory quality of life. Jacobson introduced amniocentesis for chromosome abnormalities in 1967 and ushered in our first opportunity to have a clinical impact on genetic ailments (2). Prior to this time a couple had no other alternative but to

283

take their chances or refrain from procreation. For the first time couples had a method of detection. Women felt liberated to try pregnancies that they might otherwise have foregone. Despite the simplicity of the test, it was not until 1976 that amniocentesis was used more extensively following the report of the National Institute of Child Health and Human Development's publications in the *Journal of American Medical Association* (3). While amniocentesis was gaining popularity, other investigators began looking for techniques for still earlier diagnosis. Han Anguo and colleagues from the department of Obstetrics and Gynecology, Tietung Hospital, Anshan, People's Republic of China, began in 1970 to aspirate chorionic villi in the first trimester of pregnancy and later reported it in the *Chinese Medical Journal* in 1975. Hahnemann in Demark in 1974 and Kazy in Russia in 1979 all reported on chorionic villi sampling (4,5), but it was not until Old et al. in 1982, Brambati and Samoni in 1983, and Ginsberg et al. in 1983 that this approach became noticed and rapidly developed into a common clinical alternative (6–8).

While all the methods safely and reliably provided clear genetic diagnoses, the only remedy still remained abortion for the vast majority of cases. This remedy is unacceptable for many couples who begged for another way to avoid abortion. Preimplantation genetics is the alternative to this dilemma. Patients for the first time now have the ability to begin a pregnancy without a gene disorder that they are at risk for and older women can avoid age-associated chromosome abnormalities.

INDICATIONS

The indications for preimplantation diagnosis have progressively increased with improvement in methodology and our expanding understanding of the human genome. Familial chromosome disorders such as translocations can be avoided, reducing the heartbreak of multiple spontaneous abortions and the need to actively interrupt the pregnancy. The first application of preimplantation diagnosis was directed towards Duchenne's muscular dystrophy, a common sex-linked disorder. Handyside and collaborators reported in *Nature* their initial experience with human embryo biopsy and pregnancy outcome for the first time utilizing Y specific DNA amplification on a patient at risk for X-linked disorders (9). From that time on, the list of indications has greatly increased (Table 1).

While gene disorders were the first indication, it is now utilized more frequently in the management of infertile women of advanced maternal age. Other increasingly common indications are for chromosome translocations, reducing the number of transferred embryos that lead to high order multiple gestations, human leukocyte antigen (HLA) matching of embryos to affected family members and late onset gene disorders.

PREIMPLANTATION DIAGNOSIS (PGD) AND IN VITRO FERTILIZATION—EMBRYO TRANSFER

Embryos may be obtained in natural cycle by uterine lavage or created by oocyte retrieval and fertilization. Because only one embryo at a time can be obtained by lavage, this has limited usefulness in a PGD program. Brambati and Tului were early pioneers in this approach and reported their experience in 1990 (10).

Table 1 Indications for Preimplantation Diagnosis

Cystic fibrosis
Hemophilia A and B
Retinitis pigmentosa
Sickle cell anemia
Thalassemia (alpha and beta)
Myotonic dystrophy
Huntington's disease
Fragile-X syndrome
Machado–Joseph disease
Alpha 1 antitrypsin disease
Alzheimer's disease (APP gene)
Glycogen storage disease
Choroidermia
Wiscott–Aldrich disease
Duchenne and Becker (muscular dystrophy)
Sexing for X-linked conditions
Phenylketonuria
Epidermolysis bullosa
OCT deficiency
P53 oncogene mutation
Von Hipple Lindau
LCHAD
Multiple epiphyseal dysplasia
Fanconi anemia A and C
X-linked hydrocephaly
Neurofibromatosis (NF1 and NF2)
ADA deficiency
Rhesus
Long chain acyl-CoA
Gaucher's disease
Familial posterior fossa brain tumor (HSNF5)
Myotubular myopathy
Hypophosphatasia
Familial dysautonomia
CMT 1A and 1B
Hurler's syndrome
PKD 1 and 2
Dystonia
Citrullinemia
Kell disease
Holoprosencephaly (SSH gene)
Alport disease

Most protocols today use a combination of gonadotropin-releasing hormone agonists (GNRH), purified follicle stimulating hormone, and HCG. This combination seems to be most reliable in causing super-ovulation particularly in older women.

During the administration of super-ovulating drugs, it is crucial to closely monitor the patient. This insures that the maximal number of mature oocytes can be obtained yet avoiding severe hyperstimulation syndrome. Approximately 36 hours after the administration of HCG the mature oocyte has resumed its meiotic process, which results in the extrusion of the first polar body. The mature oocyte is then ready for retrieval.

Once the ovulation induction process is begun, oocyte quality and quantity is monitored by a combination of ultrasound and plasma 17-estradiol. The diameter of the follicle may vary depending upon which stimulation protocol was used. An estradial of 250–300 pg/mL is characteristic of a mature follicle.

Each cycle is additionally monitored with determinations of lutenizing hormone (LH) and progesterone levels. Impending cycles can be detected by rising progesterone levels and the LH surge may herald ovulation. The use of GNRH agonist has been very influential in reducing the frequency of canceled cycles. The GNRH agonists have reduced the incidence of unexpected LH surges that lead to the cancellation of as much as 25 to 30% of cycles.

Transvaginal aspiration of oocytes under ultrasound guidance is now the method of choice for oocyte retrieval. In contrast to laparoscopic retrieval, this method can be done under local anesthesia with the addition of IV sedation, making it safer by eliminating general anesthesia. This process was first described by Dellenbach et al. and popularized by Feichtinger and colleges in Austria (11,12). This technique has the added benefit of not requiring an operating room. This not only reduces the cost but also eliminates competition for valuable OR time. An experienced team can be expected to accomplish oocyte retrieval this way over 98% of the time.

Follicle aspiration is generally scheduled 34 hours after the administration of HCG. The presence of an adequate number of follicles is assured by abdominal scanning, prior to prepping the patient. The bladder is emptied and vital signs are carefully monitored and recorded, while a sterile field is created. An intravenous line is started to administer analgesics just before placement of the speculum. The vagina is cleansed with sterile saline and the vaginal fornices are infiltrated with local anesthesia.

The vaginal probe with its sterile needle guide is introduced into the vagina and a 17-gauge 35 cm needle is passed through the guide. Mature follicles are targeted and aspirated. They are immediately passed on to the waiting embryologist in an adjacent room. This process is repeated until all the mature follicles have been aspirated. Follicular fluid retrieved from the mature follicles can then be returned to the cul-de-sac. The entire process is usually completed within 30 to 60 minutes. The oocytes are liberated from their cumulus and prepared for fertilization. To eliminate polyspermia and to increase the incidence of fertilization, a single sperm is selected and injected into the cytoplasm. With this technique, virtually all males can contribute their genome to the preimplantation process. It is even possible for Klenefelter fathers to have unaffected children.

Prior to discharge the patients are rescanned to assure that there is no internal bleeding. Within several hours the patients are generally ready for discharge. The number and quality of oocytes commonly varies between individuals and may vary within the same patient from cycle to cycle. Embryos may be transferred within 3 to 5 days depending upon numerous factors and the ability to accomplish the complete analysis. Two to three embryos are generally transferred to the patient. The number of embryos available for transfer may depend upon the frequency of abnormalities in the oocytes or blastomeres as well as the success of the stimulation cycle.

The success rate for IVF-ET has been slowly increasing over the years. Success rate is dependent on many patient variables and the underlying disease.

Preimplantation manipulation does not seem to reduce the success rate and may even enhance the success rate in older couples. Success is now measured by the "take home baby" rate. The Society of Assisted Reproductive Technology (SART) IVF-ET Registry now regularly reports the success rate for all the clinics in the United States on an annual basis and is available to the general public.

Preimplantation diagnosis is not associated with any more complications than IVF done for other reasons. That's not to say however, that IVF may not be linked with complications. In vitro fertilization for preimplantation diagnosis potentially requires more embryos for study than simple conception, since many of the studied embryos may be affected with the disorder of concern.

Ovarian hyperstimulation syndrome is the only reported complication related to ovulation induction agents. Although the incidence maybe less than 0.5%, it can be serious and even life threatening. This can be avoided by withholding hCG. Care is needed to avoid the complications of hypovolemia, hemoconcentration, electrolyte disturbance and hypercoagulability (13,14).

Infrequently, ultrasound-guided aspiration can lead to ovarian bleeding, which in very rare circumstance may lead to surgical intervention for control (14). Additionally rare are complications of pelvic inflammatory disease after oocyte retrieval (15).

Once pregnancy is achieved, there are other potential problems. The incidence of ectopic pregnancy is increased over that of the general population. One would expect that the rate of ectopic pregnancy would be less in preimplantation patients since they generally have healthier fallopian tubes to begin with. Supraphysiological doses of estradiol and progesterone occur with the ovulation inducing agents. These high levels have been shown to impair normal tubal ciliar motion and proper smooth muscle contractions (17). Other factors that may contribute to this higher rate may be the embryo itself or the volume of fluid required to make the transfer (18). Not only is the rate of ectopic pregnancy increased, but so also the incidence of heterotopic pregnancies. The management options are decreased in the presence of heterotopic pregnancies and the outcome for the other fetus may be compromised by general anesthesia or surgical manipulation.

Finally, success of achieving pregnancy may be tempered by the presence of twins or triplets. This is not an insignificant or rare problem. In most successful IVF programs the incidence of multiple gestations may be 20% or greater (SART). This number is no different in preimplantation patients. Multiple pregnancies are of course associated with prematurity, which increases in frequency and severity as the number of fetuses increases. Prematurity is the single most significant factor contributing to long-term morbidity. This high incidence is the greatest drawback to preimplantation genetics.

METHODS

Preimplantation genetics may be performed one of two ways. The most commonly used methodology involves removal of one or two blastomeres from a pre-embryo and then performing the analysis directly on them. The other commonly used approach is the two-step polar body analysis that is derived from the oocyte. Each polar body is sequentially evaluated and a conclusion is drawn from the results of both of them.

Cleavage cell biopsy on the embryo is generally done between the 6- and 10-cell stages. The cleavage rate is variable in human embryos. The first division generally takes 16 to 24 hours (19,20). Cell divisions are invariably asynchronous at this early stage, but by day 3 most embryos will reach the 6–10-cell stage. Human embryos that divide more rapidly are often more successful in achieving pregnancy and therefore are more desirable for study. However, this correlation is weak (21).

Removal of more cells from the embryo reduces the chance for implantation and successful pregnancy. Biopsy at the 8-cell stage allows 12 hours to perform the analysis before it is necessary to transfer the embryo. More time could be gained by freezing the embryo after biopsy, but making a hole in the zona pellucida exposes the embryo to damage from ice crystals in the freezing process and therefore is generally not done.

Once the embryo has reached the appropriate stage it is placed in media under oil and transferred to the dissecting microscope for micromanipulation. The embryos are held with a glass pipette and a hole is made in the zona pellucida. A second larger micropipette is then introduced into the hole and one or two blastomeres are aspirated. Immediately after biopsy, the embryo is transfer back to the culture media to await transfer. With experience this entire process can be accomplished in 5 to 10 minutes. Every effort is made to minimize the time that the embryo is exposed to room temperature (Fig. 1).

Polar body analysis uses nature's discarded material and therefore is nonessential to the development of the embryo. Its removal should have no effect on growth velocity or size of the ultimate baby (Fig. 2). The polar body is the reciprocal of the oocyte and therefore there are three possible combinations after meiosis I. The polar body may have the affected gene in a homozygous state, i.e., normal oocyte; the polar body might have the normal homozygous gene, i.e., the oocyte is abnormal; and finally the polar body may have a combination of both the normal and affected gene, i.e., the oocyte is heterozygous. Since the rate of crossover is determined by the distance of the gene from the centromere, first polar bodies will be heterozygous from 0% to 50% of the time. The analysis of the second polar body will be the final determining factor when the first is heterozygous. Second polar bodies with the normal gene will be associated with affected oocytes and those with abnormal genes will come from normal oocytes. It is important to analyze the second polar body to increase the number of potential embryos for transfer (Fig. 3).

The presence of a heterozygous first polar body is reassuring because it demonstrates that the system is working and potentially reduces the chance of error after

(A)   **(B)**

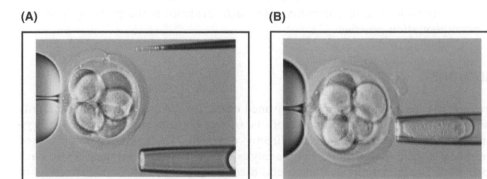

Figure 1   (**A**) An eight-cell embryo is seen before blastomere biopsy. In (**B**), a blastomere has been aspirated into the pipette. (*See color insert.*)

(A)   **(B)**

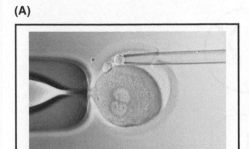
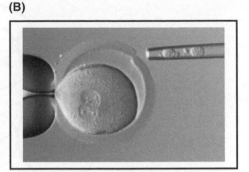

Figure 2 (**A**) Both polar bodies are seen. (**B**) Both polar bodies are seen aspirated into the pipette.

analyzing the second polar body. Each method has advantages and disadvantages. The differences can be seen in Table 2.

PROBLEMS WITH SINGLE CELL ANALYSIS

Single cell analysis of gene disorders, by the nature of the small amount of DNA available for analysis, creates unique and challenging problems. The first problem that needs to be addressed is the elimination and prevention of DNA contamination.

To prevent contamination it is very important to test all reagents and equipment for DNA contamination before beginning any evaluations. There is virtually nothing used within the lab that cannot have some DNA contamination. The only bottles to be used are those that are only touched by gloved hands. No equipment that is used or created can be touched with bare hands.

Positive displacement pipettes and laminar flow hoods are essential. Because of the rigorous controls that need to be in place, it is reasonable to separate the preimplantation laboratory from the general laboratory by freeing up personnel for easier and more efficient labor. All reagents should be separated into smaller aliquots so that if contamination is discovered another vial will be readily available. Nonspecific forms of decontamination of polymerase chain reaction (PCR) reagents by ultraviolet irradiation or psoralen treatment may be used (22). It is imperative that all diagnostic assays are run in parallel with several control assays to ensure that there is no contamination with extraneous DNA. Positive controls should contain homozygous normal, homozygous abnormal, and heterozygous DNA in all cases.

Reaction conditions will vary with the gene that needs to be analyzed as well as between patients. All reaction conditions should be individually optimized for each PCR and primer set. To obtain optimal results all the parameters need to be adjusted. In an effort to optimize results the following suggestions need to be considered. It is best to start with PCR buffers that lack Mg and then add the Mg till the optimal quantity is reached.

Finding the optimal glycerol and formamide concentration is essential to increase the specificity of the reaction by increasing the hybridization stringency (23). Glycerol is important for stabilization of the Taq polymerase that allows for better efficiency of polymerization when extended cycles of PCR are required.

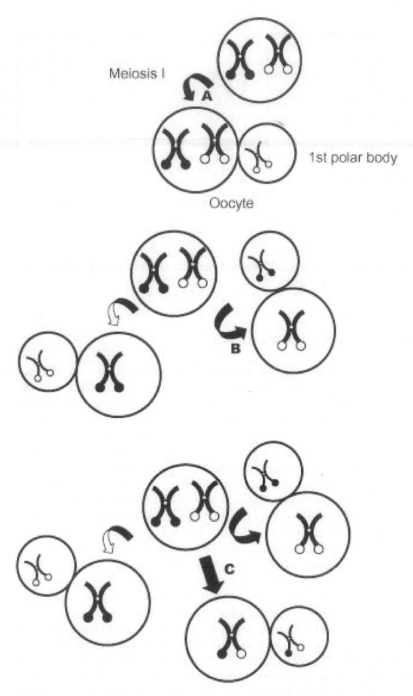

Figure 3 Analysis of the second polar body. Affected alleles are shown as dark dots. (**A**) In the absence of crossing-over if first polar body is normal, the oocyte is affected. (**B**) In the absence of crossing-over if the first polar body is affected, the oocyte will be normal. (**C**) Crossing-over occurs leading to both polar body and oocyte being heterozygous.

Table 2 Comparison between Polar Body Analysis and Blastomere Analysis

Polar body analysis	Blastomere analysis
More time for analysis	Paternal contribution analyzable
No disruption of the embryo	Detection of heterozygosity
Less allele dropout	Confirmation of polar body analysis
Avoidance of mosaicism	HLA typing

Two-temperature PCR ("turbo" PCR) appears to be just as effective as the standard three-step PCR for single-cell amplification. Using the two-temperature method allows for a reduction in the time required to complete the PCR reaction. The time for the annealing polymerization can be varied. Using these guidelines, it is possible to complete the single-cell amplification in approximately 2 hours.

To prevent nonspecific annealing of primers and subsequent chain elongation of spurious DNA, hot start PCR should be considered. Hot-start PCR is performed by withholding one or more of the required reagents until the mixture has reached a temperature of 72°C (24).

Another common problem is preferential amplification especially when using multiplex PCR. This creates shadows and faint bands as well as failure to amplify the band of interest. Shadows and faint bands lead to difficulty in interpretation of the bands. This is a result of errors in DNA processing. The reader is referred to the work of Rodriquez and colleagues for a more in depth analysis of this problem (25).

When allele-dropout or allele specific PCR failure occurs in the heterozygous cell, the cellular genotype would be misinterpreted as homozygous. This can lead to misdiagnosis in both polar bodies and blastomeres from heterozygous cells. This phenomenon occurs in all single cells and the rate may vary from 5% to 33%, which depends on the cell type as well as the methods used (26). There may be several explanations for allele dropout that include failure of cell lyses. This should lead to complete failure of any amplification. The risk of error in this setting is minimal since the embryo would never be transferred. However, this is wasteful since it may represent a perfectly normal embryo. Failure may occur secondary to loss of the DNA in the transfer process. The incidence of this is difficult to quantify. Another explanation for failure is that damage to the DNA occurs at the area of interest thereby not allowing the true structure to be amplified. The biggest potential clinical problem is the failure to detect allele dropout. When allele dropout goes undetected this can lead to the transfer of an embryo thought to be normal. PCR failure is thought to be the etiology of misdiagnosis in three cases evaluated for cystic fibrosis (27). It is generally accepted that the incidence of allele dropout varies markedly according to the cell type used for analysis. In blastomeres, some of the high level of allele dropout could be explained by a high rate of mosaicism found in blastomeres (28).

To address the problem of allele dropout or total PCR failure several approaches need to be directed to this problem. The rate of cell lyses failure needs to be reduced and when failure does occur it must be detected. Most centers use either an alkaline- or proteinase-based lysis buffer rather than collection in water followed by boiling. With regard to proteinase K enzyme, the source, length of storage, variations in fresh preparations between different batches can all contribute to lysis efficiency and are not well standardized. The alkaline lysis buffer system tends to be a more rapid lysis method but is not commercially available and often must be made in-house. When the neutralizing buffer is added the tube must be opened an additional time, creating another opportunity for contamination (29). It appears that there is no single lysis system that is uniformly superior for all cell types.

Several investigators have suggested that the use of linked markers will greatly reduce the incidence of undetected allele dropout (30,31) and simultaneously control for contamination (26). With the simple addition of one or two linked markers, undetected allele dropout can be decreased 50% and 75%, respectively, and with three linked markers it is virtually always detected (32). Reducing the incidence of undetected allele dropout has a secondary benefit of increasing the number of embryos available for transfer with the concomitant improvement in pregnancy rate per cycle. While the use of linked markers is very valuable, it is extremely labor-intensive and can be quite expensive. Another strategy to reduce allele dropout is to analyze more than one cell. Starting with polar body analysis allows for an opportunity to look at an additional cell from an embryo and limit the number of cells removed from the embryo. Removing more than one cell from the embryo may impact implantation rates.

EMBRYO MOSAICISM

Human reproduction is relatively inefficient with as much as 22% of embryos being lost before the third week after conception in natural cycles (33). In a survey reported by Plachot (34) the rate of chromosomal abnormalities in spontaneous abortions after in vitro fertilization was determined to be 60%. Additionally, Munne et al. (35) found that 37% of karyotyped preimplantation embryos were chromosomally abnormal. All of this suggests that the majority of losses is early and based on chromosome abnormalities. These results would explain the low implantation rate per embryo in in vitro fertilization programs and still lower rate found in older women.

Munne et al. (36) have used florescent in situ hybridization (FISH) studies with simultaneous multicolored probes to assess donated embryos. These embryos were allowed to cleave until they reached three days of growth. They selected for investigation those embryos that reached the 6–8-cell stage. They had to have less than 16% fragmentation, even cell size, no vacuoles, no granulations or multinucleated blastomeres. Morphologically these embryos would all have been considered prime candidates for clinical transfer. The age of the donors varied from 28 to 43 years of age with an average age of 36.7 years. The cells were individually removed by micromanipulation and fixated to glass slides. After fixation multicolor FISH probes were utilized for chromosomes 16, 18, X, and Y.

In this study, the FISH failure rate was 12%. This was made up of a combination of false negatives, false positives and lost cells. Despite this, 100% of the embryos were able to provide a result and 91% had all of their cells analyzed. Fifty-one percent of morphologically normal embryos had the expected diploid number. Several embryos had one to three cells that were tetraploid but were still considered normal. As expected aneuploidy, including triplody, polyploidy, and mosaicism were all detected. Mosaicism was differentiated from simple aneuploidy by virtue of the fact that all of the blastomeres were analyzed. This of course would be impractical in a clinical setting.

Mosaicism appears to be the most common chromosome abnormality in multiple studies (37–39). The origin of the mosaicism included mitotic nondisjunction, random karykinesis and probable anaphase lag. The origin of polyploid mosaic embryos was not clear. The presence of tetraploid cells along with normal diploid cells is normally present in human throphectoderm; its presence in cleaving embryos is not clear (40). It is likely that these tetraploid cells are destined to be trophectoderm. Mosaic embryos can likely develop into normal fetuses either because abnormal cells have proliferation disadvantage or because only a certain number of normal cells are needed. The critical balance between normal and abnormal cells is unknown.

Because of the high frequency of mosaicism present in embryos, those diagnoses made solely by embryo biopsy should be backed up by prenatal diagnosis. Analysis of gene disorders should be additionally backed up with aneuploidy studies as well.

TRANSLOCATION ANALYSIS

The evaluation of chromosome translocations may be assessed by several different methods. The method chosen will in part depend upon whether the mother or father is a carrier of the translocation. FISH can be applied to polar bodies and blastomeres; however, there are limits to this technology, being dependent on the availability of probes for a specific area of interest. Limitations of FISH require a need to do a karyotypic analysis. Karyotyping can be done by fusion techniques using the polar body when the female is the carrier or the blastomere when the male is the carrier.

Visualization of second polar body chromosomes following hybridization with a one-cell stage mouse embryo, using an electrofusion system has been demonstrated to be highly efficient (41). When the one-cell stage mouse embryos are enucleated, metaphase plate can be obtained 65% of the time. The visualized second polar body chromosomes were unichromatid G1 premature condensed chromosomes of good quality, suitable for differential staining.

The second polar body is introduced into the oocyte cytoplasts after the metaphase II nucleus is removed. The nucleus is removed after intracellular sperm injection but before fertilization. The other option is to use metaphase II oocytes that were matured 24–48 hours in vitro from immature oocytes. Because unfertilized oocytes are used, special attention is paid to remove both the meiotic metaphase II spindle and the sperm chromosomes. Then the oocyte is ready to receive the second polar body that is injected similar to the ICSI procedure.

The oocyte is activated by electrofusion with the use of custom-made electrostimulation apparatus in a fusion chamber consisting of two platinum wire electrodes glued to the bottom of a glass dish with a gap of 0.33 mm (32). Twenty-four hours after activation, the reconstructed embryos are checked every 30 minutes and then fixed 45 minutes later after the disappearance of the second polar body pronuclei. Alternatively, premature chromosome condensation of the resulting second polar body pronuclei may be induced with the use of okadaic acid. Hypotonic treatment of the embryos is avoided, to prevent overspreading of chromosomes. The whole procedure can usually be completed within two days. This allows more than sufficient time for transfer of embryos within the same stimulated cycle.

When the male is a carrier of a translocation or when confirmation of a female translocation is indicated, nuclear transplantation techniques for karyotyping a single blastomere can be done for preimplantation embryos. Blastomeres are now fused with intact or enucleated mouse zygotes at the pronuclear stage, known to be at the S phase of the cycle (42). This method is used in place of enucleated oocytes. When enucleated oocytes are used about 45% of the nuclei cannot be transformed into analyzable chromosomes by premature chromosome condensation. In order to use oocytes, the blastomere nucleus must be led into the G2 phase. Bringing the blastomere oocyte to the G2 phase requires more time than is practical. When this is done embryos need to be held to the blastocyst stage (42).

Frozen mouse zygotes, from the Charles River Laboratories (Wilmington, MA), can be conveniently used as recipient cytoplasm to induce conversion of the blastocyst nucleus into the metaphase. It is not necessary to enucleate the zygotes since the mouse chromosomes are easily differentiated from human chromosomes (32).

Precaution is taken to ensure the integrity of the blastomere plasma membrane during the biopsy. To avoid trauma, it is replaced by blastomere–zygote agglutination with phytohemagglutinin. The zygotes are prepared by removing the zona pellucida and then removing the second polar body before insertion of the blastomere.

When electrofusion is done, the blastomere–zygote pairs are oriented between electrodes by hand. Then an alternating current of 500 kHz; 0.2 kV/cm for 2 seconds is applied. The cell fusion is induced with a single pulse (1 kV/cm for 500 microseconds), and the results are assessed in 20 minutes (32).

Once the blastomeres are fused with the mouse zygote and the heterokaryons have entered into mitosis, they are identified under the dissecting microscope. The cytoplasm of the mouse cytoplasm is quite transparent. This transparency allows visualization of the disappearance of pronuclei and the formation of the joint metaphase can be clearly seen. Those heterokaryons that have a persistent pronuceleus are exposed to okadaic acid in a buffered saline solution with both bovine serum albumin and cytochalasin D. After exposure to a hypotonic solution the mitotic heterokaryons are fixed. When the cytoplasm is cleared they are then transferred to a slide for evaluation. The chromosome plates can then be assessed with a phase contrast microscope. At this stage FISH techniques can be started (32). The efficiency of this method can be improved to 100% with experience (43). Similar results can be obtained by using bovine ooplasts for fusion with humane blastomeres (44). Blastomere biopsy should be delayed for 3 to 4 days to make sure that the embryo has reached an 8-cell stage.

This method is ideal for evaluation of translocations as well as for an opportunity to look at the entire karyotype. This method may allow for still further enhanced evaluation of the embryo's chromosome constitution beyond that available from multicolor FISH analysis of selected chromosomes. Whether this method will further enhance successful outcomes of women of advanced maternal age needs further study.

SELECTED DISORDERS

Duchenne Muscular Dystrophy

Duchenne muscular dystrophy is a crippling disease that is uniformly fatal. For most patients the molecular defect can be determined, but despite that, there is no efficient treatment to prevent disability and death. Therapeutic strategies point in six different directions. The first is genetic, directed at the mutation in the dystrophin gene itself. Next is biochemical, directed to the absence of dystrophin. The cellular level centers around myofiber necrosis. The factors that lead to necrosis are: (i) susceptibility of the sarcolemma to damage; (ii) sarcolemma disruption; (iii) entry of calcium into the sarcoplasm; (iv) activation of endogenous proteases; and (v) autolysis. At the tissue level there is progressive reduction of myofiber number and size, with fibradipiotic substitution. Therapy is directed to the progressive loss of muscular function. And finally, at the clinical level there is progressive generalized paresis evolving to paralysis, column deformities, and cardiorespiratory insufficiency (45).

Palliative therapies are directed to the last two levels of the process. Corticosteroids are used to slow the progression of the disease and orthopedic surgery alleviates some of the problems associated with scoliosis. The experimental approaches are directed towards all the other levels.

Gene therapy is an attractive approach. Independent of the method chosen to introduce the normal gene, it is important that the method allows for control of production. A recent study in transgenic mice, where over expression of γ-sarcoglylcan occurred, this led to the development of muscular dystrophy and premature death (46).

Instead of introducing a healthy gene to correct the disease, other strategies are directed to gene correction or modulation of transcription translation. The methods for targeted gene correction are chimeroplasty and single-stranded short fragment homology replacement (47,48). The last approach corrected the defect in mouse myoblasts in vitro and myofiber in vivo but with very poor efficiency (49). It is known that deletion of only exon 45 leads to the development of Duchenne muscular dystrophy while deletion of both exons 45 and 46 causes a mild Becker muscular dystrophy. Antisense oligo(ribo) nucleotides can be used to interfere with processing of dystrophin RNA. Using this strategy, cells carrying a 45 exon deletion were transfected in vitro with specific antisense oligo(ribo) nucleotides which was shown to created functional short dystrphin, and was synthesized in over 75% of the myotubules. This approach could be applicable to 65% of all Duchenne muscular dystrophy patients (50). Continuous antisense oligo(ribo) nucleotide administration would be required.

Cell therapy would require the implantation of donor cells into the host. Skeletal muscle has its own stem cells called satellite cells. They are able to both fuse in myofibers and recreate new satellite cells. Myoblast transplantation was shown to produce dystrophin-positive myofibres in dy/dy mice (51). A series of myoblast transplants showed that the interinjection distance was critical to the global success. β-Galactosidase-labeled myoblasts that were injected 1 mm apart produced 25–65% β-galactosidase-positive myofibers, whereas when the interinjection distance was increased to 2 mm the production decreased to 5% to 15%. To make this practical, a tremendous number of stem cells would be required (52,53). Experiments in mice recently demonstrated that donor myoblasts not only fused with host myofibers but also formed quiescent satellite cells that were able to proliferate at a later time (54). Clearly one of the limiting factors that must be considered using this technology will be the chronic need for immune suppression.

As the proliferating potential of satellite cells is jeopardized in advanced muscular dystrophy, autotransplantation of genetically corrected cells would be beneficial. Unfortunately, at this time there are no good candidates identified.

Pharmacological therapy has been disappointing. Corticosteroids are used to slow the progression of myofiber necrosis. Anabolic agents have not had any measurable effect. However, up regulation of utropin has some promise. There is evidence that overexpression of utropin in mdx mice corrects the dystrophic phenotype, and in addition, that overexpression in nonmuscular tissues was not toxic (55).

In spite of all the encouraging progress in research in the area of muscular dystrophy it is clear that a cure is still far into the distant future. For this reason, preimplantation diagnosis is clearly a worthwhile method to avoid the disease. The results of preimplantation diagnosis for this disorder can be seen in Table 3.

Table 3 Results of Preimplantation Diagnosis

Researcher(s)	Number of live births	Year
Verlinsky et al. (56)	21	1994
Griffin et al. (57)	5	1994
Bui et al. (58)	2	1994
Liu et al. (59)	1	1995
Harper (60)	22	1996
Lee et al. (61)	1	1998
Ingerslev et al. (62)	2	2001
Papp et al. (63)	1	2002

Cystic Fibrosis

Cystic fibrosis is the most common lethal autosomal recessive disorder in the Caucasian population. There are 60,000 people worldwide who suffer from this disease. A defect in the cystic fibrosis transmembrane conductance regulator (CFTR) gene is the source of this disease (64). The clinical picture of this disease is quite varied. It may range from male infertility secondary to absence or atrophy of the epididymis, vas deferens, and seminal vesicles to chronic lung disease. Gastrointestinal problems may be apparent in utero or at birth, yet nearly 50% will have almost no problems at all. Chronic lung disease is the most important complication of this disease and the etiology for untimely deaths at a young age despite modern medical intervention.

The classically affected patient will be troubled by pancreatic dysfunction, intestinal problems, infertility, and chronic lung disease. Twenty to fifty percent of affected patients will be spared from pancreatic dysfunction. When pancreatic dysfunction is present, one can expect malabsorption and failure to thrive. Diabetes may become a later manifestation of the disease and may contribute to early death. Intestinal obstructions may occur in utero leading to multiple atresias. One can expect that 10% of newborns with cystic fibrosis will develop meconium ileus. Obstructions and perforations may lead to premature death secondary to those complications.

By far, the most significant clinical finding is a progressive deterioration in lung function, secondary to altered secretions. The secretions make the lungs more susceptible to infections by common bacterial pathogens and those pathogens not common as a cause for community disease. The lungs begin structurally normal at birth, but as a consequence of repeated infections and the abnormally thick mucus, progressive obstructive disease develops.

The classic way to make the diagnosis is the cystic fibrosis sweat test. An area of the skin is stimulated to artificially sweat. This sweat is associated with the secretion of chloride that in turn is then quantified. An abnormal result would be when the chloride concentration exceeds 60 mg/L of sweat and the sodium measures more than 70 mg/L if at least 100 mg of sweat are obtained. Today, this would likely be confirmed with DNA screening.

Specialized clinics devoted to children with cystic fibrosis have improved the longevity for many affected individuals. Although many patients still die in early childhood, about half die by the age of 26, while some may live to 40 or 50 years of age. While there is no specific medication used for cystic fibrosis children, simple aggressive attention to detail, long-term chest physiotherapy, antibiotics and vaccinations have contributed to better results. Intestinal enzymes and increased nutritional intake have all been supportive.

Since 1989, the CFTR gene has been extensively investigated and mapped. To date there are more than 1200 known mutations and sequence variants in the CFTR gene that have been linked to disease (65). The most common mutation of the gene is a deletion of three base pairs that results in the absence of the phenylalanine residue at position 508 of the cystic fibrosis protein (delta-F508). The frequency varies among the Caucasian population. Nearly 90% of carriers in Denmark have the delta-F508 mutation and in Scotland it is 75%, while in Spain and Italy it decreases to 30–49%, and finally in the Jewish population it is only 30%. Because of the wide array of probes routinely used today one may expect that 90% of at risk couples can be identified. With the wide variety of mutations that are identifiable, it is difficult to predict the significance of many of the possible heterozygotic combinations.

The recognition that the majority of cases of cystic fibrosis are the result of a defect in the biogenesis or intracellular trafficking of the protein, and that it retains at least partial function, has stimulated an intense search for therapeutic strategies aimed at rescuing the function of the mutant CFTR. The initial optimism on identifying the delta-F508 allele has been temporized by the finding that the protein is not a simple trafficking mutation, but exhibits multiple defects in folding, stability, and activation. Because the cell surface half-life of delta-F508 is so significantly reduced, it is likely that any treatment that affects folding will greatly enhance a prolongation of cell surface residence (65). There will need to be multiple simultaneous approaches to rescue the defect. Despite all of these obstacles there is reason to expect that pharmacological correction is an achievable goal. The ultimate strategy to achieve this goal will be to attack simultaneously the defects of folding, stability, and activation (65).

Because patients with cystic fibrosis develop lung involvement after birth, CFTR gene replacement during the neonatal period prior to the onset of airway damage would, in theory, significantly decrease morbidity and mortality for cystic fibrosis. An early observation that made gene therapy for cystic fibrosis a potentially achievable goal was the observation that in polarized epithelial sheets, expression of CFTR in as few as 6% to 10% of airway epithelial cells that lacked CFTR restored normal chloride transportation properties (66,67).

Several methods are currently available to transfer genetic information. In transduction, or virus mediated gene transfer, recombinant DNA techniques are used to insert the normal copy of the needed gene into the genetic information of a virus, which then acts as vector for gene transfer. The properties of the viral vector dictate the safety and efficacy of the gene transfer process. Viruses naturally contain the mechanisms that enable cell entry, integration and persistence in human cells (68).

Transfection is another method for transferring genetic material. Transfection can be accomplished in vitro in a wide range of cell types via cationic lipid DNA complexes known as liposomes or lipoplexes. Liposome delivery systems generally have been less efficient for transfer in in vitro gene delivery than viral carriers, but result in fewer inflammatory and immunologic reactions than viral vectors. There are delivery systems that show promise for in vivo gene transfer to the airway by means of tracheal injection, aerosolization, or nasal inoculation (68).

The ideal transfer agent would have the following properties: have that capacity to carry the necessary genetic information and yet go undetected by the immune system; not elicit inflammation; be safe to the human host even in the setting of lung inflammation; be able to deliver sufficient expression to correct the basic cystic fibrosis defect and not have deleterious levels of expression; have a long duration of expression; and finally have the ability to be safely readministered as many times as necessary.

Clinically speaking, the gene transfer in cystic fibrosis patients needs to be done in vivo and in situ. At the present time only a few viral vectors have been clinically studied. To date there have been nine clinical studies testing the safety and efficacy of an adenoviral vector (69–77). In these studies gene transduction was very low, generally below 1% and often associated with an inflammatory response. Dose-limiting toxicity was noted at 10^{11} viral particles (78). There were three clinical trials utilizing liposomes as vectors. Again in these studies there was some response but still less than desirable (79–81). The localized instillation of the liposome/DNA complexes seems to be well tolerated.

Gene therapy seems to have promise, but not until the distant future. Until then, it is clear that the best strategy for this disease is to avoid it. This can most safely be done in couples at risk with preimplantation genetics. To date, there have been many reports on the outcome of patients at risk for cystic fibrosis. This can be seen in Table 4.

Sickle Cell Anemia

Sickle cell anemia is one of the most common autosomal recessive hemoglobinopathies in the world. It is caused by a mutation substituting thymine for adenine in the sixth codon (GAG to GTG) of the gene for the beta-globin chain on chromosome 11p, thereby encoding valine instead of glutamic acid in the sixth position of the globin chain. The frequency of sickle cell trait that is the carrier state among the African-American population at birth is about 8%, and the incidence of sickle cell disease at birth is 0.16%, or 1 per 625 live births (92). There is a widespread presence of this gene in other ethnic groups. In urban centers in the United States, nearly 10% of patients with various sickling disorders identify themselves as non–African-American (93).

With new advances, such as early penicillin prophylaxis, pneumococcal vaccine, better blood transfusion practices, and treatment with hydroxyurea over the last 30 plus years have permitted survival of children with sickle cell disease into young adulthood. Despite this improvement in survival in developed countries, the average age of death for adult patients is 45 years of age (94,95). Children most commonly succumb to pneumococal sepsis while adults generally die from strokes,

Table 4 Outcome of Patients at Risk for Cystic Fibrosis

Researcher(s)	Number of live births	Year
Ray et al. (82)	2	2002
Moutou et al. (83)	2	2001
Goossens et al. (84)	12	2000
Verlinsky et al. (85)	8	1999
Ray et al. (86)	1	1998
Strom et al. (87)	3	1998
Ao et al. (88)	5	1996
Harper (89)	8	1996
Liu et al. (90)	1	1995
Grifo et al. (91)	4 (1 miss DX)	1994

multiorgan failure, acute chest syndrome, and recurrent pain crisis. Allogenic bone marrow transplant is the only known cure for this disease. There are less bone marrow transplants than would be expected for this disease because of several problems (96). The absence of an HLA-identical sibling is the major obstacle for expanding this curative therapy. In one study only 14% of patients had suitably matched HLA siblings to act as donors (97). The high variability of the disease and the progress in therapy has also limited the use of bone marrow stem cells. Furthermore, there are no universally accepted criteria for when to move towards bone marrow transplantation.

In a recent multicenter collaborative trial of 50 patients who underwent bone marrow transplantation, the probability of survival was 94% while the disease-free survival rate was 84% (98). Despite transplantation, 25% of patients developed neurological complications. In a Belgian study, patients who underwent bone marrow transplantation early in the course of their disease before they developed clinical complications had a better overall survival and disease-free survival as well (99).

Unlike in hematological malignancies, where mixed chimerism heralds recurrence of disease, in hemoglobinopathies stable mixed chimerism has the potential of ameliorating the disease. It appears that when stable mixed chimerism is established, even a minority of donor cells is sufficient to overcome an underlying genetic defect (96). Chimerism with HbAA is more efficient in ameliorating disease than HbAS. Donor-cell engraftment of greater than 10% is required when using a HbAA donor in contrast to 30% to 40% when a HbAS donor is used (100). These observations suggest that full-donor chimerism is not necessary to cure nonmalignant disorders, and reduced intensity regimes can induce mixed chimerism to provide an effective control on genetic defect manifestation.

The limited number of sickle cell patients with suitable HLA donors is the reason that other approaches need to be considered. One of these methods is gene therapy. The random integration of retrovirus vectors and genomic rearrangements accompanying adeno-associated viruses are the undesirable consequence of gene transfer mediated by viral vectors. Correction of the beta^S allele to beta^A through gene conversion mechanism would provide a means of gene therapy that circumvents this problem (101). The strategy used by Cole-Strauss et al. was targeted correction. Targeted correction was done with a short, double-stranded oligoneucleotide vector that is activated for recombination by incorporating RNA residues, protecting it from exonucleolytic degeneration by capping both ends. The 2'-O-methyl modification of ribose of the RNA added protection against cleavage ribonuclease (Rnase) H activities.

In this study, they corrected beta^S mutation with a chimeric oligonucleotide (SC1) as a single molecule with two sequences that were inverted and complimentary and capable of folding back on itself to form a duplex structure (101). The chimeric molecule was then introduced into lymphoblastoid cells that were homozygous for the beta^S allele by means of a commercial liposome formulation, and assayed 6 hours later. Using restriction fragment length polymorphisms (RFLPs) two fragments were observed in DNA from cells transfected with the chimeric molecule. The presence of the 1.2-kbp fragment in addition to the 1.4-kbp fragment indicates that the beta $(^S)$ allele was partially corrected in a dose-dependent fashion.

Because the beta-globulin gene is a member of a family of related genes, there was the possibility that one or more of the other globin genes might be inadvertently altered as a consequence of transfection with the chimeric molecule. The most likely candidate for alteration is the delta-globin gene because it is more than 90%

homologous to the beta-globin gene. When the cell was transfected with the chimeric molecule no change was seen in the delta-globin sequence over the region of DNA homology spanned by the chimeric molecule. While no alteration of this gene was found it is still possible that it might cause alteration in another gene. In a minimal screen for the effect on other genes, the reactivity of the hypoxathine-guanine phosphoribosyl-transferase gene was monitored. No effect of the chimeric molecule could be found on this gene. These observations suggest that treatment with a chimeric molocule in a lymphoblastoid cell can induce the desired mutation conversion but is not generally mutagenic within the limits of the aforementioned assay system. It seems that the possibility of random mutagenesis is somewhat reduced. The conversion of the globin gene was not as reliable in other cell types and therefore not ready for serious consideration.

Once again it is clear that the treatment options for most patients with sickle cell disease are still quite limited and that avoidance of the disease is still the most practical consideration. Preimplantation genetics is a valuable consideration for this disease. Xu and colleagues were the first to report preimplantation success with sickle cell disease (102). Their patient underwent two stimulatory cycles before they had a success. They used embryo biopsy and removed two cells for analysis. In their successful cycle, two blastomeres were removed on day three and three embryos were suitable for transfer on day 4. There were two embryos that were homozygous normal and one found to be a carrier. The transfer resulted in a twin pregnancy. Amniocentesis was performed and confirmed that they were both homozygous unaffected. The woman delivered them at 39 weeks of gestation.

Kuliev and colleagues reported the successful preimplantation diagnosis for sickle cell disease and delivery of an unaffected child. Their case was uniquely different from other reported cases typically done by preimplantation diagnosis because they limited the analysis to pre-embryos (103). Two different approaches have typically been used for this disease: cleavage-stage embryo biopsy and polar body sampling, both of which have resulted in live birth of unaffected children (104). In cleavage cell embryo biopsy, unaffected embryos are selected for transfer or frozen. Affected embryos are either discarded or frozen indefinitely. In standard sequential polar body analysis, the first polar body is aspirated and the second polar body is removed after fertilization. The embryos are cultured waiting for the result of the analysis. They are in turn either transferred or frozen if unaffected and discarded or indefinitely frozen if affected.

The destruction or indefinite storage of affected embryos is ethically unacceptable to some couples on ethical or religious grounds. To solve this problem, the authors developed a method to complete the removal of both the first and second polar bodies prior to fusion of the male and female pronucleus, followed by freezing all oocytes in the pronuclear phase. After analysis the unaffected oocytes are unfrozen. The thawed oocytes are cultured to the embryo stage and embryos that are predicted to be unaffected can be transferred. Since zygotes prior to pronuclear fusion are not yet considered embryos and no abnormal oocytes are thawed and cultured, no affected embryos are established, causing this technique to be ethically more acceptable to many couples. In one patient multiplex PCR was used for analysis. Twenty-eight oocytes were aspirated and 14 extruded their first polar body. Following intracytoplasmic sperm injection, the second polar body was extruded in 13 oocytes. Results were available in 12 of the 13 sequential analyses. From this analysis six oocytes were predicted to contain a normal allele. In the next cycle the patient was prepared for a frozen embryo transfer. In the first cycle, four zygotes predicted to have an unaffected allele were thawed. Of the four zygotes thawed three developed into cleavage stage embryos of acceptable quality and were transferred. The transfer resulted in a singleton pregnancy that subsequently aborted.

In the second frozen cycle, two unaffected embryos developed and were transferred. This resulted in a singleton pregnancy. A chorionic villi sampling confirmed that the fetus was unaffected and the patient delivered an unaffected child.

This case demonstrates the feasibility of performing pre-embryonic diagnosis for single gene disorders leading to the birth of an unaffected child. This method could also be applied to mothers who are translocation carriers as an alternative approach. If PCR analysis can be complete before fusion of the two pronucelei then freezing could be eliminated.

HLA Matching and Gene Disorders

Occasionally, we are faced with a family that already has a child with a genetic disorder that may be cured or ameliorated by a bone marrow transplant, but are stymied by the absence of a suitable donor. These families often would like to have another child that would be unaffected with the same disorder. When these two combinations occur we now have a method to test for the genetic disorder and select an embryo that would be a suitable donor for its sibling. With the ability to use cord blood as a source for bone marrow transplantation, the ethical issues become much less since this is a tissue that in ordinary circumstances would be discarded.

The first reported use of this technology to solve these two combined problems was reported by Verlinsky and colleges (105). Single-cell (PCR) presents the opportunity to combine preimplantation genetic diagnosis and HLA antigen testing. HLA antigen testing as a part of preimplantation diagnosis is a reasonable option, because only 2 to 3 of the 10 to 12 embryos resulting from an average hormonal stimulatory cycle in IVF are actually transferred. In this circumstance "blind" selection is changed to transfer only those embryos matching their affected sibling. Fanconi anemia (FA) is an autosomal recessive disorder, characterized by inherited bone marrow failure, congenital malformations, and an increased predisposition to the development of leukemia. It is genetically heterogeneous, involving different complementation groups (FA-A, FA-B, FA-C, FA-D, and FA-E). One of the most severe forms is the FA-C mutation leading to aberrantly spliced transcriptions (IVS4+4 A-T), which results in the inactivating FA compliment C (FANCC) protein. Bone marrow transplantation is the only treatment that definitively restores hematopoiesis in FA patients. Because modification of the conditioning by high-dose chemotherapy and ablative radiation is too toxic for these patients, the HLA antigen–identical cord blood transplantation from a sibling is particularly valuable for FA, especially in avoiding late complications due to severe graft versus host reaction (106,107).

In the study couple, both parents were unaffected carriers of IVS 4+4 A-T mutation in the FANCC gene. Their affected 6-year-old daughter had two copies of this mutation and required an HLA compatible donor for bone marrow transplantation.

Preimplantation genetic diagnosis was performed using a standard IVF protocol combined with micromanipulation procedure to biopsy a single blastomere from 3-day cleavage-stage embryos. Haplotype analysis was performed on the father, mother, and affected child. A hemi-nested PCR system was designed to study the number of short tandem repeats (STRs) in the blastomeres from different embryos.

Unaffected embryos which were HLA antigen compatible with the affected sibling, were transferred back to the patient, while the other unaffected embryos were frozen to be available for future transfer. The follow-up analysis was also performed in the established pregnancy in the last cycle, using chorionic villi sampling during the first trimester. Four cycles were required till a successful pregnancy was achieved. Thirty-three embryos underwent analysis. This resulted in 24 unaffected embryos for transfer with HLA matching of the affected sibling. Only the transfers in the fourth cycle resulted in a clinical pregnancy. In the last cycle one heterozygous embryo and two unaffected embryos, all HLA compatible, were transferred.

A healthy carrier of the FACC gene was born. At the delivery cord blood was collected and transplanted to the affected sibling. The transplantation resulted in successful hematopoietic reconstitution. The affected child remains healthy. It is likely that the success of this case will create a demand for HLA matching for siblings with leukemia that are otherwise free of any other genetic disorders and are in need of a HLA matched donor.

Late Onset Disorders

There are some genetic disorders that express themselves later in life rather than the more common genetic disorders that are expressed shortly after birth. Verlinsky and colleagues reported on the preimplantion diagnosis for the p53 tumor suppressor gene. This is a disorder that manifests itself by the patient developing multiple different malignancies. This was the first late-onset disorder where preimplantation genetic diagnosis was applied (108). Late-onset disorders have never been an indication for prenatal diagnosis because of potential pregnancy termination, which is highly controversial if performed for genetic predisposition alone. With the introduction of preimplantation diagnosis it is possible to transfer embryos that do not have this predisposed potential, thus overcoming ethical dilemmas of having children at such high risk or consideration of abortion of at-risk fetuses.

Early-onset Alzheimer's disease is a rare autosomal dominant familial predisposition to the presenile form of dementia. Three different genes have been identified and they include: presenilin 1 located on chromosome 14, presenilin 2 on chromosome 1, and amyloid precursor protein (APP) on chromosome 21, which is well known for its role in the formation of amyloid deposits found in the characteristic plaques of patients with Alzheimer's disease (109–111). Early-onset dementias that are associated with the APP mutation are nearly 100% penetrant and therefore are potential candidates for predictive testing and a clear choice for preimplantation diagnosis. There are currently 10 mutations described for APP. Mutations in exons 16 and 17 have been reported in families with the earliest onset. The onset of this disease may begin in the mid- to late 30s when exon 17 is affected by the substitution of a single G-to-C that results in a valine to leucine amino acid change at codon 717 (V717L).

Verlinsky and colleagues describe a patient for preimplantation genetic diagnosis that presented at age 30, with no sign of Alzheimer's disease, but a carrier of the V717L mutation (112). The patient was tested because her sister developed symptoms of Alzheimer's disease at age 38 and her father died at age 42 with marked memory problems. Finally, one of her brothers at age 35 had a decline in his memory. The remaining three other siblings were unaffected. Two preimplantation cycles were performed using standard IVF protocols and micromanipulation. Sequential polar body analysis was used and the oocytes were fertilized by intracytoplasmic sperm injection. Multiplex nested PCR was performed that involved the mutation simultaneously with linked polymorphic markers. In the first cycle only eight oocytes were obtained and both embryos were affected and therefore no transfer occurred. In the second cycle more oocytes were available for testing, 13 underwent polar body analysis. From the 13 embryos 7 were affected and 6 were normal. Four of the unaffected embryos developed to the cleavage-stage and all were transferred. A singleton pregnancy developed and was tested by chorionic villi sampling and a mutation free baby was delivered.

INFERTILITY AND PREIMPLANTATION GENETIC DIAGNOSIS

Infertility is generally divided into two subtypes: female associated and male associated. Now that physical barriers such as tubal disease and immobility of sperm can be overcome by IVF, one needs to address other factors that lead to failure. It is generally understood that most fetal chromosome abnormalities that are not inheritable are related to abnormalities within the oocyte.

Questions arise as to the influence of various steps in the IVF process on oocyte chromosome abnormality. The first question is, does the type of sterility lead to oocyte abnormality? In an observation by De Sutter and colleagues, and similarly by Pellestor and Sele, they reported a higher rate of aneuploidy in the oocyte in idiopathic infertility (22.5%); with male infertility the rate was (10.2%) (113,114). This suggests that male factor is not as significant a factor in IVF failure rate.

Does the stimulation protocol influence oocyte aneuploidy? Gras and colleagues determined the incidence of chromosomal aneuploidy in unstimulated uninseminated human oocytes compared to oocytes obtained by two different superovulation protocols. The frequency of aneuploidy in unstimulated oocytes was 20% that was not significantly different from a clomaphene/hMG (35%) and a buserilin-flair (32%) protocol (115). Similarly, a strong response to gonadotropin stimulation had no effect until more than 11 oocytes were recovered (116). These results demonstrate that aneuploidy rate is not affected by ordinary stimulation protocols.

Does in vitro maturation have an effect on aneuploidy? Plachot compared a series of 179 oocytes matured in vivo with 149 oocytes that matured in vitro in an ICSI program. She observed no difference in the diploidy (4%) and aneuploidy (22%) between the two groups (117).

Does the intrafollicular environment influence aneuploidy? Van Blerkom showed that dissolved oxygen in follicular fluid might differ significantly between mature and preovulatory follicules. The oxygen content in follicular fluid generally falls into two ranges, $< 1.5\%$ or 4–6%. In newly retrieved oocytes that were uninseminated, 45% of those with low follicular oxygen content were cytogenetically abnormal. This was compared to those that had high follicular oxygen content: only 7% were cytogenetically abnormal (118). This demonstrates the importance of perifollicular microvasculature expansion and oxygenation during follicular growth and preovulatory maturation. Smoking is well known to reduce fecundity and fertility, and also sets an early menopause. Zenzes and colleagues found no difference in the aneuploidy rate in oocytes from smokers versus nonsmokers, but did find a difference in the diploidy rate that would explain the previously mentioned reduction in women who smoke (119).

Advanced maternal age is the only well-documented risk factor in meiosis I and meiosis II errors, but the biological mechanism has not been well elucidated. Basal FSH levels, which reflect ovarian function increase with age. There appears to be a clear relation to the basal FSH level and chromosome abnormalities. If the basal FSH is <8 the aneulpoidy rate is 37% and when FSH is >10 it rises to 61%. This holds true until the age of 40 when the basal rate loses linear correlation. Verlinsky and colleagues found that oocytes analyzed by FISH in women aged 35 or over using probes specific for 13, 18, and 21 in polar bodies displayed aneuploidy in 40% (120).

It is a logical assumption that selecting those oocytes that are free from aneuploidy and diploidy should result in a superior implantation rate and an increased baby take home rate. To test this hypothesis, Gianaroli and colleagues offered preimplantation embryo screening to 189 women who underwent 262 IVF cycles in a nonrandomized study. Inclusion criteria were women age 36 or over ($n = 157$ cycles), previous IVF patients that had at least three previous failed IVF cycles ($n = 57$) or an altered karyotype detected in peripheral blood ($n = 51$ cycles). Preimplantation genetic diagnosis for aneuploidy screening was performed in 127 cycles, accounting for approximately half the cases in each inclusion category. Assisted hatching was performed in all cycles in which patients declined preimplantation genetic diagnosis. A doubling of the implantation rates (24% vs. 12%, $p < 0.001$) was achieved with the preimplantation genetic diagnosis group, independent of the inclusion category, and this effect was particularly pronounced in women older than 37 years of age (121). In personal communication with Verlinsky and colleagues similar results were found using polar body analysis in place of embryo biopsy. In addition, the mean number of embryos transferred was significantly reduced from 3.2 to 2.3. Moreover, although preimplantation reduced the number of cycles where embryos were transferred (78% vs. 93%), clinical pregnancy rates per cycle started were unchanged. In personal experiences at Reproductive Genetic Institute, we also had a similar experience using sequential polar body analysis and nearly identical results and additionally reduced the number of high order pregnancies as well. These results need to be reproduced in a prospective randomized study that has yet to be done.

Pregnancy Outcome After Preimplantation Genetic Diagnosis

It is clear that preimplantation genetic diagnosis now has a place in the management of infertile couples as well as those at high risk for a gene or chromosome disorder. It is important to look at the pregnancy outcome to verify that it is indeed safe for both the mother and the child and that it is acceptably reliable. At the present time there are two methods used to achieve the same end, cleavage-stage embryo biopsy and sequential polar body biopsy. There are two good reports on the outcome. The ESHRE PGD Consortium Steering Committee report their results and the diagnoses have exclusively been made from cleavage-stage embryos (122). The study by Strom and colleagues reports on a single center experience that exclusively used sequential polar body analysis (123).

The ESHRE committee reports a cumulative experience where data was collected in greater detail over the years. The total number of pregnancies was 451 (pregnancy sacs), 25 of which were subclinical, which was defined as a positive HCG only. Of 309 clinical pregnancies (426 sacs) 212 were singletons or 68.6%, 78 were twins or 25.2%, 18 were triplets or 5.8%, and 1 quadruplet or 0.3%.

First trimester loss occurred in 47 of the 426 or 11%. Vanishing twin or triplet was seen in 20 cases reducing the total number of fetuses to 359 that were equal to or greater than 12 weeks of gestation (266 pregnancies).

A pregnancy loss occurred in 10 of 266 pregnancies or 14 of 359 fetuses. Of the 14 fetuses, three underwent termination of pregnancy for misdiagnosis (four fetuses had the wrong sex) and one after an amniocentesis where the fetus had trisomy 18, but the preimplantation diagnosis was done for a parent carrier of reciprocal translocation not involving chromosome 18. There were three spontaneous losses of five fetuses during the second trimester, stillbirth occurred in two, and premature rupture of membranes in one pregnancy affected two fetuses.

Nine fetuses were reduced from multifetal pregnancies, three from triplets to twins, four from triplets to singletons, and two from quadruplets to twins. There were no losses in the pregnancies that underwent multifetal reduction.

From 309 pregnancies that included 336 fetuses a normal evaluation was found in 256 of the 309 pregnancies. Of the 256 normal evaluations 184 were singletons, 64 or 128 fetuses were in a twin gestation and 8 or 24 fetuses were in a triplet gestation. At the time of this report 215 pregnancies delivered 279 babies with 32 pregnancies and 43 fetuses still ongoing.

The mode of delivery and the prematurity rate can be seen in Table 5. Forty-four percent were delivered by cesarean; at least 17% were premature.

There was only complete information of pregnancy complications on 157 of the 215 deliveries. The absence of complete information on 27% of the pregnancies is the weakest part of the study. Despite this it is important to review the associated problems. Fifty-two of 157 pregnancies had some complication of their pregnancy. Complications occurred in 33 of 112 singletons, 16 of 45 twins, and 3 of 3 triplets. Intrauterine growth restriction occurred in only two singletons. It is likely that this problem is under reported. Hypertension occurred in six pregnancies, half divided between singletons and twins. HELLP syndrome was seen in two singletons, preeclampsia was present in four patients, one twin and three singletons. There was one case of eclampsia in a twin pregnancy. One patient had cervical insufficiency and one had a cervical cerclage, both in singleton pregnancies. The remaining complications are listed in Table 6.

From the 279 babies born, 99 had no information about malformations or complications in the neonatal period. From 180 pregnancies there were

Table 5 Mode of Delivery and Prematurity Rate

	Total	Singleton	Twins	Triplets
Number delivered	215	156	54	5
Vaginal	101	88	13	0
Cesarean	95	57	33	5
Unknown	19	11	8	0
Gestational age at delivery				
Preterm[a]	37	10	24	3
At term	163	140	21	2
Unknown	15	6	9	0

[a]Preterm was defined as less than 36 weeks.

Table 6 Pregnancy Complications

Nature of complication	Singleton	Twin	Triplet
Polyhydramnios	0	1	0
Oligohydramnios	2	0	0
Preterm contraction	7	9	3
Bleeding	8	3	0
Chorioamnionitis	1	0	0
Septic abortion	0	1	0
Placenta accreta	1	0	0
Retroplacental hematoma	1	0	0
Premature RBOW	1	5	0
Diabetes	3	0	0
Idiopathic thrombocytopenia	1	0	0
Toxoplasmosis	1	0	0

12 malformations of which 7 were categorized as major and 5 were considered to be minor. These malformations are given in Table 7.

Neonatal complications include 67 premature deliveries. Ten had complications of prematurity, two required artificial ventilation, one had persistent ductus arteriosis, one died from intracranial bleeding, one had a pneumothorax, and the remainder were minor.

When one looks at confirmation of the diagnosis only 50% of fetuses had prenatal confirmation. There were seven patients that had discordant results in the fetuses tested. When postnatal confirmation was done six more patients were found to have discordant results, five were chromosomal in karyotyped spontaneous losses and one trisomy 21 was born and found in a patient that underwent aneuploidy screening. From these data, one can compute a misdiagnosis rate of 1.8% (8/451). This was highest in the PCR group (5/145 or 3.4%) compared to the FISH group (3/305 or 0.9%).

Table 7 Malformations in the Neonatal Period

	Number
Major malformations	
Phocomelia and pulmonary deficiency	1 from a triplet gestation
Chylothorax, neonatal death	1
Congenital hip dislocation	1
Cystic mass in abdomen	1
Pes equinovarus	2
Exencephaly, neonatal death	1 from a twin gestation
Minor malformations	
Syndactyly, mother also	1
Hydrocele testis	1
Atrial septal defect	1
Mongolian spot	1
Sacral dimple	1

Table 8 Evaluation for Mendelian Disorders

Mendelian disorder	Number
Cystic fibrosis	11
Sickle cell disease	1
Long-chain acyl coenzyme A dehydrogenase deficiency	1
Beta thalassemia	5

Strom and colleagues report on the obstetrical outcome of 102 pregnancies that resulted in the birth of 114 newborns (123). In contrast to the report from the ESCHRE consortium all the patients in this group underwent their preimplantation diagnosis by sequential polar body analysis. Ninety-six babies were born after preimplantation diagnosis for chromosome disorders and 18 were evaluated for mendelian disorders (Table 8). Follow-up was available in 102 of the 114 patients for a 2% loss of follow-up rate.

The distribution of pregnancies can be seen in Table 9. As can be seen from these data, 16.6% of patients had multiple gestations and three patients chose to undergo a multifetal pregnancy reduction. Multiple gestations and particularly high-order multiple gestation is an unfortunate complication of IVF in general, but was substantially less than was seen in the ESCHRE report where the incidence was 31.4%. This difference was significant at $p = 0.005$. This difference may be explained by the difference in the proportion of patients who were tested for aneuploidy verses those tested for mendelian gene disorders. The remaining four triplets delivered between 32 and 36 weeks of gestation, none required oxygen for more than 2 hours and all were home within 1 week of delivery.

All the patients who had preimplantation genetic diagnosis for mendelian disorders had a postnatal follow-up and the predicted maternal allele was uniformly found. Additionally, those babies born after aneuploidy screenings similarly were all normal and no case of trisomy 13, 18, or 21 was found.

The cesarean rate for term singletons was 40% similar to the 37% found by the ESCHRE consortium. There are ample reports in the literature where these numbers are commonly found in patients that undergo IVF, yet there is no good explanation as to why they are so much higher than would be ordinarily expected (124,125). The indications for cesarean section can be found in Table 10.

Complications are listed in Table 11. There seems to be a similar outcome as in the ESHRE consortium report. There is no pattern of complications that is seen in preimplantation genetic diagnosis that is different from the typical IVF patient.

Table 9 Distribution of Multifetal Pregnancies

Number of fetuses	Number of pregnancies	Spontaneous abortions	Live births
1	85	4	80
2	9	1	16
3	7	0	18[a]
5	1	1	0
Total	102	7	114

[a]Three couples had multifetal pregnancy reduction to twins and four couples delivered triplets.

Table 10 Indications for Cesarean and Numbers

Singleton gestation	30
Failure to progress	7
Previous uterine scar (elective)	4
Fetal distress	4
Placenta previa (1 complete, 3 partial)	4
Failed forceps	2
Breech presentation	2
Failed vacuum	1
Abrutio placenta	1
Prolong premature ruptured membranes with failed induction	1
Postdate pregnancy with failed induction	1
HELLP syndrome	1
Extreme prematurity with poor labor pattern	1
Bicornuate uterus low placenta	1
Twin gestations	5
Malpresentation of one twin	3
Fetal distress	1
Prematurity	1
Triplet gestation	3
Elective	3

Table 11 Complications in Polar Body PGD Patients

Complication	Number
Gestational diabetes	3
Intrauterine growth restriction	3
Pregnancy-induced hypertension	3
Placenta previa	4
HELLP syndrome	1
Congestive heart failure	1
Abrutio placentea	1
Mild oligohydramnios	1

Note: All the complications listed occurred in singleton gestations.
Abbreviation: PGD, preimplantation diagnosis.

There was one neonatal death in a singleton gestation secondary to a severe abruption of the placenta. The neonate was born with multiorgan failure and quickly expired.

FUTURE CONSIDERATIONS

The promise of this technology opens up the possibility of using preimplantation genetics in nontraditional ways. One avenue of exploration will be the use of HLA matching to treat siblings with disorders requiring transplantation where there is no other alternative. The most likely use will be with children afflicted with leukemia who will ultimately require bone marrow transplantation. This issue was recently addressed by Verlinsky and colleagues (126) where preimplantation HLA matching was done to create identical matches for nine couples in the United States and one in the United Kingdom. The diseases that they addressed were acute lymphoid leukemia, acute myeloid leukemia, and Diamond–Blackfan anemia. Treating the affected children with cord blood transplantation could cure all these diseases.

Six of the 10 couples were able to reach their desired outcome. Their data showed that HLA matching with selected embryos for transfer was possible in all but one cycle. Pregnancies and birth of a HLA matched child resulted in 42% of the transferred cycles which is as good, or better than, what one might expect for IVF procedures for other indications (127). HLA typing by preimplantation genetic diagnosis is a method to avoid a highly controversial issue of cloning (128,129).

Haploidization is a technique of transforming a somatic cell to a haploid cell. It has been shown that ooplasm from a GV-stage oocyte is able to initiate a meiosis-like reduction division in mitotic nuclei originating either from germ cell lines or from differentiated somatic cells (130,131). While this process is similar to cloning, the major difference is that the resulting haploid oocyte will require the contribution of the paternal gamete to produce biparental progeny. There are still many unanswered questions associated with this technology. They include aspects of imprinting, shorter telomere length (associated with decreased lifespan) and the introduction of new mitochondria, just to mention a few. Despite all of these problems it does seem to hold promise for reproduction in couples that no longer have viable gametes.

CONCLUSION

Early prenatal diagnosis and the human genome project have improved our understanding of genetic disorders at a tremendous pace. Certainly we are on the verge of remarkable cures for many diseases. However, from a practical viewpoint, fulfillment of this promise is still well in the future.

At the present we are still limited to early diagnosis and termination when an abnormal is found. Since correction is generally not yet an option the most realistic way of complete avoidance is either to forgo reproduction or turn to preimplantation genetics. The human genome project has made it possible to apply this method to an ever-expanding number of disorders. It is anticipated that this relatively new approach will become increasingly more routine in the years to come.

REFERENCES

1. Kaback M, Lim-Steele J, Johnson D, Brown D, Levy N, Zeiger K. The control of Tay-Sach's disease (TSD): a one generation assessment. Proceedings of the 8th International Congress of Human Genetics. Am J Hum Genet 1991; (Suppl) 49, 4:42.
2. Jacobson CB, Barter RH. Intrauterine diagnosis and management of genetic defects. Am J Obstet Gynecol 1967; 99:796–807.
3. The NICHD National Registry for Amniocentesis Study Group. Midtrimester amniocentesis for prenatal diagnosis. J Am Med Assoc 1976; 236:1471–1476.
4. Hahnemann N. Early prenatal diagnosis: a study of biopsy techniques and cell culturing from extraembryonic membranes. Clin Genet 1974; 6:294–306.
5. Kazy Z, Bakharev VA, Stygar AM. Value of the ultrasonic studies in biopsy of the chorion, according to genetic indicators. Akush Ginekol (Mosk) 1979; 8:29–31.

6. Old JM, Ward RTH, Karagozlu F, Petrou M, Modell B, Weatherall DJ. First-trimesterfetal diagnosis for haemoglobinopathies; three cases. Lancet 1982; 2(8313): 1414–1416.

7. Brambati B, Simoni G. Fetal diagnosis of trisomy 21 in the first trimester of pregnancy. Lancet 1983; 1(8324):586.

8. Ginsberg NA, Pergament E, Verlinsky Y. Medical news. J Am Med Assoc 1983; 250:1249–1250.

9. Handyside AH, Koutogianni EH, Hardy K, Winston RM. Pregnancies from biopsied human preimplantation embryos sexed by Y-specific DNA amplification. Nature 1990; 344:768–770.

10. Brambati B, and Tului L. Preimplantation genetic diagnosis: a new simple uterine washing system. Hum Reprod 1990; 5:448–450.

11. Dellenbach P, Nisand I, Moreau L, et al. Transvaginal sonographically controlled ovarian follicle puncture for egg retrieval. Lancet 1984; 1:1467.

12. Feichtinger W, Kemeter P. Transvaginal sector scan sonography for needle guided transvaginal follicle aspiration and other applications in gynecologic routine and research. Fertil Steril 1986; 45:722–725.

13. Beerendonk CC, van Dop PA, Braat DD, Merkus JM. Ovarian hyperstimulation: facts and fallacies. Obstet Gynecol Surv 1998; 53:439–449.

14. Al-Shawaf T, Grudzenskas JG. Prevention and treatment of ovarian hyperstimulation syndrome. Best Pract Clin Res Clin Obstet Gnecol 2003; 17:249–261.

15. Azem F, Wolf Y, Botchan A, Amit A, Lessing JB, Kluger Y. Massive retroperitoneal bleeding: a complication of transvaginal-guided oocyte retrieval for in vitro fertilization-embryo transfer. Fertil Streil 2000; 74:405–406.

16. Askenazi J, Farhi J, Dicker D, Feldberg D, Shalev J, Ben-Rafael J. Acute pelvic inflammatory disease after oocyte retrieval: adverse effects on the result of implantation. Fertil Steril 1994; 61:526–528.

17. Doyle M, DeCherney A, Diamond M. Epidemiology and etiology of ectopic pregnancy. Obstet Gynecol Clin North Am 1991; 18:1–17.

18. Elias S, LeBeau M, Simpson JL, Maryian AO. Chromosomal analysis of ectopic human conceptuses. Am J Obstet Gynecol 1981; 141:698–703.

19. Edwards RG, Purdy JM, Steptoe PC, Walters DE. The growth of the human preimplantation embryo in vitro. Am J Obstet Gynecol 1981; 141:408 416.

20. Sundstrom P, Nilsson O, Liedholm P. Cleavage rate and the morphology of early human embryos obtained after artificial fertilization and culture. Acta Obstet Gynecol Scand 1981; 60:109–120.

21. Bolton VN, Hawes SM, Taylor TC, Parsons JH. Development of spare embryos in vitro: an analysis of the correlations among gross morphology, cleavage rates and the development to the blastocyst. J In Vitro Fertil Embryo Transf 1989; 6:30–35.

22. Verlinsky Y, Kuliev AM. Preimplantation Diagnosis of Genetic Diseases: A New Technique in Assisted Reproduction. New York: Wiley-Liss, 1993.

23. Pomp D, Medrano JF. Organic solvents as facilitators of polymerase chain reaction. Biotechniques 1991; 10:58–59.

24. Faloona F, Weiss S, Ferre F, Mulliis K. "PCR." Paper presented at the Sixth International Conference on AIDS, June 20–24, San Francisco, CA, 1990.

25. Rodriquez S, Visedo G, Zapata C. Detection of errors in denucleotide repeat typing by denaturing electrophoresis. Electrophoresis 2001; 13:2656–2664.

26. Findlay I, Matthews P, Quirke P. Multiple genetic diagnosis from single cells using multiplex PCR: reliability and allele dropout. Prenat Diagn 1998; 18:1413–1421.

27. Wells D, Sherlock JK. Strategies for preimplantation genetic diagnosis of single gene disorders by DNA amplification. Prenat Diagn 1998; 18:1389–1401.

28. Munne S, Weier HU, Grifo J, Cohen J. Chromosome mosaicism in human embryos. Biol Reprod 1994; 51:373–379.

29. Thornhill AR, McGath JA, Eady RAJ, Braude PR, Handyside AH. A comparison of different lysis buffers to asses allele dropout from single cells for preimplantation genetic diagnosis. Prenat Diagn 2001; 21:490–497.

30. Ao A, Wells D, Handyside AH, Winston RM, Delhanty JD. Preimplantation genetic diagnosis of inherited cancer: familial adenomatous polyposis coli. J Assist Reprod Genet 1998; 15:140–144.

31. Rechitsky S, Strom C, Verlinsky O, et al. Allele dropout in polar bodies and blasto-meres. J Assist Reprod Genet 1998; 15:253–257.

32. Verlinsky Y, Kuliev A. An Atlas of Preimplantation Genetic Diagnosis. New York: Parthenon, 2000.

33. Wilcox AJ, Weinberg CR, O'Coonor JF, et al. Incidence of early loss of pregnancy. N Engl J Med 1988; 319:189–194.

34. Plachot M. Chromosome analysis of spontaneous abortions after IVF: a European survey. Hum Reprod 1989; 5:425–429.

35. Munne S, Grifo J, Cohen J, Weir HUB. Chromosome abnormalities in human arrested preimplantation embryos: a multi-probe FISH study. Am J Hum Genet 1994; 55:150–159.

36. Munne S, Sulta KM, Weier HU, Grifo JA, Cohen J, Rosenwaks Z. Assessment of numeric abnormalities of X, Y, 18 and 16 chromosomes in preimplantation human embryos before transfer. Am J Obstet Gynecol 1995; 172:1191–1201.

37. Pellestor F, Dufour MC, Arnal F, Humaeu C. Direct assessment of the rate of chromo-some abnormalities in grade IV human embryos produced by in-vitro fertilization procedure. Hum Reprod 1994; 9:293–302.

38. Plachot M, Junca AM, Mandelbaum J, de Grouchi J, Salat-Baroux J, Cohen J. Chro-mosome investigations in early life: human preimplantation embryos. Hum Reprod 1987; 2:29–35.

39. Bongso A, Fong CH, Ng SC, Ratman S, Lim J. Preimplantation genetics: chromosomes of the fragmented human embryos. Fertil Steril 1991; 56:66–70.

40. Benkhalifa M, Janny L, Vye P, Malet P, Bloucher D, Menezo Y. Assessment of ploidy in human morulae and blastocysts using co-culture and florescent in-situ hybridization. Hum Reprod 1993; 8:895–902.

41. Verlinsky Y, Dozortsev D, Evsikov S. Visualization and cytogenetic analysis of second polar body chromosomes following its fusion with a one-cell mouse embryo. J Assist Reprod Genet 1994; 11:123–131.

42. Evsikov S, Verlinsky Y. Visualization of chromosomes in single human blastomeres. J Assist Reprod Genet 1999; 16:133–137.

43. Verlinsky Y, Evsikov S. A simplified and efficient method for obtaining metaphase chromosomes from individual human blastomeres. Fertil Steril 1999; 72:1–6.

44. Willadsen S, Levron J, Munne S, et al. Rapid visualization of metephase chromosomes in single human blastomeres after fusion with in-vitro mature bovine eggs. Hum Reprod 1999; 14:470–474.

45. Skuk D, Vilquin JT, Tremblay JP. Experimental and therapeutic approaches to muscu-lar dystrophies. Curr Opin Neurol 2002; 15:563–569.

46. Zhu X, Hadhazy M, Grom ME, Wheeler MT, Wollman R, Mc Nally EM. Over expres-sion of gamma-sarcoglycan induces severe muscular dystrophy. Implications for the regulation of sarcoglycan assembly. J Biol Chem 2001; 276:21785–21790.

47. Yoon K, Cole-Strauss A, Kmiec EB. Targeted gene correction of episomal DNA in mammalian cells mediated by a chimeric RNA, DNA oligonucleotide. Proc Natl Acad Sci USA 1996; 93:2071–2076.

48. Kunzelmann K, Legendre JY, Knoell DL, Escobar LC, Xu Z, Gruenert DC. Gene targeting of CFTR DNA in CF epithelial cells. Gene Ther 1996; 3:859–867.

49. Kapsa R, Quigley A, Lynch GS, et al. In-vivo and in-vitro correction of the mdx dystrophin gene nonsense mutation by short-fragment homologous replacement. Hum Gene Ther 2001; 12: 629–642.

50. VanDeutekom JC, Bremmer-Bout M, Janson AA, et al. Antisense-induced exon skipping restores dystrophin expression in DMD patient derived muscle cells. Hum Mol Genet 2001; 10:1547–1554.
51. Leriche-Guerin K, Anderson LV, Roy B, Goulet M, Tramblay JP, Wrogemann K. Dysferlin expression after normal myoblast transplantation in SCID and SJL mice. Neuromusc Disord 2002; 12:167–173.
52. Skuk D, Tremblay JP. Engineering myoblast transplantation. Graft 2001; 4:558–570.
53. Skuk D, Goulet M, Roy B, Tremblay JP. Efficiency of myoblast transplantation in nonhuman primates following simple intramuscular cell injections: toward defining strategies applicable to humans. Exp Neurol 2002; 175:112–126.
54. Heslop L, Beauschamp JR, Tajbakhsh S, Buchingham ME, Partidge TA, Zammet PS. Transplanted primary neonatal myoblasts can give rise to functional cells as identified using the Myf5(nlacZl+) mouse. Gene Ther 2001; 8:778–783.
55. Fisher R, Tinsly JM, Phelps SR, et al. Non-toxic ubiquitous over-expression of utropin in the mdx mouse. Neuromusc Disord 2001; 11:713–721.
56. Verlinsky Y, Handyside A, Grifo J, et al. Preimplantation diagnosis of genetic and chromosome disorders. J Assist Reprod Genet 1994; 11:236–243.
57. Griffin DK, Handyside AH, Harper JC, et al. Clinical experience with preimplantation diagnosis of sex by dual fluorescent in situ hybridization. J Assist Reprod Genet 1994; 11:132–143.
58. Bui TH, Anvret M, Dahl N, Garoff L, Sjoblom P, Hillensjo T. Complex genetic counseling and exclusion of Duchenne muscular dystrophy in a twin pregnancy after in vitro fertilization. J Assist Reprod &Genet 1994; 11:144–148.
59. Lui J, Lissen W, Van Broeckhoven C, et al. Normal pregnancy after preimplantation DNA diagnosis of a dystrophin gene deletion. Prenat Diagn 1995; 15:351–358.
60. Harper JC. Preimplantation diagnosis of inherited disease by embryo biopsy: an update of the world figures. J Assist Reprod &Genet 1996; 13:90–95.
61. Lee SH, Kwak IP, Cha KE, Park SE, Kim NK, Cha KY. Preimplantation diagnosis of non-deletion Duchenne muscular dystrophy by linkage polymerase chain reaction analysis. Mol Hum Reprod 1998; 4:345–349.
62. Ingerslev HJ, Hindkjaer J, Jespersgaard C, Lind MP, Kolvraa S. Preimplantation genetic diagnosis. The first experience in Denmark. Ugeskr Laeger 2001; 163:5525–5528.
63. Papp Z, Fancsovits P, Ban Z, To the GZ Urbancsck J. First case of successful pregnancy after preimplantation genetic diagnosis. Orvosi Hetilap 2002; 143:2281–2883.
64. Riorddan JM, Rommens JM, Kerem B, et al. Identification of the cystic fibrosis gene: cloning and characterization of complimentary DNA. Science 1989; 245:1066–1073.
65. Gelman MS, Kopito RR. Rescuing protein confirmation: prospects for pharmacological therapy in cystic fibrosis. J Clin Invest 2002; 110:1591–1597.
66. Johnson LG, Olsen JC, Sarkadi B, Moore KL, Swanstrom R, Boucher RC. Efficiency of gene transfer for restoration of normal airway epithelial function in cystic fibrosis. Nat Genet 1992; 2:21–25.
67. Johnson LG, Boyles SE, Wilson J, Boucher RC. Normalization of raised sodium absorption and raised calcium-mediated chloride secretion by adenovirus-mediated expression of cystic fibrosis transmembrane conductance regulator in primary human cystic fibrosis airway epithelial cells. J Clin Invest 1995; 95:1377–1382.
68. Flotte TR, Laube BL. Gene therapy in cystic fibrosis. Chest 2001; 1120:124S–131S.
69. Zabner J, Couture LA, Gregory RJ, Graham SM, Smith AE, Welsh MJ. Adenovirus-mediated gene transfer transiently corrects the chloride transport defect in nasal epithelia of patient with cystic fibrosis. Cell 1993; 75:207–216.
70. Crystal RG, McElvaney NG, Rosenfeld MA, et al. Administration of an adenovirus containing the human CFTR cDNA to the respiratory tract of individuals with cystic fibrosis. Nat Genet 1994; 8:42–51.
71. Hay JG, McElvaney NG, Herena J, Crystal RG. Modification of nasal epithelial potential differences of individuala with cystic fibrosis consequent to local administration

of a normal CFTR cDNA adenovirus gene transfer vector. Hum Gene Ther 1995; 6:1487–1496.

72. Knowles MR, Hohneler KW, Zhou Z, et al. A controlled study of adenovirus-vector-mediated gene transfer in the nasal epithelium of patients with cystic fibrosis. N Engl J Med 1995; 333:823–831.

73. Zabner J, Ramsey BW, Meeker DP, et al. Repeat administration of an adenovirus vector encoding cystic fibrosis transmembrane conductance regulator to the nasal epithelium of patient with cystic fibrosis. J Clin Invest 1996; 97:1504–1511.

74. Bellon G, Michel-Calemard L, Thouvenot D, et al. Aerosol administration of a recombinant adenovirus expressing CFTR to cystic fibrosis patients: a phase I clinical trial. Hum Gene Ther 1997; 8:15–25.

75. Zuckerman JB, Robinson CB, McCoy KS, et al. A phase I study of adenovirus-mediated transfer of the human cystic fibrosis transmembrane conductance regulator gene to a lung segment of individuals with cystic fibrosis. Hum Gene Ther 1999; 10:2973–2985.

76. Wagner JA, Moran ML, Messner AH, et al. A phase I/II study of tgAAV-CF for the treatment of the chronic sinusitis in patients with cystic fibrosis. Hum Gene Ther 1998; 9:889–909.

77. Wagner JA, Reynolds T, Moran ML, et al. Efficiency and persistent gene transfer of AAV-CFTR in the maxillary sinus. Lancet 1998; 351:1702–1703.

78. Albelda SM, Wiewrodt R, Zuckerman JB. Gene therapy for lung disease: hype or hope. Ann Intern Med 2000; 132:649–660.

79. Caplen NJ, AltonEW, Middleton PG, et al. Liposome-mediated CFTR gene transfer to the nasal epithelium of patients with cystic fibrosis. Nat Med 1995; 1:39–46.

80. Gill DR, Southern KW, Mofford KA, et al. A placebo-controlled study of liposome-mediated gene transfer to the nasal epithelium of patients with cystic fibrosis. Gene Ther 1997; 4:199–209.

81. Porteous DJ, Dorin JR, McLachlan G, et al. Evidence for safety and efficacy of DOTAP cationic liposome mediated CFTR gene transfer to the nasal epithelium of patients with cystic fibrosis. Gene Ther 1997; 4:210–218.

82. Ray PF, Frydman N, Attic T, et al. Birth of healthy and female twins after preimplantation genetic diagnosis of cystic fibrosis combined with gender determination. Mol Hum Reprod 2002; 8:688–694.

83. Moutou C, Ohl J, Wittemer C, Nisand I, Gerlinger P, Viville S. Twin birth after preimplantation diagnosis for cystic fibrosis. Gynecol Obstet Fertil 2001; 10:668–672.

84. Goossens V, Sermon K, Lissens W, et al. Clinical application of preimplantation genetic diagnosis for cystic fibrosis. Prenat Diagn 2000; 20:571–581.

85. Verlinsky Y, Rechisky S, Verlinsky O, et al. Prepregnancy testing for single-gene disorders by polar body analysis. Genet Test 1999; 3:185–190.

86. Ray PF, Ao A, Taylor DM, Winston RM, Handyside AH. Assessment of the reliability of single blastomere analysis for preimplantation diagnosis of the delta F508 deletion causing cystic fibrosis in clinical practice. Prenat Diagn 1998; 18:1402–1412.

87. Strom CM, Ginsberg N, Rechitsky S, et al. Three births after preimplantation genetic diagnosis for cystic fibrosis with sequential first and second polar body analysis. Am J Obstet Gynecol 1998; 178:1298–1306.

88. Ao A, Handyside A, Winston RM. Preimplantation genetic diagnosis of cystic fibrosis (delta F508). Eur J Obstet Gynecol Reprod Biol 1996; 65:7–10.

89. Harper JC. Preimplantation diagnosis of inherited diseases by embryo biopsy: an update of the world figures. J Assist Reprod Genet 1996; 13:90–95.

90. Liu J, Lissens W, Silber SJ, Devroey P, Liebaers I, Van Steirtegham A. Birth after preimplantation diagnosis of the cystic fibrosis delta F508 mutation by polymerase chain reaction in human embryos resulting from intracytoplasmic sperm injection with epididiymal sperm. J Am Med Assoc 1995; 274:126–127.

91. Grifo JA, Tang YX, Munne S, Alikani M, Cohen J, Rosenwaks Z. Healthy deliveries from biopsied human embryos. Hum Reprod 1994; 9:912–916.

92. Motulsky AG. Frequency of sickle cell disorders in US blacks. N Engl J Med 1973; 288:31–33.
93. Powars DR. Sickle cell disease in nonblack persons. J Am Med Assoc 1994; 271:1885.
94. Platt OS, Brambilla DJ, Rosse WF, et al. Mortality in sickle cell disease: life expectancy and risk factors for early death. N Engl J Med 1994; 330:1639–1644.
95. Serjeant GR. Natural history and determinants of clinical severity of sickle cell disease. Curr Opin Hematol 1995; 2:103–108.
96. Gaziev J, Lucarelli G. Stem cell transplantation for hemoglobinopathies. Curr Opin Pediatr 2003; 15:24–31.
97. Walters MC, Patience M, Leisenring W, et al. Barriers to bone marrow transplantation for sickle cell anemia. Biol Blood Marrow Transplant 1996; 2:100–104.
98. Walters MC, Strob R, Patience M, et al. Impact of bone marrow transplantation for symptomatic sickle cell disease: an interim report. Blood 2000; 95:1918–1924.
99. Vermylen C, Cornu G, Ferster A, et al. Hematopoietic stem cell transplantation for sickle cell disease: the first 50 patients transplanted in Belgium. Bone Marrow Transplant 1998; 22:1–6.
100. Woodard P, Cunningham MJ. Remeasurement of chimerism after hematopoietic stem cell transplantation. Biol Blood Marrow Transplant 2002; 8:170.
101. Cole-Strauss A, Yoon K, Xiang Y, et al. Correction of the mutation responsible for sickle cell anemia by an RNA–DNA oligonucleotide. Science 1996; 273:1386–1389.
102. Xu K, Shi ZM, Veeck LL, Hughes MR, Rosenwaks Z. First unaffected pregnancy using preimplantation genetic diagnosis for sickle cell anemia. J Am Med Assoc 1999; 281:1701–1706.
103. Kuliev A, Rechitsky S, Verlinsky O, Strom C, Verlinsky Y. Preembryonic diagnosis for sickle cell diagnosis. Mol Cell Endocrinol 2001; 183:s19–s22.
104. International Working Group on Preimplantation Genetics, 1998. Preimplantation diagnosis: an alternative to prenatal diagnosis of genetic and chromosomal disorders. Report of the 8th Annual Meeting in Association with International Conference on Prenatal Diagnosis and Therapy, Los Angles. J Assist Reprod Genet 1998; 16:161–164.
105. Verlinsky Y, Rechitsky S, Schoolcraft W, Strom C, Kuliev A. Preimplantation diagnosis for Fanconi anemia combined with HLA matching. J Am Med Assoc 2001; 285:3130–3133.
106. Gluckman E, Devergie A, Schaison G, et al. Bone marrow transplantation for Fanconi anemia. Br J Haematol 1980; 45:557–564.
107. Wagner JE, Davies SM, Auerbach AD. Hematopoietic stem cell transplantation in the treatment of Fanconi anemia. In: Forman SJ, Blum KG, Thomas ED, eds. Hematopoietic Cell Transplantation. 2nd ed. Maldin, MA: Blackwell Science Inc, 1999:1204–1219.
108. Verlinsky Y, Rechisky S, Verlinsky O. Preimplantation diagnosis for p53 tumor suppressor gene mutations. Reprod Biomed Online 2001; 3:49–53.
109. Sherington R, Rogaev EI, Liang Y, et al. Cloning of the gene bearing missense mutations in early onset familial Alzheimer disease. Nature 1995; 375:754–760.
110. Levy-Lehad E, Wasco W, Poorkaj P. Candidate gene for the chromosome 1 familial Alzheimer's disease locus. Science 1995; 269:973–977.
111. Goate AM, Chanrier-Harlin MC, Mullan M, et al. Segregation of missense mutation in the amyloid precursor protein gene with familial Alzheimer disease. Nature 1991; 349:704–706.
112. Verlinsky Y, Rechitsky S, Verlinsky O, Masciangelo C, Lederer K, Kuliev A. Preimplantation diagnosis for early-onset Alzheimer disease caused by V717L mutation. J Am Med Assoc 2002; 278:1018–1021.
113. De Sutter P, Dhont M, Vanluchene E, Vandekerckhove D. Correlation between follicular fluid steroid analysis and maturity and cytogenetic analysis of human oocytes that remain unfertilized after in vitro fertilization. Fertil Steril 1991; 55:958–963.

114. Pellestor F, Sele B. Assessment of aneuploidy in the human female by using cytogenetics of IVF failures. Am J Hum Genet 1988; 42:274–283.

115. Gras L, McBain J, Trouson A, Kola I. The incidence of chromosomal aneuploidy in stimulated and unstimulated (natural) uninseminated human oocytes. Hum Reprod 1992; 7:1396–1401.

116. Tarin JJ, Pellicer A. Consequences of high ovarian response to gonadotropins: a cytogenetic analysis of unfertilized human oocytes. Fertil Steril 1990; 54:665.

117. Plachot M. Chromosomal abnormalities in oocytes. Mol Cell Endocrinol 2001; 183:S59–S63.

118. Van Blerkom J. The influence of intrinsic and extrinsic factors on the development potential and chromosomal normality of the human oocyte. J Soc Gynecol Investig 1996; 3:1–11.

119. Zenzes MT, Wang P, Casper RF. Cigarette smoking may affect meiotic maturation of human oocytes. Hum Reprod 1995; 10:3213–3217.

120. Verlinsky Y, Cieslak J, Ivakhnenko V, et al. Preimplantation diagnosis of common aneulpoidies by the first and second polar body FISH analysis. J Assist Reprod Genet 1998; 15:285–289.

121. Gianaroli L, Magli MC, FerrarettiAP, Munne S. Preimplantation diagnosis for aneupoidy in patients undergoing in vitro fertilization with a poor prognosis; identification of the categories that it should be proposed. Fertil Steril 1999; 72:837–844.

122. ESHRE PGD Consortium Steering Committee. ESHRE Preimplantation Genetic Diagnosis Consortium: data collection III (May 2001). Hum Reprod 2002; 17:233–246.

123. Strom CM, Strom S, Levine E, Ginsberg N, Barton J, Verlinsky Y. Obstetrical outcome in 102 pregnancies after preimplantation genetic diagnosis. Am J Obstet Gynecol 2000; 182:1629–1632.

124. Reubinoff BE, Sameuloff A, Ben-Haim M, Freidler S, Schenker J, Lewin A. Is the obstetrical outcome of in vitro fertilized singleton gestations different from natural ones? A controlled study. Fertil Steril 1997; 67:1077–1083.

125. Maman E, Lunenfeld E, Levy A, Vardi H, Potashnik G. Obstetrical outcome of singleton pregnancies conceived by in vitro fertilization and ovulation induction compared with those conceived spontaneously. Fertil Steril 1998; 70:240–245.

126. Verlinsky Y, Rechitsky S, Sharapova T, Morris R, Taranissi M, Kuliev A. Preimplantation HLA testing. J Am Med Assoc 2003; 291:2079–2085.

127. Assisted reproductive technology in the United States; 1997 results generated from the American Society for Reproductive Medicine/Society for Assisted Reproductive Technology Registry. Fertil Steril 2000; 74:641–654.

128. Damewood MD. Ethical implications of preimplantation diagnosis. J Am Med Assoc 2001; 285:3143–3144.

129. Edwards RG. Ethics of preimplantation diagnosis. Recordings from the Fourth International Symposium on Preimplantation Genetics. Reprod BioMed Online 2003; 6:170–180.

130. Kubelka M, Moor RM. The behavior of mitotic nuclei after transplantation of early meiotic ooplasts or mitotic cytoplasts. Zygote 1997; 5:219–227.

131. Takeuchi MCT, Bedford MJ, Reis MM, Rosenwaks Z, Palermo GD. Alternative sources of gametes: reality or science fiction? Hum Reprod 2000; 15:988–999.

18

Fetal Anomaly Scan

Melanie A. J. Engels and John M. G. van Vugt
*Department of Obstetrics and Gynecology, VU University Medical Center,
Amsterdam, The Netherlands*

INTRODUCTION

In the last two decades, considerable advances have been made in obstetric ultrasonography due to improved equipment and expertise. Routine ultrasonography is of value in determination of gestational age and placental localization, diagnosis of multiple pregnancies, and evaluation of fetal growth. The value of routine ultrasonography in screening for fetal malformations has been the subject of debate in recent years. It is imperative that such a screening in an unselected population of pregnant women should have high sensitivity and specificity and should have a high predictive value even when the prevalence of the conditions is low. Despite their low prevalence (ranging from 2% to 4%) fetal structural malformations are responsible for approximately 20% to 30% of perinatal mortality in developed countries (1–3). The vast majority of these malformations occur in low-risk pregnancies (4). The ideal timing for screening in a low-risk population seems to be a compromise between obtaining adequate images for diagnosis in the majority of routine patients, scanning sufficiently late not to miss late-developing lesions, and yet offering diagnosis as early as possible for parents to consider their options.

Routine Fetal Anomaly Screening vs. Indication-based Ultrasonography

Fetal anomaly screening in the midtrimester of pregnancy is now a routine part of antenatal care in most European countries. In the United States, however, the National Institutes of Health agreed only on indication-based ultrasonography and refused the principle of screening. It is important whether the performance of fetal anomaly screening and the gestational age at diagnosis is of value for decisions on management during pregnancy and for appropriate care and treatment of the newborn at birth. Several randomized European studies in low-risk populations showed benefits of ultrasound screening for the management of pregnancy and fetal outcome (5–7). Contradictory to these findings were the results of the Routine Antenatal Diagnostic Imaging with Ultrasound (RADIUS) trial (8) carried out in the United States. They concluded that routine ultrasound screening, compared with selective use of ultrasonography, did not improve perinatal outcome. The most controversial result of this study was the poor detection rate of fetal abnormalities with routine ultrasound screening (35% overall and 17% before 24 weeks' gestation). Analysis afterward showed that the reasons that perinatal outcome was similar in the screened and the nonscreened groups were based on poor training of some sonographers, different criteria for defining major malformations, and differences in detection and documentation of congenital malformations in the neonatal period from one center to the next. Although the RADIUS study showed low detection rates of routine ultrasound screening, more congenital abnormalities were detected by fetal anomaly screening than by indication-based ultrasonography. The results of another, retrospective, study of fetal anomaly screening in high-risk pregnancies carried out in the United States (9) are also in favor of routine ultrasound screening. This study reported a detection rate of congenital abnormalities of 53%, which is similar to the sensitivity of fetal anomaly screening found in low-risk pregnancies in the Belgian Multicentric Study (10). From the Eurocat register (11) data are available on areas with and without routine fetal anomaly screening. Congenital abnormalities like bilateral renal agenesis, spina bifida, ventriculomegaly, cystic kidney disease, and omphalocoele were detected in 50% to 70% of the screened cases versus 2% to 4% in the nonscreened cases.

Sensitivity and Specificity of Fetal Anomaly Scan

The overall sensitivity of antenatal ultrasonography for correctly identifying fetuses with structural defects varies widely (10,12–18). However, differences in the criteria used for recording malformations, different screening populations, and screening policies make it difficult to compare the different studies. An overview of fetal anomaly screening in Europe, given by Levi (19), showed that clinical trials of routine ultrasonography reported before 1985 usually showed benefits in pregnancy outcome, although not significant because of the low prevalence of abnormalities and the small size of the samples. From the early 1990s, systematic routine ultrasound examinations for detection of congenital abnormalities were performed in larger populations. Since health insurance systems in Europe support fetal anomaly screening, approximately 98% of pregnant women have ultrasound examinations and, frequently, two to three times. An important conclusion is that effectiveness of screening is increased where experienced sonographers do the scanning. Therefore, training in ultrasound is imperative in making prenatal diagnosis. Particular certification, however, is in most countries not yet required. Notwithstanding, programs for qualification in obstetrical ultrasound are organized everywhere in Europe, but are not compulsory.

For evaluation of fetal anomaly screening in Europe, two main databases can be used: the Eurocat (16) and the Eurofetus (18) databases. Eurocat is a register that records congenital abnormalities in 30 geographical areas from 15 countries for the epidemiological surveillance of births with defects. The Eurofetus study is the largest prospective study to date on the evaluation of fetal anomaly screening. In this study three ultrasound investigations per pregnancy were done, which is regarded as the norm for ultrasonographic screening in most countries in Europe. About 4600 congenital abnormalities were recorded. An overall sensitivity of fetal anomaly screening was found to be 61.4%. The most common fetal structural abnormalities found were abnormalities of the musculoskeletal system, urinary tract system, central nervous system (CNS), and cardiac abnormalities. Overall, 44% of structural abnormalities were detected before 24 weeks' gestation, and 38.5% after 29 weeks' gestation. Of the major abnormalities, 55% were detected before 24 weeks' gestation. The gestational age at diagnosis depended on the type of malformation. Diagnosis was made earlier for minor and major musculoskeletal abnormalities, CNS abnormalities, and major abnormalities of the urinary tract system. Cardiac abnormalities, cleft lips and palates, minor urinary tract system abnormalities, and digestive system abnormalities were detected later in pregnancies. In contrast to sensitivity, the specificity of routine ultrasonography for detecting fetal malformations is very good and appears to be consistently higher than 99% (Table 1) (13,15–17).

Table 1 Detection of Fetal Abnormalities in Routine Ultrasound Screening

	Chitty et al. (1991)	Belgian multicentric study/Levi et al. (1991)	Luck (1992)	RADIUS/ Crane et al. (1994)	Eurofetus/ Grandjean et al. (1999)
Central nervous system abnormalities					
Anencephaly	6/6	6/6	7/7	3/3	156/157
Spina bifida, meningocele	5/5	4/7	2/2	4/5	146/181
Encephalocele	2/2		1/1		41/48
Ventriculomegaly	3/3	4/15			188/201
Holoprosencephaly	2/3	0/1			
Others	2/2	3/7	1/1	2/2	121/151
Total	20/21	17/36	11/11	9/10	652/738
Cardiovascular system abnormalities					
Atrial and/or ventricular septal defects	1/2	0/27	2/3	0/21	55/462
Univentricular heart	1/3	2/5	4/8		10/22
Complex heart abnormalities	5/6	1/40	3/14	5/19	132/344
Others					67/125
Total	7/11	3/72	9/25	5/40	264/953
Thoracic abnormalities					
Cystic adenomatoid malformation	4/4		1/1		11/11
Diaphragmatic hernia	2/2	1/2	2/5	1/1	51/88
Pleural effusion	1/3				
Others				1/4	10/19
Total	7/9	1/2	3/6	2/5	72/118
Abdominal and abdominal wall abnormalities					
Abdominal wall defects	4/4	4/4	4/4	1/1	129/158
Exomphalos	3/3	2/2	2/2	1/1	
Gastroschisis	1/1	2/2	2/2		
Esophageal atresia	0/2	1/7	1/2	0/3	29/58
Bowel obstruction/atresia	0/1	0/1	1/1	1/1	76/129
Others		1/14	1/1		18/42
Total	4/7	6/33	7/8	2/5	254/387

(Continued)

Table 1 Detection of Fetal Abnormalities in Routine Ultrasound Screening (*Continued*)

	Chitty et al. (1991)	Belgian multicentric study/Levi et al. (1991)	Luck (1992)	RADIUS/ Crane et al. (1994)	Eurofetus/ Grandjean et al. (1999)
Urinary tract abnormalities					
Obstructive uropathy	10/10	2/25	99/99	28/29	523/561
Cystic renal disease	5/8	4/11	4/4		164/179
Renal agenesis	5/5	3/4	2/2		75/92
Unilateral	1/1				39/49
Bilateral	4/4		2/2		36/43
Others	1/2	3/4		6/6	7/30
Total	21/25	12/44	105/105	34/35	769/862
Facial abnormalities					
Facial clefting	2/7			3/10	113/560
Skeletal abnormalities					
Dwarfism	2/2	0/2	2/2		39/43
Limb deficiency	2/5	0/1	1/2	2/5	29/110
Deformities of feet					48/279
Talipes	6/12	3/14	2/2	2/24	
Others	3/4	1/1	0/1		86/365
Total	13/23	4/18	5/7	4/29	202/797

Note: The above table lists selected abnormalities and does not give all the abnormalities reported in the studies.

FETAL STRUCTURAL ABNORMALITIES

The detection of fetal structural defects depends mainly on the severity and size of the abnormality and the gestational age at scanning. Furthermore, some defects are detected more easily because they are visible in the standard scanning planes, while others are only suspected by detection of associated sonographic features. In this chapter, the normal ultrasound appearances of the different tracti will be discussed, and an overview will be given of the most common abnormalities detected with fetal anomaly screening.

CENTRAL NERVOUS SYSTEM ABNORMALITIES

The incidence of abnormalities of the fetal CNS has been estimated at approximately 5–6 per 1000. Overall, the best detection rates are found for CNS abnormalities; sensitivity of detecting CNS abnormalities is approximately 90% (12,13,15–18).

Normal Ultrasound Appearances

Scanning of the CNS involves assessment of the fetal head and the spine. Examination of the fetal head can essentially be carried out by two transverse planes, commonly referred to as the transventricular and the transcerebellar plane. In the transventricular plane, the fetal head shape and size, the cavum septum pellucidum, the lateral ventricles and choroid plexuses, and the Sylvian fissures can be assessed.

The transventricular plane is used for measurement of the biparietal diameter and the head circumference, and the diameter of the atrium of the lateral ventricles. The transcerebellar plane allows examination of the midbrain and the posterior fossa; this view is used for measurement of the cerebellum and the cisterna magna. Due to reverberation artifacts, usually the cerebral hemisphere close to the transducer is not clearly visualized. Unilateral cerebral lesions, however, are rare and are often associated with a shift in the midline echo. Therefore, examination of only one hemisphere in routine scanning is sufficient to exclude major abnormalities. The spine should be assessed in the transverse, coronal, and sagittal planes. The transverse plane shows all three ossification centers of a vertebra on one image. In the coronal plane, the posterior centers are visualized, showing a characteristic railtrack appearance with the centers gradually widening toward the head, together with a slight expansion in the lumbar region before the centers converge in the sacrum. The coronal image also allows determination of the level, as the 12th rib can be seen adjacent to the 12th thoracic vertebra, and the first sacral vertebra is level with the top of the iliac wing. The sagittal view shows the normal steady curvature of the spine as well as a gradual tapering toward the sacrum. The transverse and sagittal planes allow assessment of the overlying skin.

Neural Tube Defects

Neural tube defects are the most common CNS abnormalities likely to be diagnosed by a sonographer, and they include anencephaly, spina bifida, and encephalocele. The prevalence is subject to large geographical and temporal variations (20). Anencephaly and spina bifida, with an approximately equal prevalence, account for 95% of the cases and encephalocele for the remaining 5%.

Anencephaly is recognized by failure of development of the fetal skull vault with secondary degeneration of the brain. The incidence of anencephaly is approximately 1 per 1000. At 12 weeks of gestation, ossification of the skull vault is complete. In the first trimester, the pathognomonic feature of anencephaly is acrania with the brain being either entirely normal or disorganized and incompletely formed. It has been demonstrated that there is progression from acrania to exencephaly and finally anencephaly (21). Sonographic features of anencephaly in the second trimester are absence of the skull vault and the hemispheres. However, the facial bones, brain stem, and portions of the occipital bones and midbrain are usually present. Associated spinal defects are found in about 50% of cases.

A high detection rate of up to 99% is reported for anencephaly (10,12–18).

Spinal defects occur in approximately 1–2 in 1000 live births. In spina bifida, the neural arch, usually in the lumbosacral region, is incomplete with secondary damage to the exposed spinal cord. In a transverse plane, a normal neural arch appears as a closed circle with an intact skin covering, whereas in spina bifida the neural arch is U-shaped, and there is an associated bulging meningocele or myelomeningocele (Fig. 1). Most lesions occur in the lumbosacral and sacral region, less in the thoracolumbar region and only few in the cervical region (22). The effectiveness of ultrasound in diagnosing spinal defects has improved greatly by the recognition of associated intracranial abnormalities. First, the shape of the skull vault changes from egg-shaped to lemon-shaped with indentation of the frontal bones bilaterally (23). The positive predictive value of this "lemon" sign for neural tube defects in a low-risk population is approximately 6%. Second, changes can be seen in the posterior fossa with an alteration of the shape of the cerebellum

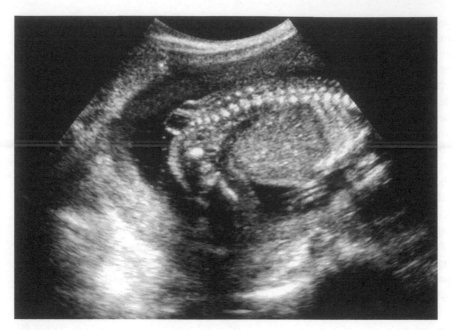

Figure 1 Spina bifida. Sagittal view of the fetus showing a cystic structure extending posteriorly from the sacral spine.

from a typical dumb-bell shape to a "banana" shape (23), due to compression of the cerebellum in the posterior fossa. The lemon sign and banana sign are seen in most of the cases with an open spina bifida before 24 weeks of gestation. The lemon sign disappears in later pregnancy. Third, there may be associated ventriculomegaly. The prevalence of ventriculomegaly varies, depending on the gestational age at scanning; before 24 weeks' gestation about three-quarters of fetuses will have ventriculomegaly; after 24 weeks' gestation ventriculomegaly has been reported as high as 100% (24).

The second trimester fetal anomaly scan is accurate in diagnosing spinal defects; detection rate of spina bifida with and without ventriculomegaly is about 95% and 66%, respectively (17).

An *encephalocele* is characterized by a defect in the skull and dura through which the meninges herniate with or without skin covering. The meningeal sac can contain brain tissue (encephalocele) or only cerebrospinal fluid (meningocele). In the majority of the cases a bone defect of the skull can be recognized. Encephaloceles are detected in about 85% of cases. The incidence of encephalocele is approximately 0.5 per 1000. Encephaloceles may be part of a genetic syndrome of which Meckel–Gruber syndrome and Walker–Warburg syndrome are the most common ones.

Cerebral Abnormalities

Ventriculomegaly is a descriptive term for enlargement of the intracranial ventricular system. It is distinct from hydrocephalus that implies not only enlargement but also raised pressure within the system. Ventriculomegaly is defined as dilated lateral cerebral ventricular atria of >10 mm, at any gestation, measured in an axial plane at the level of the cavum septum pellucidum (25). Ventriculomegaly is found in about 0.3% of all pregnancies (26). In most cases, ventriculomegaly is caused by an obstruction

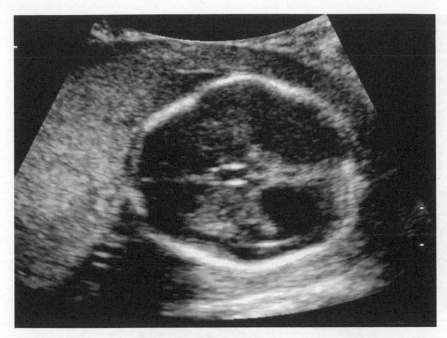

Figure 2 Ventriculomegaly. Transverse scan of the fetal head showing enlargment of both lateral and third ventricles. There is "dangling" of the choroid plexus in the dependent lateral ventricle. Note the lemon-shaped skull ("lemon" sign).

in the circulation of the cerebrospinal fluid. "Dangling" of the choroid plexus and enlargement of the third ventricle are associated sonographic features (Fig. 2). Ventriculomegaly, however, may not be apparent until the late second or early third trimester. While significant dilatation of the lateral and third ventricles can be easily demonstrated, borderline ventriculomegaly in the second trimester can be more difficult to assess.

Agenesis of the corpus callosum occurs in approximately 3 to 7 in 1000 live births. The corpus callosum is a bundle of fibers that connects the two cerebral hemispheres across the midline. Agenesis of the corpus callosum may be either complete or partial. The corpus callosum can be visualized on ultrasound in the midline sagittal and coronal planes but is not visible in the standard transverse scanning planes of the brain. In routine scanning, agenesis of the corpus callosum, however, is suspected by detection of associated sonographic features like focal dilatation of the posterior horns of the lateral ventricles (teardrop configuration), absent cavum septum pellucidum—seen to be absent on the transventricular image plane, and a high-riding third ventricle—filling the void left by the absent cavum septum pellucidum and corpus callosum (27). The corpus callosum has formed entirely by 20 weeks of gestation. Accurate diagnosis of agenesis of the corpus callosum can only be made after this gestation.

Holoprosencephaly is a spectrum of cerebral abnormalities due to incomplete cleavage of the forebrain and resulting in failure of development of midline structures and the cerebral mantle. The incidence of holoprosencephaly varies between 0.6 and 1.9 per 10,000. The disorder is classified into three groups depending on the severity of the intracranial findings: alobar, semilobar, and lobar holoprosencephaly. In the alobar form, the sonographic features are a monoventricular cavity,

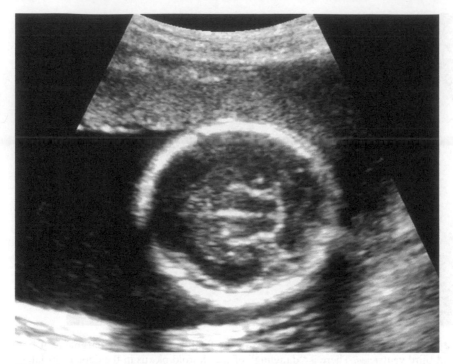

Figure 3 Alobar holoprosencephaly. Transverse scan through the fetal head showing fusion of the thalami, a large monoventricle, and absence of the midline structures anteriorly. Note the microcephaly.

fused thalami, and absence of midline structures such as the corpus callosum and the falx cerebri (Fig. 3). In the semilobar form, there is partial segmentation of the ventricles and cerebral hemispheres posterior, with incomplete fusion of the thalami. In lobar holoprosencephaly, there is normal separation of the ventricles and thalami but absence of the cavum septum pellucidum. There is often brachycephaly, microcephaly, and abnormal facial development (most commonly hypotelorism or cyclopia, facial cleft, and nasal hypoplasia or proboscis) (28). The detection rate by routine fetal anomaly scan is high for both the alobar and semilobar form; even in the first trimester, these forms can be detected with confidence.

Schizencephaly is a condition in which there is a complete cleft through the cerebral hemispheres, resulting in a free communication between the ventricular system and the subarachnoid space. On ultrasound, the bilateral clefts can be seen as hypoechoic areas extending from the dilated lateral ventricles to the subarachnoid space. Usually, there is associated absence of the cavum septum pellucidum.

Choroid plexus cysts are the most common intracerebral cystic lesions. The prevalence in a low-risk population is approximately 1% to 2%. Choroid plexus cysts contain cerebrospinal fluid and cellular debris. They are detected on ultrasound as hypoechoic structures within the body of the choroid plexus with a variable diameter, to be found uni- or bilateral and with or without septation. Most of the cysts are seen in the second trimester. The majority (80%) will resolve on scan by 24 weeks of gestation, and approximately 95% will be resolved by 28 weeks of gestation. It is generally accepted that choroid plexus cysts reflect a normal variation of the intracranial anatomy.

The *Dandy-Walker complex* refers to a spectrum of abnormalities of the cerebellar vermis, the fourth ventricle, and the cisterna magna (29). The condition is classified as Dandy-Walker malformation, Dandy-Walker variant, and mega cisterna magna. Dandy-Walker malformation is characterized by failure of development of the cerebellar vermis with a midline cyst in the posterior fossa resulting in communication between the fourth ventricle and the enlarged cisterna magna. In Dandy-Walker variant (inferior vermian agenesis) there is partial agenesis of the cerebellar vermis without enlargement of the posterior fossa. Both conditions are recognized in the standard transcerebellar plane as an (partial) absence of the echogenic vermis of the cerebellum. In about one-third of cases, there is associated ventriculomegaly. Mega cisterna magna is diagnosed if the distance from the vermis to the inner border of the skull measures >10 mm with no identifiable structural abnormality in the posterior fossa.

An *aneurysm of the vein of Galen* is a rare vascular malformation of the choroid plexus within the roof of the third ventricle. Arteriovenous fistulas from the choroid arteries, anterior cerebral arteries, and other arteries to the vein of Galen lead to the aneurysmal dilatation of the vein. On ultrasound, a large midline cystic structure superior to the thalamus can be seen. With color Doppler investigation, a turbulent blood flow can be demonstrated. The actual incidence of aneurysm of the vein of Galen is unknown, but the prevalence is 1% of all neonatal intracranial vascular malformations.

Porencephaly is a smooth-walled cavity within the cerebral cortex that usually communicates with the ipsilateral lateral ventricle and/or the subarachnoid space. The cavity is lined with white matter, filled with cerebrospinal fluid, and exerts no mass effect. Porencephaly most commonly occurs secondary to an intrauterine insult to the brain, but cases of familial porencephaly have been described.

Abnormalities of the Fetal Head Size and Shape

Microcephaly means small head and brain. The incidence of microcephaly varies from 1.6 to 4 per 10,000. Microcephaly is a heterogenous condition with many different causes. It is commonly found in the presence of other brain abnormalities, such as encephalocele or holoprosencephaly. Microcephaly is diagnosed when with advancing gestation a progressive decrease in the head circumference below the third percentile is demonstrated. Furthermore, there is a typical disproportion between the size of the skull and the face. Microcephaly is most often diagnosed after 24 weeks of gestation. Serial scans are necessary for appropriate diagnosis. Therefore, the detecting rate for microcephaly with routine fetal anomaly screening is poor.

Macrocephaly is diagnosed when the head circumference is found to be >97th percentile. This disproportion may arise from a fundamental abnormality of the fetus such as dwarfism or underlying structural abnormalities like ventriculomegaly and brain tumors that may cause the disproportional large head.

Dolicocephaly, elongation of the skull in the axial section, is most commonly seen in cases with oligohydramnios or breech position. *Brachycephaly* occurs when the biparietal diameter is large in comparison to the head circumference. It is observed in normal fetuses, but there may be underlying structural abnormalities.

Other head shapes like *cloverleaf- and strawberry-shaped head* can be seen in chromosomal abnormalities, in skeletal dysplasia, and in craniosynostosis (premature fusion of the sutures). Craniosynostosis produces a characteristic appearance with increased growth of the skull parallel to the fused suture. Sonographically, the sutures appear as linear translucencies within the skull with a characteristic location and distribution. The *lemon-shaped* skull is seen in association with neural tube defects (see section "Neural tube defects").

SPINAL ABNORMALITIES

Sacral agenesis and *caudal regression syndrome* are related disorders; the latter syndrome has variable spinal anomalies varying from partial sacral agenesis to complete absence of the lumbosacral spine. On ultrasound, sacral agenesis is visualized in a sagittal plane: the normal curve of the sacrum is lost and the spine appears shortened with an abrupt termination. If there is caudal regression, the lower limbs may be hypoplastic, and the bladder may be large. In more severe cases, the bones of the pelvis may be absent. Both conditions are strongly associated with maternal diabetes (30).

Scoliosis of the fetal spine is often caused by structural abnormalities of the vertebrae. A hemivertebra results from failure of formation of a part of the vertebra, and it can act as a wedge in the spinal column. Failure of segmentation of a vertebra produces a blocked or fused vertebra, which in turn can cause kyphosis, scoliosis, and shortening of the spine. Kyphosis is best demonstrated in a sagittal plane and scoliosis in a coronal plane. Axial section may show the partial absence of a vertebra, and a coronal section, the displacement of one of the ossification centers. If a vertebral abnormality is found, a search should be done for the components of the VACTERL complex (vertebral defects, anal atresia, cardiovascular abnormalities, tracheoesophageal fistula, esophageal atresia, renal abnormalities, and radial ray limb abnormalities).

Spina Bifida

See the section on Neural Tube Defects.

CARDIOVASCULAR SYSTEM ABNORMALITIES

Cardiac abnormalities are the most common congenital abnormalities and are found in 5–10 in 1000 live births. The etiology of heart defects is heterogenous and probably depends on the interplay of multiple genetic and environmental factors, including maternal diabetes mellitus or collagen disease, exposure to drugs such as lithium, and viral infections such as rubella. The majority of fetuses with a chromosomal disorder have a heart defect. Cardiac defects are not well detected on fetal anomaly scanning, whether major (38.8%) or minor (20.8%) defects (18). The presence of associated abnormalities increases the detection rate. Cardiac defects affecting the size of the ventricles have the highest detection rate. Prenatal detection of congenital heart defects increases with gestational age and by including routine examination of the four-chamber view and of the inflow and outflow tracts of the fetal heart. Evaluation of the cardiac inflow and outflow tracts, however, is at present not considered a part of the standard examination of the fetal heart.

Normal Ultrasound Appearances

Scanning of the fetal heart should begin with the assessment of the disposition of abdominal and thoracic organs, as an abnormal disposition is frequently associated with complex cardiac anomalies. A transverse plane of the abdomen, the same plane used for the measurement of the abdominal circumference, allows identification of the position of liver, stomach, and great abdominal vessels. A transverse plane of the thorax reveals the four-chamber view. Detailed descriptions of the four-chamber view and improved equipment allow a high degree of diagnostic accuracy in the detection of fetal cardiac defects (31). Probably, about 90% of ultrasonographically detectable fetal cardiac defects demonstrate some abnormalities in this view. The heart occupies about one-third of the thorax and is shifted to the left side of the chest, with the apex pointing to the left. The axis of the interventricular septum is about 45–20° to the left of the anteroposterior axis of the fetus. In the four-chamber view, the ventricles, atria, atrio-ventricular valves, ventricular and atrial septa, and foramen ovale flap can be identified. There are two atria of approximately equal size. There are two ventricles of approximately equal size and thickness. Identification of the cardiac chambers is done by reference to the spine. Opposite the spine is the anterior chest wall, and beneath this is the right ventricle. The descending aorta is seen as a circular structure lying anterior to the spine, and anterior to this is the left atrium. The confluence of the pulmonary veins into the left atrium also serves to identify it as such. The right atrium and the left ventricle can then also be identified. In the apex of the right ventricle, the moderator band can be visualized. In contrast, the left ventricle has a smooth inner wall. The atrial and ventricular septa are assessed. The foramen ovale flap is visible in the left atrium, beating toward the left side. The atrial and ventricular septa meet the two atrioventricular valves at the crux of the heart. The insertion of the tricuspid valve along the interventricular septum is positioned more apical than the insertion of the mitral valve.

Septal Defects

Septal defects represent about half of all congenital heart defects. Overall, small isolated atrial and ventricular septal defects are difficult to detect with detection rates reported of about 13% and 11%, respectively (18). Sonographic diagnosis of a septal defect depends on the demonstration of a dropout of echoes in the septum. Septal defects do not cause an impairment of cardiac function in utero. At the level of the atria, the large right-to-left shunt is a physiological condition in the fetus. In case of a ventricular septal defect, the right and left ventricular pressures are very similar, and the degree of shunting will be minimal. In atrioventricular septal defects, however, atrioventricular valve insufficiency may lead to intrauterine heart failure.

Atrial septal defects involve either the septum primum (the portion of the atrial septum below the foramen ovale) or the septum secundum (the portion of the atrial septum above the foramen ovale).

Secundum atrial septal defects are found in approximately 1 in 3000 live births and are usually isolated defects. Diagnosis remains difficult because of the physiological presence of the foramen ovale.

Ventricular septal defects are either isolated (approximately 50%) or they are part of a complex heart defect. Ventricular septal defects represent approximately 30% of all congenital heart defects. Depending on the location in the septum, the septal defects are classified into perimembranous defects (involves the perimembranous septum below the aortic valve), inlet defects (on the inflow tract of the right ventricle), trabecular defects (involves the muscular portion of the septum), and the outlet defects (in the infundibular portion of the right ventricle). Most defects are perimembranous defects (80%) and are best visualized in the view of the left outflow tract. Trabecular and inlet defects will be seen in the four-chamber view; in case of inlet defects, there is loss of the insertion of the atrioventricular valves to the septum.

Atrioventricular septal defects will be usually encountered either in fetuses with chromosomal abnormalities or in fetuses with cardiosplenic syndromes (left or right isomerism). Atrioventricular septal defects are found in about 1 in 3000 live births. Two forms are recognized: the incomplete and the complete atrioventricular septal defect. In the complete form, the tricuspid and mitral valve are fused in a large single atrioventricular valve. The incomplete forms are more difficult to recognize. The main clue is the absence of the atrial septum below the level of the foramen ovale and the demonstration that the tricuspid and mitral valves attach at the same level at the crest of the septum.

Heart Defects Associated with Ventricular Septal Defects

In tetralogy of Fallot a ventricular septal defect can be demonstrated in a four-chamber view as well as right ventricular hypertrophy; the other components of this condition are overriding aorta and pulmonary stenosis. Some major heart defects will only be recognized by detection of a septal defect. In transposition of the great arteries, the aorta arises from the right ventricle and the pulmonary artery from the left ventricle. The abnormal position of the great arteries is not found in a four-chamber view. Only in case of an associated ventricular septal defect, further investigation may show the parallel position of both arteries. In double outlet right ventricle, both great arteries arise predominantly from the right ventricle. The position of the two great arteries is usually variable and either artery can be obstructed. If the aorta and the pulmonary artery are not obstructed, only the presence of the ventricular septal defect can be seen in a four-chamber view.

Asymmetric Four-Chamber View

The appearance of the four-chamber view will vary according to the orientation of the fetus to the ultrasound beam. The same method of orientation should always be used to identify the cardiac chambers. An asymmetric appearance of the four-chamber view should prompt a search for cardiac anomalies.

Univentricular Heart

This term defines a group of abnormalities characterized by the presence of an atrioventricular junction that is entirely connected to only one chamber in the ventricular mass. Univentricular heart includes both those cases in which two atrial chambers are connected to a main ventricular chamber, by either two distinct atrioventricular valves or by a common one (double-inlet single ventricle), as well as those cases in which one of the ventricular chambers is either absent or rudimentary with absence of one atrioventricular connection (tricuspid or mitral atresia). In all cases, the four-chamber view will be abnormal. Mitral atresia most commonly occurs in association with aortic atresia in the hypoplastic left heart syndrome.

Right Heart Dominance

Obstruction to the right ventricle outflow tract is commonly manifest as pulmonary atresia or stenosis. Severe pulmonary stenosis will show the same ultrasound

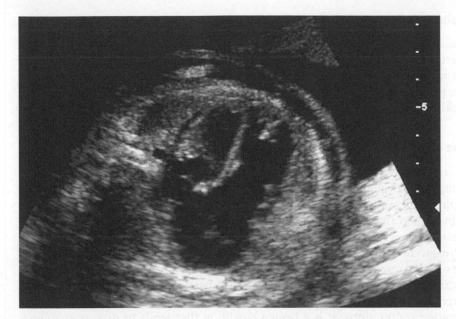

Figure 4 Ebstein's malformation. Transverse scan of the fetal chest, showing displacement of the tricuspid valve into the right ventricle with enlargement of the right atrium. The right ventricle is also dilated due to volume overload. Note the increased cardiothoracic ratio.

appearances as pulmonary atresia. In pulmonary atresia, the right ventricle is hypertrophied and contracts poorly. In case of pulmonary atresia with an intact interventricular septum, tricuspid incompetence can be seen. Significant tricuspid incompetence results in progressive right ventricular and right atrial enlargement due to volume overload. Tricuspid incompetence is also seen in tricuspid valve dysplasia; on ultrasound, the tricuspid valve appears thickened and nodular. In Ebstein's malformation, the attachment of the septal leaflet of the tricuspid valve is displaced into the right ventricle (Fig. 4). With a variable degree of displacement, the tricuspid incompetence and right atrial enlargement are variable. Right ventricular enlargement is seen as well if significant tricuspid incompetence is present. Due to an increased cardiothoracic ratio, secondary pulmonary hypoplasia can occur.

In case of coarctation of aorta, the right ventricle is enlarged relative to the left ventricle, and the pulmonary artery is relatively dilated compared with the aorta. The coarctation itself is not seen in utero, so the diagnosis can only be suspected on the associated signs.

Left Heart Dominance

A dilated, poorly contracting left ventricle with increased echogenicity of the ventricular walls is seen in cases of critical aortic stenosis.

Pericardial Effusion

It is common to see a rim of fluid around the ventricles in utero. In pericardial effusion, >2 mm of fluid around the heart is measured. Isolated pericardial effusions can be a marker of chromosomal abnormalities, in particular trisomy 21 (32).

Golfballs

These are bright echogenic lesions within the ventricular cavities. Echogenic foci in the heart are found in approximately 4% of pregnancies and are most commonly seen as a single lesion in the left ventricle. These lesions are usually of no consequence, provided that the structure of the heart is normal (33). The risk of a chromosomal abnormality in the absence of any other ultrasound marker is low (34).

Cardiac Dysrhythmias

Irregularity of the heart rhythm can be detected easily. Dysrhythmias are classified according to the origin and the number of beats per minute (bpm). M-mode echocardiography (preferably examining atrial and ventricular wall motion simultaneously) is used in order to assess atrioventricular synchrony as well as heart rate. M-mode echocardiography, however, is not a part of the standard examination of the fetal heart.

Premature contractions are the most common cause of fetal arrhythmia and may be of atrial (most common) or ventricular origin. They may present as irregular fetal heartrate, tachycardia, or as bradycardia caused by the compensatory pauses after premature contractions. Immaturity of the conducting system may be the origin of premature contractions. It is a benign condition that tends to disappear spontaneously in utero, and only rarely persists after birth.

Tachyarrhythmias (heart rate >200 bpm). A regular atrial rate of 200–300 bpm with a one-to-one atrioventricular conduction suggests supraventricular tachycardia. A regular atrial rate ≥300 bpm suggests atrial flutter with an atrioventricular block (e.g., 2:1 or 3:1). An irregular atrial rate suggests atrial fibrillation with a completely irregular ventricular rhythm.

Ventricular tachycardias are rare, and have typically a ventricular frequency of ≤200 bpm. Persistent tachycardia is commonly associated with fetal hydrops as a consequence of low cardiac output. Maternal drug therapy may be successful in controlling fetal tachyarrhythmias (35).

Bradyarrhythmias (heart rate <80 bpm) are almost always due to fetal heart block. Regular atrial premature contractions may mimic a sinus bradycardia owing to the ventricular compensatory pauses. Fetal heart block may be complete with total dissociation of atrial and ventricular contraction, or with lesser degrees of block. Complete atrioventricular block is mainly caused by structural cardiac defects, or it is related to maternal autoimmune disease (36).

THORACIC ABNORMALITIES

Normal Ultrasound Appearances

Examination of the lungs can be done in the same transverse plane used for the four-chamber view of the fetal heart. Under normal conditions, the fetal lungs are uniformly echogenic, and they occupy about two-thirds of the thoracic area. A sagittal plane of the fetal trunk allows identification of the diaphragm as a thin sonolucent line separating the abdominal from the thoracic cavity.

Lung Abnormalities

Echogenic lungs can be caused by any condition that prevents the normal circulation of lung fluid. In tracheal and laryngeal atresia, uniform increased echogenicity of both lungs is seen. Lung volume is enlarged with a displacement of the diaphragm downward. Bronchial atresia results in uniform echogenicity of a single lung with increase in volume. Uniform increased echogenicity of a part of one of the lungs can be seen in bronchopulmonary sequestration (37). In this condition, a part of the lung is disconnected to the bronchial tree during development.

Congenital cystic adenomatoid malformation (CCAM) is a rare condition with a variable sonographic appearance. CCAM is a developmental abnormality arising from an overgrowth of the terminal respiratory bronchioles. In most cases, the condition is unilateral and involves a single lung or lobe. Based on the sonographic appearance, three types are recognized. Type 1 is predominantly macrocystic; type 2 is mixed; and type 3 is microcystic that appears predominantly echogenic (Fig. 5). Lesions may change in character during pregnancy; resolution is described in about 20% of cases. All types may be associated with deviation of the mediastinum. Fetal hydrops develops when there is compression of the heart and the major blood vessels in the thorax.

Pulmonary hypoplasia is defined as an absolute decrease in lung volume and lung weight for gestational age. Pulmonary hypoplasia is usually secondary to

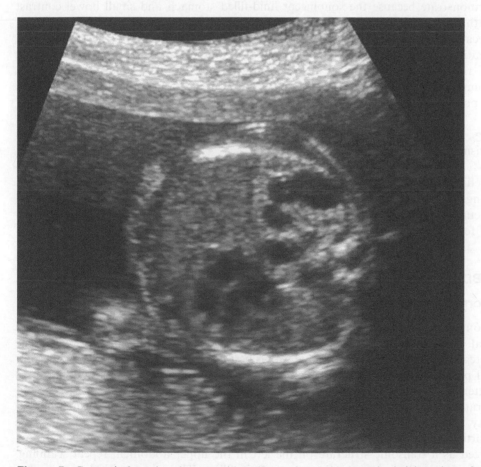

Figure 5 Congenital cystic adenomatoid malformation (mixed type). Axial section of the fetal chest, showing echogenic lung tissue with multiple cystic lesions situated in the right upper lobe. There is a moderate displacement of the heart to the left.

oligohydramnios or compression (e.g., pleural effusions, diaphragmatic hernia, CCAM, cardiomegaly, skeletal dysplasia). On ultrasound, pulmonary hypoplasia is suspected when chest volume is considerably reduced with the heart appearing relatively enlarged. The chest shape can become typically "bell-shaped." Measurement of thoracic circumference and cardiac diameters will help to differentiate reduced chest volume from increased cardiac size (38). Measuring fetal lung length and comparing the thoracic circumference with other body parameters are methods used to predict pulmonary hypoplasia. A more accurate method to predict pulmonary hypoplasia in utero is measuring fetal lung volume with 3D ultrasonography (39). The ultimate diagnosis of pulmonary hypoplasia, however, can only be made at postmortem.

Mediastinal Shift

In case of *diaphragmatic hernia*, there is herniation of the abdominal viscera into the thorax. A defective diaphragm can be left-sided (most common) or right-sided. In left-sided hernia, there is herniation of stomach and intestines with an associated mediastinal shift to the right. Herniated abdominal contents are easy to demonstrate because the sonolucent fluid-filled stomach and small bowel contrast with the more echogenic lung. Right-sided hernia is more difficult to detect because the echogenicity of the herniated liver is similar to that of the lung. Visualization of the gall bladder in the right side of the thorax may be the only sign of right-sided hernia. Large defects cause a considerable mediastinal shift with compression of the contralateral lung. A late complication of diaphragmatic hernia is polyhydramnios.

Mediastinal shift may also be seen in cases of *cystic lesions* in the mediastinum, e.g., bronchogenic cysts and thymic cysts; they appear as thoracic sonolucent lesions arising near the midline.

Large fetal *pleural effusions* can cause depression of the diaphragm and mediastinal shift. Pleural effusion is seen as a sonolucent area around one or both lungs (Fig. 6). Chylothorax and transudate can cause both unilateral and bilateral pleural effusions. Bilateral pleural effusions are also seen as part of the spectrum of fetal hydrops.

ABDOMINAL AND ABDOMINAL WALL ABNORMALITIES

Normal Ultrasound Appearances

Routine scanning of the abdomen involves assessment of the anterior abdominal wall and the presence, size, and position of the different abdominal organs. The integrity of the anterior abdominal wall is best demonstrated in transverse and sagittal planes. The anterior abdominal wall is clearly outlined by amniotic fluid on its external surface with the site of the umbilical cord insertion being clearly demonstrated. In the upper abdomen, the liver can be visualized; it has a uniform echodensity and contains a number of transonic structures, most notably the intrahepatic portion of the umbilical vein and the gall bladder. The stomach can usually be recognized as a transonic structure on the left in the upper abdomen; repeat scanning, however, can be necessary to demonstrate its filling. The spleen, with the same echogenicity as the liver, is positioned dorsally of the stomach and is more difficult to assess. Small bowel can often be identified in the second trimester as small fluid-filled

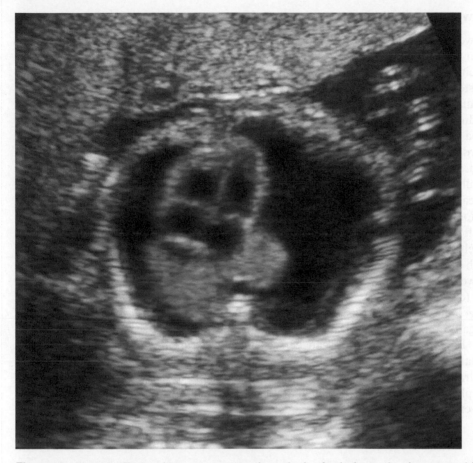

Figure 6 Pleural effusion. Transverse scan through the fetal chest, showing severe bilateral pleural effusion with a displacement of the heart to the right and compression of the lungs.

loops. Large bowel becomes apparent only in the third trimester; it is recognized by its haustral appearance and its position in the abdomen. The kidneys should be visualized, as well as the adrenal glands situated above the kidneys. The bladder is variable in size and transonic in appearance. Around the bladder, both umbilical arteries can be demonstrated using color Doppler.

ABDOMINAL ABNORMALITIES

Intra-Abdominal Cysts

Cystic abdominal lesions in the fetus are quite common. Cysts can originate from all abdominal organs. In female fetuses, the most common cause of a transonic abdominal structure is an ovarian cyst. Vaginal atresia or an imperforate hymen may present in utero as a cystic pelvic lesion (hydrometrocolpos). Duplication cysts of the bowel are the second commonest cause. These cysts are usually unilocular. Mesenteric cysts may also be seen in utero, but they are usually multilocular. Transonic structures in the liver can represent lymphangiomas, choledochal cysts, or varices of the umbilical vein. Cysts, hemorrhage, and neuroblastoma in the adrenal glands can also appear as hypoechoic structures. In the spleen, cysts have been described as isolated findings.

Bowel Abnormalities

Bowel atresias are the most common bowel abnormalities. *Esophageal atresia* is seen in approximately 1 in 3000 live births and is suspected if the fetal stomach is either small or not easily demonstrated on serial scanning in the second trimester. However, esophageal atresia can appear with and without tracheoesophageal fistula. Many cases with tracheoesophageal fistula will have normal ultrasound findings in the second trimester, because fluid can pass into the stomach via the trachea and the distal tracheoesophageal fistula. Developing polyhydramnios in the third trimester should raise the possibility of the diagnosis again. In cases of polyhydramnios with absent stomach, other conditions should be considered (e.g., poor swallowing due to neuromuscular or craniofacial disorders; misplaced stomach in case of diaphragmatic hernia or situs inversus). In *duodenal atresia* the typical sonographic appearance is a "double bubble" with the stomach and duodenum each forming similarly sized, fluid-filled structures (Fig. 7). This diagnosis is rarely made before the last part of the second trimester. It is often associated with polyhydramnios. *Small bowel atresia* is suspected when multiple fluid-filled bowel loops are seen. The obstruction can be intrinsic (atresia or stenosis) or extrinsic (e.g., malrotation). Multiple atresias are well described. Differentiation from *large bowel atresia* is possible considering the position and the haustral pattern of large bowel. Large bowel atresia is usually seen in the late second or third trimester. Large bowel dilatation can be seen in *imperforate anus*, but this condition is usually diagnosed postnatal following a normal antenatal scan. Associated polyhydramnios in bowel atresias is common. Dilated ureters can mimic the sonographic appearances of bowel dilatations; ureters, however, usually present with lower echogenicity.

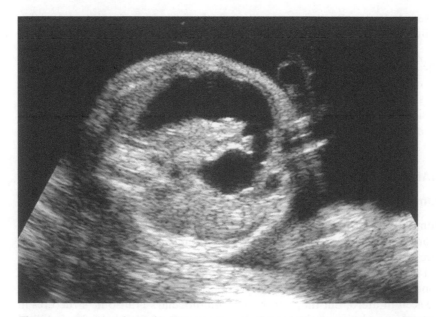

Figure 7 Duodenal atresia. Transverse scan through the fetal abdomen showing the typical appearance of a "double bubble," with the stomach and duodenum both visible as fluid-filled structures.

The observation of *hyperechoic bowel* is a nonspecific finding. Bowel is considered hyperechogenic when it appears as "bright as bone." This appearance is associated in some cases with Down syndrome, intrauterine growth restriction, cystic fibrosis, swallowed blood, and viral infections, but in the majority of cases no underlying cause is found (40).

Ascites

Any fluid seen in the abdomen is abnormal. A very thin black line around the inner aspect of the abdomen is, however, a normal appearance. Isolated ascites is a frequent, early manifestation of fetal hydrops.

Intra-Abdominal Tumors

Intra-abdominal masses are not frequently seen. *Neuroblastoma* of the adrenal glands appears as a suprarenal mass that increases in size with time. The appearance is variable; some will have a cystic component, others will be solid isoechoic or complex.

Sacrococcygeal teratoma is the most common congenital tumor with an incidence of 1 in 40,000 live births. The condition originates from an area of primitive streak called the Hensen's node. In case this node does not degenerate, it may give rise to a sacrococcygeal teratoma. The condition is classified into four types depending on the location and the amount of tumor that is intra-abdominal (41). Hydrops can occur as a result of high output cardiac failure secondary to the vascular nature of some of these tumors. On ultrasound, the tumors can be solid, cystic, or mixed (Fig. 8). Demonstration of the intra-abdominal form can be difficult but may be suspected if the bladder is displaced.

ABDOMINAL WALL ABNORMALITIES

Abdominal wall abnormalities are one of the more common fetal abnormalities demonstrated on ultrasound. The spectrum of anterior wall defects extends from the very minor exomphalos with bowel herniation into the base of the umbilical cord to the most major defects, including the pentalogy of Cantrell and body stalk anomaly.

Exomphalos is an incomplete return of the abdominal contents to the abdominal cavity in early pregnancy. At 8 to 10 weeks of gestation, all fetuses show herniation of the midgut, visible as a hyperechogenic mass in the base of the umbilical cord; retraction into the abdominal cavity occurs at 10 to 12 weeks. Exomphalos is found in about 1 in 4000 live births. On ultrasound, the sac of the exomphalos is clearly visible in the amniotic fluid. The sac consists of peritoneum and amnion and may contain any of the abdominal organs; bowel is most commonly present (Fig. 9). The umbilical vein is seen coursing through the sac and its contents. Exomphalos is frequently associated with other abnormalities. Chromosomal abnormalities are more frequently associated with small exomphalos containing only bowel. A high detection rate is reported for exomphalos.

In *gastroschisis*, there is a herniation of abdominal contents usually to the right of the umbilical cord insertion. Gastroschisis never has a surrounding membrane and usually contains only bowel, predominantly small bowel. The multiple loops of bowel can be seen outlined by the amniotic fluid. Later in pregnancy, complications can occur such as bowel wall thickening and bowel dilatations. The thickening is suggested to

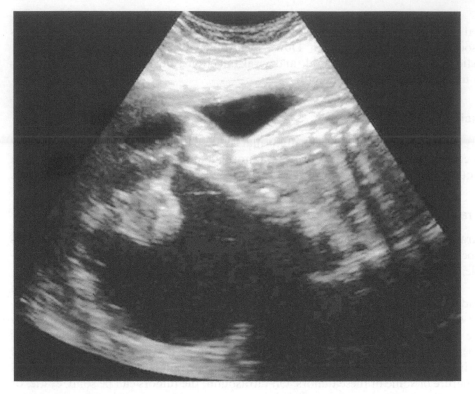

Figure 8 Sacrococcygeal teratoma. A mixed cystic and solid tumor.

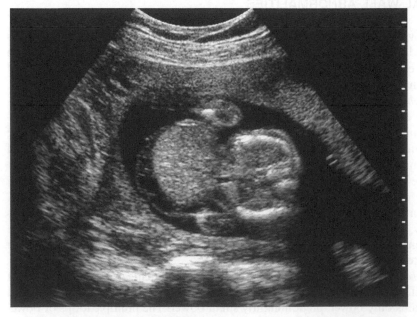

Figure 9 Exomphalos. Transverse section of a fetus with exomphalus showing the large sac containing loops of bowel and liver.

result from a chemical peritonitis due to exposure of the bowel to fetal urine in the amniotic fluid (42). Intestinal atresias or stenosis can be seen secondary to intestinal ischemia. Rarely gastroschisis is associated with other abnormalities.

Bladder exstrophy is a defect of the caudal fold of the anterior abdominal wall; a small defect may cause epispadias alone, while a large defect leads to exposure of the posterior bladder wall. Bladder exstrophy should be suspected when, in the presence of normal amniotic fluid, the fetal bladder cannot be visualized. Sonographically, an echogenic mass can be seen protruding from the lower abdominal wall, in close association with the umbilical arteries. Associated abnormalities are uncommon.

Cloacal exstrophy is thought to represent maldevelopment of the cloacal membrane and defective subumbilical abdominal wall development. Both the urinary and gastrointestinal tracts are involved. There is bladder exstrophy, epispadias, and imperforate anus. Other associated abnormalities may be spinal defects, exomphalos, talipes, vertebral abnormalities, and single umbilical artery. The association of exomphalos, bladder exstrophy, imperforate anus, and spinal defect is referred to as OEIS complex.

In *body stalk anomaly*, there is a large abdominal wall defect. Pathogenesis is uncertain, but different theories are suggested, including early amnion rupture, abnormal folding of the trilaminar embryo in early development, and amniotic band syndrome. The sonographic features are extensive facial, thoracic, and abdominal abnormalities entangled with the membranes. Usually, there is severe kyphoscoliosis, a short umbilical cord, and spinal defects.

In *ectopia cordis*, the fetal heart is herniated through a defect in the chest or the thoracoabdominal wall. Ectopia cordis is diagnosed on ultrasound when the heart is visible outside the chest in the amniotic fluid. The association of ectopia cordis, diaphragmatic hernia, exomphalos, sternal cleft, and a cardiac defect is known as *pentology of Cantrell.*

URINARY TRACT ABNORMALITIES

Congenital abnormalities of the urinary tract are common, and the incidence appears to vary between 2 and 5 per 1000. Overall sensitivity of ultrasound in detecting abnormalities of the urinary tract is reportedly good (15,17,18). In the third trimester, more urinary tract abnormalities are detected than in the second trimester.

Normal Ultrasound Appearances

Scanning of the urinary tract involves assessment of both kidneys, bladder, and amniotic fluid volume. The presence, size, and echogenicity of both kidneys should be assessed. In the first trimester, the kidneys appear as bilateral parasagittal echogenic structures; the bladder is situated in the pelvis as a well-defined sonolucent structure. In the second trimester, the kidneys appear less echogenic, and the pyramids become more prominent. The renal pelves can be visualized centrally. The adrenal glands are seen as triangular hypoechoic structures outlining the upper poles of the kidneys. Bladder size and bladder wall thickness can be assessed. Bladder wall is best measured at the point where the umbilical artery separates around the bladder. Bladder filling and emptying can normally be demonstrated over a period of 30 to 40 minutes.

Amniotic fluid is produced by the amnion, fetal urine, and fetal lung fluid. From 16 weeks' gestation, urine production is the most important factor of amniotic fluid production. Regulation of the amniotic fluid volume within limits of 0.5–2.0 L in pregnancy is thought to include alterations in chorioamniotic membrane permeability, alterations of fetal urine regulation (via hormones), and alterations in fetal swallowing. Maternal osmolality may also affect amniotic fluid volume.

The standard technique of assessing amniotic fluid volume is the amniotic fluid index (AFI) (43) that measures the amniotic fluid in four quadrants of the uterus. Subjective assessment of amniotic fluid volume, however, remains an important and reliable method. Amniotic fluid is usually transonic. In case the amniotic fluid in the third trimester has a more echoic aspect, the most common cause is the presence of vernix instead of meconium.

Obstruction of the Urinary Tract System

There are a number of different structural abnormalities producing obstruction of the urinary tract system. The level of the obstruction can usually be suggested by the degree of dilatation of renal pelves, ureters, and bladder. But also nonobstructing conditions such as vesicoureteric reflux and prune belly syndrome can cause dilatation of the urinary tract system. In early severe obstruction, signs of cystic renal dysplasia can be seen.

Renal pelvic dilatation is referred to as hydronephrosis. Hydronephrosis is seen in almost all cases of urinary tract system obstruction. The most common causes are pelvic–ureteric junction obstruction, vesicoureteric reflux, vesicoureteric junction obstruction, posterior urethral valves, and obstruction in duplex kidneys. Pelvic–ureteric junction obstruction typically presents with dilatation of the pelves and the calyces without ureteric dilatation. With increasing degree of obstruction, the collecting system becomes effaced with thinning of the renal cortex. The degree of renal pelvic dilatation appears to have a correlation with outcome. Cutoff values for the anteroposterior diameter of the renal pelves are used in order to predict significant renal pathology. Renal pelvec diameters >10 mm in the second trimester have a high incidence of significant renal pathology (44). Follow-up and investigation in the neonatal period is necessary in these cases. Mild renal pelvic dilatation (renal pelvic diameters between 5 and 10 mm) in the second trimester can progress in utero to produce significant renal pathology. Furthermore, mild renal pelvic dilatation is associated with vesicoureteric reflux in the neonatal period (44). So, follow-up scans are advised at around 28 weeks of gestation. Renal pelvic dilatation <5 mm in the second trimester often resolves after delivery (45). Extrarenal pelves can also be the cause of renal pelvic dilatation without significant renal pathology.

A *megaureter* is defined as a dilated ureter visible on ultrasound. It usually appears unilateral. A megaureter can be caused by vesicoureteric junction obstruction, vesicoureteric reflux, and by an obstruction secondary to an ureterocele. Also, ectopic ureters are usually dilated. On ultrasound, a megaureter appears as a serpiginous transsonic tubular structure and communicates with the renal pelves that is usually also dilated. A megaureter is seen in vesicoureteric obstruction, vesicoureteric reflux, and in obstruction secondary to an ureterocele. In case of vesicoureteric reflux, the degree of dilatation of the ureter is variable and changes with bladder volume. In vesicoureteric junction obstruction, there is no evidence of reflux or bladder outlet obstruction. An ureterocele can be demonstrated as a cystic dilatation of the intravesical segment of the distal ureter (46) and is often associated with a duplex kidney. Visualization of the ureterocele, however, can be difficult; if the bladder is empty, the uterocele can be mistaken for the bladder, and if the bladder is full, the ureterocele can be obscured. Megaureters are in most cases related to significant renal pathology. They are amenable to prenatal diagnosis, but it may be difficult to differentiate it from fluid-filled bowel.

Megacystis is defined as massive bladder extension; the bladder extends above the crista iliaca. Urethral posterior valves are the most common cause leading to severe obstructive uropathy in boys. On ultrasound, a dilated thick-walled bladder with a dilated posterior urethra is found, usually associated with dilated ureters and hydronephrosis due to vesicoureteric reflux. Amniotic fluid volume is variable; oligohydramnios is possible. Megacystis is also seen in severe bilateral vesicoureteric reflux with a thin-walled bladder and normal amniotic fluid volume (Fig. 10). Massive bladder extension in combination with dilatation of the upper urinary tract and abdominal wall distension is referred to as *prune belly syndrome*.

Cystic Renal Disease

Cystic renal disease covers a wide range of conditions with differing antenatal appearances and modes of inheritance.

Multicystic renal dysplasia is the most common form of cystic renal disease in childhood (47) and has an incidence of 1 in 3000 live births. It is usually unilateral and more common in boys. On ultrasound, the affected kidney contains noncommunicating cysts of variable size and number. The stroma is often dense without normal renal tissue recognizable (Fig. 11). Usually, multicystic dysplasia affects the

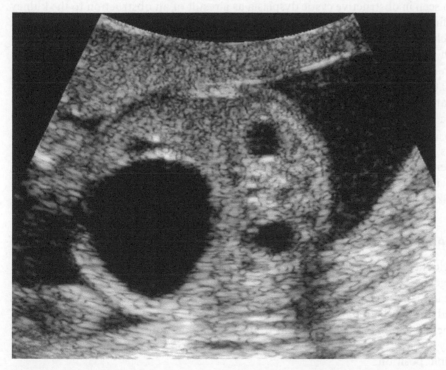

Figure 10 Megacystis. Transverse scan through the fetal abdomen with a distended bladder and bilateral renal pelvic dilatation due to vesicoureteric reflux.

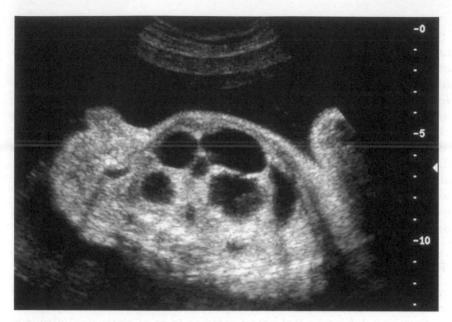

Figure 11 Unilateral multicystic kidney. Transverse scan through the fetal kidneys showing unilateral multiple cysts of varying sizes with dense renal stroma.

whole kidney, but it may affect only a part of it, particularly the upper pole of a duplex kidney. Most cases of multicystic renal disease are sporadic. Renal cysts are also seen in obstructive cystic dysplasia as a result of an obstruction to the kidney in the first or early second trimester. The typical sonographic appearance is of a small echogenic kidney with peripheral cortical cysts.

Of *polycystic renal disease*, two distinct types are recognized. Infantile polycystic renal disease (autosomal recessive) has an incidence of approximately 1 to 40 in 50,000 live births and affects both kidneys (48). The typical ultrasound appearances are of enlarged echogenic kidneys associated with oligohydramnios or anhydramnios. This form of polycystic renal disease is associated with hepatic portal fibrosis (48). The adult form of polycystic renal disease (autosomal dominant) presents with the same sonographic features of the kidneys as the infantile form. However, in the adult form the condition can be unilateral. Both forms may appear normal in the early second trimester, and so follow-up scans are essential in the high-risk group.

Renal Agenesis

The incidence of *unilateral renal agenesis* is 1 in 1000 live births (49). In unilateral renal agenesis, there is a compensatory enlargement of the opposite kidney. Sonographically, the affected renal fossa is empty. However, the adrenal gland can be flattened and fill the renal fossa and may be confused with a kidney. Unless a careful assessment is made of each kidney at routine scanning, unilateral renal agenesis can be easily missed. The absence of one kidney should prompt a search for the kidney in an ectopic position.

Bilateral renal agenesis has an incidence of 1 in 4000 (50). On ultrasound, bilateral renal agenesis is associated with severe oligohydramnios, absence of the kidneys and the bladder. However, until 17 weeks of gestation amniotic fluid volume can be normal. Using color Doppler, absence of both renal arteries can be demonstrated. Intra-amniotic infusion of fluid can be used for a better visualization of the fetus and for assessment of the renal fossae. The severe oligohydramnios produces the typical Potter's sequence of low set ears, wide set eyes, micrognathia, limb contractures, talipes, and pulmonary hypoplasia (51).

Renal Ectopia

An ectopic kidney lies outside its normal position in the renal fossa. Most ectopic kidneys are pelvic or at the opposite site (crossed renal ectopia), but they can also be positioned lumbar or even thoracic (52). Ectopic kidneys appear in 1 in 1200 live births.

Horseshoe Kidney

Horseshoe kidney is a common abnormality with an incidence of 1 in 400 live births. It is usually the result of fusion of the lower poles of both kidneys. On ultrasound, the horseshoe kidney can be demonstrated on a standard transverse plane, where, at the inferior poles of the kidneys renal tissue will be seen to cross the midline joining both kidneys.

Disorders of the Amniotic Fluid

If the amount of the amniotic fluid volume is abnormal, ultrasonographic examination should be focused on causes of disturbed production or resorption.

Oligohydramnios is defined as an AFI <5 cm or as a vertical length of the largest cord-free pool of amniotic fluid <2 cm. The most common causes are urinary tract abnormalities, intrauterine growth restriction, rupture of membranes, and post-term pregnancy. Oligohydramnios can result in secondary pulmonary hypoplasia. Oligohydramnios has been shown to be an important predictor of perinatal outcome (53).

Polyhydramnios is defined as an AFI >25 cm or as a vertical length of the largest cord-free pool of amniotic fluid >8 cm. Bowel abnormalities and CNS abnormalities can result in problems in fetal swallowing. Congenital heart defects, diabetes mellitus, fetal hydrops, and twin-to-twin transfusion syndrome can result in increased diuresis. Polyhydramnios in the second trimester resolves spontaneously in up to 50% of cases with normal perinatal outcome (54).

FACIAL ABNORMALITIES

Detection rates for fetal facial abnormalities vary, ranging from 25% to 43% in low-risk populations. Facial abnormalities are often associated with genetic syndromes and chromosomal abnormalities.

Normal Ultrasound Appearances

Routine scanning of the fetal face should involve scanning in the three scanning planes. In a midsagittal plane, the profile can be assessed. The profile view should form a smooth curve running from forehead, nose, lips, and chin. In successive transverse planes, the orbits with the lenses, the nasal bone, the maxilla, and the mandible can be demonstrated. The distances between the orbits should be taken into account, and both lenses should be visible. Both lips and nostrils should be visualized using coronal and transverse scans. In a coronal scan, the ears can be visualized, but visualization of the ears is not part of routine assessment of the fetus.

Facial clefting is the most common congenital facial abnormality with an overall incidence of approximately 1 in 1000 live births. There is, however, a wide racial variation. Unilateral cleft lip is more common than bilateral cleft lip. Most cases of cleft lip and/or palate are idiopathic, but some drugs (e.g., antiepileptic drugs) are known to be associated with facial clefting (55). Sonographically, a vertical hypoechoic area within the upper lip can be demonstrated on coronal scanning (Fig. 12). With involvement of the palate, the hypoechoic area will extend into the nose. Bilateral cleft lip and palate are recognized in a sagittal or transverse plane by the presence of a central echodense mass in the region of the upper lip. This premaxillary protrusion can be large and can obscure the clefts. Median clefts are demonstrated as a wide central gap in the upper lip involving the palate.

Frontal bossing is a very prominent forehead with depression of the nasal bridge (Fig. 13). This feature is seen in achondroplasia.

Marked *micrognathia* is seen in a large number of chromosomal and genetic syndromes and in some skeletal dysplasias. Mild micrognathia may be a normal variant and is probably overlooked during routine scanning.

Cyclopia is seen in 10% to 20% of fetuses with holoprosencephaly and represents varying degrees of ocular fusion. In most cases, the fusion is not complete and two fused eyes can be seen within a single orbit (56). The nose is situated above the eye in the form of a proboscis. The mouth may be small or absent and the ears are often low set.

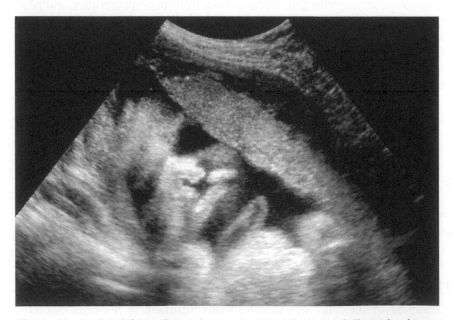

Figure 12   Facial clefting. Coronal scan, showing bilateral cleft lip and palate.

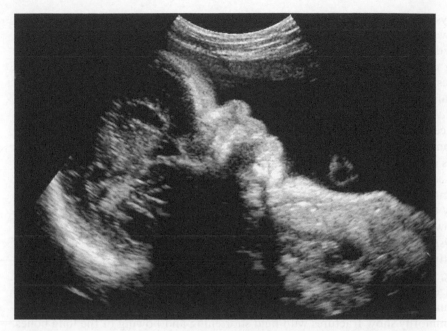

Figure 13 Frontal bossing. The facial profile shows a prominent forehead with a depression of the nasal bridge.

SKELETAL ABNORMALITIES

Abnormalities of the fetal skeleton have a heterogenous etiology and are relatively common with an incidence of 2 in 1000 live births. However, true skeletal dysplasias are less common.

Normal Ultrasound Appearances

Skeletal abnormalities are amenable to antenatal diagnosis as bone is a reflector of ultrasound. A structured approach to the routine ultrasound scanning of the fetal skeleton includes a careful survey of many bony structures. Biparietal diameter, head circumference, and femur length are routinely measured. The ribs are imaged on the four-chamber view; normal ribs extend two-thirds around the thorax. The assessment of the spine includes the vertebral bodies and the appendages. The three segments of all extremities should be visualized, but it is only necessary to measure the length of the femur. The long bones should be appropriately modeled—straight and in proportion; the lengths of all long bones are approximately similar and increase linearly with gestation. The position of the feet is checked. Ossification of the bone can be assessed by posterior acoustic shadowing, and by reference to the fetal falx and intracranial structures; in the normally ossified skull vault, the bones are more reflective than the falx and midline structures. This relationship is lost or reversed when ossification is deficient. An abnormality of bone morphology or length on a screening survey should always promote a more extensive survey of the fetal skeleton with assessment of all long bones.

The most common skeletal abnormalities will be addressed and classified according to the most striking ultrasound features (57). The majority of lethal, short limb dysplasias will show marked shortening of the long bones (micromelia) by 18–20 weeks of gestation, and are often associated with a small thorax; chest restriction leads to pulmonary hypoplasia and finally death. Associated features may be bowing of the long bones (campomelia), undermineralization of the skeleton, and fractures. Nonlethal, short limb dysplasias will often show normal ultrasound appearances in the second trimester.

Achondroplasia is the most common nonlethal skeletal dysplasia with an incidence of 1 in 50,000 live births. Although the condition is transmitted as autosomal dominant, most cases represent sporadic new mutations. The sonographic features are mild micromelia, lumbar lordosis, short hands and fingers, and narrow thorax secondary to rib shortening. Associated macrocephaly and frontal bossing are common. The sonographic features may be apparent only in the late second or early third trimester. The homozygous form of achondroplasia is associated with a narrow thorax and is a lethal condition.

Osteogenesis imperfecta is a clinically and genetically diverse disorder of connective tissue, presenting with fragility of the bones, blue sclerae, impaired hearing, defective dentition, loose joints, and growth deficiency. Four types are recognized (58–60). Type I has a birth prevalence of about 1 in 30,000. Affected individuals have fragile bones, blue sclerae, and progressive deafness. On ultrasound, only a minority show fractures with mild shortening and bowing of the long bones. Type IV is comparable to type I, but without deafness and blue sclerae and with defective dentition. Usually, the onset is in childhood or puberty, but both types can be symptomatic at birth and in utero.

Type II is lethal in utero or early in the neonatal period for most cases. The incidence is approximately 1 in 60,000. The main sonographic features are bent, shortened long bones. Three separate variants are recognized. Type IIA presents with shortened and broad long bones with low echogenicity with beading (string of fractures) of the ribs and long bones. In type IIB, there is moderate shortening of the long bones with usually single fractures. The ribs are rather small and irregular with only a few fractures. Type IIC shows moderately shortened long bones with almost normal echogenicity, but with multiple fractures, causing angulation of the bone. The ribs are thin.

Type III has a variable expression, but the majority will have severe short stature with progressive deformity of long bones and spine, often leading to death in early adulthood. The main ultrasound feature is of shortening of the long bones that have fractured.

The most common lethal skeletal dysplasia is *thanatophoric dysplasia* with an incidence of 1 in 30,000 (61). The condition is sporadic. It can be detected in the early second trimester. The main sonographic features are of severe micromelia with bowing associated with a narrow, shortened thorax with short ribs. Two types are recognized. Type 1 is seen more frequently and has a typical telephone receiver aspect of the femora (Fig. 14). Type 2 shows cloverleaf skull with less long bone shortening and bowing. In most cases, there is associated polyhydramnios.

Achondrogenesis is a lethal condition with an incidence of approximately 1 in 50,000 live births. Two distinct types of achondrogenesis are recognized (62). On ultrasound, type I presents with skin edema, severe micromelia, poor mineralization of both the skull and the vertebral bodies, and short ribs, often fractured. Associated polyhydramnios is often seen.

Type II shows variable shortening of the long bones, short ribs without fractures, and hypomineralization of only the vertebral bodies. This type usually presents with frontal bossing and depression of the nose. The mild form, known

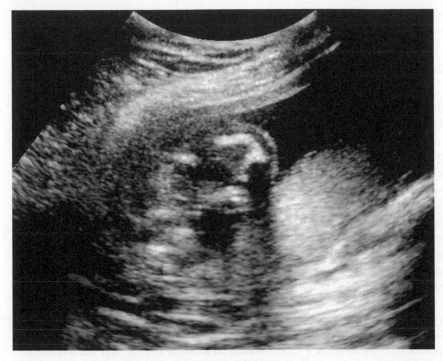

Figure 14 Typical short and bent femur ("telephone receiver") in thanatophoric dysplasia.

as hypochondrogenesis, shows a continuous spectrum of severity in which the limbs are longer and less bowed.

Short rib polydactyly is a group of disorders characterized by severe micromelia, short horizontal ribs, and postaxial polydactyly, and frequently cardiac and renal abnormalities are seen. There are four distinct subgroups; they are rare disorders with lethal outcome. The distinguishing features between the different subgroups are the presence of facial clefting, tibial length, and metaphyseal morphology (63).

Campomelic dysplasia is a skeletal dysplasia with mild to severe micromelia but with marked bowing of the femur and tibia. Hypoplasia of the fibula and scapula are associated features. These ultrasound appearances are apparent at 18 to 20 weeks of gestation. Campomelic dysplasia is lethal in most cases; survival is dependent on the degree of respiratory failure due to pulmonary hypoplasia and tracheobronchial malacia.

Diastrophic dysplasia is a skeletal dysplasia with a variable phenotypic expression and variable outcome. It can be lethal in the neonatal and early childhood caused by respiratory failure due to tracheobronchial malacia. It is a generalized destructive disorder of cartilage with contractures as a result. The typical features are of micromelia with flexion limitations at the elbows, hips, and finger joints, resulting in the classical hitchhiker thumb owing to fixed lateral position. There is a progressive scoliosis that may be apparent antenatal.

Hypophosphatasia is characterized by lack of alkaline phosphatase resulting in undermineralization of the fetal skeleton. On ultrasound, the skeleton is hardly visible and usually there is extreme bowing of the long bones. Fractures can be seen antenatal. Hypophosphatasia has a variable outcome; antenatal detected hypopho-sphatasia, however, is lethal in most cases.

Limb Abnormalities

In *limb reduction deformities*, there is absence of an extremity or a segment of an extremity. The prevalence of limb reduction deformities is approximately 1 in 20,000 live births. In about 50% of cases, there are simple transverse reduction defi-ciencies of one forearm or hand without other anomalies. Isolated amputation of an extremity can be due to amniotic band syndrome, exposure to a teratogen or a vas-cular accident. In the remainder, there are multiple reduction deficiencies and internal or craniofacial abnormalities (64).

In *sirenomelia*, the characteristic feature is the presence of single or fused lower limbs. Other features include renal agenesis, a single umbilical artery, anal atresia, and absence of the lower part of the spine. It has been proposed that the condition is caused by a vascular steal phenomenon with the single, aberrant, umbilical artery stealing blood supply from the lower torso and limbs.

Split hand and foot syndrome refers to a group of disorders characterized by splitting of the hand and the foot into two parts; other terms include lobster-claw deformity and ectrodactyly. The conditions are classified into typical and atypical varieties. The typical variety consists of absence of both the middle digit and the metacarpal bone, resulting in a deep V-shaped central defect that clearly divides the hand and foot into a lateral and a medial part. The atypical variety is character-ized by a much wider cleft formed by a defect of the metacarpals and the middle digits; the cleft is U-shaped, with only the most lateral and medial digits remaining. Split hand and foot deformities can occur as isolated anomalies, but more commonly they are part of a more complex syndrome.

Clubhand deformities are classified into two main categories: radial and ulnar. Radial clubhand includes a wide spectrum of disorders that encompass absent thumb, thumb hypoplasia, thin first metacarpal, and absent radius. Ulnar clubhand, which is less common, ranges from mild deviations of the hand on the ulnar side of the forearm to complete absence of the ulna. Ulnar clubhand is usually an isolated anomaly. Radial clubhand is frequently associated with chromosomal abnormalities, hematological abnormalities (Fanconi's pancytopenia), or genetic syndromes.

Polydactyly is the presence of an additional digit, which may range from a fleshy nubbin to a complete digit with controlled flexion and extension. Postaxial polydactyly is the most common form and occurs on the ulnar side of the hand and the fibular side of the foot. Preaxial polydactyly is present on the radial side of the hand and the tibial side of the foot. The majority conditions are isolated with an autosomal dominant mode of inheritance. Some are part of a syndrome. Central polydactyly, which consists of an extra digit usually hidden between the long and the ring finger, is often bilateral and is associated with other hand and foot malformations.

Fetal akinesia deformity sequence is a heterogenous group of disorders with a birth prevalence of approximately 1 in 3000. Neurological, muscular, skeletal, and connective tissue abnormalities can result in multiple joint contractures including bilateral talipes and fixed flexion or extension deformities of the hips, elbows, and wrists. The deformities are usually symmetric and, in most cases, all four extremities are involved. The severity of the deformities increases distally in the involved limb, with the hands and feet typically being the most severely affected. The condition is commonly associated with polyhydramnios (usually after 25 weeks), narrow chest, micrognathia, and nuchal edema.

ABNORMALITIES OF THE PLACENTA, MEMBRANES, AND UMBILICAL CORD

Normal Ultrasound Appearances

Fetal anomaly scan should also involve examination of the placenta, the membranes, and the umbilical cord. The texture of the placenta, its size, its position, and the presence of abnormalities should be examined. Until 20 weeks' gestation, the placenta appears as a homogenous low-echoic mass with a small hypoechoic retroplacental zone as the separation between decidua and myometrium. With increasing gestation, echoic spots and hypoechoic areas will appear in the placenta. This process of placental maturation has been described in four stages by Grannum et al. (65). Before 20 weeks' gestation, the upper limit of normal placenta size is 3 cm and between 4 and 5 cm up to 40 weeks' gestation. Ultrasound examination does not usually involve a formal measurement of placental thickness. Placental position should be checked; when the placenta is found to be covering the internal os at 20 weeks' gestation, repeat examination should be performed after 34 weeks' gestation to demonstrate whether there is a placenta previa. At 32 to 34 weeks' gestation, the lower uterus segment is formed from the isthmus; the placenta will then be positioned away from the internal os.

In singleton pregnancies, chorioamniotic membranes are not visible on ultrasound scanning. However, chorioamniotic separation prior to the fusion of the membranes is a normal finding until 16 weeks' gestation.

The umbilical cord consists of the central umbilical vein and the two umbilical arteries spiraling around it. A transverse section of the umbilical cord will show the three vessels. The umbilical arteries can also be visualized with color Doppler showing the abdominal portion of the umbilical arteries beside the bladder.

Placental Abnormalities

Abnormal Placenta Size or Shape

A smaller than average placenta may be seen in pregnancies complicated by pregnancy-induced hypertension, intrauterine growth restriction, fetal trisomies, and in insulin-dependent diabetes with vascular pathology. A thickened placenta can be seen in different disorders like diabetes gravidarum, maternal anemia, hydrops fetalis, aneuploidies, intrauterine infections, placental bleeding, and hydatidiform mole (66).

A succenturiate lobe is an accessory lobe of the placenta attached to the main body of the placenta by blood vessels that pass through the membranes. Its presence should be reported as this accessory lobe may be retained following delivery resulting in postpartum hemorrhage or infection.

Placental Tumors

Hydatidiform mole is a trophoblastic tumor of the placenta and is the most common placental anomaly. On ultrasound, a classic "snowstorm" appearance is visible with multiple hypoechoic areas. No fetus is present. In partial mole (commonly a triploid pregnancy) a fetus is present.

The most common nontrophoblastic tumor is a chorioangioma. On ultrasound, it appears as a hypoechoic encapsulated mass, usually lying within the body of the placenta or close to, or protruding from, the cord insertion (Fig. 15). Color Doppler will show vessels within the tumor with usually high arterial flow. Large tumors are associated with fetal nonimmune hydrops, intrauterine growth restriction, and antepartum hemorrhage. Placental teratomas may also occur but are rare. Myometrial contractions or uterine fibroids may mimic placental tumors.

Placental "Lakes"

After 28 weeks' gestation, hypoechoic areas may be seen in the placenta. These blood-filled cavities are devoid of villi. These placental "lakes" are of no clinical significance, unless they are large and widespread.

Retroplacental Hematoma

Retroplacental hematoma can be seen in case of placental abruption or a threatened miscarriage. Ultrasound appearances are dependent on the stage of the hemorrhage. Acute hemorrhage is seen as a hypoechoic area, later becoming more inhomogenous and hyperechoic. Retroplacental veins, the most common finding in the retroplacental area, may mimic the ultrasound appearances of an acute hemorrhage. Hematoma may also occur subchorial.

Abnormalities of the Membranes

The presence of chorioamniotic membranes within the uterine cavity may be due to chorioamniotic separation, chorioamniotic elevation (in case of hemorrhage), or amniotic bands. The most widely held theory for the formation of a band within the uterine cavity is early amnion rupture. Amniotic bands may cause severe fetal

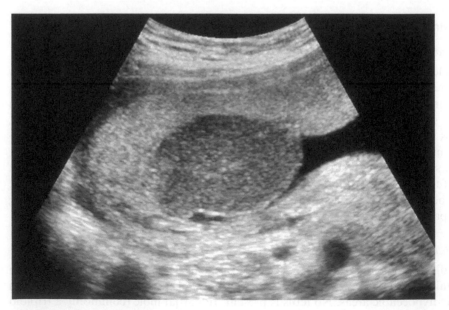

Figure 15   Chorioangioma. A hypoechoic encapsulated tumor of the placenta.

abnormalities as they become attached to the developing fetus. These abnormalities include limb defects, craniofacial abnormalities, and abdominal wall defects.

Umbilical Cord Abnormalities

Abnormal Number of Cord Vessels

Single umbilical artery is the most common abnormality of the umbilical cord; it occurs in 1% of all pregnancies. Single umbilical artery is associated with fetal structural abnormalities, aneuploidies, intrauterine growth restriction, and stillbirths. Four-vessels cord results from the persistence of the right umbilical vein or a vitelline artery. Allantoic or omphalomesenteric duct remnants may appear similar on ultrasound; distinction between duct remnants and vessels using color Doppler may be difficult since flow in small vessels may not always be detected. Cords with five and more vessels are associated with conjoined twins. Occasionally, the original primordial umbilical artery fails to divide longitudinally into two umbilical arteries. These cords present with three vessels at the placental end and two vessels at the fetal end.

Abnormal Cord Insertion and Vasa Previa

In velamentous insertion, the cord inserts on the chorioamniotic membranes rather than on the placental plate. A variable segment of the umbilical vessels runs between the amnion and the chorion, losing the protection of the Wharton's jelly. Velamentous insertion is eight to nine times more common in twin pregnancies than in singleton pregnancies. The most significant clinical problem arising from a velamentous insertion of the umbilical cord is vasa previa, a condition in which the velamentous umbilical vessels traverse the fetal membranes in the lower uterine segment below the presenting part. These unprotected vessels may rupture at any time during pregnancy, causing fetal exsanguination and death.

Abnormalities of the Umbilical Cord

Umbilical cord cysts developing from the remnants of the allantoic or omphalomesenteric duct are rare, and are of no clinical relevance. Hemangiomas formation of the umbilical cord is also a rare condition. It can be mistaken for an omphalocele if its location is near the fetal cord insertion. Occasionally, hemangiomas may impair the umbilical circulation and cause fetal demise.

In patent urachus, there is persistence of the communication between the fetal bladder and the umbilicus. In this case, the cord can be dilated due to urine absorption by Wharton's jelly. When no other structural abnormalities are found, prognosis is good.

Hematomas of the umbilical cord most often appear after funipuncture for diagnostic means.

REFERENCES

1. Alberman E. Perinatal mortality. In: Turnbull A, Chamberlain G, eds. Obstetrics. Edinburgh: Churchill Livingstone, 1989:1111–1119.
2. Kalter H, Warkany J. Congenital malformations (first of two parts). N Engl J Med 1983; 308:424–431.

3. Kalter H, Warkany J. Congenital malformations (second of two parts). N Engl J Med 1983; 308:491–497.
4. Kalter H. Five-decade international trends in the relation of perinatal mortality and congenital malformations: stillbirth and neonatal death compared. Int J Epidemiol 1991; 20:173–179.
5. Bucher HC, Schmidt JG. Does routine ultrasound scanning improve outcome in pregnancy? Meta-analysis of various outcome measures. Br Med J 1993; 307:13–17.
6. Saari-Kemppainen A, Karjalainen O, Ylostalo P, Heinonen P. Ultrasound screening and perinatal mortality: Controlled trial of systematic one-stage screening in pregnancy. Lancet 1990; 336:387–391.
7. Waldenstrom U, Nilsson S, Fall O, Axelsson O, Eklund G, Lindeberg S. Effects of routine one-stage ultrasound screening in pregnancy: A randomized controlled trial. Lancet 1988; 2:585–588.
8. Ewigman BG, Crane JP, Frigoletto FD, Lefevre ML, Bain RP, McNellis D and the RADIUS Study Group. Effect of prenatal ultrasound screening on perinatal outcome. N Engl J Med 1993; 329:821–827.
9. Goncalves FL, Jeanty P, Piper JC. The accuracy of prenatal ultrasonography in detecting congenital anomalies. Am J Obstet Gynecol 1994; 171:1606–1612.
10. Levi S, Hyjazi Y, Schaaps JP, Defoort P, Coulon R, Buekens P. Sensitivity and specificity of routine antenatal screening for congenital anomalies by ultrasound: The Belgian Multicentric Study. Ultrasound Obstet Gynecol 1991; 1:102–110.
11. EUROCAT Working Group. Surveillance of congenital anomalies in Europe 1980–1992 (report 6). 1995. European Union Project, Institute og Hygiene and Epidemiology, Brussels.
12. Ewigman B, Lefèvre M, Hesser J. A randomized trial of routine prenatal ultrasound. Obstet Gynecol 1990; 76:189–194.
13. Chitty LS, Hunt GH, Moore J, Lobb MO. Effectiveness of routine ultrasonography in detecting fetal structural abnormalities in a low risk population. BMJ 1991; 303: 1165–1169.
14. Carrera JM, Torrents M, Mortera C, Cusi V, Munez A. Routine prenatal ultrasound screening for fetal abnormalities: 22 years' experience. Ultrasound Obstet Gynecol 1995; 5:174–179.
15. Luck CA. Value of routine ultrasound scanning at 19 weeks: a four year study of 8849 deliveries. BMJ 1992; 304:1474–1478.
16. Shirley IM, Bottomley F, Robinson VP. Routine radiographer screening for fetal abnormalities in an unselected low risk population. Br J Radiol 1992; 65:564–569.
17. Crane JP, LeFevre ML, Winborn RC, et al. A randomized trial of prenatal ultrasonographic screening: Impact on the detection, management and outcome of anomalous fetuses. Am J Obstet Gynecol 1994; 171:392–399.
18. Grandjean H, Larroque D, Levi S, and the Eurofetus Study Group. The performance of routine ultrasonographic screening of pregnancies in the Eurofetus Study. Am J Obstet Gynecol 1999; 181:446–454.
19. Levi S. Routine ultrasound screening of congenital anomalies. An overview of the European experience. Ann N Y Acad Sci. 1998; 847:86–898. Review.
20. EUROCAT Working Group. Prevalence of neural tube defects in 20 regions of Europe and the impact of prenatal diagnosis, 1980–1986. J Epidemiol Community Health 1991; 45:52–58.
21. Wilkins-Haug L, Freedman W. Progression of exencephaly to anencephaly in the human fetus – an ultrasound perspective. Prenat Diagn 1991; 11(1):227–233.
22. Van den Hof MC, Nicolaides KH, Campbell J, Campbell S. Evaluation of the lemon and banana signs in one hundred and thirty fetuses with open spina bifida. Am J Obstet Gynecol 1990; 162:322–327.
23. Nicolaides KH, Campbell S, Gabbe SG, Guidetti R. Ultrasound screening for spina bifida: cranial and cerebellar signs. Lancet 1986; ii:72–74.

24. Nyberg DA, Mack LA, Hirsch J, Pagon RO, Shepard TH. Fetal hydrocephalus: sonographic detection and clinical significance of associated anomalies. Radiology 1987; 163:187–191.

25. Cardoza JD, Goldstein RB, Filly RA. Exclusion of fetal ventriculomegaly with a single measurement: the width of the lateral ventricular atrium. Radiology 1988; 169:711–714.

26. Serlo W, Kirkinen P, Jouppila P, Herva R. Prognostic signs in fetal hydrocephalus. Child's Nerv Syst 1986; 2:93–97.

27. Parrish M, Roessmen U, Levinsohn M. Agenesis of the corpus callosum: a study of the frequency of associated malformations. Ann Neurol 1979; 6:349–352.

28. McGahan JP, Nyberg DA, Mack LA. Sonography of facial features of alobar and semilobar holoprosencephaly. Am J Roentgenol 1990; 154(1):143–148.

29. Barkovich AJ, Kjos BO, Norman D, Edwards MS. Revised classification of posteroir fossa cysts and cystlike malformations based on the results of multiplanar MR imaging. Am J Roentgenol 1989; 153(6):1289–1300.

30. Goto MP, Goldman AS. Diabetic embryopathy. Curr Opin Paediatr 1994; 6:486–491.

31. Allan LD, Hornberger L, Sharland G. Textbook of fetal cardiology. London: Greenwich Medical Media Limited, 2000.

32. Sharland GK, Allan LD. Isolated pericardial effusion: an indication for fetal karyotyping?. Ultrasound Obstet Gynecol 1995; 6:29–32.

33. How HY, Villafane J, Parihus RR, Spinnato JA. Small hyperechogenic foci of the fetal cardiac ventricle: a benign sonographic finding?. Ultrasound Obstet Gynecol 1994; 4:205–207.

34. Simpson JM, Rowlands ML, Sharland GK. The significance of echogenic foci ('golfballs') in the fetal heart: a prospective study of 147 cases. (Abstract) BMUS meeting, Torquay;1995.

35. Allan L, Chita S, Maxwell D, Priestley K, Sharland G. Use of flecainide in fetal atrial tachycardia. Br Heart J 1991; 65:46–48.

36. Gembruch U, Hanasmann M, Redel DA, Bald R, Knopfle G. Fetal complete heart block: antenatal diagnosis, significance and management. Eur J Obst Gynecol 1989; 31:9–22.

37. Romero R, Chervenak FA, Kotzen J, et al. Antenatal sonographic findings of extralobular pulmonary sequestration. J Ultrasound Med 1982; 1:131–132.

38. De Vore GR, Hovenstein J, Platt LD. Fetal echocardiography: Assessment of cardiothoracic disproportion – A new technique for the diagnosis of thoracic hypoplasia. Am J Obstet Gynecol 1986; 155:1066–1071.

39. Gerards et al.

40. Sipes SL, Weiner CP, Wenstrom KD, et al. Fetal echogenic bowel on ultrasound – is there clinical significance? Fetal Diagn Ther 1994; 9:38–43.

41. Altman RP, Randolph JG, Lilly JR. Sacrococcygeal teratoma. American Academy of Pediatrics surgical section survey – 1973. J Pediatr Surg 1974; 9:389–398.

42. Kluck P, Tibboel D, Van der Kamp AWM, et al. The effect of fetal urine on the development of bowel in gastroschisis. J Pediatr Surg 1983; 18:47–50.

43. Phelan JP, Ahn MO, Smith CV. Amniotic Fluid Index measurements during pregnancy. J Reprod Med 1987; 32:627.

44. Barker AF, Cave MM, Thomas DFM, Lilford RJ,Irvine HC, Arthur RJ, Smith SEW. Fetal pelvi-ureteric junction obstruction: predictions of outcome. BR J Urol 1995; 76:649–652.

45. James CA, Watson AR, Twining P, Rance CH. Antenatally detected urinary tract abnormalities: changing incidence managment. Eur J Pediatr 1998; 157:508–511.

46. Cremin BJ. A review of the ultrasonic appearances of posterior urethral valve and ureterocoeles. Pediatr Radiol 1986; 16:357–364.

47. Al-Khaldi N, Watson AR, Zuccollo J, Twining P, Rose DH. Outcome of antenatally detected cystic dysplastic kidney disease. Arch Dis Child 1994; 70:520–522.

48. Zerres K. Autosomal recessive polycystic kidney disease. Clinical Investigator 1992; 70:794–901.
49. Hitchcock R, Burge DM. Renal agenesis: an acquired condition?. J Pediatr Surg 1994; 29:454–455.
50. Bronshtein M, Amil A, Achiron R, Noy I, Blumenfeld Z. The early prenatal diagnosis of renal agenesis: techniques and possibl pitfalls. Prenat Diagn 1994; 14:291–297.
51. Potter EL. Bilateral absence of ureters and kidneys: report of fifty cases. Obstet Gynecol 1965; 25:3–12.
52. Hill L, Peterson CS. Antenatal diagnosis of fetal pelvic kidneys. J Ultrasound Med 1987; 6:393–396.
53. Rutherford SE, Phelan JP, Smith CV. The four quadrant assessment of amniotic fluid volume: an adjunct to antepartum fetal heart rate testing. Obstet Gynecol 1987; 70:533.
54. Zamah NM, Gillieson MS, Walters JH, Hall PF. Sonographic detection of polyhydramnios: A five year experience. Am J Obstet Gynecol 1982; 143:523.
55. Koren G, Edwards MB, iskin M. Antenatal sonography for fetal malformations associated with drugs ad chemicals: a guide. Am J Obstet Gynecol 1987; 176:79–84.
56. McGahan JP, Nyberg DA, Mack LA. Sonography of facial features of alobar and semilobar holoprosencephaly. Am J Radiol 1990; 154:143–148.
57. Romero R, Pilu G, et al. Skeletal Dysplasias. In: Prenatal diagnosis of congenital anomalies (chapter 10). Norwalk: Appleton & Lange, 1988.
58. Genetic heterogeneity in osteogenesis imperfecta. J Med Genet 1979 Apr; 16(2):101–116.
59. Osteogenesis imperfecta type II delineation of the phenotype with reference to genetic heterogeneity. Am J Med Genet 1984 Feb; 17(2):407–423.
60. Maroteaux P, Frézal J, Cohen-Solal L, Bonaventure J. Les formes antenatles de l'ostéogenése imparfaite. Arch Fr Pediatr 1986; 43:235–241.
61. Saunders RC, Blaemore K. Lethal fetal anomalies. Sonographic demonstration. Radiology 1989; 172:1–6.
62. Achondrogenesis-hypochondrogenesis: the spectrum of chondrogenesis imperfecta. A radiological, ultrasonographic, and histopathologic study of 23 cases. Pediatr Pathol 1988; 8(6):571–597.
63. International classification of osteochondrodysplasias. International Working Group on Constitutional Diseases of Bone. Am J Med Genet. 1992 Sep 15; 44(2):223–229.
64. Firth HV, Boyd PA, Chamberlain P, et al. Severe limb abnormalities after chorionic villus sampling at 56–66 days gestation. Lancet 1991; 377:762.
65. Grannum PAT, Berkowitz RL, Hobbins JC. The ultrasonic changes in the maturing placenta and their relation to fetal pulmonic maturity. Am J Obstet Gynecol 1995; 5: 353–357.
66. Hoddick WK, Mahony BS, Callen PW, et al. Placental thickness. J Ultrasound Med 1985; 4:479–482.

19

The Role of Three-Dimensional Ultrasound in Prenatal Diagnosis

Leeber Cohen
Department of Obstetrics and Gynecology, Division of Reproductive Genetics,
Feinberg School of Medicine, Northwestern University, Chicago, Illinois, U.S.A.

INTRODUCTION

Surface rendering of the fetus from three-dimensional (3-D) volume sets was first reported by Baba and Sato in the mid-1980s (Figs. 1 and 2) (1). This was followed by reconstruction of a 3-D volume set as three orthogonal sections in the early 1990s (Fig. 3) (2). Widespread usage of the 3-D technique was initially hindered by the very slow processing speeds of the computers used to coordinate the reconstruction of the visual sections and by the need for these computer work stations to be separate from the ultrasound machine.

A variety of techniques have been used for acquiring 3-D volume sets. These include, but are not limited to, free-hand manual sweeps of traditional probes, mechanized probes championed commercially on the Kretz Voluson 530 in the mid-1990s, and matrix array electronically steered probes primarily used for adult cardiology. Real-time 3-D rendering with refresh rates of four frames per second became available on the Voluson 530 in the late 1990s and was rapidly followed by a much higher quality 16 frames per second on the Voluson 730. Mechanized probes have now been licensed from Kretz (now owned by General Electric) or separately developed by other ultrasound vendors.

Although sales of 3-D machines are rapidly increasing all over the world, there is little evidence that obstetric outcomes are affected by its use. There is also little evidence that the detection rate for fetal anomalies is improved in comparison to images obtained from 2-D technology. There are some preliminary data that suggest that counseling of patients with certain anomalies such as spina bifida and facial clefting is facilitated by being able to more carefully illustrate the anomaly to them. That being said, the increasing popularity of 3-D ultrasound is currently focused on the beauty and seductiveness of the fetal 3-D images for patients and clinicians alike. However, the potential of 3-D imaging as an important advancement in ultrasonographic diagnostics is likely to be lost on those who solely concentrate on rendered images. Multiplanar imaging with simultaneous display of three orthogonal planes, whether static or real time, has great potential to alter our abilities to diagnose

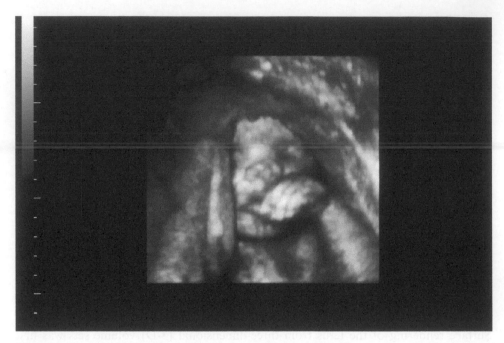

Figure 1 A typical rendering of a fetal face and hand at 30-weeks gestation obtained on the Voluson 530 in the late 1990s. (*See color insert.*)

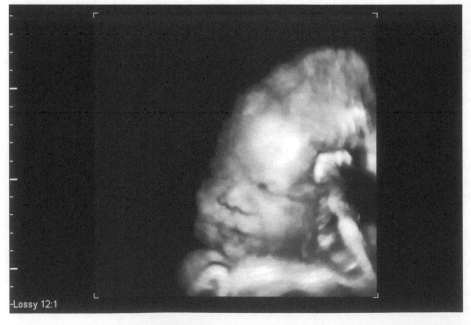

Figure 2 Another rendered fetal face obtained at 30 weeks. High quality rendering and real-time rendering are now available on mid-price machines.

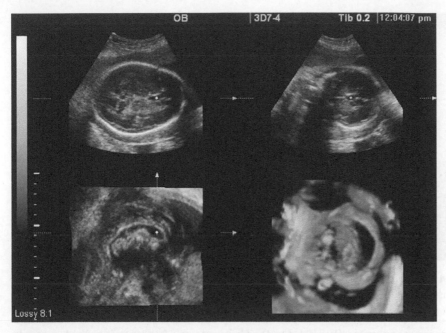

Figure 3 This 3-D study is displayed in three orthogonal planes. The volume was acquired in the axial plane at the level of the standard BPD. It is easy to scroll through all the axial cuts until the cavum is identified. The cavum can easily be identified in the coronal and midline sagittal planes by moving the marker dot into the cavum septum pellucidum in the axial cut. The midline sagittal cut can be further rotated to give routine visualization of the cavum, corpus callosum, third, and fourth ventricles.

pathology in pregnancies as well as adults. Essentially, the box of voxels (the volume equivalent of pixels in a flat plane) can be rotated and sliced in almost any direction with each of the planes able to be scrolled through from front to back, top to bottom, or side to side. Such capabilities allow the ultrasonographer to obtain multiple views of a particular organ, allowing for a more detailed assessment of fetal anatomy. An example of this is the determination of the volume obtained at the level of the standard biparietal diameter (BPD). Multiple axial, coronal, and sagittal planes can be obtained of the brain from a 1 to 2 second volume sweep from this volume assessment (Fig. 3), allowing for a detailed assessment of the fetal brain from a simple measurement of BPD and calculation of intracranial volume.

This chapter will thus seek to present the clinical potential of 3-D ultrasound by reviewing the current application of this technology in obstetrics and women's health care.

CONGENITAL UTERINE ANOMALIES

Jurkovic and colleagues in 1995 demonstrated that 3-D ultrasound clearly helped to differentiate arcuate from septate uteri (3). A more recent study by Woelfer and colleagues screened 1089 low-risk women and found 106 uterine anomalies (72 arcuate, 29 subseptate , and five bicornuate). The reconstructed coronal plane clearly allows for the differentiation of arcuate, thin membranous septums, thick vascular septums,

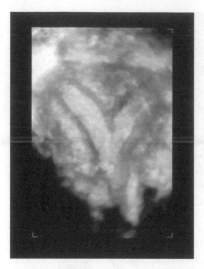

Figure 4 This coronal reconstruction illustrates a septated uterus. The contour of the uterine fundus is smooth. The initial volume was obtained from a midline sagittal cut.

and bicornuate uteruses (Figs. 4–6) (4). The contour of the uterine fundus can be clearly seen in contrast to X-ray fluoroscopy and this technique is clearly less expensive than magnetic resonance imaging and less invasive than endoscopy. In our own center, 3-D vaginal imaging without contrast has largely replaced X-ray fluoroscopy in the evaluation of the uterine cavity in women with repeated first trimester losses or

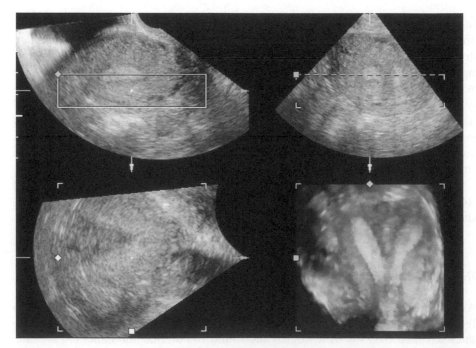

Figure 5 This coronal reconstruction reveals complete septation of the endometrial cavity and cervix. The contour of the uterine fundus is smooth.

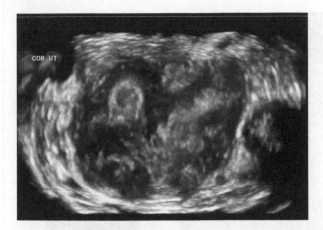

Figure 6 This coronal reconstruction displays a bicornuate uterus. The fundus is clearly notched more than 1 cm.

unexplained second trimester pregnancy loss. This subject is more thoroughly reviewed in a recent review article by Puscheck and Cohen (5).

FIRST TRIMESTER FETUS

The April 1995 issue of the *Journal of Ultrasound in Obstetrics and Gynecology* (Parthenon Publishing) is a nice starting place for those interested in the early developments and applications of 3-D ultrasound for prenatal diagnosis. Two editorials, the first by Kosoff and the second by Pretorius and Nelson, take a conservative and optimistic view of the potential of 3-D ultrasound (6,7). An article by Blaas et al. clearly illustrates the potential of 3-D ultrasound to provide beautiful reconstructions of the early embryonic brain cavity between 7 and 10 menstrual weeks that are strikingly similar to the illustrations from standard embryology textbooks (8). Merz et al. reviewed 204 fetal anomalies that had been detected by conventional ultrasound between 13 and 40 weeks gestation and evaluated with 3-D ultrasound. The 3-D views provide more detailed information concerning the malformations (9).

Despite the presence of many case reports and descriptive studies of early diagnosis of fetal anomalies evaluated with 3-D in the literature, there is little strong scientific evidence to suggest that this technology is superior to that of conventional ultrasound for the detection of first-trimester anomalies. Indeed, the advocacy of the 12 to 14 transvaginal 3-D anatomic survey is exemplified in the editorial by Bonilla-Musoles in 1996 (10), the initial detailed 3-D reconstructions of the fetal embryo starting at 7 weeks were described by Blaas et al. in 1999 (Figs. 7 and 8) (11).

The first study, by Hull et al. (12), directly comparing early transvaginal 2-D and 3-D images with independent review was not published until 2001. The authors compared biometry, nuchal measurements, and anatomy in 32 patients scanned at 12 to 14 weeks using the Medison 530D. Two-Dimensional and 3-D transvaginal studies were performed by the same examiner using the identical probe and then all films and volumes were independently reviewed. Satisfactory biometry measurements were obtained more frequently in 3-D than 2-D (HC-84% vs. 50%, AC-72% vs. 16%).

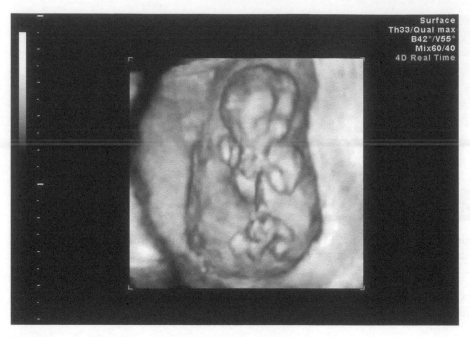

Figure 7 A rendered 12-week fetus is displayed. (*See color insert.*)

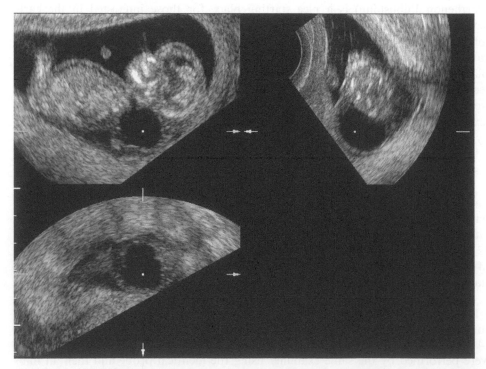

Figure 8 A cystic hygroma is displayed orthogonally. *Source*: Courtesy of GE Healthcare, Milwaukee, Wisconsin.

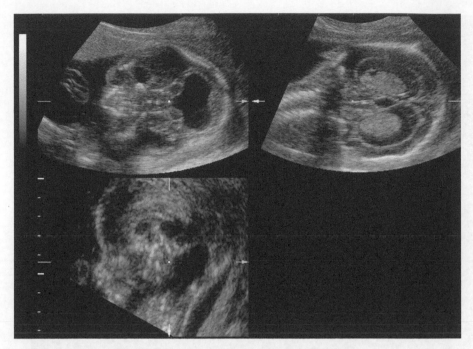

Figure 9 This third trimester 3-D orthogonal display clearly demonstrates a fetus with a Dandy–Walker malformation. *Source*: Courtesy of GE Healthcare, Milwaukee Wisconsin.

Nuchal measurements were obtained in 31 of 32 fetuses by 3-D transvaginal sonography (TVS) versus 12 of 32 fetuses by 2-D TVS. The authors state that stomach, cord insertion, choroid plexus, cerebral ventricles, and hands were seen in significantly more subjects among the 2-D cohort, with another major advantage of the 2-D approach being the significantly shorter time in which the vaginal probe must remain inserted in the patient. Unfortunately, the study was small and was not performed with one of the newer and higher resolution 3-D machines.

Despite the possible advantages of early 12 to 14 weeks' 3-D TVS studies, there has been minimal advocacy of this technique in the United States. As noted by Timor-Tritsch and Copel in two separate editorials discussing pros and cons from 2001, the United States has been very slow to adapt or explore the 14 to 16 weeks' transvaginal 2-D anatomic surveys despite their increasing use in Europe and Asia (13). Articles by Broshtein et al. and Harnandi et al. have shown that many of the birth defects detectable at 20 to 22 weeks can be identified earlier by transvaginal scans (14,15). The notable exceptions are cardiac anomalies, and brain and renal defects manifesting themselves in the late second and third trimester. Clearly, with the increasing interest in nuchal screening at 12 to 14 weeks' gestation, the 12 to 14 week anatomic survey with either 2-D or 3-D technique needs to be carefully investigated.

Brain

Timor-Tritsch and Monteagudo in 1996 described the technique of prenatal transvaginal neurosonography using the anterior fontanelle as acoustic window (16). The high resolution transvaginal imaging and the minimal acoustic attenuation provided

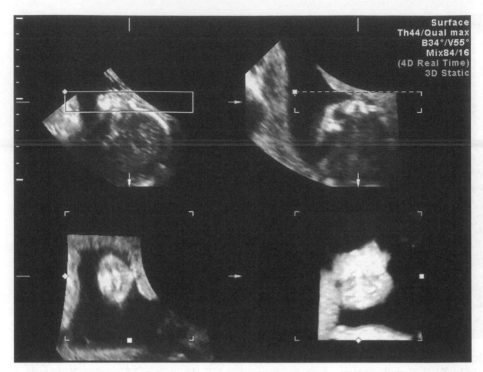

Figure 10 This 3-D rendering of a 20-week fetus illustrates a normal nose and lip. Improved resolution at 20 weeks will be needed for this technique to be more clinically useful earlier in gestation.

high quality images resembling the images seen with the imaging of neonatal crania. The major disadvantage of the technique was that it required the fetal head to be centrally located in the occiput position. This 3-D transvaginal neurosonographic technique was subsequently reported by the initial investigators to be applicable to a wider spectrum of cranial anatomic assessment (17,18). Cohen et al. in 1999 evaluated the technique of transabdominal 3-D volume acquisition at the level of the standard axial BPD (Fig. 3) (19). Satisfactory visualization of the midline sagittal cut including the cavum septum pellucidum and overlying corpus callosum was possible in approximately 50% of cases at 20 to 22 weeks gestation using the transabdominal technique. The image quality of the 530D was felt to be a major limiting parameter in not obtaining a higher rate of satisfactory images.

Whether done by TVS or transabdominal sonography (TAS), 3-D offers obvious advantages for those performing neurosonography (Fig. 9). The third missing set of planes in 2-D imaging is automatically reconstructed and, with minimal rotation, exact standard anatomic cuts can be displayed. Each plane can be navigated through and the location in the other planes is immediately displayed by a marker dot. Endres and Cohen in 2000 published a 3-D study looking at normative cross-sectional brain volumes during the second and third trimester and found that the 3-D approach was characterized by excellent intraobserver and interobserver reliability with brain volumes that correlated well with standard BPD and head circumference measurements. Accordingly, brain volumes could be used to accurately estimate gestational age with similar accuracy currently observed with conventional measurements of BPD and head circumference (20).

Cleft Lip and Palate

Potential advantages of 3-D ultrasound in evaluating the fetal face and cleft lip and palate were offered by Pretorius et al. in 1995 (21). Lee et al. in 2000 confirmed that 3-D allowed better prenatal classification of the extent of clefting (22). An editorial by Carlson found that 3-D was clearly more satisfactory for assessing the extent of a cleft lip and or palate and that it allowed for improved counseling (23). Unfortunately, both the above studies were performed with fetuses above 24 weeks (Fig. 10) and there are few data to suggest that 3-D visualization improves the ability to detect fetal lip or palatal clefting earlier in gestation.

Cardiac Anomalies

Initial papers by Zosmer et al., Nelson et al., Sklansky et al., and Deng et al., as well as others in the mid-1990s, suggested that 3-D ultrasound might be helpful in the evaluation of the anatomy and function of the fetal heart (24–27). All papers suggested that it might be easier to obtain standard cardiac views from navigation and rotation through a volume set. However, the lack of a good technique for gating and less than optimal image quality were major concerns. Efforts at the end of the 1990s centered around development of fetal cardiac gating so that accurate calculations of chamber volumes and ejection fractions could be obtained.

The last few years have generated a great deal of excitement regarding the potential applications of 3-D color and power Doppler imaging to provide a more detailed assessment of the fetal heart. Studies by Devore et al., Vinals et al., and Chaoui et al. appeared in 2003 and 2004 regarding the use of spatiotemporal image correlation (color Doppler) technology for the evaluation of the fetal heart (Figs. 11 and 12) (28–30). This technology allows for the acquisition of a volume of data from a single cardiac cycle and allows a combination of color Doppler with multiplanar imaging. The ability to navigate and rotate through the various planes at varying points during the cardiac cycle theoretically should allow experts to better evaluate fetal cardiac anomalies. As this technology permits not just an improved view of fetal cardiac anatomy but also provides an assessment of cardiac function, it is possible that a routine 3-D cine-clip volume of the fetal heart may eventually become part of a standard fetal anatomic examination. With the expanding availability of telemedicine ultrasound practices, this technology would also allow for routine assessment of cardiac outflow tracts by the attending physician reading the scan and a telemedicine review by subspecialists. Nonetheless, large series will be required to demonstrate an outcome or economic benefit of this technology before it is incorporated into routine obstetrical care.

Sklansky et al. in 2004 described an initial series of fetuses with cardiac anomalies scanned with real-time instantaneous cardiac rendering (31). The probes in this study used a matrix-phased array that had been previously developed for adult cardiac images. Many expect that this probe technology represents a marked improvement over current motor-driven probes now used for both static and live 3-D. Advancements such as these will invariably make the prenatal assessment of fetal cardiac

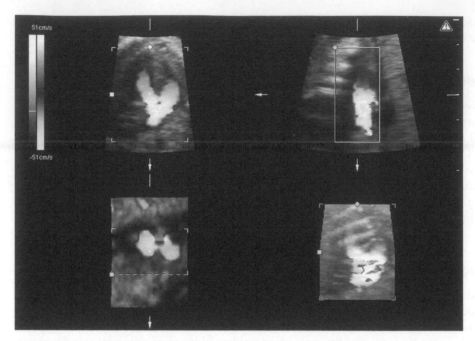

Figure 11 A third-trimester study of a fetus with transformation of the major vessels. *Source*: Courtesy of GE Healthcare, Milwaukee, Wisconsin. (*See color insert*.)

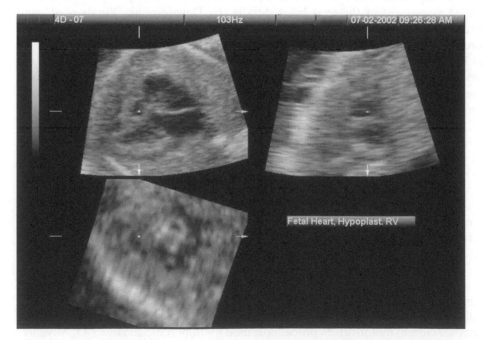

Figure 12 A third-trimester study revealing a hypoplastic right heart. *Source*: Courtesy of GE Healthcare, Milwaukee, Wisconsin.

structure and function available to a wider number of people and provide for a more accurate examination that will allow for more accurate counseling of women found to be carrying fetuses with cardiac anomalies.

Nuchal Translucency Testing

Kurjak et al. in 1999 suggested that 3-D imaging may improve the measurement of the nuchal translucency (Fig. 13A,B) (32). Another article by Chung et al. in 2000 also reported on the potential of 3-D technology to provide important and accurate information concerning first-trimester fetal nuchal translucency (33). Much larger controlled studies with newer equipment, by both TAS and TVS, will be needed to assess the potential of 3-D ultrasound to more accurately measure the nuchal translucency for calculating risks for fetal Down syndrome and trisomy 18 in first- and second-trimester screening protocols.

Neural Tube Defects

In a series of nine fetuses ranging from 18 to 26 weeks, Lee and colleagues (2002) described the potential advantages of characterizing neural tube defects with 3-D multiplanar imaging (Fig. 14) (34). The authors found that multiplanar views were generally more informative than rendered views for localizing bony defects of the fetal spine but that the level of the defect on 3-D ultrasound correlates well with conventional 2-D views. The authors further felt that although 3-D ultrasound did not provide considerable improvement over 2-D scans for the delineation of second trimester neural tube defects, the ability of 3-D ultrasound to provide complementary information after the initial detection of the neural tube defect by 2-D scanning may provide benefit in some cases. However, a more likely advantage of 3-D ultrasound for the detection of fetal neural tube defects may be in the ability to detect these lesions earlier than is currently feasible with conventional 2-D technology. Blaas et al. have described early detection of spina bifida in three fetuses prior to 10 weeks using transvaginal ultrasound (35), thus creating the possibility of using 3-D ultrasound to provide an accurate determination of the presence of fetal neural tube defects during the first trimester in women at increased risk for having affected fetuses.

Organ Volume

The measurement of fetal organ volumes may provide a new approach to the detection of anomalies as well as the monitoring of fetal growth and development. Fetal lung volume measurements have been described using a multiplanar technique and with rotational (vocal) pathology. These two techniques and a review of the literature can be found in a recent article by Kalache et al. (36). Fetal liver volume normative values using 3-D have been published by Kuno et al. (37).

Power Doppler Mapping

The ability of 3-D ultrasound to assess Doppler wave forms in fetal and placental circulations represents another potential advancement in prenatal diagnosis. Measuring these wave forms by 3-D ultrasound provides a unique assessment of

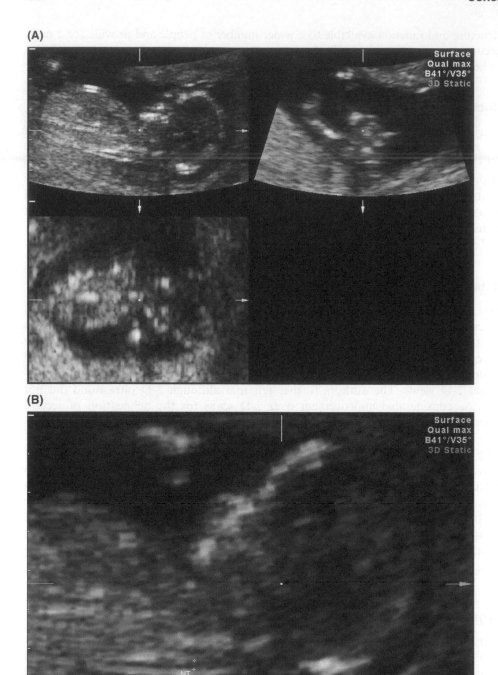

Figure 13 (A) A 13-week fetus is displayed orthogonally. The nuchal could not be measured in 2-D due to axis of fetus. (B) The fetus was rotated using the above volume set and the nuchal measurement easily obtained. This technique may improve visualization of both the nuchal area and nasal bone, and allow for scrolling through the data set to obtain other fetal anatomy.

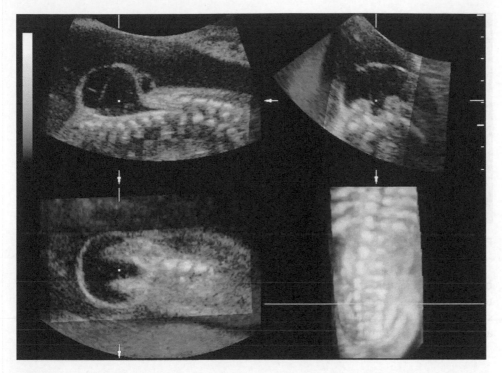

Figure 14 This third trimester 3-D orthogonal study of a spina bifida clearly demonstrates the location and number of affected vertebral processes. *Source*: Courtesy of GE Healthcare, Milwaukee, Wisconsin.

blood flow patterns in a variety of vessels and organ systems, potentially providing new and unique information concerning vasculature structure, function, and fetal well-being. The emerging role of 3-D power Doppler in mapping the fetal and placental circulation has been well illustrated and reviewed by Lee and colleagues (38), who found that this approach was an important adjunctive method for the characterization of normal vascular development and circulatory anomalies of the fetus.

SUMMARY

Three-dimensional ultrasound technological advancements as well as the novel clinical prenatal applications utilizing this technology, continue to progress. In particular, the use of mechanized probes rather than free sweeps has made volume acquisition, and thus structural organic evaluation, much simpler. The further development of phased-array matrix probes should theoretically allow for improvement in volume set data acquisition, further simplifying and accelerating the 3-D ultrasound examination. As with any new technology, clinical advancements are unfortunately associated with unscrupulous uses and applications. To this end, the use and misuse of 3-D ultrasound has been well reviewed by Benacerraf (39). Three-dimensional ultrasonography represents technical and clinical advancements in the field of prenatal ultrasonography. Nonetheless, no matter how impressive initial reports of this technology may be (Fig. 15), the promise of 3-D ultrasound can only be evaluated

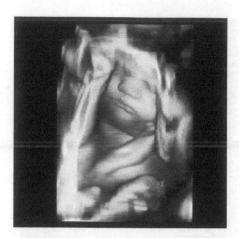

Figure 15 A 36-week rendered face.

by rigorous scientific trials and clinically relevant cost-effectiveness studies. Indeed, until the benefits and cost effectiveness of 3-D ultrasound have been well demonstrated (40), this technology will largely remain an experimental and adjunctive assessment of fetal anatomy, function, and well-being.

REFERENCES

1. Baba K, Satoh K. Development of the system for ultrasonic fetal three-dimensional reconstruction. Acta Obstet Gynaecol Jpn 1986; 38:1385.
2. Riccabona M, Pretorius DH, Nelson TR, Johnson D, Budorick NE. Three-dimensional ultrasound: display modalities in obstetrics. J Clin Ultrasound 1997; 25:157–167.
3. Jurkovic D, Geipel A, Gruboeck K, Jauniaux E, Natucci M, Campbell S. Three-dimensional ultrasound for the assessment of uterine anatomy and the detection of congenital anomalies. Ultrasound Obstet Gynecol 1995; 5:233–237.
4. Woelfer B, Salim R, Banerjee S, Elson J, Regan L, Jurkovic D. Reproductive outcomes in women with congenital anomalies detected by three-dimensional ultrasound screening. Obstet Gynecol 2001; 98:1099–1103.
5. Puscheck E, Cohen L. The diagnosis of congenital uterine anomalies: the role of 3-D ultrasonography. Female Patient 2004; 29:7–15.
6. Kossoff G. Three dimensional ultrasound-technology push or market pull? Ultrasound Obstet Gynecol 1995; 5:217–218 (Editorial).
7. Pretorius DH, Nelson TR. Three-dimensional ultrasound. Ultrasound Obstet Gynecol 1995; 5:219–221.
8. Blaas HG, Eik-Nes SH, Kiserud T, Berg S, Angelsen B, Olstad B. Three dimensional imaging of the brain cavities in human embryos. Ultrasound Obstet Gynecol 1995; 5:228–232.
9. Merz E, Bahlmann F, Weber G. Volume scanning in the evaluation of fetal malformations: a new dimension in prenatal diagnosis. Ultrasound Obstet Gynecol 1995; 5:222–228.
10. Bonilla-Musoles F. Three dimensional visualization of the human embryo: a potential revolution in prenatal diagnosis. Ultrasound Obstet Gynecol 1996; 7:393–397.
11. Blaas HG, Eik-Nes SH, Berg S, Torp H. In vivo three-dimensional ultrasound reconstructions of embryos and early fetuses. Lancet 1998; 352:1182–1186.

12. Hull AD, James J, Salerno CS, Nelson T, Pretorius DH. Three-dimensional ultrasonography and assessment of the first-trimester fetus. J Ultrasound Med 2001; 20: 287–294.
13. Timor-Tritsch I, Copel J. Point/counterpoint. Transvaginal sonographic evaluation of fetal anatomy at 14–16 weeks. J Ultrasound Med 2001; 20:705–712.
14. Broshstein M. Fetal scanning between 18 and 22 weeks is passé. Ultrasound Obstet Gynecol 2000; 16:69.
15. Harnandi L, Torocsik M. Screening for fetal anomalies in the 12th week of pregnancy by transvaginal sonography in an unselected population. Prenat Diagn 1997; 17:753–759.
16. Timor-Tritsch IE, Monteagudo A. Transvaginal fetal neurosonography: standardization of planes and sections using anatomic landmarks. Ultrasound Obstet Gynecol 1996; 8:42–47.
17. Timor-Tritsch IE, Montageudo A, Mayberry P. Three-dimensional ultrasound evaluation of the fetal brain: the three horn view. Ultrasound Obstet Gynecol 2000; 16:302–306.
18. Montageudo A, Timor-Tritsch IE, Mayberry P. Three-dimensional neurosonography of the fetal brain: "navigating" in the volume scan. Ultrasound Obstet Gynecol 2000; 16:307–313.
19. Cohen LS, Sankpal R, Endres L. Transabdominal three-dimensional volume imaging of the fetal brain at 18–24 weeks gestation. Int J Obstet Gynecol 2001; 72:145–150.
20. Endres L, Cohen L. Reliability and validity of 3-D fetal brain volumes. J Ultrasound Med 2001; 20:1265–1270.
21. Pretorius DH, House M, NelsonTR, Hollenbach KA. Evaluation of normal and abnormal lips in fetuses: comparison between three-and two-dimensional sonography. AJR Am J Roentgenol 1995; 165:1223–1227.
22. Lee W, Kirk JS, Shaheen KW, Romeo R, Hodges AN, Comstock CH. Fetal cleft lip and palate detection by three-dimensional ultrasonography. Ultrasound Obstet Gynecol 2000; 16:314–320.
23. Carlson DE. Opinion. The ultrasound evaluation of cleft lip and palate—a clear winner for 3D. Ultrasound Obstet Gynecol 2000; 16:299–301.
24. Zosmer N, Jurkovic D, Jauniaux E, Gruboeck K, Lees C, Campbell S. Selection and identification of standard cardiac views from three-dimensional volume scan of the fetal thorax. J Ultrasound Med 1996; 15:25–32.
25. Nelson TR, Pretorius DH, Sklansky M, Hagen-Ansert S. Three-dimensional echocardiographic evaluation of the fetal heart anatomy and function. J Ultrasound Med 1996; 15:1–9.
26. Sklansky MS, Nelson TR, Pretorius DH. Usefulness of gated three-dimensional fetal echocardiography to reconstruct and display structures not seen with two-dimensional imaging. Am J Cardiol 1997; 80:665–668.
27. Deng J, Gardener JE, Rodeck CH, Lees WR. Fetal echocardiography in three and four dimensions. Ultrasound Med Biol 1996; 22:979–986.
28. Devore GR, Falkensammer P, Sklansky MS, Platt LD. Spatio-temporal image correlation (STIC): new technology for evaluation of the fetal heart. Ultrasound Obstet Gynecol 2003; 22:380–382.
29. Vinals F, Poblete P, Guliano A. Spatio-temporal image correlation (STIC): a new tool for screening of congenital heart defects. Ultrasound Obstet Gynecol 2003; 22: 388–394.
30. Chaoui R, Hoffman J, Heling KS. Three-dimensional (3D) and 4D color Doppler fetal echocardiography using spatio-temporal image correlation (STIC). Ultrasound Obstet Gynecol 2004; 23:535–545.
31. Sklansky MS, Devore G, Wong PC. Real-time 3-dimensional fetal echocardiography with instantaneous volume-rendered display. J Ultrasound Med 2004; 23:283–289.
32. Kurjak A, Kupesic S, Ivancic-Kosuta M. Three-dimensional transvaginal ultrasound improves measurement of the nuchal translucency. J Perinat Med 1999; 27:97–102.

33. Chung BL, Kim HJ, Lee KH. The application of three-dimensional ultrasound to nuchal translucency measurement in early pregnancy (10–14 weeks); a preliminary study. Ultrasound Obstet Gynecol 2000; 15:122–125.

34. Lee W, Chaiworapongsa T, Romero R, et al. A diagnostic approach for the evaluation of spina bifida by three-dimensional ultrasonography. J Ultrasound Med 2002; 21:619–626.

35. Blaas HG, Eik-Nes SH, Isaksen CV. The detection of spina bifida before 10 gestational weeks using two and 3-dimensional ultrasound. Ultrasound Obstet Gynecol 2000; 16: 25–29.

36. Kalache KD, Espinoza J, Chaiworapongsa T, et al. Three dimensional ultrasound fetal lung volume measurement: a systematic study comparing the multiplanar method with rotational (vocal) technique. Ultrasound Obstet Gynecol 2003; 21:111–118.

37. Kuno A, Hayashi Y, Akiyama M, et al. Three-dimensional sonographic measurement of liver volume in small for gestational age fetus. J Ultrasound Med 2002; 21:361–366.

38. Lee W, Karache K, Chaiworapongsa T, et al. Three-dimensional power Doppler ultrasonography during pregnancy. J Ultrasound Med 2003; 22:91–97.

39. Benacerraf B. Three-dimensinoal fetal sonography: use and misuse. J Ultrasound Med 2002; 21:1063–1068 (Editorial).

40. Filly RA, Crane JP. Routine obstetric sonography. J Ultrasound Med 2002; 21:713–718.

20

Fetal Magnetic Resonance Imaging

Deborah Levine

*Department of Radiology, Beth Israel Deaconess Medical Center,
Boston, Massachusetts, U.S.A.*

INTRODUCTION

Ultrasonography is the method of choice for imaging the fetus. However, there are instances when additional information is helpful in counseling and managing the pregnant patient. In the past, pelvic magnetic resonance imaging (MRI) was used during pregnancy to evaluate maternal abnormalities such as adnexal masses, that required further characterization beyond that available with ultrasound. Although adnexal structures could be visualized with conventional techniques, fetal anatomy typically could not be adequately assessed due to degradation of image quality by fetal motion during the relatively long acquisition times (1–3).

In order to decrease fetal motion, recommendations were made to limit imaging to late pregnancy or to cases of oligohydramnios (4,5). Other investigators used benzodiezepines to sedate the pregnant patient, or curarization by direct fetal injection to decrease fetal motion (6,7). Subsequently, echo planar imaging was advocated for obstetric MRI since its short (100 milliseconds) scan time makes fetal paralysis unnecessary (8). However, echo planar imaging has several disadvantages including susceptibility artifacts, chemical shift artifacts, and limited availability due to special hardware requirements (9). Despite these limitations, fetal MRI was suggested as an important technique to evaluate anomalous fetuses.

In the past decade, fast scan techniques have been developed that allow for visualization of fetal anatomy in a manner not possible previously. Using fast scan techniques, images can be obtained in less than 1 second, allowing for imaging the fetus without maternal or fetal sedation. MRI is typically utilized for evaluation of the anomalous fetal central nervous system (CNS), for further characterization of complex fetal anomalies that are not fully characterized by ultrasound, and for evaluation of patients desiring fetal surgery. In these cases, MR imaging may provide additional information that can aid in pregnancy management.

This chapter covers techniques for performing fetal MRI and current applications in imaging the pregnant patient.

SAFETY OF MRI IN PREGNANCY

MRI is felt to be safe for use in pregnancy. As for all patients, there are absolute contraindications to MRI (e.g., a ferromagnetic cerebral aneurysm clip) and some patients are too claustrophobic to undergo the examination. While the use of short bore magnets makes claustrophobia less of a concern, an additional problem is that pregnant patients may have difficulty lying on their backs, especially in the third trimester.

There are no known biological risks from MRI. No delayed sequelae from MRI examination have been encountered, and it is expected that the potential risk for any delayed sequelae is extremely small or nonexistent (10–16). According to the Safety Committee of the Society for Magnetic Resonance Imaging (17), MRI procedures are indicated for use in pregnant women if other nonionizing forms of diagnostic imaging are inadequate, or if the examination provides important information that would otherwise require exposure to ionizing radiation (i.e., X-ray, CT, etc.). It is required that pregnant patients be informed that, to date, although there is no indication that the use of clinical MRI procedures during pregnancy produces deleterious effects, according to the Food Drug Administration, the safety of MRI procedures during pregnancy has not been definitively proven (14).

Also, it is well known that dividing cells, as in the case of the developing embryo during the first trimester, are susceptible to injury from a variety of physical agents. Because of limited data, we avoid MRI in the first trimester whenever feasible. For fetal imaging, this typically is not an issue since the small fetal size in the first trimester is difficult to evaluate with MRI. However, when there is a maternal condition that requires imaging with a modality other than ultrasound, MRI is a reasonable alternative, regardless of the trimester of pregnancy (18).

Gadolinium, the contrast agent used for MRI, is not recommended for use in pregnancy (19). It is considered a pregnancy category C drug (meaning that it should be given only if potential benefit outweighs the risk) since animal studies have revealed adverse effects, but no controlled studies have been performed in humans (19).

Gadolinium has been shown to cross the placenta and appear within the fetal bladder only moments after intravenous administration (20). From the fetal bladder, the contrast is excreted into the amniotic fluid where it is then swallowed, and potentially reabsorbed from the gastrointestinal tract. Because of this reabsorption, the half-life of gadolinium in the fetal circulation is not known (20). Therefore, for fetal imaging, gadolinium is not utilized.

CONDITIONS UNIQUE TO PREGNANCY THAT
MAY REQUIRE MRI

Pelvimetry

In the past, methods to perform pelvimetry involved exposure of the patient to ionizing radiation. Although pelvimetry is no longer commonly performed, it is beneficial in patients who desire a trial of labor when the fetus is in breech presentation (21–23). In cases where pelvimetry is requested, MRI offers the benefit of accurate measurement of the bony structures in the pelvis without ionizing radiation.

For MRI pelvimetry, gradient echo techniques are utilized, with scan times of less than 5 minutes (23,24). A midline sagittal view is obtained for assessment of the fetal presentation and for measurement of the anteroposterior pelvic inlet diameter (from the sacral promontory to the posterosuperior margin of the pubic symphysis). Oblique coronal views (parallel to the anteroposterior pelvic inlet) are obtained for measurement of the pelvic inlet (maximum distance between the arcuate lines of the iliac bones on either side) and bispinous diameter (23).

Using acceptable values of >11.0 cm for the anteroposterior pelvic inlet, >9.5 cm for the transverse midpelvic distance (interspinal distance), and >11.0 cm for the pelvic outlet, van Loon et al. (23) showed that while use of MRI pelvimetry in breech presentation at term did not reduce the overall cesarean-section rate, it allowed better selection of the delivery route with a significantly lower emergency cesarean-section rate.

Placental Evaluation

A number of case reports have recommended MRI for the evaluation of placenta accreta (25–28), however, one case series showed that transvaginal sonography with a partially full bladder was best for most cases of suspected accreta, with MRI being helpful in a case with a posterior placenta accreta after myomectomy (Fig. 1) (29). MRI findings of placenta accreta or one of its variants include focal exophytic masses and absence of visualized myometrium.

MRI can be utilized to assess placental abnormalities such as placenta previa, succenturiate lobe, vasa previa, and chorioangioma (2,30–34).

Ectopic Pregnancy

Ectopic pregnancy is typically diagnosed sonographically. At times, the diagnosis is uncertain, or additional questions regarding anatomy require further imaging. Figure 2 illustrates the appearance of an abdominal ectopic at term.

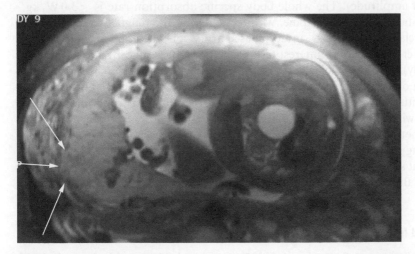

Figure 1 Axial view of the uterus in a patient with placenta accreta after myomectomy. Note the small region where the placenta extends out of the confines of the myometrium (*arrows*). This region was not adequately assessed on ultrasound, and was only visible on the MRI. Placenta accreta was found at the time of cesarean section. *Abbreviation*: MRI, magnetic resonance imaging.

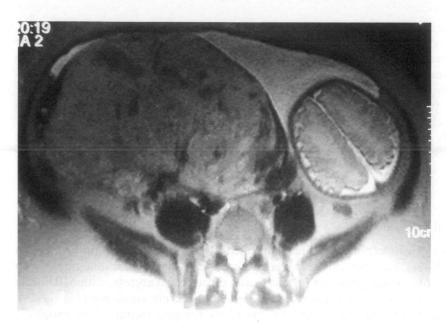

Figure 2 Transverse view of the maternal pelvis in a patient with an abdominal ectopic pregnancy at 35-weeks gestation. Note the lack of myometrium surrounding the pregnancy. Delivery was performed by laparotomy, and the placenta was left in situ. *Source*: Courtesy of Sue Ulrich, Perth, Australia.

FETAL IMAGING TECHNIQUES

The MR images in this chapter were obtained with a 1.5 T superconducting system (Siemens Vision, Erlangen, Germany or General Electric Signa Excite Twin Speed (Milwaukee, WI). The minimum gradient rise time is 600 microseconds (for a 25 mT peak gradient amplitude). The whole body specific absorption rate is <3.0 W/kg.

We position the patient supine, with feet entering the magnet to minimize the possibility of claustrophobia. A surface phased array coil with four or eight elements is centered over the region of interest (established on ultrasound performed prior to the MRI study). A pillow is placed below the patient's knees. If the patient is uncomfortable lying on her back for prolonged periods, then the patient is imaged in the lateral decubitus position. For women with a history of claustrophobia, sedation can be given with sublingual benzodiazepines.

Fetal motion presents a challenge for MRI. Since the fetus is commonly moving during the examination, it is best to have each sequence serve as a scout for subsequent sequences. Sequences are repeated as needed when fetal motion limits evaluation of the region of interest.

T2 Weighted Imaging

Most fetal imaging is performed with half Fourier single shot rapid acquisition with relaxation enhancement (RARE) technique (Fig. 3). With this T2 weighted sequence fluid is bright. Since the fetus has a large amount of water in the soft tissues, there is excellent soft tissue contrast (35).

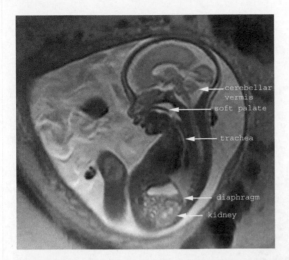

Figure 3 Sagittal T2 weighted image of fetus at 26-weeks gestational age. The heterogeneous signal intensity in the fluid surrounding the fetus is due to motion artifact. Note that although the amniotic fluid is moving (as demonstrated by regions of lower signal intensity), the fetal anatomy is well visualized.

After a three-dimensional (3D) scout is obtained, and T2 weighted imaging is performed in the fetal sagittal, coronal, and axial planes. A typical sequence for fetal imaging uses an echo spacing of 4.2 milliseconds, a $TE_{effective}$ of 60 milliseconds, an echo train length of 72, 1 acquisition, and a 4 mm section thickness. The field of view (FOV) is tailored to fetal and patient size such that the smallest FOV is utilized that allows for fetal imaging without overlap of maternal structures into the region of interest. A 192×256 or 256×512 acquisition matrix is utilized. A 130–155° refocusing pulse is used to minimize the amount of radiofrequency power deposition. The slice thickness can be decreased to 3 mm when the fetus is of early gestational age or if the structure being evaluated is small. Alternatively, in large patients in the third trimester, slices of 5 mm thickness often give better signal to noise ratio.

The acquisition time per image is 300–1400 milliseconds. A 1 second or greater delay between image acquisitions minimizes the specific absorption rate and allows for improved signal to noise ratio in adjacent slices. As the RARE sequence is a single slice acquisition technique, it limits artifacts related to maternal and fetal motion (35), since only the slice in which the motion occurred will be affected. This will generally lead to nonvisualization of a portion of the fetal anatomy, but may lead to repeated visualization of a fetal part (35). For example, if an extremity moves in plane with the sequence, it may be visualized more than once during a series of images.

T1 Weighted Imaging

T1 weighted imaging (Fig. 4) is more difficult than T2 weighted imaging of the fetus since there is less inherent soft tissue contrast. In addition, since most T1 weighted sequences are not single shot, the images are degraded by motion that occurs during the breath-hold. We currently employ spoiled gradient echo technique in and out of phase with the following parameters: TR = 180; TE = 2.2 and 4.5; Flip angle = 80°; 5 mm slice thickness; FOV = 36 cm; Matrix = 160×256; Scan time = 17 seconds

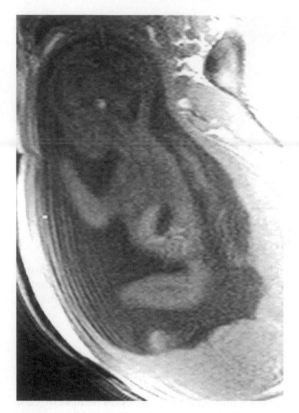

Figure 4 Sagittal T1 weighted image of fetus at 24-weeks gestational age. Note the motion that degrades the image, and overall poor contrast in the image.

(breath-hold). T1 weighted imaging is used to assess for hemorrhage or fat in a lesion, and to assess the liver position in cases of congenital diaphragmatic hernia.

FETAL ANOMALIES

CNS Anomalies

One area where MRI has proven to be especially beneficial is in evaluation of the fetal CNS. Whereas ultrasound can assess the ventricular size and contour, it can be difficult to obtain adequate visualization of the cortex on the side of the brain closest to the transducer due to shadowing from the skull. While transvaginal scanning is helpful in fetuses in cephalic presentation, the head is not always in optimal position for this technique. Small cortical abnormalities can be missed with ultrasound, and are more easily detectable by MRI. MRI also allows for obtaining images in the true sagittal plane of the fetus, which allows for improved diagnosis of callosal abnormalities, and abnormalities in the Dandy-Walker spectrum (36). Many case reports and series reports detail the potential of MR imaging to improve upon the sonographic diagnosis of CNS anomalies (37–47).

We always perform an ultrasound prior to MRI to ensure that a high quality study is available for comparison. Results from our study comparing ultrasound to MR imaging demonstrated that of 124 fetuses with CNS anomalies confirmed at our institution, there were 86 changes in counseling, 49 major changes in diagnosis, and 27 clear changes in management (Table 1) (47). MRI findings not visualized by ultrasound include porencephaly, partial or complete agenesis of the corpus callosum, cortical gyral abnormality (Fig. 5), tethered cord, cortical clefts, midbrain abnormalities, partial or complete agenesis of the septi pellucidi, holoprosencephaly, cerebellar hypoplasia, subependymal and cortical tubers in association with tuberous sclerosis, vascular malformation, and hemorrhage and vermian cysts. Abnormalities better defined by MRI than ultrasound include encephaloceles, arteriovenous malformations, and the mass effect of arachnoid cysts (48–50). We found that MR imaging was least helpful in patients with a normal confirmatory sonogram and myelomeningocele.

The information provided by MRI allows for improved patient counseling, which may be used to assist patients in the decision to continue or discontinue a pregnancy, or may be used to facilitate planning the mode of delivery and perinatal

Table 1 MRI Changes in Counseling, Diagnosis, and Management

US CNS diagnosis	N	MRI-changed counseling	MRI-changed diagnosis	MRI-changed management
Normal	69	13	3	2
Normal, but CNS anomaly suspected by US findings	9	7	4	3
Mild ventriculomegaly	28	5	5	1
Moderate ventriculomegaly	18	8	7	1
Severe ventriculomegaly	9	6	5	3
Arachnoid cyst	14	12	5	3
Spinal neural tube defect	21	5	2	1
Encephalocele	9	7	5	4
Dandy-Walker variant/ malformation	16	8	4	3
Small head	4	4	4	3
Vascular malformation	3	3	1	3
Holoprosencephaly	4	1	1	0
Megacisterna magna	2	2	0	0
Miscellaneous	8	5	3	2
Total	214	86	49	29

Abbreviations: US, ultrasound; MRI, magnetic resonance imaging; CNS, central nervous system.
Source: From Ref. 47.

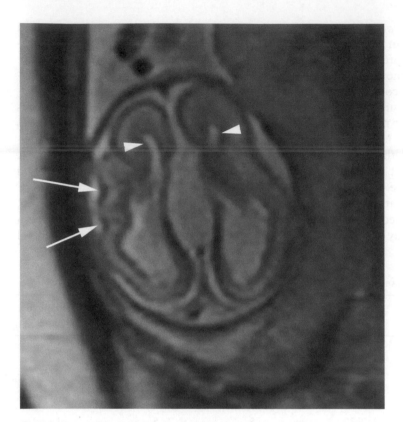

Figure 5 Axial view of the brain of a fetus at 21-weeks gestational age with Aicardi syndrome. Agenesis of the corpus callosum, and an irregular ventricular contour was visualized on sonography. The MRI shows the parallel orientation of the frontal horns (*arrowheads*), an interhemispheric cyst, and absence of the corpus callosum. In addition, an abnormal cortical gyral pattern is present (*arrows*), which was not adequately characterized by sonography. Note that the hemisphere with the cortical gyral abnormality is closest to the maternal anterior abdominal wall. This side of the brain was obscured by shadowing from the skull at the time of sonography. The fetus was in breech presentation so vaginal scanning was unhelpful. *Abbreviation*: MRI, magnetic resonance imaging.

care. The types of management changes were correlated with gestational age, with decisions to terminate/continue a pregnancy being made at early gestational ages, and decisions regarding mode of delivery, location of delivery, and perinatal care being made late in gestation (47). At times, MRI in the third trimester can obviate the need for postnatal MRI (which may require neonatal sedation and its associated risks).

We have found MRI to be especially useful in fetuses with ventriculomegaly. The degree of ventriculomegaly, the cause of ventriculomegaly, and any associated findings are important in providing a management plan and prognosis for the fetus (51–54). We are currently following a cohort of fetuses with ventriculomegaly to assess how MRI measurements of cortical volume, ventricular volume, and cortical development correlate with postnatal outcome.

Prenatal counseling is frequently performed by pediatric specialists such as pediatric neurosurgeons who have experience reading MRI examinations but limited ability to interpret sonograms. At times the benefit of performing a fetal MRI is that a specialist can feel more confident about a specific diagnosis and can, therefore, better counsel the patient.

One question that remains to be evaluated with respect to fetal counseling is how the MRI findings in utero correlate with MRI findings postnatally. For example, we know that the degree of hydrocephalus is a less important factor than the intrinsic parenchymal damage (55). However, it is possible that the consequences of parenchymal damage in utero may not be the same as parenchymal damage postnatally. Just as it is difficult to assess the amount of residual normal cortex in fetuses with severe ventriculomegaly prior to shunting, the same may be true in our assessment of porencephaly. While there is no doubt that the visualization of parenchymal damage portends worse for the outcome than nonvisualization of cortical destruction, we must temper our counseling of patients since our knowledge of the natural history of prenatally diagnosed porencephaly with postnatal correlation is still limited.

Non-CNS Anomalies

MR imaging is contributive in defining fetal abdominal, lung, and pelvic masses (36,56,57). MRI is helpful in the documentation of liver position in fetuses with congenital diaphragmatic hernia (58,59). The liver position is important for prognosis since isolated "liver-up" and "liver-down" congenital diaphragmatic hernia have a respective mortality of 57% and 7% (58,60,61). MRI is also helpful in fetuses with hernias in the assessment of the amount of normal appearing lung remaining since the lung is poorly visualized with sonography but is well-depicted with MR imaging (Fig. 6) (58). MRI volumetry of the fetal lungs may be more predictive of outcome than sonographic measurements (62). Multiple reports in the literature have documented the use of MRI in aiding in the diagnosis of fetal non-CNS anomalies such as autosomal recessive polycystic kidney disease (63), and lung masses (64,65). Further studies will be needed to assess how additional information from MR imaging of abnormalities in the fetal chest and abdomen affect patient management and outcome.

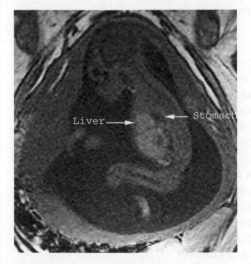

Figure 6 Sagittal T1 weighted image in a 27-week-gestational-age fetus shows a congenital diaphragmatic hernia with the stomach and liver in the chest.

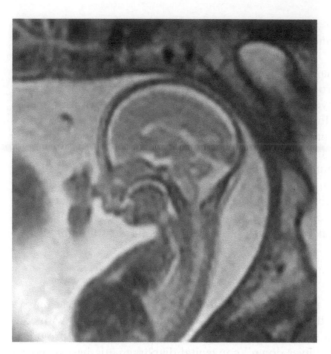

Figure 7 Profile view of face of fetus at 19 weeks with micrognathia and cleft soft palate. Ultrasound (not shown) demonstrated micrognathia. MRI also shows absence of the soft palate, visible as communication of the oro- and nasopharyx, and high position of the tongue. Note the absent soft tissue band of the soft palate (compare with Fig. 3). *Abbreviation*: MRI, magnetic resonance imaging.

Fetal cleft lip and palate is an area where MRI shows potential. It is difficult to directly visualize the soft palate with ultrasound. However, MRI can clearly demonstrate the region of the cleft soft palate in both normal (Fig. 3) and abnormal fetuses (Fig. 7). This has important implications in patient counseling, since clefts in the soft palate are associated with speech and hearing difficulties.

The Fetal Surgery Patient

A rapidly expanding area for MRI is the evaluation of fetuses that potentially will undergo in utero surgery and in fetuses being assessed for potential ex utero intrapartum treatment (EXIT) procedure. In this procedure, while still attached to umbilical blood circulation, the appropriate diagnostic and therapeutic maneuvers are undertaken to either provide ventilation or put the fetus on extra corporeal membrane oxygenation prior to clamping the umbilical cord. Assessment of airway obstruction is thus an important indication for prenatal MRI. This, typically undertaken, defines the extent of a cervical teratoma and lymphatic malformation (66,68). It is increasingly common for fetuses with proven or suspected airway obstruction to undergo the EXIT procedure (68,69). In patients being evaluated for EXIT procedure, MRI is helpful for visualizing potential airway obstruction, and in planning for intervention at the time of delivery (Fig. 8) (56,70).

For all fetal surgery patients, MRI is very helpful to ensure that unexpected anomalies are not present prior to undertaking the morbidity of fetal surgery

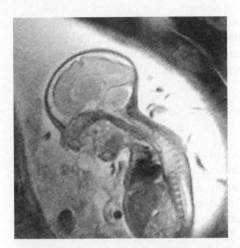

Figure 8 Sagittal view of face at 28-weeks gestational in fetus with oropharyngeal teratoma. The large tumor is visualized distending the oropharynx. Both ultrasound (not shown) and MRI showed the trachea to be patent in the lower neck, allowing for surgical planning for trachostomy at the time of EXIT procedure. *Abbreviations*: EXIT, ex utero intrapartum treatment; MRI, magnetic resonance imaging.

(71,72). In patients undergoing surgery for neural tube defects, MRI is helpful in characterizing the Chiari malformation, since the amount of cerebellar herniation is easily followed on serial MRI examinations.

MRI Volumetry

The data obtained from fast scan techniques can be used to assess the volume of the fetus and supporting structures. The expectation is that fetal weight estimates based on fetal volume determinations will be more accurate than those obtained with ultrasound. While sonographic estimates of fetal weight are reasonably accurate for the majority of the fetal population, at the extremes of weight, in the intrauterine growth restricted (IUGR) and in the macrosomic fetus, where accuracy is most important, sonographic biometry is frequently limited. MRI has the promise of being less affected by patient body habitus (unless the patient cannot fit into the magnet bore), and instead of 2D measurements being used for estimation of weight, a true fetal mass can be assessed (73). A number of different methods have been described for obtaining the data upon which fetal volumetry can be performed (74–79).

MRI measurements of liver show that a single fetal liver volume measurement, performed several weeks before delivery can distinguish fetuses subsequently diagnosed as being growth restricted with greater accuracy than ultrasound (80,81).

Oligohydramnios is another finding in IUGR. Variations in technique for assessing amniotic fluid volume, typically by use of the amniotic fluid index, hamper our ability to standardize assessment of oligohydramnios. It is possible that MRI will allow for a more reliable means of assessing amniotic fluid volume. Information regarding fetal fat (82), functional evaluation of the placenta (83,84), and placental volume assessments will likely be used in combination with other data to better distinguish between the constitutionally small but appropriately grown fetus and the fetus at risk due to placental insufficiency.

Similarly, additional features of the macrosomic fetus will be information regarding pelvimetry (85), fetal shoulder width (85), and fetal fat (82). The incremental benefit of MRI beyond that of ultrasound in the assessment of fetuses at the extremes of fetal growth remains to be determined in clinical practice.

SUMMARY

Ultrasound continues to be the screening modality of choice in the evaluation of the fetus due to its relatively low cost and real-time capability. However, there are many cases in which alternative imaging is useful as an adjunct to ultrasound. Fast MRI techniques allow for superb imaging of fetal anatomy. In the future, faster imaging, 3D volumetry, and functional imaging will add to our ability to better assess the fetus and optimize patient care. As our experience with fast MRI techniques increases, we will continue to identify patients in whom MRI contributes to patient evaluation.

ACKNOWLEDGMENTS

The studies of fetal CNS in this paper were supported by an NIH grant, NS 37945 and EB 001998.

REFERENCES

1. Weinreb JC, Lowe T, Cohen JM, Kutler M. Human fetal anatomy: MR imaging. Radiology 1985; 157:715–720.
2. Antuaco TL, Shah HR, Mattison DR, Quirk JG Jr. MR imaging in high-risk obstetric patients: a valuable complement to US. Radiographics 1992; 12:91–109.
3. Powell MC, Worthington BS, Buckley JM, Symonds EM. Magnetic resonance imaging (MRI) in obstetrics. II. Fetal anatomy. Br J Obstet Gynaecol 1988; 95:38–46.
4. Williamson RA, Weiner CP, Yuh WT, Abu-Yousef MM. Magnetic resonance imaging of anomalous fetuses. Obstet Gynecol 1989; 73:952–956.
5. Stark DD, McCarthy SM, Filly RA, Callen PW, Hricak H, Parer JT. Intrauterine growth retardation: evaluation by magnetic resonance. Work in progress. Radiology 1985; 155:425–427.
6. Lenke RR, Persutte WH, Nemes JM. Use of pancuronium bromide to inhibit fetal movement during magnetic resonance imaging. A case report. J Reprod Med 1989; 34: 315–317.
7. Horvath L, Seeds JW. Temporary arrest of fetal movement with pancuronium bromide to enable antenatal magnetic resonance imaging of holoprosencephaly. Am J Perinatol 1989; 6:418–420.
8. Mansfield P, Stehling MK, Ordidge RJ, et al. Echo planar imaging of the human fetus in utero at 0.5 T. Br J Radiol 1990; 63:833–841.
9. Edelman RR, Wielopolski PA. Fast MRI. 2nd ed. Philadelphia, PA: Saunders Publishing, 1996:302–352.
10. Schwartz JL, Crooks LE. NMR imaging produces no observable mutations or cytotoxicity in mammalian cells. AJR Am J Roentgenol 1982; 139:583–585.
11. Wolff S, Crooks LE, Brown P, Howard R, Painter RB. Tests for DNA and chromosomal damage induced by nuclear magnetic resonance imaging. Radiology 1980; 136: 707–710.

12. Baker PN, Johnson IR, Harvey PR, Gowland PA, Mansfield P. A three-year follow-up of children imaged in utero using echo planar magnetic resonance. Am J Obstet Gynecol 1994; 170:32–33.
13. Kanal E, Gillen J, Evans JA, Savitz DA, Shellock FG. Survey of reproductive health among female MR workers. Radiology 1993; 187:395–399.
14. U.S. Food and Drug Administration. Guidance for content and review of a magnetic resonance diagnostic device 510 (k) application. Washington, DC: U.S. Food and Drug Administration, August 2, 1988.
15. Myers C, Duncan KR, Gowland PA, Johnson IR, Baker PN. Failure to detect intrauterine growth restriction following in utero exposure to MRI. Br J Radiol 1998; 71:549–551.
16. Levine D, Zuo C, Faro CB, Chen Q. Potential heating effect in the gravid uterus during MR HASTE imaging. J Magn Reson Imaging 2001; 13:856–861.
17. Shellock FG, Kanal E. Policies, guidelines, and recommendations for MR imaging safety and patient management. SMRI Safety Committee. J Magn Reson Imaging 1991; 1:97–101.
18. Shellock FG, Crues JV. MR procedures: biologic effects, safety, and patient care. Radiology 2004; 232:635–652.
19. Product Information. Magnevist. Berlex Laboratories, 2000.
20. Shellock FG, Kanal E. Bioeffects and safety of MR procedures. In: Edelman RR, Hesselink JR, Zlatkin MB, eds. Clinical Magnetic Resonance Imaging. Philadelphia: W.B. Saunders, 1996:429.
21. van Loon AJ, Mantingh A, Thijn CJ, Mooyaart EL. Pelvimetry by magnetic resonance imaging in breech presentation. Am J Obstet Gynecol 1990; 163:1256–1260.
22. Stark DD, McCarthy SM, Filly RA, Parer JT, Hricak H, Callen PW. Pelvimetry by magnetic resonance imaging. AJR Am J Roentgenol 1985; 144:947–950.
23. van Loon AJ, Mantingh A, Serlier EK, Kroon G, Mooyaart EL, Huisjes HJ. Randomised controlled trial of magnetic-resonancy pelvimetry in breech presentation at term. Lancet 1997; 350:1799–1804.
24. Wright AR, Cameron HM, Lind T. Magnetic resonance imaging pelvimetry: a useful adjunct in the management of the obese patient. Br J Obstet Gynaecol 1992; 99:852–853.
25. Kirkinen P, Helin-Martikainen HL, Vanninen R, Partanen K. Placenta accreta: imaging by gray-scale and contrast-enhanced color Doppler sonography and magnetic resonance imaging. J Clin Ultrasound 1998; 26:90–94.
26. Ha TP, Li KC. Placenta accreta: MRI antenatal diagnosis and surgical correlation. J Magn Reson Imaging 1998; 8:748–750.
27. Fejgin MD, Rosen DJ, Ben-Nun I, Goldberger SB, Beyth Y. Ultrasonic and magnetic resonance imaging diagnosis of placenta accreta managed conservatively. J Perinat Med 1993; 21:165–168.
28. Thorp JMJ, Councell RB, Sandridge DA, Wiest HH. Antepartum diagnosis of placenta previa percreta by magnetic resonance imaging. Obstet Gynecol 1992; 80:506–508.
29. Levine D, Hulka CA, Ludmir J, Li W, Edelman RR. Placenta accreta: evaluation with color Doppler, power Doppler and fast MR imaging. Radiology 1997; 205:773–776.
30. McCarthy SM, Stark DD, Filly RA, Callen PW, Hricak H, Higgins CB. Obstetrical magnetic resonance imaging: maternal anatomy. Radiology 1985; 154:421–425.
31. Weinreb JC, Lowe TW, Santos-Ramos R, Cunningham FG, Parkey R. Magnetic resonance imaging in obstetric diagnosis. Radiology 1985; 154:157–161.
32. Powell MC, Buckley J, Price H, Worthington BS, Symonds EM. Magnetic resonance imaging and placenta previa. Am J Obstet Gynecol 1986; 154:565–569.
33. Nimmo MJ, Kinsella D, Andrews HS. MRI in pregnancy: the diagnosis of vasa previa by magnetic resonance imaging. Bristol Med Chir J 1988; 103:12.
34. Mochizuki T, Nishiguchi T, Ito I, et al. Case report. Antenatal diagnosis of chorioangioma of the placenta: MR features. J Comput Assist Tomogr 1996; 20:413–416.
35. Levine D, Barnes PD, Sher S, et al. Fetal fast MR imaging: reproducibility, technical quality, and conspicuity of anatomy. Radiology 1998; 206:549–554.

36. Levine D. MR imaging of fetal central nervous system abnormalities. Brain Cogn 2002; 50:432–448.

37. Dinh DH, Wright RM, Hanigan WC. The use of magnetic resonance imaging for the diagnosis of fetal intracranial anomalies. Childs Nerv Syst 1990; 6:212–215.

38. Guibaud L, Champion F, Buenerd A, Pelizzari M, Bourgeois J, Pracros JP. Fetal intraventricular glioblastoma: ultrasonographic, magnetic resonance imaging, and pathologic findings. J Ultrasound Med 1997; 16:285–288.

39. Kultursay N, Gelal F, Mutluer S, Senrecper S, Oziz E, Oral R. Antenatally diagnosed neonatal craniopharyngioma. J Perinatol 1995; 15:426–428.

40. Campi A, Scotti G, Filippi M, Gerevini S, Strigimi F, Lasjaunias P. Antenatal diagnosis of vein of Galen aneurysmal malformation: MR study of fetal brain and postnatal follow-up. Neuroradiology 1996; 38:87–90.

41. Reid A, Smith FW, Hutchinson JM. Nuclear magnetic resonance imaging and its safety implications: follow-up of 181 patients. Br J Radiol 1982; 55:784–786.

42. Thickman D, Mintz M, Mennuti M, Kressel HY. MR imaging of cerebral abnormalities in utero. J Comput Assist Tomogr 1984; 8:1058–1061.

43. Fusch C, Ozdoba C, Kuhn P, et al. Perinatal ultrasonography and magnetic resonance imaging findings in congenital hydrocephalus associated with fetal intraventricular hemorrhage. Am J Obstet Gynecol 1997; 177:512–518.

44. Koga Y, Tahara Y, Kida T, Matumoto Y, Negishi H, Fujimoto S. Prenatal diagnosis of congenital unilateral hydrocephalus. Pediatr Radiol 1997; 27:319–320.

45. Sonigo PC, Rypens FF, Carteret M, Delezoide AL, Brunelle FO. MR imaging of fetal cerebral anomalies. Pediatr Radiol 1998; 28:212–222.

46. Rypens F, Sonigo P, Aubry MC, Delezoide AL, Cessot F, Brunelle F. Prenatal MR diagnosis of a thick corpus callosum. AJNR Am J Neuroradiol 1996; 17:1918–1920.

47. Levine D, Barnes PD, Robertson RR, Wong G, Mehta TS. Fast MRI of fetal central nervous system abnormalities. Radiology 2003; 229:51–61.

48. Levine D, Mehta T, Trop I, Barnes P. Fast MRI of fetal CNS anomalies with prenatal MRI: results of 149 cases. Radiology 2000; 217:101.

49. Levine D, Barnes PD, Madsen JR, Li W, Edelman RR. Fetal central nervous system anomalies: MR imaging augments sonographic diagnosis. Radiology 1997; 204: 635–642.

50. Levine D, Barnes PD, Madsen JR, Abbott J, Mehta T, Edelman RR. Central nervous system abnormalities assessed with prenatal magnetic resonance imaging. Obstet Gynecol 1999; 94:1011–1019.

51. Vergani P, Locatelli A, Strobelt N, et al. Clinical outcome of mild fetal ventriculomegaly. Am J Obstet Gynecol 1998; 178:218–222.

52. Patel MD, Filly AL, Hersh DR, Goldstein RB. Isolated mild fetal cerebral ventriculomegaly: clinical course and outcome. Radiology 1994; 192:759–764.

53. Bloom SL, Bloom DD, Dellanebbia C, Martin LB, Lucas MJ, Twickler DM. The developmental outcome of children with antenatal mild isolated ventriculomegaly. Obstet Gynecol 1997; 90:93–97.

54. Nicolaides KH, Berry S, Snijders RJ, Thorpe-Beeston JG, Gosden C. Fetal lateral cerebral ventriculomegaly: associated malformations and chromosomal defects. Fetal Diagn Ther 1990; 5:5–14.

55. Giudetti B, Occhipinti E, Riccio A. Ventriculo-atrial shunt in 200 cases of nontumoroural hydrocephalus in children: remarks on the diagnostic criteria, postoperative complications and long-term results. Acta Neurochir 1969; 21:295–308.

56. Quinn TM, Hubbard AM, Adzick NS. Prenatal magnetic resonance imaging enhances fetal diagnosis. J Pediatr Surg 1998; 33:553–558.

57. Levine D, Barnes PD, Edelman RR. State of the art: obstetric MR imaging. Radiology 1999; 211:609–617.

58. Leung JW, Coakley FV, Hricak H, et al. Prenatal MR imaging of congenital diaphragmatic hernia. AJR Am J Roentgenol 2000; 174:1607–1612.

59. Hubbard AM, Adzick NS, Crombleholme TM, Haselgrove JC. Left-sided congenital diaphragmatic hernia: value of prenatal MR imaging in preparation for fetal surgery. Radiology 1997; 203:636–640.

60. Metkus AP, Filly RA, Stringer MD, Harrison MR, Adzick NS. Sonographic predictors of survival in fetal diaphragmatic hernia. J Pediatr Surg 1996; 31:148–152.

61. Adzick SN, Harrison MR, Glick PL, Nakayama DK, Manning FA, deLorimier AA. Diaphragmatic hernia in the fetus: prenatal diagnosis and outcome in 94 cases. J Pediatr Surg 1985; 20:357–361.

62. Coakley FV, Lopoo JB, Lu Y, et al. Normal and hypoplastic fetal lungs: volumetric assessment with prenatal single-shot rapid acquisition with relaxation enhancement MR imaging. Radiology 2000; 216:107–111.

63. Nishi T. Magnetic resonance imaging of autosomal recessive polycystic kidney disease in utero. J Obstet Gynaecol 1995; 21:471–474.

64. Hubbard AM, Adzick NS, Crombleholme TM, et al. Congenital chest lesions: diagnosis and characterization with prenatal MR imaging. Radiology 1999; 212:43–48.

65. Dhingsa R, Coakley FV, Albanese CT, Filly RA, Goldstein RB. Prenatal sonography and MR imaging of pulmonary sequestration. AJR Am J Roentgenol 2003; 180:433–437.

66. Kaminopetros P, Jauniaux E, Kane P, Weston M, Nicolaides KH, Campbell DJ. Prenatal diagnosis of an extensive fetal lymphangioma using ultrasonography, magnetic resonance imaging and cytology. Br J Radiol 1997; 70:750–753.

67. Tsuda H, Matsumoto M, Yamamoto K, et al. Usefulness of ultrasonography and magnetic resonance imaging for prenatal diagnosis of fetal teratoma of the neck. J Clin Ultrasound 1996; 24:217–219.

68. Hubbard AM, Crombleholme TM, Adzick NS. Prenatal MRI evaluation of giant neck masses in preparation for the fetal EXIT procedure. Am J Perinatol 1998; 15:253–257.

69. Morof D, Grable I, Fishman S, et al. Oropharyngeal teratoma: prenatal diagnosis and assessment using ultrasound, MRI, and CT with management by EXIT procedure. Am J Roentgenol 2004; 183:493–496.

70. Levine D, Jennings R, Barnewolt C, Mehta T, Wilson J, Wong G. Progressive fetal bronchial obstruction caused by a bronchogenic cyst diagnosed by prenatal MR imaging. AJR Am J Roentgenol 2001; 176:49–52.

71. Coakley FV. Role of magnetic resonance imaging in fetal surgery. Top Magn Reson Imaging 2001; 12:39–51.

72. Coakley FV, Hricak H, Filly RA, Barkovich AJ, Harrison MR. Complex fetal disorders: effect of MR imaging on management—preliminary clinical experience. Radiology 1999; 213:691–696.

73. Levine D. 3D fetal MRI—will it fulfill its promise? [Editorial]. Radiology 2001; 219: 313–315.

74. Uotila J, Dastidar P, Heinonen T, Ryymin P, Punnonen R, Laasonen E. Magnetic resonance imaging compared to ultrasonography in fetal weight and volume estimation in diabetic and normal pregnancy. Acta Obstet Gynecol Scand 2000; 79:255–259.

75. Roberts N, Garden AS, Cruz-Orive LM, Whitehouse GH, Edwards RH. Estimation of fetal volume by magnetic resonance imaging and stereology. Br J Radiol 1994; 67:1067–1077.

76. Garden AS, Roberts N. Fetal and fetal organ volume estimations with magnetic resonance imaging. Am J Obstet Gynecol 1996; 175:442–448.

77. Qong QY, Roberts N, Garden AS, Whitehouse GH. Fetal and fetal brain volume estimation in the third trimester of human pregnancy using gradient echo MR imaging. Magn Reson Imaging 1998; 16:235–240.

78. Kubik-Huch RA, Wildermuth S, Cettuzii L, et al. Ultrafast magnetic resonance imaging of the fetus and uteroplacental unit: 3-dimensional reconstruction and volumetry—feasibility study. Radiology 2001; 219:567–573.

79. Baker PN, Johnson IR, Gowland PA, et al. Fetal weight estimation by echo-planar magnetic resonance imaging. Lancet 1994; 343:644–645.

80. Duncan KR. Fetal and placental volumetric and functional analysis using echo-planar imaging. Top Magn Reson Imaging 2001; 12:52–66.
81. Baker PN, Johnson IR, Gowland PA, et al. Measurement of fetal liver, brain and placental volumes with echo-planar magnetic resonance imaging. Br J Obstet Gynaecol 1995; 102:35–39.
82. Deans HE, Smith FW, Lloyd DJ, Law AN, Sutherland HW. Fetal fat measurement by magnetic resonance imaging. Br J Radiol 1989; 62:603–607.
83. Francis ST, Duncan KR, Moore RJ, Baker PN, Johnson IR, Gowland PA. Non-invasive mapping of placental perfusion. Lancet 1998; 351:1397–1399.
84. Duncan KR, Gowland P, Francis S, Moore R, Baker PN, Johnson IR. The investigation of placental relaxation and estimation of placental perfusion using echo-planar magnetic resonance imaging. Placenta 1998; 19:539–543.
85. Kastler B, Gangi A, Mathelin C, et al. Fetal shoulder measurements with MRI. J Comput Assist Tomogr 1993; 17:777–780.

21

Prenatal Therapy—Prevention of Labor

Susan E. Gerber

Department of Obstetrics and Gynecology, Division of Maternal Fetal Medicine,
Feinberg School of Medicine, Northwestern University, Chicago, Illinois, U.S.A.

Labor is the physiologic process in which the uterine cervix progressively dilates and effaces in the presence of regular uterine contractions, ultimately resulting in the delivery of a fetus or fetuses. The ability to prevent this process is most important in the setting of preterm labor, or labor that begins prior to 37 completed weeks of gestation.

Preterm birth is the leading cause of perinatal mortality and morbidity in industrialized nations. Preterm birth, and especially extreme preterm birth, is associated with high rates of impaired long-term health outcomes such as neurosensory deficits, cognitive delay, and chronic lung disease, as well as infant death (1–3). In 2003, the rate of preterm birth in the United States was 12.3% (4). This rate has risen gradually over the past two decades from 9.4% in 1981 to 10.6% in 1990 (Fig. 1) (5). With some exceptions, reports from most other developed nations demonstrate a similar increase in the rate of preterm birth (6).

Forty to fifty percent of preterm births are the result of spontaneous preterm labor. The failure of medical technology to reduce preterm delivery rates is due, in part, to a lack of understanding of the cause of spontaneous labor. The exact physiologic mechanisms that lead to both term and preterm parturition remain incompletely elucidated. Most believe that parturition is a multifactorial process, rather than the result of a single trigger (7). Similarly, preterm labor likely has multiple disparate causes that result in the common pathway of preterm labor.

ETIOLOGY OF PRETERM BIRTH

While there are many theories, the exact etiology or etiologies of preterm birth remain unknown. Preterm birth may be the result of the pathologic activation of the normal labor process; it may result from an alternate pathway, or a combination of the two possibilities. The triggers of preterm labor are often thought to be different from those that lead to birth at term, but this remains unproven.

One clear association is that between intrauterine infection and preterm birth. Preterm labor is often associated with high levels of cytokines and matrix metalloproteinases, indicating an inflammatory response possibly secondary to infectious

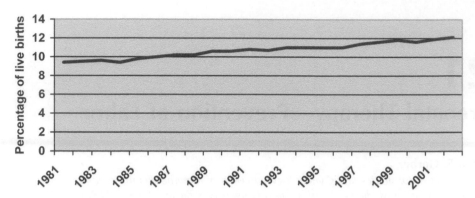

Figure 1 Preterm birth rates in the United States from 1981 to 2002. *Source*: From Ref. 5.

processes (7). The presumed mechanism involves bacterial invasion of the choriode-cidual space associated with endotoxin and/or exotoxin release stimulating decidua and fetal membrane production of cytokines. Endotoxins, exotoxins, and cytokines stimulate the production of prostaglandins, which in turn lead to uterine con-tractions (8). Decidual bleeding has also been implicated in preterm birth. Women destined to deliver preterm have been found to have elevated levels of thrombin–antithrombin III complex, suggesting a role for intrauterine bleeding such as that seen with placental abruption (9).

PRIMARY PREVENTION

Prevention of labor may be categorized as primary prevention or secondary preven-tion. Primary prevention requires identification of risk factors and causes to address the source of labor and prevent its occurrence. Secondary prevention assumes the occurrence of labor, with preventive efforts directed at aborting the process in order to prevent preterm birth.

Prenatal Care

Pregnancies delivered prematurely are often associated with a reduced number of prenatal visits. In part, this is due to the abbreviated gestation. It is also true that the absence of prenatal care is closely associated with other risk factors for preterm birth such as low socioeconomic status and maternal substance abuse. What is unclear is whether increased prenatal care would decrease the rate of preterm birth. Studies of programs designed to increase access to prenatal care have not demon-strated a significant reduction in the rate of preterm birth (10). Similarly, studies of increased prenatal care compared to standard care have also not demonstrated significant decreases in preterm birth rates (10,11).

Identification and Modification of Risk Factors

Clinical risk assessment and scoring systems have been developed to estimate the risk of preterm delivery based upon historical risk factors. These systems have been suc-cessful in identifying women whose risk of preterm delivery is three to four times that

Table 1 Risk Factors Associated with Preterm Birth

Prior preterm birth
Multiple gestation
Uterine anomalies
African–American race
Maternal age <15 or >45 years
Maternal smoking
Low socioeconomic status
No prenatal care
Maternal BMI <19.8
Infection
Polyhydramnios
Positive fetal fibronectin assay
Short cervical length
Bacterial vaginosis

seen in the general population. However, these systems are limited by poor sensitivities and positive predictive values (12). Whereas numerous risk factors have been associated with an increased risk of spontaneous preterm birth (Table 1), some of these risk factors are modifiable, such as maternal smoking and low body mass index (BMI), while others, such as race, are not.

Maternal Race/Ethnicity

In the United States, preterm birth rates are higher among African–American mothers (17.5% in 2002) than among non-Hispanic Whites (11.0% in 2002) (5). Evidence of this racial disparity remains despite controlling for sociodemographic differences as well as receipt of prenatal care (13). There is considerable evidence of an increased risk of adverse health outcomes in general among non-Caucasian Americans. The mechanisms that result in this disparity remain unclear, but are currently the subject of increased research focus (14).

Maternal Age

Preterm birth rates are highest at the extremes of maternal age. Among American women with singleton deliveries in 2002, the rate of preterm delivery was 9% for those aged 30–34, 17% for those 45 and older, and 21% for mothers under age 15 (5). Rates of teen pregnancy have been on the decline since the 1990s, but pregnancies at advanced maternal age continue to rise (5).

Maternal Weight

Underweight women (BMI < 19.8) have been shown to have a twofold increased risk of preterm birth (15). Inadequate weight gain in the third trimester is also associated with preterm birth (15).

To date, no nutritional supplementation plan has been demonstrated to significantly reduce the rate of preterm birth. Protein, calcium, iron, folate, and zinc are among the supplements that have been studied. Studies evaluating the use of fish oil have demonstrated a possible role for this treatment in the prevention of preterm birth, but large well-designed randomized trials remain to be done (16).

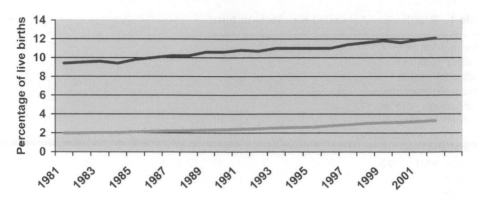

Figure 2 Multiple gestation and preterm birth rates in the United States from 1981 to 2002. *Dark line*—proportion of all live births born preterm (prior to 37 completed weeks of gestation). *Light line*—proportion of all live births that are multiple gestation. *Source*: From Refs. 5, 17.

Multiple Gestation

Multiple gestation accounts for 3% of all live births, but 16% of all preterm births, and 22% of births at <32 weeks' gestation. Sixty percent of all multiple births are delivered preterm (5). The rates of multiple gestations in the United States have steadily risen and this rise is closely linked to the rise in preterm births (Fig. 2).

This increase is largely due to the increased utilization of assisted reproductive technologies (ART). With growing awareness of the increased morbidity and mortality associated with multiple gestations, there have been efforts on the part of the medical community to reduce the rate of multiple gestations. A study of the use of ART in the United States between 1995 and 2001 demonstrated a steady increase in the number of embryo transfers annually. However, since 1997, there has been a decrease in the number of embryos transferred per cycle as well as the resulting number of pregnancies with three or more fetuses (18). In Europe, further efforts are addressing the number of twin births. A Swedish randomized trial of single- versus double-embryo transfer demonstrated a dramatic decrease (33.1–0.8%) in multiple gestation with only a slight decrease (42.9–38.8%) in live birth rate (19).

Maternal Smoking

The prevalence of maternal cigarette smoking during pregnancy varies between countries, but remains one of the most important modifiable risk factors for preterm birth. In the United States, 11.4% of women delivering in 2002 reported smoking during pregnancy (5). The odds ratios for the association between smoking and preterm birth have been reported to be in the order of 1.1–1.8. This effect appears to be dose-dependent, is similar for preterm and very preterm (<32 week) births, and is found in both singleton and twin pregnancies (20–23). This association is, in part, due to the increased risk of placental abruption and fetal growth restriction associated with maternal smoking. However, the association remains even when controlling for these factors.

In the United States, efforts to reduce cigarette smoking in pregnancy have been successful, with the rate of 11.4% in 2002 representing a decline of 42% from 1989 (5). However, smoking cessation programs have been hampered by a high rate of recidivism and have not yet clearly demonstrated a beneficial impact on perinatal outcomes (24).

Maternal Alcohol and Drug Use

Maternal substance abuse has been associated with increased rates of preterm labor and delivery. Multiple confounding factors may account for this association in this population, as the direct effect does not appear to be large (25). However, cocaine use in particular is associated with an approximately fourfold increased risk of abruptio placentae, presumably due to the vasoconstrictive effects of this agent (26). This may lead to both an increase in spontaneous as well as indicated preterm birth.

Identification and Treatment of Infection

It has long been recognized that preterm delivery is often associated with intrauterine infection (8,27). This infection may occur within the choriodecidual space, the placenta, the amniotic fluid, the umbilical cord, or the fetus. Lower genital tract infection has also been associated with an increased risk of preterm birth. The presence of bacterial vaginosis in the lower genital tract is associated with a twofold increased risk of spontaneous preterm delivery (8,28,29). Infection with *Trichomonas vaginalis* has also been associated with an increased risk of preterm birth (30). There is some evidence that a subgroup of women at increased risk for spontaneous preterm birth may benefit from treatment of bacterial vaginosis (31). However, large randomized controlled trials have not demonstrated a reduction in preterm birth with the treatment of asymptomatic bacterial vaginosis in pregnancy (32), or the treatment of asymptomatic trichomoniasis (33). Others have demonstrated no benefit from treatment of bacterial vaginosis even in high-risk groups (34).

Infection distant from the pelvis has also been implicated in preterm labor. While the exact mechanism is unknown, release of cytokines or endotoxins by nongenital tract infections may result in a local inflammatory response within the genital tract, thereby leading to preterm labor (26). Studies have demonstrated increased rates of periodontal disease in women with spontaneous preterm birth, while controlling for maternal characteristics such as age, race, prior preterm birth, and smoking (35,36). Urinary tract infection, both symptomatic and asymptomatic, has been associated with an increased risk of preterm birth. Randomized controlled trials have demonstrated a reduced incidence of preterm delivery with treatment of asymptomatic bacteriuria (37).

Fetal Fibronectin

In addition to demographic characteristics, biophysical characteristics have been discovered that are associated with an increased risk of spontaneous preterm birth.

Biochemical markers such as fetal fibronectin, salivary estriol, and relaxin have been described that identify women at increased risk of preterm delivery. Fetal fibronectin is a high molecular-weight extracellular matrix glycoprotein normally found in fetal membranes, placental tissues, and amniotic fluid. Between 22 and 37 weeks of gestation, the presence of fetal fibronectin in cervicovaginal secretions in concentrations >50 ng/mL is unusual, and associated with an increased risk of spontaneous preterm delivery (38). However, the clinical utility of this test lies more in its negative predictive value than its positive predictive value. While a positive test is of limited value due to a positive predictive value of ≤20%, 98% of women with a negative test will not deliver in the week following the test (39,40). Intervention trials have not demonstrated significantly improved outcomes following identification of a positive assay. A randomized controlled trial of 715 women with positive fetal fibronectin assays demonstrated no difference in preterm birth rates between women receiving metronidazole and erythromycin and women receiving placebo (41).

Cervical Length Assessment

In 1996, Iams et al. published an observational trial demonstrating that women with short cervices on transvaginal ultrasound examination are at greater risk of spontaneous preterm delivery, with a relative risk of 6.2 for cervical lengths <10th percentile at 24 weeks (26 mm) and a relative risk of 14.0 for cervical lengths <1st percentile at 24 weeks (13 mm) (42). This association has been demonstrated for singleton as well as for multiple gestations (43,44). In addition to cervical length, other ultrasonographic characteristics of the cervix such as cervical funneling have demonstrated increased risk of preterm birth (44,45).

As with nearly all screening tools that identify women at increased risk for preterm birth, the controversy lies in the response to this elevated risk. Multiple studies have addressed the efficacy of cervical cerclage in patients with abnormal cervices to prevent preterm birth. While there have been some contradictory results, the current evidence does not support a reduction in preterm birth or adverse neonatal outcome with cerclage placement in singleton or twin pregnancies (46–50).

Progesterone Therapy

Progesterone supplementation has long been studied as a potential therapy to prevent preterm labor due to the "progesterone withdrawal" theory of labor. In some mammals, although not in humans, a decrease in plasma progesterone precedes the onset of labor (51). Most recently, Meis et al. (52) conducted a double-blinded randomized controlled trial of weekly injections of 17 α-hydroxyprogesterone caproate (17P) in 463 women with a history of spontaneous preterm birth. 17P is a weakly active, naturally occurring progesterone metabolite. Results of this trial demonstrated a significant decrease (54.9–36.3%) in the rate of recurrent preterm birth <37 weeks. In another recent trial, a reduction in recurrent preterm birth was demonstrated using progesterone vaginal suppositories (53).

SECONDARY PREVENTION

Bedrest

Bedrest is used in approximately 20% of pregnancies to prevent a variety of adverse outcomes, including preterm birth. However, review of the literature reveals no evidence as to the effectiveness of this intervention in either the primary or secondary prevention of preterm birth or perinatal mortality. Considerable cost is associated with it in terms of both money and disruption of family life (54–56).

Hydration

Dehydration has been associated with an increase in uterine contractility, theoretically due to an increase in pituitary secretion of antidiuretic hormone and oxytocin. Increased hydration is often recommended in cases of threatened preterm delivery.

However, studies evaluating intravenous hydration compared to bedrest or tocolytic agents have found no significant difference in preterm birth rates or neonatal outcome (57–59).

Uterine Activity Monitoring

Ambulatory (or home) uterine activity monitoring was developed to identify women with asymptomatic but increased uterine activity. This theoretically presents an opportunity to intervene early in the process of preterm labor, when there might be a greater opportunity to halt the progression of labor. Iams et al. (60) studied 306 women with singleton gestations at low and high risk for preterm delivery. Increased frequency of uterine contractions was found to be associated with an increased risk of preterm birth. However, this measurement had poor sensitivity and poor positive predictive value, making it an unacceptable screening test. Furthermore, its use has not been demonstrated to decrease the incidence of preterm birth. In a large randomized controlled trial, Dyson et al. (61) randomized 2422 women at risk for preterm labor to receive education and to have either weekly contact with a nurse, daily contact with a nurse, or daily contact with a nurse and home uterine monitoring. No significant difference in outcome was detected between the three groups.

Antibiotic Therapy

As preterm labor is thought to be due to infection in a large subset of cases, antibiotic use has been studied in the setting of preterm labor. Multiple studies have demonstrated a significant association between silent upper genital tract infection and risk of preterm labor. Positive amniotic fluid cultures were found in 19% of women with intact membranes, idiopathic preterm labor, and no overt clinical signs of intra-amniotic infection (27). In a multicenter trial of women in preterm labor with intact membranes, the use of routine amniocentesis demonstrated an incidence of intra-amniotic infection of 5.8% (62). Trials of antibiotic use to prevent preterm birth once preterm labor occurs have demonstrated mixed results, but ultimately the evidence at this time does not support the use of antibiotics in the setting of preterm labor (62–65). Not surprisingly, the routine use of amniocentesis to detect intrauterine infection has also not been demonstrated to decrease the rate of preterm birth.

Tocolytic Therapy

Tocolytic drugs are the mainstay of the pharmacologic management of preterm labor. Tocolytics, by definition, inhibit myometrial contractions, and are used both in an acute episode of preterm labor as well as prophylactically to maintain uterine quiescence. Agents have included ethanol, magnesium sulfate, calcium channel blockers, beta mimetics, oxytocin antagonists, prostaglandin synthetase inhibitors, cyclo-oxygenase 2 inhibitors, and oxytocin antagonists. Commonly used tocolytics are listed in Table 2 along with their mechanism of action and side effects.

The efficacy of tocolytic agents has long been debated, with the preponderance of evidence indicating a small (2–7 days), but significant prolongation of pregnancy for all drugs except ethanol when compared to placebo (67–69). While the data are less conclusive regarding the impact on neonatal outcome, it is generally believed to be of benefit in order to allow for administration of antenatal corticosteroids.

Table 2 Tocolytics Commonly Used to Arrest Preterm Labor

Tocolytic agent	Dosage and administration	Contraindications	Maternal side effects	Fetal/neonatal side effects
Betamimetic	Terbutaline 0.25 mg subcutaneous every 20 min to 3 hrs (hold for pulse >120 beats per minute)	Cardiac arrhythmias	Cardiac or cardiopulmonary arrhythmias, pulmonary edema, myocardial ischemia, hypotension, tachycardia	Fetal tachycardia, hyperinsulinemia, hyperglycemia, myocardial and septal hypertrophy, myocardial ischemia
	Ritodrine initial dose 50–100 µg/min, increase 50 µg/min every 10 min until contractions cease or side effects develop. Maximum dose = 350 µg/min	Poorly controlled thyroid disease	Metabolic hyperglycemia, hyperinsulinemia, hypokalemia, antidiuresis, altered thyroid function	Neonatal tachycardia, hypoglycemia, hypocalcemia, hyperbilirubinemia, hypotension, intraventricular hemorrhage
		Poorly controlled diabetes mellitus	Physiologic tremor, palpitations, nervousness, nausea/vomiting, fever, hallucinations	
Magnesium sulfate	4.0–6.0 g bolus for 20 min, then 2–3 g/hr	Myasthenia gravis	Flushing, lethargy, headache, muscle weakness, diplopia, dry mouth, pulmonary edema, cardiac arrest	Lethargy, hypotonia, respiratory depression, demineralization with prolonged use
Calcium channel blockers	30 mg loading dose, then 10–20 mg every 4–6 hrs	Cardiac disease	Flushing, headache, dizziness, nausea, transient hypotension	None noted as yet
		Use caution with renal disease, maternal hypotension (<90/50 mmHg) Avoid concomitant use with $MgSO_4$		

Prostaglandin synthetase inhibitors	Indomethacin loading dose of 50 mg rectally or 50–100 mg orally, then 25–50 mg orally every 6 hrs × 48 hrs	Significant renal or hepatic impairment	Nausea, heartburn	Constriction of ductus arteriosus, pulmonary hypertension, reversible decrease in renal function with oligohydramnios, intraventricular hemorrhage, hyperbilirubinemia, necrotizing enterocolitis
	Ketorolac loading dose 60 mg intramuscularly, then 30 mg intramuscularly every 6 hrs × 48 hrs	Active peptic ulcer disease		
	Sulindac 200 mg orally every 12 hrs × 48 hrs	Coagulation disorders or thrombocytopenia NSAID-sensitive asthma Other sensitivity to NSAIDs		

Abbreviation: NSAIDs, nonsteroidal anti-inflammatory drugs.
Source: From Ref. 66.

The utility of long-term tocolytic therapy is less clear and generally believed to be of little benefit over short-term therapy (67,70). Studies of maintenance tocolysis demonstrate no evidence of decreased uterine activity, reduced rates of preterm birth, or improved neonatal outcome (71).

It is also important to recognize the adverse maternal and neonatal outcomes caused by tocolytic therapy. Beta mimetics are associated with maternal cardiac arrhythmias, heart failure, and chest pain. Pulmonary edema is associated with the use of tocolytic agents together with corticosteroids. Use of nonsteroidal anti-inflammatory drugs is associated with premature constriction of the ductus arteriosus as well as decreased amniotic fluid volume (67,72).

CONCLUSION

Despite a plethora of research, limited progress has been made in the search for a "cure" for preterm labor. While the rate of preterm birth has risen over the past two decades, the good news is that neonatal mortality rates have fallen. The decrease in neonatal mortality is largely due to improvements in neonatal medicine and improved ventilatory technology. Advances in obstetric care that have also contributed to the improved outcomes include perinatal regionalization efforts and the widespread use of antenatal corticosteroids. Despite the inability to stop a preterm birth, obstetricians now have more techniques by which to identify the women destined to deliver preterm. Identification of the at-risk pregnancy allows for the administration of corticosteroids and for the delivery of the preterm neonate at a tertiary care hospital, where he or she may benefit from the advanced expertise and technology.

REFERENCES

1. Hack M, Flannery DJ, Schluchter M, Cartar L, Borawski E, Klein N. Outcomes in young adulthood for very-low-birth-weight infants. N Engl J Med 2002; 346:149–157.
2. Kramer MS, Demissie K, Yang H, Platt RW, Sauve R, Liston R. The contribution of mild and moderate preterm birth to infant mortality. J Am Med Assoc 2000; 284:843–849.
3. McCormick MC. The contribution of low birth weight to infant mortality and childhood morbidity. N Engl J Med 1985; 312:82–90.
4. Hamilton BE, Martin JA, Sutton PD. Births: preliminary data for 2003. Natl Vital Stat Rep 2004; 53:1–18.
5. Martin JA, Hamilton BE, Sutton PD, Ventura SJ, Menacker F, Munson ML. Births: final data for 2002. Natl Vital Stat Rep 2003; 52:1–114.
6. Joseph KS, Kramer MS, Marcoux S, et al. Determinants of preterm birth rates in Canada from 1981 through 1983 and from 1992 through 1994. N Engl J Med 1998; 339:1434–1439.
7. Norwitz ER, Robinson JN, Challis JRG. The control of labor. N Engl J Med 1999; 341:660–666.
8. Goldenberg RL, Hauth JC, Andrews WW. Intrauterine infection and preterm delivery. N Engl J Med 2000; 342:1500–1507.
9. Elovitz MA, Baron J, Phillippe M. The role of thrombin in preterm parturition. Am J Obstet Gynecol 2001; 185:1059–1063.
10. Fiscella K. Does prenatal care improve birth outcomes? A critical review. Obstet Gynecol 1995; 85:468–479.

11. Collaborative Group on Preterm Birth Prevention. Multicenter randomized, controlled trial of a preterm birth prevention program. Am J Obstet Gynecol 1993; 169:352–366.
12. Mercer BM, Goldenberg RL, Das A, et al. The preterm prediction study: a clinical risk assessment system. Am J Obstet Gynecol 1996; 174:1885–1893.
13. Collins JW, Hammond NA. Relation of maternal race to the risk of preterm, non-low birth weight infants: a population study. Am J Epidemiol 1996; 143:333–337.
14. Iyasu S, Tomashek K, Barfield W. Infant mortality and low birth weight among black and white infants—United States, 1980–2000. MMWR Morb Mortal Wkly Rep 2002; 51:589–592.
15. Siega-Riz AM, Adair LS, Hobel CJ. Maternal underweight status and inadequate rate of weight gain during the third trimester of pregnancy increases the risk of preterm delivery. J Nutr 1996; 126:146–153.
16. Villar J, Merialdi M, Metin Gulmezoglu A, et al. Nutritional interventions during pregnancy for the prevention or treatment of maternal morbidity and preterm delivery: an overview of randomized controlled trials. J Nutr 2003; 133:1606S–1625S.
17. Martin JA, Park MM. Trends in twin and triplet births: 1980–1997. Natl Vital Stat Rep 1999; 47:1–20.
18. Jain T, Missmer SA, Hornstein MD. Trends in embryo-transfer practice and in outcomes of the use of assisted reproductive technology in the United States. N Engl J Med 2004; 350:1639–1645.
19. Thurin A, Hausken J, Hillensjo T, et al. Elective single-embryo transfer versus double-embryo transfer in in vitro fertilization. N Engl J Med 2004; 351:2392–2402.
20. Burguet A, Kaminski M, Abraham-Lerat L, et al. The complex relationship between smoking in pregnancy and very preterm delivery. Results of the Epipage study. Br J Obstet Gynaecol 2004; 111:258–265.
21. Kyrklund-Blomberg, Cnattingius S. Preterm birth and maternal smoking: risks related to gestational age and onset of delivery. Am J Obstet Gynecol 1998; 179:1051–1055.
22. Shah NR, Bracken MB. A systematic review and meta-analysis of prospective studies on the association between maternal cigarette smoking and preterm delivery. Am J Obstet Gynecol 2000; 182:465–472.
23. Wisborg K, Henriksen TB, Secher NJ. Maternal smoking and gestational age in twin pregnancies. Acta Obstet Gynecol Scand 2001; 80:926–930.
24. Lawrence T, Aveyard P, Evans O, Cheng KK. A cluster randomized controlled trial of smoking cessation in pregnant women comparing interventions based on the transtheoretical (stages of change) model to standard care. Tob Control 2003; 12:168–177.
25. Bauer CR, Shankaran S, Bada HS, et al. The maternal lifestyle study: drug exposure during pregnancy and short-term maternal outcomes. Am J Obstet Gynecol 2002; 186:487–495.
26. Hladky K, Yankowitz J, Hansen WF. Placental abruption. Obstet Gynecol Surv 2002; 57:299–305.
27. Watts DH, Krohn MA, Hillier SL, Eschenbach DA. The association of occult amniotic fluid infection with gestational age and neonatal outcome among women in preterm labor. Obstet Gynecol 1992; 79:351–357.
28. Hillier SL, Nugent RP, Eschenbach DA, et al. Association between bacterial vaginosis and preterm delivery of a low-birth-weight infant. N Engl J Med 1995; 333:1737–1742.
29. Leitich H, Bodner-Adler B, Brunbauer M, et al. Bacterial vaginosis as a risk factor for preterm delivery: a meta-analysis. Am J Obstet Gynecol 2003; 189:139–147.
30. Cotch MF, Pastorek JG, Nugent RP, et al. Trichomonas vaginalis associated with low birth weight and preterm delivery. The Vaginal Infections and Prematurity Study Group. Sex Transm Dis 1997; 24:353–360.
31. Hauth JC, Goldenberg RL, Andrews WW, DuBard MB, Copper RL. Reduced incidence of preterm delivery with metronidazole and erythromycin in women with bacterial vaginosis. N Engl J Med 1995; 333:1732–1736.
32. Carey JC, Klebanoff MA, Hauth JC, et al. Metronidazole to prevent preterm delivery in pregnant women with asymptomatic bacterial vaginosis. N Engl J Med 2000; 342:534–540.

33. Klebanoff MA, Carey JC, Hauth JC, et al. Failure of metronidazole to prevent preterm delivery among pregnant women with asymptomatic trichomonas vaginalis infection. N Engl J Med 2001; 345:487–493.

34. Riggs MA, Klebanoff MA. Treatment of vaginal infections to prevent preterm birth: a meta-analysis. Clin Obstet Gynecol 2004; 47:796–807.

35. Goepfert AR, Jeffcoat MK, Andrews WW, et al. Periodontal disease and upper genital tract inflammation in early spontaneous preterm birth. Obstet Gynecol 2004; 104: 777–783.

36. Radnai M, Gorzo I, Nagy E, Urban E, Novak T, Pal A. A possible association between preterm birth and early periodontitis. J Clin Periodontol 2004; 31:736–741.

37. Romero R, Oyarzun E, Mazor M, Sirtori M, Hobbins JC, Bracken M. Meta-analysis of the relationship between asymptomatic bacteriuria and preterm delivery/low birth weight. Obstet Gynecol 1989; 73:576–582.

38. Lockwood CJ, Senyei AE, Dische MR, et al. Fetal fibronectin in cervical and vaginal secretions as a predictor of preterm delivery. N Engl J Med 1991; 325:669–674.

39. Iams JD, Casal D, Mac Gregor JA, et al. Fetal fibronectin improves the accuracy of diagnosis of preterm labor. Am J Obstet Gynecol 1995; 173:141–145.

40. Iams JD, Goldenberg RL, Mercer BM, et al. The preterm prediction study: can low-risk women destined for spontaneous preterm birth be identified? Am J Obstet Gynecol 2001; 184:652–655.

41. Andrews WW, Sibai BM, Thom EA, et al. Randomized clinical trial of metronidazole plus erythromycin to prevent spontaneous preterm delivery in fetal fibronectin-positive women. Obstet Gynecol 2003; 101:847–855.

42. Iams JD, Goldenberg RL, Meis PJ, et al. The length of the cervix and the risk of spontaneous premature delivery. N Engl J Med 1996; 334:567–572.

43. Gibson JL, Macara LM, Owen P, Young D, Macauley J, Mackenzie F. Prediction of preterm delivery in twin pregnancy: a prospective, observational study of cervical length and fetal fibronectin testing. Ultrasound Obstet Gynecol 2004; 23:561–566.

44. Vayssiere C, Favre R, Audibert F, et al. Cervical length and funneling at 22 and 27 weeks to predict spontaneous birth before 32 weeks in twin pregnancies: a French prospective multicenter study. Am J Obstet Gynecol 2002; 187:1596–1604.

45. Andrews WW, Copper R, Hauth JC, Goldenberg RL, Neely C, Dubard M. Second-trimester cervical ultrasound: associations with increased risk for recurrent early spontaneous delivery. Obstet Gynecol 2000; 95:222–226.

46. Althsuisius SM, Dekker GA, Hummel P, Bekedam DJ, van Geijn HP. Final results of the cervical incompetence prevention randomized cerclage trial (CIPRACT): therapeutic cerclage with bed rest versus bed rest alone. Am J Obstet Gynecol 2001; 185:1106–1112.

47. Berghella V, Odibo AO, Tolosa JE. Cerclage for prevention of preterm birth in women with a short cervix found on transvaginal ultrasound examination: a randomized trial. Am J Obstet Gynecol 2004; 191:1311–1317.

48. Newman RB, Krombach RS, Myers MC, McGee DL. Effect of cerclage on obstetrical outcome in twin gestations with a shortened cervical length. Am J Obstet Gynecol 2002; 186:634–640.

49. Rust OA, Atlas RO, Reed J, van Gaalen J, Balducci J. Revisiting the short cervix detected by transvaginal ultrasound in the second trimester: why cerclage therapy may not help. Am J Obstet Gynecol 2001; 185:1098–1105.

50. To MS, Alfirevic Z, Heath VC, et al. Cervical cerclage for prevention of preterm delivery in women with short cervix: randomised controlled trial. Lancet 2004; 363:1849–1853.

51. Challis JRG. Sharp increases in free circulating oestrogens immediately before parturition in sheep. Nature 1971; 229:208.

52. Meis PJ, Klebanoff M, Thom E, et al. Prevention of recurrent preterm delivery by 17 Alpha-Hydroxyprogesterone Caproate. N Engl J Med 2003; 348:2379–2385.

53. Da Fonseca EB, Bittar RE, Carvalho MH, Zugaib M. Prophylactic administration of progesterone by vaginal suppository to reduce the incidence of spontaneous preterm

birth in women at increased risk: a randomized placebo-controlled double-blind study. Am J Obstet Gynecol 2003; 188:419–424.

54. Crowther CA. Hospitalisation and bed rest for multiple pregnancy. Cochrane Database Syst Rev 2001; 1:CD000110.

55. Goldenberg RL, Cliver SP, Bronstein J, Cutter GR, Andrews WW, Mennemeyer ST. Bed rest in pregnancy. Obstet Gynecol 1994; 84:131–136.

56. Sosa C, Althabe F, Belizan J, Bergel E. Bed rest in singleton pregnancies for preventing preterm birth. Cochrane Database Syst Rev 2004; CD003581.

57. Freda MC, DeVore N. Should intravenous hydration be the first line of defense with threatened preterm labor? A critical review of the literature. J Perinatol 1996; 16: 385–389.

58. Guinn DA, Goepfert AR, Owen J, Brumfield C, Hauth JC. Management options in women with preterm uterine contractions: a randomized controlled trial. Am J Obstet Gynecol 1997; 177:814–818.

59. Stan C, Boulvain M, Hirsbrunner-Amagbaly P, Pfister R. Hydration for treatment of preterm labour. Cochrane Database Syst Rev 2002; CD003096.

60. Iams JD, Newman RB, Thom EA, et al. Frequency of uterine contractions and the risk of spontaneous preterm delivery. N Engl J Med 2002; 346:250–255.

61. Dyson DC, Danbe KH, Bamber JA, et al. Monitoring women at risk for preterm labor. N Engl J Med 1998; 338:15–19.

62. Romero R, Sibai B, Caritis S, et al. Antibiotic treatment of preterm labor with intact membranes: a multicenter, randomized, double-blinded, placebo-controlled trial. Am J Obstet Gynecol 1993; 169:764–774.

63. Cox SM, Bohman VR, Sherman ML, Leveno KJ. Randomized investigation of antimi-crobials for the prevention of preterm birth. Am J Obstet Gynecol 1996; 174:206–210.

64. Goldenberg RL. The management of preterm labor. Obstet Gynecol 2002; 100:1020–1037.

65. King J, Flenady V. Prophylactic antibiotics for inhibiting preterm labour with intact membranes (Cochrane Review). In: The Cochrane Library, Issue 1. Oxford: Update Software, 2003.

66. Hearne AE, Nagey DA. Therapeutic agents in preterm labor: tocolytic agents. Clin Obstet Gynecol 2000; 43:787–801.

67. Berkman ND, Thorp JM, Lohr KN, et al. Tocolytic treatment for the management of preterm labor: a review of the evidence. Am J Obstet Gynecol 2003; 188:1648–1659.

68. Goldenberg RL, Rouse DJ. Prevention of premature birth. N Engl J Med 1998; 339:313–320.

69. Gyetvai K, Hannah ME, Hodnett ED, Ohlsson A. Tocolytics for preterm labor: a sys-tematic review. Obstet Gynecol 1999; 94:869–877.

70. Agency for Healthcare Research and Quality. Management of preterm labor. Evidence Report/Technology Assessment No. 18. Rockville (MD): AHRQ, 2000. AHRQ Publica-tion No. 01-E021.

71. Rust OA, Bofill JA, Arriola RM, Andrew ME, Morrison JC. The clinical efficacy of oral tocolytic therapy. Am J Obstet Gynecol 1996; 175:838–842.

72. Moise KJ, Huhta JC, Sharif DS, et al. Indomethacin in the treatment of premature labor: effects on the fetal ductus arteriosus. N Engl J Med 1988; 319:327–331.

22

Pharmacological Therapy

Jay J. Bringman and Owen P. Phillips
*Department of Obstetrics and Gynecology, University of Tennessee Health Sciences
Center, Memphis, Tennessee, U.S.A.*

INTRODUCTION

Advances in genetics and prenatal diagnosis have increased our understanding of anatomic, physiologic, and molecular disorders of the fetus. This has enabled researchers to pursue the ultimate goal of treating fetal disorders in utero in order to optimize neonatal health. This chapter will deal with the medical treatments of the fetus currently in practice and those with potential, including genetic disorders and medical disorders of the fetus. Surgical therapies and ethical considerations surrounding prenatal treatments are discussed elsewhere in this text.

PREREQUISITES FOR FETAL THERAPY

Certain prerequisites must be satisfied prior to undertaking fetal therapy (1). First, an accurate diagnosis of the fetal abnormality must be established. High resolution ultrasound to assess fetal anatomy has made accurate diagnoses possible. Fetal echocardiography can accurately diagnose cardiac arrhythmias. Chorionic villus sampling (CVS) (2) can be performed at 11 to 12 weeks' gestation, allowing for earlier diagnosis for many genetic disorders than the more traditional midtrimester amniocentesis. For example, CVS has proven particularly valuable in the management of fetal 21-hydroxylase deficiency (3), which will be discussed later in this chapter. And finally, preimplantation diagnosis may one day move routine diagnosis and treatment of genetic disease back even further.

Second, an understanding of the disorder and its pathophysiology is necessary prior to initiating fetal therapy. Because many genetic diseases vary widely in their severity, the clinical consequences and natural history of a disease must be known and conveyed to the couple prior to considering therapy.

Third, whether there is need for treatment must be considered. The following principles should apply: (i) the disorder must be severe enough that therapy is justified; (ii) consideration must be given as to whether the fetus will benefit more from antenatal therapy than from treatment after delivery. Thus, the justification for fetal therapy should be that the condition of the fetus will deteriorate and irrevocable damage or death will ensue if antenatal treatment is not undertaken.

Lastly, the risks of treatment both to mother and fetus must be known. After having established that fetal therapy is necessary, a risk–benefit analysis should be undertaken. Investigational fetal therapy should be performed only with prior approval of an Institutional Review Board (IRB) and in all cases only with the informed consent of the parents.

GENETIC DISORDERS AFFECTING THE FETUS

Inborn errors of metabolism are devastating genetic diseases that are often fatal in childhood. These disorders are predominantly inherited in autosomal recessive fashion. Treatment is usually palliative and seldom curative. However, fetal therapy may offer successful treatment for some of these disorders. It may be necessary to begin therapy in early gestation or preconceptionally in order to prevent untoward effects that occur during organogenesis. Therefore, diagnosis will be required as early in pregnancy as possible; prenatal testing by CVS or in the preimplantation embryo will become increasingly important. In some disorders, treatment may have to be initiated before a definitive diagnosis is made.

Congenital Adrenal Hyperplasia

Congenital adrenal hyperplasia (CAH) caused by 21-hydroxylase deficiency (classical CAH) or 11 β-hydroxylase deficiency causes virilization of the affected female fetus because of an overproduction of adrenal androgens by the fetal adrenal gland. Clitoromegaly or a urogenital sinus results and gender assignment may be difficult at birth; surgical treatment is usually required. However, antenatal treatment of the mother with glucocorticoids has been successful in suppressing the fetal adrenal gland and preventing virilization in affected females. Dexamethasone is currently the corticosteroid of choice because it is not readily deactivated when it crosses the placenta (3,4).

Candidates for treatments are usually ascertained because the couple has had an affected offspring. As an autosomal recessive disorder, the recurrence risk is 25% or one in four. The risk for an affected female is one in eight. In order to prevent virilization of a subsequent female offspring, dexamethasone is administered to the mother when the pregnancy is confirmed. Prenatal diagnosis is carried out as soon as feasible, preferably by CVS at 11 weeks' gestation or at 14 weeks by amniocentesis. If the fetus is male, dexamethasone is discontinued. If the fetus is female, diagnosis for affected status is performed by mutation analysis. If the fetus is unaffected, the drug is discontinued. If the female fetus is affected, dexamethasone is continued until delivery.

Mercado et al. (5) published a cohort of 176 pregnancies in which the index case was an affected female sibling. Dexamethasone 20 μg/kg prepregnancy weight per day in three divided doses was begun before the ninth week gestation in 101 cases. Prenatal diagnosis was performed, and 13 affected females were diagnosed. Treatment was effective in preventing virilization or in significantly reducing virilization compared to their affected, untreated female siblings. Antenatal treatment begun after the 10th week gestation had little or no effect on preventing virilization.

In this study (5), there were no significant side effects to the children born. The treated newborns did not differ from untreated in weight, length, or head circumference. No birth defects occurred. Maternal complications were noted in six cases.

Cushingoid facies and excessive weight gain occurred in two women. Another woman experienced an increase in blood pressure and headache. Mood fluctuations, edema, striae, and general discomfort were reported as well. All symptoms were relieved when the medication was stopped.

Long-term studies of children treated prenatally with dexamethasone have been performed as well. A multicenter study in France (6) found normal growth, development, and intelligence in children followed beyond 10 years of age.

Another cause of CAH and virilization in female offspring is 11 β-hydroxylase deficiency. Cerame et al. (7) reported on the successful antenatal treatment in pregnancies of two families, both with affected children. Treatment was begun by the fifth week and prenatal diagnosis was performed by CVS. The protocol followed was identical to that of accepted treatment plans for 21-hydroxylase deficiency (see earlier). In this case series, a treated female was born with 11 β-hydroxylase deficiency but with normal genitalia. There were no adverse effects reported in the mother or in the offspring.

Despite these obvious successes, there is still controversy over antenatal treatment of CAH (8,9). Prenatal diagnosis of 21-hydroxylase deficiency is about 95% accurate; there have been false-negative and false-positive results reported in many studies. Furthermore, because males and unaffected females will not benefit from treatment, theoretically eight fetuses will be exposed to treat one. There may be an increased risk of pregnancy loss in treated women. And finally, a Swedish study (8) found abnormalities in several unaffected but antenatally treated children. The abnormalities were varied and, therefore, less likely to be secondary to a drug effect. But several children had developmental problems and growth disturbances. Further, controlled studies on the minimal dose necessary for benefit and long-term and short-term safety need to be conducted.

Smith–Lemli–Opitz Syndrome

Smith–Lemli–Opitz syndrome (SLOS) is an autosomal recessively inherited congenital anomaly syndrome caused by an abnormality in cholesterol metabolism. It is characterized by prenatal and postnatal growth restriction, mental retardation, microcephaly, and in boys, hypospadias. Other malformations may include cardiac defects, cleft palate, distinctive facial features, polydactaly, and syndactaly. A deficiency of the enzyme 7-dehydrocholesterol reductase is responsible for the features. Cholesterol supplementation beginning in the neonatal periods appears to improve growth in children with SLOS (10,11) as well as improving developmental progress and behavior (10). Because prenatal diagnosis can be made by finding abnormally high levels of 7-dehydrocholesterol levels in amniotic fluid or in tissue obtained from CVS (12,13), and by molecular diagnosis if mutational analysis delineates the parental mutations (14), it seems possible that antenatal treatment with cholesterol supplementation might also be efficacious.

In one case published by Irons et al. (15), treatment with cholesterol was administered by fetal intravenous and intraperitoneal transfusions of fresh frozen plasma with a cholesterol concentration of 219 mg/dL. Follow-up cordocentesis was performed and found that fetal plasma cholesterol levels increased as did the fetal red blood cell volume (indicating incorporation of cholesterol into fetal erythrocytes). The diagnosis and treatment were performed in the third trimester and, clearly, would not have prevented congenital malformations. And although no postnatal follow-up was reported, the case illustrates that increasing cholesterol levels is possible antenatally, which may provide some benefit.

Women carrying offspring with SLOS have low serum unconjugated estriol levels detected on maternal serum screening for Down syndrome (16). Women carrying a pregnancy with low unconjugated estriol levels and characteristic ultrasound findings should be offered prenatal diagnosis for SLOS.

Disorders of Vitamin Metabolism

Several inborn errors of metabolism cause relative deficiencies of vitamins required for neonatal development. Treatment with large maternal vitamin administration has been tried as fetal treatment. These include methylmalonic acidemia (MMA) (vitamin B12), multiple carboxylase deficiency (biotin), and the possible treatment options for glutathione synthetase deficiency (vitamin E) and abetalipoproteinemia (vitamin E). Folic acid plays a role in neural tube defects (NTDs), and this condition will be considered here as well.

Methylmalonic Acidemia

MMA was the first vitamin responsive inborn error of metabolism to be treated prenatally (17). Coenzymatically active vitamin B12 is necessary for the conversion of methylmalonyl CoA to succinyl CoA, an essential step in the degradation of several amino acids and fatty acids. At least six different genetically determined biochemical defects (all autosomal recessive) can result in accumulation of methylmalonic acid. Affected newborns present with vomiting, failure to thrive, developmental retardation, intermittent neutropenia, and hepatomegaly; acidosis ensues and is often life threatening.

Prenatal diagnosis has been achieved by the detection of maternal urinary excretion of methylmalonate, which should not otherwise be present (17). More recently, however, the human methylmalonic CoA mutase has been localized to the short arm of chromosome 6 (18); a highly informative restriction fragment length polymorphism has been identified at this gene locus and should be very useful for prenatal diagnosis (19). Ampola et al. (17) reported a case in which maternal urinary excretion of methylmalonate was used to diagnose this disorder in a fetus at risk and to monitor antenatal treatment. Because the mother did not excrete methylmalonate when she was not pregnant, the appearance of this compound in her urine was used as a biochemical index of fetal status. Large doses of vitamin B12 (5 mg/day) were administered intravenously to the mother during the third trimester. Maternal serum B12 levels increased to six times normal levels without ill effects, and maternal urinary excretion of methylmalonate correspondingly decreased. Following birth, umbilical cord blood levels of B12 were markedly elevated and the neonatal course was uncomplicated. The diagnosis of MMA was confirmed, and the infant did well, thereafter, on a protein-restricted diet without the need for continuous vitamin therapy. This outcome was in marked contrast to that of an untreated affected sibling who died at three months of age of severe acidosis and dehydration.

There are now other cases of prenatal treatment of MMA with vitamin B12 (20) with results similar to those of Ampola et al. (17). However, further studies will be necessary to completely assess the risks and benefits of this therapy.

Multiple Carboxylase Deficiency

Three biotin-dependent mitochondrial enzymes (pyruvate carboxylase, proprionyl-CoA carboxylase, and β-methylcrotonyl CoA carboxylase) are deficient in multiple carboxylase deficiency, a rare autosomal recessive disorder. Infants present in the first few weeks of life with severe metabolic acidosis, vomiting, hypertonia, irritability, seizures, and dermatitis. Left untreated, they become lethargic, lapse into coma, and die.

In a case reported by Packman et al. (21), a woman who had one child affected with multiple carboxylase deficiency underwent prenatal diagnosis by enzyme assay of cultured amniotic fluid cells obtained at 17 weeks' gestation; the fetus was determined to be affected. Maternal biotin therapy, 10 mg/day, was instituted orally at 23 weeks' gestation and continued until delivery. Postnatally, the diagnosis was confirmed by enzyme assay of skin fibroblasts and the child was continued on biotin therapy, with normal subsequent development. In another case of a twin gestation reported by Roth et al. (22), treatment was initiated without a prenatal diagnosis having been made first. This patient had two previous infants who had died from unremitting metabolic acidosis due to multiple carboxylase deficiency. She presented at 34 weeks' gestation; biotin therapy was begun empirically at the same dose described previously and continued until delivery. Nonidentical twins were delivered at term, one affected, and one unaffected. Cord blood levels of biotin were several-fold the normal range, indicating therapeutic levels. The affected twin did well on continued postnatal therapy, and at the four year follow-up, neither twin showed evidence of adverse affects from the prenatal biotin therapy.

More recently, a pregnancy at risk for holocarboxylase synthetase deficiency was diagnosed and treated prenatally; this enzyme disorder is an early-onset, biotin-responsive form of multiple carboxylase deficiency (23,24). Thuy et al. (23) described a family with two affected offspring, products of a consanguineous relationship. CVS was performed at 11 weeks. Holocarboxylase synthetase levels were low, consistent with affected status when compared to normal controls. The mother was begun on 10 mg oral biotin per day and maintained on this dose for the duration of her pregnancy. The diagnosis was confirmed and the child has been continuously treated on biotin and has done well.

Considering the above case reports, several questions about prenatal therapy in multiple carboxylase deficiency appear to have been answered. First, high levels of biotin do not appear to have any untoward effects on an unaffected fetus or the mother. It also suggests that therapy begun late in gestation is effective; therefore, administration of the vitamin during early fetal development may not be necessary. Diagnosis can be made by amniocentesis as well as CVS. Because there is no apparent benefit to starting prenatal treatment early in pregnancy and there is currently no information available on the teratogenicity of biotin, beginning therapy after organogenesis may be preferable.

Glutathione Synthetase Deficiency and Abetalipoproteinemia

Both of these rare autosomal recessive disorders are associated with vitamins. In glutathione synthetase deficiency, vitamins E and A function as antioxidants and when administered postnatally result in improvement in red cell survival and prevention of abnormalities in leukocyte function (25). Postnatal treatment with vitamins may inhibit the development of the progressive neurological impairment that occurs in most patients with this disease.

In abetalipoproteinemia, supplementation with high doses of vitamins E and C has been shown to retard or prevent the severe and fatal neurological damage (26). Therefore, it is possible that prenatal therapy with vitamin E may be beneficial in fetuses, although no clinical studies have been performed to test this hypothesis.

Neural Tube Defects

NTDs, particularly anencephaly and spina bifida, have a familial predisposition and can be prevented by folic acid supplementation (27–29). However, it does not appear that folic acid supplementation simply corrects a vitamin deficiency; most women carrying affected fetuses have folic acid in the normal range (30). The enzyme 5,10 methylenetetrahydrofolate reductase is a folate-dependent enzyme that regulates the conversion of homocysteine to methionine (31). The thermolabile isoform (T genotype) of this enzyme in the mother has been associated with NTDs in the offspring. However, there is evidence that it is the genotype in the fetus that is important in causing the pathology (32). The TT homozygous genotype in the fetus in the presence of low folate levels is pathogenic and causes a certain percentage of NTDs.

Regardless of the precise pathogenesis, NTDs can be prevented with maternal folic acid supplementation. The Centers for Disease Control (CDC) recommends that all women take folic acid supplementation preconceptually and during the early part of pregnancy (33). To prevent occurrence, 400 µg a day is recommended. For the prevention of recurrence of NTDs, 4 mg daily is recommended.

Disorders of Diet

Maternal Phenylketonuria

There are now hundreds of women with phenylketonuria (PKU) who have received dietary restriction therapy and who are in the reproductive years (34,35). In late childhood, these patients invariably abandon the phenylalanine-restricted diet to a more palatable diet with little to no harm to themselves. However, the high maternal levels of phenylalanine affect fetal brain development causing mental deficiencies, microcephaly, cardiac defects, and intrauterine growth restriction.

That offspring of women with classical PKU have abnormalities was first noted in 1956 and initially the children were thought to have an aberrant form of PKU. Lenke and Levy (36) clarified that it was maternal disease having an effect on fetal development. They found that in mothers who have PKU and whose phenylalanine levels are >20 mg/dL, 90% of their offspring had intelligent quotients (IQs) <75, 73% were microcephalic, 17% had congenital heart disease, and about 50% had low birth weight. They found no consistent relationship between treatment initiated during pregnancy and prevention of abnormalities; when phenylalanine levels were lowered to 3–10 mg/dL (normal <2 mg/dL), 33% had an IQ <75 and 44% were microcephalic. Even when dietary treatment was initiated in the first trimester, 4 of 11 offspring died of congenital heart disease. However, in two of three cases in which treatment was initiated before conception, the offspring were apparently normal; the third case had an IQ of 80 and microcephaly.

Murphy et al. (37) reported two cases in which diet was initiated prior to conception and maintained throughout pregnancy; in both cases the offspring showed normal development at four and five years of age, respectively. In an international study by Drogari et al. (38), no cases of mental deficiency, congenital heart disease, or low birth weight was seen in 17 women who began strict diet restriction prior to conception and whose blood phenylalanine levels were <6 mg/dL; the rates of malformations in women who began strict diets during pregnancy were similar to those of women who received no treatment during pregnancy. Therefore, dietary treatment in women with PKU must begin preconceptionally and maintained through pregnancy to have maximal benefit for their offspring (34,37,38); treatment delayed until the second and third trimesters may be of no benefit (34).

On the other hand, fetuses of women with atypical PKU or non-PKU mild hyperphenylanemia are probably at no increased risk of adverse effects (34). This is important because at some centers, these cases comprise 50% of hyperphenylalanemic patients. It also illustrates the point that the nature of the toxic agent in maternal PKU and pathogenesis of fetal damage is unclear.

Galactosemia

Affected individuals with galactosemia show growth deficiency, cataracts, ovarian failure, and mental retardation. It is an autosomal recessive condition that results in diminished activity of the enzyme galactose-1-phosphate uridyl transferase. The sequelae can largely be ameliorated by elimination of galactose from the diet; early neonatal treatment with a low galactose diet may not ensure normal development. The damage to oocytes in humans may occur before birth (39–41). Subtle abnormalities may be present in the male gonads as well (41). Abnormal neurological development and cataract formation may also result from prenatal damage in galactosemic fetuses (41,42).

Galactose restriction during pregnancy may be beneficial when the fetus is affected with galactosemia. Prenatal diagnosis of galactosemia is possible by enzyme assay of cultured amniocytes or chorionic villi. However, ovarian meiosis begins at 12 weeks and is complete by 28 weeks; neurological and lens abnormalities may occur this early as well. Therefore, it may be necessary to begin treatment early in gestation or perhaps preconceptionally. Although there are no studies that have assessed the impact of prenatal dietary restriction of galactose, both normal and galactosemic fetuses are capable of some endogenous galactose synthesis; therefore, galactose restriction should not be harmful to unaffected fetuses and beneficial to those affected.

MEDICAL DISORDERS OF THE FETUS

Fetal Therapy for Cardiac Arrhythmias

Fetal cardiac arrhythmias occur in up to 2% of pregnancies and the vast majority of these are benign in nature (43). They are usually brought to the attention of the physician after detection of an irregular fetal heart rate during routine auscultation. Of those fetuses referred for irregular beats, <2% will have a clinically significant arrhythmia (44).

With the use of such techniques as M-mode echocardiography and Doppler ultrasound, correct diagnosis of fetal cardiac arrhythmias may be accomplished. M-mode echocardiography can provide ventricular and atrial wall motion during an arrhythmia, while Doppler ultrasound can provide information as to the timing of atrial and ventricular events. Although a detailed ultrasound is required for the diagnosis of the arrhythmia, there appears to be no increase in the rate of structural cardiac defects in fetuses referred because of a benign irregular heart rate on auscultation (44). However, fetuses diagnosed with cardiac arrhythmias do have a higher rate of structural cardiac defects (45).

Hydrops fetalis can result from fetal arrhythmias, especially persistent fetal tachycardias. The associated risk can be as high as 64% (46). Hydrops carries a substantial mortality rate and clearly requires in utero treatment. However, hydrops may adversely affect placental transport of antiarrhythmic medications. Distinguishing those fetuses that will develop hydrops from those that will not is difficult because of the lack of reliable predictors for hydrops (47). Therefore, treating fetuses with sustained tachycardia is appropriate.

In treating the fetus, one must remember the risks associated with antiarrhythmic use in the mother. All antiarrhythmics can be proarrhythmic; therefore, close observation of the mother is mandatory. Certain laboratory tests should be performed prior to administration, such as an electrocardiogram, serum electrolytes, blood urea nitrogen, and creatinine to establish a baseline for the mother. Treatment of tachyarrythmias and heart block will be discussed specific to the type of disorder. Tachyarrythmias include superventricular tachycardia (SVT), atrial flutter, atrial fibrillation, and ventricular tachycardia (VT).

Superventricular Tachycardia

SVT is the most common tachyarrhythmia. First-line treatment for SVT is digoxin, a cardiac glycoside. Digoxin given intravenously may be more successful in restoration of sinus rhythm than if given orally (48,49). Success rates for conversion to sinus rhythm when digoxin is used alone are different in the nonhydropic and hydropic fetus. A retrospective review by Krapp et al. (50) reports success rates of 65% when hydrops is absent, compared to 24.6% when hydrops is present.

Schmolling et al. (51) compared the maternofetal transplacental transfer of digoxin, flecainide, and amiodarone and also assessed the effect of an elevated umbilical venous pressure on the transfer rate. This perfusion method suggested that transplacental digoxin transfer is greater than that of flecainide. With the elevation of umbilical venous pressure (similar to that seen in hydrops), digoxin and flecainide transfer decreased.

Frohn-Mulder et al. (52) compared flecainide with digoxin in fetuses with SVT. Digoxin was the first-line agent in fetuses with SVT and no hydrops. In fetuses with hydrops, digoxin was the first-line agent up to 1991; subsequently, flecainide was the agent used as the first-line agent in hydrops. Digoxin was effective in restoring sinus rhythm in 55% of the nonhydropic fetuses and 8% of the hydropic fetuses. In contrast, flecainide restored sinus rhythm in 43% of hydropic fetuses. As a second-line agent, it was effective in restoring sinus rhythm in all nonhydropic fetuses where digoxin treatment failed. Also, the administration of flecainide resulted in a significantly reduced mortality rate compared with digoxin treatment.

Flecainide use is not without maternal risks. In the Cardiac Arrhythmia Suppression Trial (53), the use of flecainide and/or encainide after myocardial infarction was associated with a significant increase in sudden arrhythmia death among postmyocardial infarction patients. The population in this study consisted mostly of older male patients that had suffered a myocardial infarction.

Hohnloser et al. (54) reviewed their experience with oral sotalol as first-line therapy for the treatment of fetal SVT. Sotalol, a beta-blocker, was successful in converting 6 of 10 (60%) of fetuses with SVT. Three of four fetal deaths occurred in fetuses treated with sotalol as a first-line agent and the fourth had significant neurologic morbidity after birth.

There is some controversy over what constitutes second-line therapy. Certain authors suggest that propranolol should be the drug of choice (55). However, in the review by Krapp et al. (50), flecainide was added to the digoxin regimen most often, followed by verapamil (a calcium channel blocker), amiodarone, and propafenone. While the success rate for flecainide (alone or in combination) was 87%, there were not enough cases to prove one drug superior to the others. Amiodarone has been investigated as a second-line agent. Jouannic et al. evaluated the role of amiodarone for the prenatal treatment of hydropic fetuses with SVT. In nine fetuses with hydrops where either digoxin or flecainide failed as first-line agents, five were converted to sinus rhythm with the addition of amiodarone as a second-line agent (56).

Regardless of the agent added as a second-line agent, one must take into account certain pharmacokinetic properties of the medication being used. Amiodarone can decrease clearance of digoxin; therefore, the digoxin dose should be halved (57). Flecainide and propranolol can potentiate the proarrhythmic effects of amiodarone; therefore, these drugs should be discontinued for 48 hours prior to the administration of amiodarone (58). Prior to the use of sotalol, procainamide and flecainide must be discontinued for 72 hours in order for clearance of these drugs to take place (57). Also, amiodarone has been associated with transient fetal hypothyroidism (59).

Maternal administration of antiarrhythmics for fetal arrhythmias is best done on an inpatient basis. Treatment also should be done in collaboration with a pediatric cardiologist. The fetus should be monitored by way of electronic fetal heart rate monitoring so that the time spent in tachycardia can be determined. Because all antiarrhythmics are potentially proarrhythmic, electrocardiographic observation of the mother should be considered. And finally, certain medications can cause maternal side effects. It is imperative for the physician administering these medicines to be familiar with these side effects.

Atrial Flutter and Atrial Fibrillation

Fetuses with atrial flutter and atrial fibrillation have a relatively high incidence of structural heart disease (49). Diagnosis of atrial flutter involves identifying an atrioventricular heart block, which will be absent in SVT. In atrial fibrillation, there is no relationship between the erratic atrial activity and the ventricular contractions. This results in an irregular ventricular rhythm (58). Control of the atrial impulse is critical for management of this arrhythmia.

Treatment of atrial flutter and atrial fibrillation is usually initiated by first controlling the ventricular response with digoxin or propranolol. After the ventricular rate has been controlled with either digoxin or propranolol, attention is then turned to restoration of sinus rhythm (58). There does not appear to be widespread acceptance of one drug or another as a first-line agent in the restoration of sinus rhythm. Krapp et al. published a retrospective review of the diagnosis, treatment, and outcome of fetal atrial flutter versus SVT (50). In this review, digoxin was used as first-line therapy in fetuses with atrial flutter and was successful in restoring sinus rhythm in 45% of these fetuses. However, the difference in success rate for digoxin in fetuses with hydrops (6.3%) versus fetuses without hydrops (51.7%) failed to reach significance due to the low number of fetuses in the study group. There was a wide range of second-line agents used. Flecainide, amiodarone, and propafenone were used most often, with conversion rates of 5/6, 3/7, and 1/3, respectively.

Ventricular Tachycardia

Fetal VT is relatively rare. In seven cases reported by Kleinman et al. (47), one fetus had hydrops. In two fetuses, the arrhythmia was successfully controlled and two had persistent tachycardia after birth. Treatment for VT is usually initiated if there is a rapid ventricular rate (>200 bpm), if VT is associated with structural heart disease, or if hydrops is present (55). Information concerning treatment of VT is scarce. The first-line drug is usually propranolol. If this is ineffective, then direct umbilical venous administration of lidocaine to the fetus may be warranted (55).

Complete Heart Block

Atrioventricular conduction disturbances can occur in the fetus. These conduction disturbances can either be partial (first- or second-degree heart block) or complete. Diagnosis of first-degree heart block is done by measuring the time interval from the onset of the mitral A wave (atrial systole) to the onset of the aortic pulsed Doppler tracing (ventricular systole) within the same ventricular cardiac cycle (60). This interval is the mechanical PR interval. In fetuses with first-degree heart block, this mechanical PR interval is increased, with normal values being less than 150 ms (60,61). In fetuses with second-degree atrioventricular block, some atrial impulses fail to conduct to the ventricles. Third-degree block or complete heart block occurs when no atrial impulses conduct to the ventricles. It may be that third-degree heart block represents an end-point in immune-mediated destruction of the conduction system.

Fetuses with complete heart block appear to have either structural heart disease or heart block associated with immune complex–mediated destruction of the conduction system and the myocardium (62). Schmidt et al. reported 55 cases of complete fetal heart block (62). Twenty-nine fetuses had heart block associated with structural heart disease, while 26 fetuses had normal cardiac anatomy. Of these 26 fetuses, 21 were positive for anti-Ro and/or anti-La antibodies which have been associated with congenital complete heart block (63). These IgG antibodies cross the placenta and react with all myocardial tissue, including the myocardium and the conduction system.

Fetuses with heart block associated with hydrops fetalis, structural heart disease or ventricular rates below 55 bpm carry a poor prognosis (62). In fetuses with partial heart block associated high anti-Ro/anti-La titers, maternally administered fluorinated steroids may improve the prognosis. Copel et al. (64) reported five fetuses with heart block and either anti-Ro or anti-La antibodies in which the mothers were treated with dexamethasone 4 mg daily. In two patients, the degree of heart block was reduced with treatment and hydrops resolved in three patients with complete heart block.

The Retrospective Review of a Research Registry for Neonatal Lupus studied 47 mothers with maternal autoantibodies and their 50 offsprings with heart blocks. There were no cases of third-degree block reduced with the use of either dexamethasone or betamethasone (65). In four fetuses with second-degree block, there was reversal to first-degree block in all four; all remained in an incomplete block after birth. Fetal hydrops and ascites resolved in the majority of fetuses after treatment with maternal steroids. Steroids should be considered when fetuses are diagnosed with partial heart block or hydrops.

Fetal Thyroid Disorders

Fetal thyroid dysfunction usually goes undetected in utero. However, fetal hypo- and hyperthyroidism may be suspected by eliciting a careful maternal history of thyroid disease, use of thionamides (propylthiouracil [PTU] and methimazole) or amiodarone, iodine exposure, or a family history of neonates with thyroid dysfunction. Maternal thyroid disease such as Graves' disease and Hashimoto's thyroiditis should alert the physician to possible fetal thyroid dysfunction.

Fetal Hyperthyroidism

Fetal and neonatal hyperthyroidism is usually caused by transplacental passage of maternal thyroid-stimulating immunoglobulin (TSI). These antibodies are present in Graves' disease, but can be seen in Hashimoto's thyroiditis (66). Even a maternal history of Graves' disease that has been successfully treated with surgery or radioactive iodine places the fetus at risk for thyrotoxicosis because antibodies continue to circulate.

Fetuses with thyrotoxicosis can present with elevated heart rates, growth retardation, advanced bone age, craniosynostosis, goiter, and hydrops. Fetal mortality rates as high as 16% have been reported with fetal thyrotoxicosis (67). Neonatal effects include hyperkinesis, diarrhea, goiter, exopthalmos, weight loss, hypertension, and irritability. It is estimated that approximately 1% to 12% of neonates born to mothers with Graves' disease will show some evidence of thyrotoxicosis at delivery (68,69).

Clinically, tachycardia is the most common presenting sign for fetal thyrotoxicosis. However, normal fetal heart rates have been reported. Stillbirth without any other signs of morbidity has also been reported (70,71). High maternal levels of TSIs usually correlate with fetal hyperthyroidism; nevertheless, there are many different ways to measure TSIs with no international standard for the TSI assay (72). Therefore, correlating the levels with the thyroid status of the fetus can be difficult, and fetal thyroid function does not necessarily mimic maternal thyroid function (69).

Amniotic fluid measurements of thyroid function tests do not correlate with disease activity in the fetus; however, accurate fetal thyroid status can be determined by cordocentesis (71,73). Several cases of the use of cordocentesis in the diagnosis of fetal hyperthyroidism have been reported (69,74,75) and normal fetal thyroid values have been established (76).

Many case reports in the literature report successful in utero treatment of fetal thyrotoxicosis (69,71,74,75,77). Maternally administered PTU is considered the drug of choice in the treatment of fetal thyrotoxicosis. While PTU has a better safety profile in pregnancy than either methimazole or carbimazole, these latter two medications have a more rapid and complete transplacental transfer than PTU (78). In certain cases, it may be necessary to provide thyroid hormone replacement to the mother if she becomes hypothyroid from the PTU (78). Doses of PTU used in studies range from 100 mg/day to 200 mg three times a day.

The fetal response to treatment may be followed by the fetal heart rate. Restoration of a normal fetal heart rate may show adequate fetal treatment. Repeat cordocentesis may also be performed for direct fetal thyroid activity measurement.

Fetal Hypothyroidism

Fetal hypothyroidism is most commonly caused by thyroid dysgenesis with a reported incidence of 1 in 4000 (79). Maternal ingestion of antithyroid drugs or chemicals can also cause fetal thyroid dysfunction, affecting approximately 1 in 40,000 pregnancies (79). The majority of fetuses affected by hypothyroidism will not be detected in utero and will develop normally because of the low thyroxine requirement in the fetus and the maternal transfer of T_4 from a euthyroid mother. Routine neonatal screening for congenital hypothyroidism is mandatory in most states. Neonates with congenital hypothyroidism will be detected by screening programs and treated. Normal IQs at ages 5–7 years, as well as normal growth and development usually result (80,81).

Several case reports exist describing the in utero treatment of hypothyroidism (82–86). In the majority of these cases, fetal hypothyroidism is suspected by a fetal goiter on ultrasound or a maternal history of antithyroid medication use. Once hypothyroidism is diagnosed, thyroid hormone replacement is accomplished by intra-amniotic injections of levothyroxine. Animal models have shown that 90% of levothyroxine injected into the amniotic fluid is absorbed within 24 hours of instillation (83). Doses of levothyroxine have ranged from 250 to 500 µg. This intra-amniotic treatment can be repeated weekly until the fetal goiter resolves or cordocentesis shows normalization of fetal thyroid function.

Congenital Infections

Of the congenital infections, only syphilis and toxoplasmosis are amenable to in utero treatment. Parvovirus may cause fetal hemolysis and the fetus can be treated with transfusions.

Toxoplasmosis

Clinically significant congenital toxoplasmosis infection occurs in approximately 1 in 10,000 deliveries, with an estimated 400 to 4000 cases in the United States each year (87,88). Toxoplasmosis is caused by the protozoan parasite, *Toxoplasma gondii*. It can be transmitted to a pregnant woman through ingestion or handling of infected meats or contamination of food from infected cat feces. The incidence of seroprevalence of *Toxoplasma* in the United States for women of childbearing age is 14% (89).

Transmission to the fetus in the third trimester is associated with the highest rates of fetal infection, while infection in the first trimester has a greater likelihood of severe postnatal sequelae. During the first, second, and third trimester, the rates of fetal infection are 15%, 30%, and 60%, respectively (90). Approximately 40% of neonates born to mothers with acute primary infection will show evidence of infection, with less than half of these infants showing signs of infection at birth.

The diagnosis of maternal toxoplasmosis infection is usually suspected through serologic testing. The presence of toxoplasma-specific IgG indicates that infection has occurred, but does not distinguish between recent or past maternal infection. Detection of a high toxoplasma-specific IgM antibody titer combined with a high IgG titer most likely indicates infection within the last three months. If the IgM is a low to medium titer, then infection may have occurred in the last three to six months. However, IgM can stay positive for up to 18 months (89). Testing for toxoplasma-specific IgM and IgG is not well-standardized and samples should be sent to a well-established reference laboratory (e.g., Palo Alto Medical Foundation research division) (55).

The diagnosis of fetal congenital toxoplasmosis relies upon ultrasound and invasive prenatal diagnosis. Ultrasound findings suggestive of toxoplasmosis infection in the fetus include periventricular calcifications, ventriculomegaly, microcephaly, hepatic calcifications, and ascites/hydrops. If toxoplasmosis infection in the fetus is suspected, an amniocentesis or CVS should be considered. Polymerase chain reaction specific for toxoplasma DNA can be performed on amniotic fluid or villi. The overall sensitivity and specificity for this test is 64% and 100%, respectively, with positive and negative predictive values 100% and 88%, respectively (91,92). Cordocentesis is reserved for cases where diagnosis is not confirmed by testing with amniocentesis.

Acute toxoplasmosis in the mother warrants prompt treatment. Treatment is with spiramycin, a macrolide antibiotic. Spiramycin is used in Europe; but in the United States, approval must be granted through the CDC in order to obtain this drug for treatment. The drug does not cross the placenta; however, it appears to inhibit transplacental crossage of the protozoa to the fetus. If the fetus is found to be infected, pyrimethamine plus either sulfadoxine or sulfadiazine should be added (93). This treatment regimen has been reported to reduce the risk of congenital infection by approximately 70% (93).

Syphilis

Syphilis results from infection caused by the spirochete *Treponema pallidum*. The maternal disease is divided into primary, secondary, latent, and tertiary stages. *T. pallidum* is able to cross the placenta and infect the fetus in all trimesters and intrapartum; however, infection late in pregnancy is associated with higher rates of congenital syphilis (55). Other factors associated with transmission to the fetus include primary or secondary infection in the mother and inadequate or no treatment of maternal syphilis (94,95).

During 2000–2002, rates of congenital syphilis have decreased 21.1%, from 14.2 to 11.2 cases per 100,000 live births. This rate of decline occurred in all racial/ethnic minority populations in the United States (96).

Darkfield examinations and direct fluorescent antibody tests of lesion exudates or tissue are the definitive methods for diagnosing syphilis. A presumptive diagnosis can be made with the use of nontreponemal and treponemal tests. The nontreponemal tests include the Venereal Disease Research Laboratory (VDRL) test and the rapid plasma reagin (RPR). The treponemal tests include the fluorescent treponemal antibody absorbed (FTA-ABS) and the *T. pallidum* particle agglutination (TP-PA) (97).

The diagnosis of congenital syphilis may be difficult. Ultrasonographic findings associated with congenital syphilis include dilated bowel segments, hepatomegaly, hydrops, and placentomegaly (98). A confirmation of congenital syphilis requires the detection of *T. pallidum* by darkfield microscopy, fluorescent antibody, or other specific stains in specimens from lesions, placenta, umbilical cord, or autopsy material. A presumptive case is defined as any infant whose mother had untreated or inadequately treated syphilis at delivery, regardless of the signs or symptoms. In addition, a presumptive case can be any infant who has a reactive treponemal test for syphilis and any one of the following: evidence of congential syphilis on physical examination or long-bone X-ray, reactive cerebrospinal fluid (CSF) VDRL, elevated CSF cell count, or protein or reactive test for FTA-ABS-IgM antibody (99).

Once a pregnant patient is diagnosed with syphilis, treatment should ensue. The preferred treatment is penicillin. Erythromycin use in pregnancy is inadequate and tetracycline use should be avoided in pregnancy. Penicillin is effective for preventing maternal transmission to the fetus and for treating fetal infection. The treatment regimen should be according to the patient's stage of syphilis infection. In patients with primary, secondary, or early latent syphilis (<1 year), the treatment consists of benzathine penicillin G, 2.4 million units IM in a single dose. For latent syphilis, benzathine penicillin G, 7.2 million units, administered as three doses of 2.4 million units IM at 1-week intervals is recommended. For patients with neurosyphilis, aqueous penicillin G, 18–24 million units/day, administered as 3–4 million units IV every 4 hours for 10–14 days or procaine penicillin, 2.4 million units IM daily, plus probenecid 500 mg PO QID, should be administered for 10–14 days. In patients who are penicillin-allergic, penicillin desensitization should be done (97).

Several reports have brought to light the possibility of treatment failures in pregnancy (100,101). Factors associated with higher rates of treatment failure for congenital syphilis include women with a high VDRL titer at diagnosis, unknown duration of disease, ultrasonographic findings of congenital syphilis, and treatment within four weeks of delivery. Because of this, an additional dose of benzathine penicillin 2.4 million units IM may be administered one week after the initial dose for women who have primary, secondary, or early latent syphilis (<1 year) or ultrasonographic findings consistent with congenital syphilis (93).

Obstetricians should be aware of the Jarisch–Herxheimer reaction. This reaction is an acute systemic reaction seen in patients being treated for syphilis. Klein et al. (102) reported 33 gravidas that were monitored with hourly vital signs and examinations for 24 hours after treatment with benzathine penicillin G. All of the patients with primary syphilis (3 of 3), 12 of 20 (60%) with secondary syphilis, and 0 of 10 (0%) with latent syphilis had the reaction. The most common symptoms observed were fever (73%), uterine contractions (67%), and decreased fetal movement (67%). Three of the 11 (27%) monitored patients experienced transient late decelerations.

In this review, treatment consisted of benzathine penicillin G, 2.4 million units IM for primary, secondary, and early latent syphilis. Patients with latent disease of unknown or over one year's duration were treated with the same dose of penicillin weekly for two additional weeks. Three cases of congenital syphilis were identified; two cases in patients identified as having secondary syphilis and one case in a patient with primary syphilis. Although the number of cases was small, treatment failed to prevent congenital syphilis in one of three patients with primary syphilis and 2 of 20 patients with secondary syphilis using the treatment regimen above. Finally, there were no cases of congenital syphilis in the group of patients that did not experience the Jarisch–Herxheimer reaction.

CONCLUSION

There are two requirements for pursuing fetal therapy. First, is there reasonable scientific evidence to believe that it will cure or prevent a disabling disease; and second, is the intervention done with the informed, voluntary, competent, and understanding consent of the individuals involved? Many advances are occurring in fetal diagnostics and in therapies for genetic disease. Therefore, more treatments for fetal disease should be anticipated.

REFERENCES

1. Johnson JM, Elias S. Prenatal treatment. Medical and gene therapy in the fetus. Clinc Obstet Gynecol 1988; 31(2):390–407.
2. Elias S, Simpson JL, Shulman LP, Emerson D, Tharapel A, Seely L. Transabdominal chorionic villus sampling for first-trimester prenatal diagnosis. Am J Obstet Gynecol 1989; 160:870–884.
3. New MI. Prenatal treatment of congenital adrenal hyperplasia. The United States Experience. Endocrinol Metab Clin North Am 2001; 30:1–13.
4. Speiser PW, Laforgia N, Kato K, et al. First trimester prenatal treatment and molecular genetic diagnosis of congenital adrenal hyperplasia (21-hydroxylase deficiency). J Clin Endocrinol Metab 1990; 70:838–848.
5. Mercado AB, Wilson RC, Cheng KC, Wei J. Prenatal treatment and diagnosis of congenital adrenal hyperplasia owing to steroid 21-hydroxylase deficiency. J Clin Endocrinol Metab 1995; 80:2014–2020.
6. Forrest MG, David M, Morel Y. Prenatal treatment and diagnosis of congenital adrenal hyperplasia. J Steroid Biochem Mol Biol 1993; 45:75–82.
7. Cerame BI, Newfield RS, Pascoe L, et al. Prenatal diagnosis and treatment of 11 beta hydroxylase deficiency congenital adrenal hyperplasia resulting in normal female genitalia. J Clin Endocrinol Metab 1999; 84:3129–3134.

8. Lagic S, Wedell A, Bui T-H, Ritzen EM, Hoist M. Long term somatic followup of prenatally treated children with CAH. J Clin Endocrinol Metab 1998; 83:3872–3880.
9. Brook CGD. Antenatal treatment of a mother bearing a fetus with congenital adrenal hyperplasia. Arch Dis Child Fetal Neonatal Ed 2000; 82:F176–F181.
10. Elias ER, Irons MB, Hurley AD, Tint GS, Salen G. Clinical effects of cholesterol supplementation in six patients with the Smith–Lemli–Opitz syndrome (SLOS). Am J Med Genet 1997; 68:305–310.
11. Irons M, Elias ER, Abuelo D, et al. Treatment of Smith–Lemli–Opitz syndrome: results of a multicenter trial. Am J Med Genet 1997; 68:311–314.
12. Rossiter JP, Hofman KJ, Kelley RI. Smith–Lemli–Opitz syndrome: prenatal diagnosis by quantification of cholesterol precursors. Am J Med Genet 1998; 56:272–275.
13. Mills K, Mandel H, Montemagno R, Soothill P, Gershoni-Baruch R, Clayton PT. First trimester prenatal diagnosis of Smith–Lemli–Opitz syndrome (7-dehydrocholesterol reductase deficiency). Pediatr Res 1996; 39:816–819.
14. Loeffler J, Utermann G, Witsch-Baumgartner M. Molecular prenatal diagnosis of Smith–Lemli–Opitz syndrome is reliable and efficient. Prenat Diagn 2002; 22:827–830.
15. Irons MB, Nores J, Stewart TL, et al. Antenatal therapy of Smith–Lemli–Opitz syndrome. Fetal Diagn Ther 1999; 14:133–137.
16. Palomaki GE, Bradley LA, Knight GJ, Craig WY, Haddow JE. Assigning risk for Smith–Lemli–Opitz syndrome as part of 2nd trimester screening for Down's syndrome. J Med Screen 2002; 9:43–44.
17. Ampola MG, Mahoney MJ, Nakamura E, Tanaka K. Prenatal therapy of a patient with vitamin B12-responsive methylamalonic acidemia. N Engl J Med 1975; 293:313–317.
18. Zoghbi HY, O'Brien WE, Ledley FD. Linkage relationships of the human methylmalonyl CoA mutase to the HLA and D654 loci on chromosome 6. Genomics 1988; 3:396–398.
19. Ledley FD, Lumetta MR, Zoghbi HY, Van Tuinen P, Ledbetter SA, Ledbetter DH. Mapping of human methylmalonyl CoA mutase (MUT) locus on chromosome 6. Am J Hum Genet 1988; 42:839–846.
20. Rosenblatt DS, Cooper BA, Schmutz SM, Zaleski WA, Casey RE. Prenatal vitamin B12 therapy of a fetus with methylcobalamin deficiency (cobalamin E disease). Lancet 1985; 1:1127–1129.
21. Packman S, Cowan MJ, Golbus MS, et al. Prenatal treatment of biotin-responsive multiple carboxylase deficiency. Lancet 1982; 1:1435–1438.
22. Roth KS, Yang W, Allan L, Saunders M, Gravel RA, Dakshinamurti D. Prenatal administration of biotin in biotin-responsive multiple carboxylase deficiency. Pediatr Res 1982; 16:126–129.
23. Thuy LP, Jurecki E, Nemzer L, Nyhan WL. Prenatal diagnosis of holocarboxylase synthetase deficiency by assay of the enzyme in chorionic villus material followed by prenatal treatment. Clin Chim Acta 1999; 284:59–68.
24. Burri BJ, Sweetman L, Nyhan WL. Heterogeneity of holocarboxylase synthetase in patients with biotin-responsive multiple carboxylase deficiency. Am J Hum Genet 1985; 37:326–337.
25. Ristoff E, Mayatepek E, Larsson A. Long-term clinical outcome in patients with glutathione synthetase deficiency. J Pediatr 2001; 139:79–84.
26. Granot E, Kohen R. Oxidative stress in abetalipoproteinemai patients receiving long-term vitamin E and vitamin A supplementation. Am J Clin Nutr 2004; 79:226–230.
27. Czeizel AE, Dudas I. Prevention of the first occurrence of neural tube defects by periconceptual vitamin supplementation. N Engl J Med 1992; 327:1832–1835.
28. Laurence KM, James N, Miller MH, Tennant GB, Campbell H. Double-blind randomized controlled trial of folate treatment before conception to prevent recurrence of neural-tube defects. Br Med J 1981; 282:1509–1511.
29. Smithells RW, Nevin NC, Seller MJ, et al. Further experience of vitamin supplementation for prevention of neural tube defect recurrences. Lancet 1983; 1:1027–1031.

30. Shields DC, Kirke PN, Mills JL, et al. The thermolabile variant of methylenetetra-hydrofolate reductase and neural tube defects: an evaluation of genetic risk and the relative importance of the genotypes of the embryo and the mother. Am J Hum Genet 1999; 64:1045–1055.

31. Kirke PN, Mills JL, Brody LC, et al. Impact of the MTHFR C677T polymorphism on risk of neural tube defects: case–control study. Br Med J 2004; 328:1535–1536.

32. Scott JM, Weir DG. Folate/vitamin B12 inter-relationships. Essays Biochem 1994; 28: 63–72.

33. Centers for Disease Control (CDC). Knowledge and use of folic acid by women of childbearing age—United States, 1995. MMWR Morb Mortal Wkly Rep 1995; 44:716–718.

34. Hanley WB, Clarke JTR, Schoonheyt W. Maternal phenylketonuria (PKU)—a review. Clin Biochem 1987; 20:149–155.

35. Levy HL. Historical background for the maternal PKU syndrome. Pediatrics 2003; 112:1516–1518.

36. Lenke R, Levy HL. Maternal phenylketonuria and hyperphenylalaninemia. N Engl J Med 1980; 303:1202–1208.

37. Murphy D, Saul I, Kirby M. Maternal PKU and phenylalanine-restricted diet: studies of seven pregnancies and of offspring produced. Ir J Med Sci 1985; 154:66–70.

38. Drogari E, Smith I, Beasley M, Lloyd JK. Timing of strict diet in relation to fetal damage in maternal phenylketonuria. An international collaborative study by the MRC/DHSS Phenylketonuria Register. Lancet 1987; 2:927–930.

39. Harley JD, Mutton P, Irvine S, Gupta JD. Maternal enzymes of galactose metabolism and the "inexplicable" infantile cataract. Lancet 1974; 2:259–261.

40. Chen YT, Mattison DR, Feigenbaum L, Fukui H, Schulman JD. Reduction in oocyte number following prenatal exposure to a high galactose diet. Science 1981; 214: 1145–1147.

41. Segal SS. Disorders of galactose metabolism. In: Stanbury JB, Wyngaarden JB, Fredrickson DS, eds. The Metabolic Basis of Inherited Disease. 5th ed. New York: McGraw Hill, 1983:167.

42. Vannas A, Hogan MJ, Golbus MS, Wood I. Lens changes in a galactosemic fetus. Am J Ophthalmol 1975; 80:726–733.

43. Friedman AH, Copel JA, Kleinman CS. Fetal echocardiography and fetal cardiography: indications, diagnosis and management. Semin Perinatol 1993; 17:76–88.

44. Copel JA, Liang RI, Demasio K, Ozeren S, Kleinman CS. The clinical significance of the irregular heart rhythm. Am J Obstet Gynecol 2000; 182:813–819.

45. Boldt T, Eronen M, Andersson S. Long-term outcome in fetuses with cardiac arrhythmias. Obstet Gynecol 2003; 102:1372–1379.

46. Andersen HM, Drew JH, Beischer NA, Hutchison AA, Fortune DW. Non-immune hydrops fetalis: changing contribution to perinatal mortality. Br J Obstet Gynaecol 1983; 90:636–639.

47. Kleinman CS, Donnerstein RL, Jaffe CC, et al. Fetal echocardiography. A tool for evaluation of in utero cardiac arrhythmias and monitoring of in utero therapy: analysis of 71 patients. Am J Cardiol 1983; 51:237–243.

48. Azancot-Benisty A, Jacqz-Aigrain E, Guirgis NM, Decrepy A, Oury JF, Blot P. Clinical and pharmacologic study of fetal supraventricular tachyarrhythmias. J Pediatr 1992; 121:608–613.

49. Wiggins JW, Bowes W, Clewell W, et al. Echocardiographic diagnosis and intravenous digoxin management of fetal tachyarrhythmias and congestive heart failure. Am J Dis Child 1986; 140:202–204.

50. Krapp M, Kohl T, Simpson JM, Sharland GK, Katalinic A, Gembruch U. Review of diagnosis, treatment and outcome of fetal atrial flutter compared with supraventricular tachycardia. Heart 2003; 89:913–917.

51. Schmolling J, Renke K, Richter O, Pfeiffer K, Sohlebusch H, Holler T. Digoxin, flecainide, and amiodarone transfer across the placenta and the effects of an elevated umbilical venous pressure on the transfer rate. Ther Drug Monit 2000; 22:582–588.

52. Frohn-Mulder IM, Stewart PA, Witsenburg M, Den Hollander NS, Wladimiroff JW, Hess J. The efficacy of flecainide versus digoxin in the management of fetal supraventricular tachycardia. Prenat Diagn 1995; 15:1297–302 (Comment, 1995; 15:1209–1213).

53. The Cardiac Arrhythmia Suppression Trial (CAST) Investigators. Preliminary report: effect of encainide and flecainide on mortality in a randomized trial of arrhythmia suppression after myocardial infarction. N Engl J Med 1989; 321:406–412.

54. Hohnloser SH, Woosley RL. Sotalol. N Engl J Med 1994; 331:31–38.

55. Creasy RK, Resnik R, Iams JD, eds. Maternal–Fetal Medicine: Principles and Practice. 5th ed. Philadelphia, PA: Saunders, 2004.

56. Jouannic JM, Delahaye S, Fermont L, et al. Fetal supraventricular tachyardia: a role for amiodarone as second-line therapy? Prenat Diagn 2003; 23:152–156.

57. Copel JA, Kleinman CS. Fetal arrhythmias. In: Wladimiroff JW, Pilu G, eds. Ultrasound and the Fetal Heart. New York, NY: Parthenon Publishing Group, 1996:93–106.

58. Simpson LL. Fetal supraventricular tachycardias: diagnosis and management. Semin Perinatol 2000; 24:360–372.

59. Vanbesien J, Casteels A, Bougatef A, et al. Transient fetal hypothyroidism due to direct fetal administration of amiodarone for drug resistant fetal tachycardia. Am J Perinatol 2001; 18:113–116.

60. Glickstein JS, Buyon J, Friedman D. Pulsed Doppler echocardiographic assessment of the fetal PR interval. Am J Cardiol 2000; 86:236–239.

61. Andelfinger G, Fouron JC, Sonesson SE, Proulx F. Reference values for time intervals between atrial and ventricular contractions of the fetal heart measured by two Doppler techniques. Am J Cardiol 2001; 88:1433–1436.

62. Schmidt KG, Ulmer HE, Silverman NH, Kleinman CS, Copel JA. Perinatal outcome of fetal complete atrioventricular heart block: a multicenter experience. J Am Coll Cardiol 1991; 17:1360–1366.

63. Taylor PV, Scott JS, Gerlis LM, Esscher E, Scott O. Maternal antibodies against fetal cardiac antigens in congenital complete heart block. N Engl J Med 1986; 315:667–672.

64. Copel JA, Buyon JP, Kleinman CS. Successful in utero therapy of fetal heart block. Am J Obstet Gynecol 1995; 173:1384–1390 (Comment, Am J Obstet Gynecol 1996; 75: 502–503.

65. Saleeb S, Copel J, Friedman D, Buyon JP. Comparison of treatment with fluorinated glucocorticoids to the natural history of autoantibody-associated congenital heart block: retrospective review of the research registry for neonatal lupus. Arthritis Rheum 1999; 42:2335–2345.

66. Volpe R, Ehrlich R, Steiner G, Row VV. Graves' disease in pregnancy years after hypothyroidism with recurrent passive-transfer of neonatal Graves' disease in offspring. Therapeutic considerations. Am J Med 1984; 77:572–578.

67. Zimmerman D, Lteif AN. Thyrotoxicosis in children. Endocrinol Metab Clin North Am 1998; 27:109–126.

68. Choppra IJ. Fetal and neonatal hypothyroidism. Thyroid 1992; 2:161–163.

69. Wenstrom KD, Weiner CP, Williamson RA, Grant SS. Prenatal diagnosis of fetal hyperthyroidism using funipuncture. Obstet Gynecol 1990; 76:513–517.

70. Page DV, Brady K, Mitchell J, Pehrson J, Wade G. The pathology of intrauterine thyrotoxicosis: two case reports. Obstet Gynecol 1988; 72:479–481.

71. Nachum Z, Rakover Y, Weiner E, Shalev E. Graves' disease in pregnancy: prospective evaluation of a selective invasive treatment protocol. Am J Obstet Gynecol 2003; 189:159–165 (Comment, Am J Obstet Gynecol 2003; 189:1–2).

72. Zimmerman D, Lfeif AN. Thyrotoxicosis in children. Endocrinol Metab Clin North Am 1998; 27:109–127.

73. Sack J, Fisher DA, Hobel CJ, Lam R. Thyroxine in human amniotic fluid. J Pediatr 1975; 87:364–368.

74. Porreco RP, Bloch CA. Fetal blood sampling in the management of intrauterine thyrotoxicosis. Obstet Gynecol 1990; 76:509–512.

75. Heckel S, Favre R, Schlienger JL, Soskin P. Diagnosis and successful in utero treatment of a fetal goitrous hyperthyroidism caused by maternal Graves' disease: A case report. Fetal Diagn Ther 1997; 12:54–58.

76. Thorpe-Beeston JG, Nicolaides KH, Felton CV, Butler J, McGregor AM. Maturation of the secretion of thyroid hormone and thyroid-stimulating hormone in the fetus. N Engl J Med 1991; 324:532–536 (Comment, N Engl J Med 1991; 324:559–561).

77. Hatjis CG. Diagnosis and successful treatment of fetal goitrous hyperthyroidism caused by maternal Graves' disease. Obstet Gynecol 1993; 81:837–879.

78. Bianchi DW, Crombleholme TM, D'Alton ME. Fetology: Diagnosis and Management of the Fetal Patient. New York: McGraw-Hill Medical Publishing Division, 2003.

79. Fisher DA. Fetal thyroid function: diagnosis and management of fetal thyroid disorders. Clin Obstet Gynecol 1997; 40:16–31.

80. Burrow GN, Fisher DA, Larsen PR. Maternal and fetal thyroid function. N Engl J Med 1994; 331:1072–1078.

81. Fisher DA. Screening for congenital hypothyroidism. Trends Endocrinol Metab 1991; 2:129–133.

82. Vicens-Calvet E, Potau N, Carreras E, Bellart J, Albisu MA, Carrascosa A. Diagnosis and treatment in utero of goiter with hypothyroidism caused by iodide overload. J Pediatr 1998; 133:147–148.

83. Noia G, DeSantis M, Tocci A, et al. Early prenatal diagnosis and therapy of fetal hypothyroid goiter. Fetal Diagn Ther 1992; 7:138–143.

84. Bruner JP, Dellinger E. Antenatal diagnosis and treatment of fetal hypothyroidism. A report of two cases. Fetal Diagn Ther 1997; 12:200–204.

85. Davidson KM, Richards DS, Schatz DA, Fisher DA. Successful in utero treatment of fetal goiter and hypothyroidism. N Engl J Med 1991; 324:543–536 (Comment, N Engl J Med 1991; 324:559–561).

86. Van Loon AJ, Derksen JT, Bos AF, Rouwe CW. In utero diagnosis and treatment of fetal goitrous hypothyroidism, caused by maternal use of propylthiouracil. Prenat Diagn 1995; 15:599–604.

87. Guerina NG, Hsu H-W, Meissner H, et al. Neonatal serologic screening and early treatment for congenital *Toxoplasma gondii* infection. The New England Regional Toxoplasma Working Group. N Engl J Med 1994; 330:1858–1863 (Comment, N Engl J Med 1994; 331:1458–1459).

88. Lopez A, Dietz VJ, Wilson M, Navin TR, Jones JL. Preventing congenital toxoplasmosis. MMWR Morb Mortal Wkly Rep 2000; 49:57–75.

89. National Center for Health Statistics. Plan and operation of the Third National Health and Nutrition Examination Survey, 1988–94. Series 1: Programs and collections procedures. Vital Health Stat 1 1994; 32:1–407.

90. Beazley DM, Egerman RS. Toxoplasmosis. Semin Perinatol 1998; 22:332–338.

91. Hohlfeld P, Daffos F, Costa JM, Thulliez P, Forestier F, Vidaud M. Prenatal diagnosis of congenital toxoplasmosis with a polymerase-chain reaction test on amniotic fluid. N Engl J Med 1994; 331:695–699.

92. Romand S, Wallon M, Franck J, Thulliez P, Peyron F, Dumon H. Prenatal diagnosis using polymerase chain reaction on amniotic fluid for congenital toxoplasmosis. Obstet Gynecol 2001; 97:296–300.

93. Daffos F, Forestier F, Capella-Pavlovsky M, et al. Prenatal management of 746 pregnancies at risk for congenital toxoplasmosis. N Engl J Med 1988; 318:271–275.

94. Fiumara NJ, Fleming WL, Downing JG, Good FL. The incidence of prenatal syphilis at the Boston City Hospital. N Engl J Med 1952; 247:48–52.

95. Fiumara NJ, Lessell S. Manifestations of late congenital syphilis. An analysis of 271 patients. Arch Dermatol 1970; 102:78–83.

96. Centers for Disease Control and Prevention (CDC). Congenital Syphilis—United States, 2002. MMWR Morb Mortal Wkly Rep 2004; 53:716–719.

97. Centers for Disease Control and Prevention (CDC). Sexually transmitted diseases guidelines 2002. MMWR Morb Mortal Wkly Rep 2002; 51:26–30.

98. Nyberg DA, Mahony BS, Pretorius D, eds. Diagnostic Ultrasound of Fetal Anomalies: Text and Atlas. Chicago, IL: Year Book Medical Publishers, 1990.

99. Centers for Disease Control and Prevention (CDC). Congenital syphilis case definition 1998. MMWR Morb Mortal Wkly Rep 1999; 48:757–761.

100. McFarlin BL, Bottoms SF, Dock BS, Isada NB. Epidemic syphilis: maternal factors associated with congenital infection. Am J Obstet Gynecol 1994; 170:535–540 (Comment, Am J Obstet Gynecol 1994; 170:705).

101. Sanchez PJ, Wendel GD. Syphilis in pregnancy. Clin Perinatol 1997; 24:71–90.

102. Klein VR, Cox SM, Mitchell MD, Wendel GD Jr. The Jarisch-Herxheimer reaction complicating syphilotherapy in pregnancy. Obstet Gynecol 1990; 75:375–380.

23

Intrauterine Intravascular Treatment

Phebe Nanine Adama van Scheltema and Dick Oepkes
Department of Obstetrics, Leiden University Medical Center, Leiden, The Netherlands

BACKGROUND

Fifty years ago, hemolytic disease of the newborn was one of the most common causes of perinatal mortality. Early delivery and neonatal exchange transfusions were the only treatment options, until in the 1960s, intrauterine transfusion became possible. Freda and colleagues performed open fetal surgery, transfusing the fetus using a vein in the exteriorized leg (1,2). A major breakthrough was the development of percutaneous intraperitoneal transfusion under X-ray guidance by Sir William Liley (3). However, hydropic fetuses did not take up the transfused blood from the peritoneal cavity very well. In addition, the technique was not feasible before 27 weeks' gestation (4). In the 1980s, Sir Charles Rodeck introduced the technique of intravascular transfusion by needling the umbilical artery under direct fetoscopic guidance (5). Shortly afterwards, Jens Bang in Denmark and Fernand Daffos in France both pioneered fetal blood sampling under ultrasound guidance. In the last two decades, their approach is still used worldwide as the technique for intrauterine transfusions (6,7).

The main indication for intrauterine blood transfusion still is fetal anemia due to red cell alloimmunization. However, in any fetal disease with severe anemia, intrauterine blood transfusion can be considered. Successful fetal treatment has been reported in human parvovirus infection (8,9), severe fetomaternal hemorrhage (10), placental chorioangiomas (11), homozygous α-thalassemia (12,13), and others. Intravenous access to the fetus also allows treatment of other conditions, including alloimmune thrombocytopenia (AITP) by platelet transfusions, and cardiac arrhythmias by injecting antiarrhythmic agents. The procedure of intrauterine transfusion is identical in all these diseases, independent of the indication. In this chapter, we will, therefore, focus on intrauterine transfusion for red cell alloimmunization, and touch briefly on a few particular aspects of transfusion for other reasons.

WHEN TO TRANSFUSE: MONITORING A PREGNANCY AT RISK

As in all surgical procedures, the technical details are only part of the clinicians' skills. The correct indication and timing are as also equally important. Especially in invasive procedures in obstetrics, in which any complication is potentially lethal

419

for the fetus, a careful individual risk–benefit analysis must be made each time. In red cell alloimmunization, maternal serum antibody levels and obstetric history help to identify fetuses at risk for anemia. However, not all fetuses in alloimmunized pregnancies develop severe anemia. Serial assessment of signs of anemia is necessary to enable optimal timing of intervention. The goal and the challenge are to transfuse only in case of severe anemia, but before the fetus develops hydrops. In all series, survival of hydropic fetuses after intrauterine transfusion is significantly lower compared to nonhydropic fetuses (14). Several studies have shown that hydrops only develops when the fetal hemoglobin drops to levels 6–7 SD below the mean for the gestational age. Ideally, a transfusion is given when the fetal hemoglobin level is between 4 and 6 SD below the mean. In such cases, one can transfuse a relatively large amount of O-negative donor blood, which is not hemolyzed by the red cell antibodies. The next transfusion can then be given several weeks later. Transfusion intervals will be discussed in more detail later in this chapter.

As timing of transfusion is such an important issue, we will briefly describe the currently used diagnostic tests for evaluation of red cell alloimmunized pregnancies.

Ultrasound Assessment

Weekly ultrasonographic evaluation is important for early detection of fetal hydrops. Hydrops is a sign of severe fetal anemia and, as mentioned before, associated with adverse outcome. The first signs of hydrops due to anemia are ascites and pericardial effusion, practically always in conjunction with cardiomegaly. Skin edema develops later, and pleural effusions are only apparent in advanced stages. The latter is also true for increased placental thickness and polyhydramnios. Some severely hydropic anemic fetuses even have oligohydramnios. Fetal movements are sometimes remarkably normal despite severe anemia.

There are other, less specific signs that indicate anemia: enlargement of the heart, spleen, and liver due to cardiovascular adaptation and increased extramedullary erythropoiesis, respectively.

Doppler Studies

Progressive anemia leads to an elevated cardiac output and decreased blood viscosity. This results in an increased maximum or systolic flow velocities in various parts of the fetal venous and arterial circulation (15–19). For clinical practice, the most reliable and reproducible of these Doppler parameters is the middle cerebral artery peak velocity (20,21). In comparative studies, Doppler parameters have been shown to be more useful in the prediction of fetal anemia than liver and spleen measurements (16,21,22).

Amniotic Fluid

The end product of fetal red cell destruction is bilirubin. Most bilirubin is removed from the fetus via the placenta but small amounts enter the amniotic fluid in the second and third trimester and increases in bilirubin level in amniotic fluid correlate with the fetal red cell destruction (23). The amniotic bilirubin concentration can be quantified spectrophotometrically by assessing the change in optical density at a specific wavelength (24). In 1961, Liley devised a system for managing pregnancies complicated by rhesus alloimmunization based on the correlation of bilirubin levels in amniotic fluid and neonatal outcome (24). This Liley chart, or an extended version, is still in use for predicting fetal anemia. An alternative chart was produced by Queenan et al. (25), based on a reference range of bilirubin levels in normal pregnancies. There is no evidence that one of these methods is superior to the other. A large prospective study has recently shown that middle cerebral artery Doppler measurement provides a higher sensitivity and specificity than amniotic fluid analysis in the prediction of fetal anemia (Diamond study group, personal communication).

THE TECHNIQUE

In most centers, the procedure is performed by a team consisting of at least three or four members: one operator to actually put the needle in the fetal vessel of choice, either using a free hand technique or with an ultrasonographer to guide the procedure, to monitor the transfusion site and the fetal condition, one nurse with sterile gloves on to assist with the various medications and syringes, and one assistant to perform the on-site blood tests and calculations (26,27). The use of a fixed needle guide technique has been advocated by some (28). However, we feel that the disadvantage of not being able to move the ultrasound transducer for Doppler assessment or fetal cardiac function evaluation is an important one. In general, fetal blood transfusions including all preparations take 40 to 60 minutes, and can be done as outpatient procedure or with an overnight stay. In our unit, we plan these procedures in the afternoon and we discharge the patient either the same evening or the next morning.

Premedication

Some sedation may be useful for anxious patients, as it is important that they lie quietly on the operating table for about 30 minutes. Maternal pain relief by local anesthetic injection at the puncture site is usually sufficient, but painful contractions are sometimes problematic. Routinely, in our center the patient receives pethidine/promethazine i.m. and indomethacin pr. 30 minutes prior to the procedure. Others administer midazolam orally (29,30) or intravenously, or give no premedication at all (31). Some operators administer fentanyl to the fetus in case of transfusion through the intrahepatic vein, to avoid fetal stress and pain (30,32). There is no evidence that prophylactic antibiotics are beneficial. In a recent series describing over 750 transfusions without the use of antibiotics, one case was found of an *Escherichia coli* infection in both fetus and mother (33).

Fetal Paralysis

Fetal movements during the procedure can cause needle displacement, hematomas or even tearing of the vessel wall with life-threatening bleeding as a result. The routine administration of muscle relaxants such as pancuronium or atracurium to achieve fetal paralysis, either intravenously or intramuscularly, was suggested to be the preferred policy in a recent study by Van Kamp et al. (33). Others only administer these substances when the fetus is very active and the extremities are in close proximity of the transfusion site.

Site for Transfusion

Depending on both fetal position and placenta localization, the operator chooses the site for transfusion, either the intrahepatic umbilical vein or the umbilical cord at placental insertion. Some operators prefer the placental cord insertion, because transfusion in the intrahepatic vein has been reported to be associated with an increase in fetal stress hormones (34–37). Others prefer the intrahepatic vein because this technique minimizes blood loss from the cord puncture site, as the blood is absorbed from the peritoneal cavity (38). If the placenta lies anterior, we consider the umbilical cord at placenta insertion to be the safest choice, unless the fetus is blocking the view and/or insertion. If the placenta lies posterior, we consider the intrahepatic vein to be the safest choice. Puncturing a free loop of the umbilical cord has the risk of tearing during fetal movement, and "jet" with an unknown amount of blood loss in the amniotic cavity after removal of the needle post procedure. Accessing or transfusing in the umbilical artery has a high complication risk, because the artery is smaller in diameter than the vein and is more likely to go into spasm during the procedure and cause a fetal bradycardia (33,39). Cardiac punction is rarely used because of the potential hazards such as cardiac tamponade, hemopericardium, and arrhythmia including asystole (40).

Intravascular vs. Intraperitoneal Approach

Intraperitoneal transfusion relies on placing the donor cells into the peritoneal cavity so that they become absorbed into the fetal circulation via the subdiaphragmatic lymphatics and thoracic duct. This absorption is somewhat unpredictable, and may be impaired in case of severe hydrops. Apart from the fact that intravascular transfusion delivers the donor cells immediately where they should be, the other major advantage is that the fetal hemoglobin levels can be obtained before and after the transfusion. The amount of blood (V) that needs to be transfused can be calculated using the following formula:

$$V = \frac{\text{Fetoplacental volume} \times (\text{Ht post} - \text{Ht pre})}{\text{Ht donor blood}}$$

Commonly, the donor blood has a hematocrit of around 80%. Fetoplacental volume has been estimated by several authors, either based on gestational age (41) or estimated fetal weight (42). The aim for posttransfusion hematocrit, in case of complete intravascular transfusion, is generally set at 40% to 50%. This slightly supranormal value allows for a longer transfusion interval, minimizing procedure-related risks. Welch et al. (43) warned of serious adverse effects when transfusing to a hematocrit above 50%. The volume given when intraperitoneal transfusion alone is performed has traditionally been calculated as follows:

IPT $V = (\text{gestational age in weeks} - 20) \times 10$

Intravascular transfusion is considerably more successful at reversing hydrops than is intraperitoneal transfusion (44), possibly because hydrops reduces the absorption of red cells from the lymphatic system.

A few studies show considerable advantages of a combined technique of intravascular and intraperitoneal transfusion (45,46). With this method, the aim of the final hematocrit after the intravascular part must be adapted to a maximum of 35% to 40%, followed by the standard amount for the intraperitoneal transfusion.

This should result in considerably longer transfusion intervals, although in one study the mean gain was only three days (26,45).

One remaining indication for intraperitoneal transfusion could be a high likelihood of severe anemia in the very early (e.g., before 18–20 weeks) gestational age fetus, although experienced operators are usually able to access the cord or intrahepatic vein from 17 weeks' gestation onward. Sometimes such cases, especially if associated with maternal obesity, can be a real challenge. We recommend watchful waiting, monitoring twice weekly if needed, and only attempt to transfuse at the first signs of hydrops. In very severely affected pregnancies, e.g., with previous fetal loss or hydrops before 20 weeks' gestation, this policy can be combined with maternal intravenous immunoglobulin (IVIG) administration, plasmapheresis, or both. For details, we refer to an excellent review of these options by Moise (34).

Volume and Rate of Transfusion

On obtaining access to the fetal circulation, a 1 mL sample of fetal blood is obtained in order to determine the fetal hematocrit and hemoglobin level. Most centers have a Coulter counter in the procedure room so that the result is available in a few seconds. Verification of correct placement of the needle is done by injecting a small amount of saline, followed by a fetal weight adjusted dose of muscle relaxant. The needle is connected, preferably via a short flexible tube, to a three-way tap, which is in turn connected to a sac with donor blood. The blood is guided through a heater, which warms the blood to body temperature. The volume to be transfused has been discussed above. After transfusing the estimated amount of blood, the needle is flushed with some saline and left in place for one to two minutes to allow mixing of blood in the fetoplacental unit. Then, a 1 mL sample is taken for immediate assessment, and if the desired hematocrit is not yet reached, more blood is given. At the end of the procedure, a final sample is taken again after one to two minutes mixing time.

The blood is transfused at a rate of 5–10 mL per minute. During the procedure, the blood flow is continuously visualized on the ultrasound screen to confirm the needle position. Periodically, the fetal heart rate is checked for arrhythmias, especially bradycardia. If a bradycardia occurs, we wait with further transfusing until the heart rate has normalized. The procedure is performed using a 20 or 22 gauge needle, depending on gestational age.

Donor Blood

The primary source of blood for intrauterine transfusion is O-negative unrelated donor blood. The blood has to be collected within 24 hours and cross-matched with the maternal blood. It should have been screened for hepatitis B and C, cytomegalovirus, and human immunodeficiency virus as well as irradiated to remove the white blood cells to avoid "graft-versus-host"–like complications in the fetus. The blood is packed to a hematocrit of 75% to 85% to minimize the volume of blood that needs to be transfused.

Maternal blood is also a good source of blood for intrauterine transfusions. It has the theoretical advantage of decreasing the risk for sensitization to new red cell antigens. In addition, a longer circulating half-life can be expected because of the fresh source of cells. Parents seem to have some preference for the use of mothers' own blood to donate to the fetus. However, the blood must undergo rigorous testing for antibodies against the infectious diseases mentioned above. For logistic reasons, we have, therefore, chosen to use unrelated donor blood. A study comparing the fetal effects of maternal red cells versus unrelated donor cells showed no significant differences in decline rate of red blood cells until 33 weeks gestation (47).

TOP-UP VS. EXCHANGE TRANSFUSION

Concern has been raised that directly transfusing blood into the fetus without removing any blood (the top-up procedure) may lead to volume overload and cardiac compromise. Some operators aspirate small amounts of blood from the fetus at regular intervals during the transfusion with the intention of preventing hypervolemia (the exchange procedure) (48,49). Others suggest that the umbilical venous pressure should be routinely monitored and if the change in pressure exceeds 10 mmHg, then blood should be removed and replaced with an equal volume of saline (50). In practice, with many centers performing top-up transfusions for 20 years now, the fetus appears to tolerate the top-up transfusion without any adverse effects.

TIMING OF SUBSEQUENT TRANSFUSIONS

The second transfusion usually has to be performed two to three weeks after the first transfusion, or earlier if the desired posttransfusion hematocrit has not been reached. The mean fall in hematocrit is around 1% per day, but there is a wide variation (SD 0.44) (45). This donor cell fall is due mainly to growth of the fetus with increasing fetoplacental volume and only partly due to actual destruction of red cells. This rate of fall is quite unpredictable between the first and second transfusion, because at this stage the percentage of fetal erythrocytes in the fetal circulation and the suppression of erythropoiesis are variable. After the second transfusion, the mean fall in hematocrit is generally easier to predict, because at this stage almost all of the fetal erythrocytes are replaced with donor erythrocytes and the erythropoiesis is almost completely suppressed. After the second transfusion, the interval can safely be 4 or even 5 weeks if the hematocrit after transfusion is at least 45%. In general, transfusions are performed until the gestational age of 35 weeks is reached (51). This means that a pregnancy in which transfusions are performed can be continued until approximately 37 weeks, thereby reducing the risks of respiratory and other prematurity problems. The chances for a successful induction and vaginal delivery obviously also increase with advancing gestation.

Several groups have published their experience showing that repeated intravascular transfusions throughout pregnancy are associated with survival rates ranging from 76% to 96% (41,48,52–54).

COMPLICATIONS

Intrauterine transfusion is a safe procedure with a relatively low procedure-related complication and perinatal loss rate. However, complications do sometimes occur. Fetal complications during or after an invasive procedure may either result from the procedure or from the underlying pathologic condition necessitating treatment.

This means that not all complications are due to the procedure, but some are a consequence of the compromised fetal condition.

Transient fetal bradycardia during transfusion is the most common complication, occurring in 8% of procedures (54). Fetal distress during or after transfusion is the most feared complication and may result in fetal death or emergency delivery with the risk of neonatal asphyxia and death. Fetal distress can occur after cord accidents (rupture, spasm, and tamponade from a hematoma), hemorrhage from the puncture site, volume overload, chorioamnionitis, preterm rupture of membranes, or preterm labor. Fortunately, all these complications are rare. Between 1988 and 2001 our center has systematically scored all procedure-related complications (33). These were rupture of membranes (0.1%), intrauterine infection (0.3%), emergency cesarean section (2.0%), fetal death (0.9%), and neonatal death (0.7%). Fetal death occurred in 19 cases and was considered to be procedure-related in seven cases. In six cases the fetal distress originated from local cord complications or inadvertent arterial puncture. In one case an infection with *E. coli* resulted in fetal death. Neonatal death occurred in 10 cases and was considered to be procedure-related in five cases. All five fetuses were delivered by emergency cesarean section because of fetal distress during the procedure as a result of local cord complications or excessive bleeding from the puncture site but died, nonetheless, shortly after birth. The total procedure-related complication rate was 2.9% in the absence of hydrops and 3.9% in the presence of hydrops. The risk of procedure-related perinatal death was 1.6% per procedure (33).

POSTTRANSFUSION CARE

After the transfusion, the woman is advised to rest on her left side for half an hour, to optimize blood flow to and from the uterus, during which time the fetal heart rate is monitored by cardiotocography. She then remains in bed until all effects of the sedatives have gone, usually two to four hours. Before discharge, the same or the next day, an ultrasonographic evaluation is done to reassure the patient, and ourselves, on the fetal condition. She is discharged home. A follow-up appointment is typically scheduled for 10 to 12 days afterward.

OUTCOME OF TREATMENT

Survival after intrauterine transfusion varies with center, experience, and the presence of fetal hydrops. At Leiden University Medical Center, between January 1988 and January 2001, 740 intrauterine procedures were performed in 254 fetuses with a median of three transfusions per fetus. The perinatal loss rate was 1.4% in the absence of fetal hydrops and 2.6% in the presence of hydrops (55). Other groups report a fetal loss rate per intravascular transfusion ranging from 0.6% to 4% (44,45).

Several groups have studied the long-term outcome for children treated with intrauterine transfusions with follow-up ranging from six months to six years (56,57). The neurodevelopmental outcome of these children is normal, even for the children who initially presented with fetal hydrops. Hearing deficits in the neonate have been reported in association with high serum bilirubin levels (58,59). However, a study by Janssens et al. did not show any permanent hearing problems in children treated with intrauterine transfusions (56).

TRANSFUSION IN OTHER DISEASES

Parvovirus B19 infection during pregnancy causes up to 27% of cases of nonimmune hydrops in fetuses. Fetal infection is especially damaging between 10 and 20 weeks of gestation, although hydrops has been reported up to 40 weeks of gestation (60). In this period, the development of the erythroid precursors take place. Parvovirus B19, with its preference for rapidly dividing cells, causes arrest of maturation of these cells. Extremely low hemoglobin levels have been reported (61). In many cases, the diagnosis of fetal parvovirus B19 infection is usually made only after the finding of fetal hydrops (60). However, increasingly pregnant women are referred following contact with a child with "fifth disease" and seroconversion for parvovirus B19 (62). In our center, in case of fetal parvovirus infection, we perform ultrasonographic checkups on a weekly basis until 10 to 12 weeks after initial seroconversion. In case of fetal hydrops or elevated middle cerebral artery peak velocity, an intrauterine transfusion is performed. Usually one intrauterine transfusion is enough. A review article by von Kaisenberg et al. (60) describes 705 cases of fetal parvovirus infection. There seems to be a benefit of transfusion therapy over conservative management in infected fetuses: 230 fetuses received intrauterine transfusion, with 82% survival, as apposed to 435 fetal parvovirus infections that were conservatively managed with 55% survival. However, because spontaneous resolution has been described and every procedure has its risks, we only perform an intrauterine transfusion if the fetus has signs of anemia. Apart from severe anemia, parvovirus B19 infection also causes thrombocytopenia. If the fetal platelet count drops $<30 \times 10^9/L$, an increased risk of hemorrhage may complicate cordocentesis and transfusion. For this reason, we recommend having platelets available for transfusion as well in all cases of hydrops caused by parvovirus B19.

Massive fetomaternal hemorrhage is a rare but serious complication in pregnancy, which may result in severe fetal anemia, hydrops, and death. It mostly occurs unexpectedly, and clinical symptoms are often nonspecific. A combination of reduced fetal movements and sinusoidal fetal heart rate pattern may raise suspicion. Increased blood flow velocities in the middle cerebral artery can be found (63). The diagnosis is confirmed by a Kleihauer–Betke test. If the fetus is preterm, intrauterine transfusion can be preferable over delivery.

Placental chorioangiomas occur in 1% of pregnancies. Large chorioangiomas may cause serious complications such as fetal anemia, hydrops, and fetal death. Haak et al. have described successful intrauterine transfusion in a case of fetal anemia due to a placental chorioangioma (11).

α-Thalassemia is due to the defective synthesis of alphaglobin chains, principally because of a deletion of one, two, three, or four genes. Homozygous α-thalassemia-1 results from a deletion of all four genes. The total hemoglobin concentration may not be very low, but most of the hemoglobin consists of nonfunctional gamma-chains. The functional result is fetal hydrops, cardiomegaly, placentomegaly, and often a maternal hydrops or "mirror" syndrome. It is considered a lethal disease (64). In countries with a high prevalence, screening may be performed using maternal mean corpuscular volume as a first test. Testing both parents is the next step. In experienced hands, fetal cardiothoracic ratio assessment and doppler measurements are reliable tests (65). The diagnosis can be made by chorionic villus sampling. Most commonly, once the diagnosis is made, the pregnancy is terminated. Intrauterine transfusion is not a standard treatment for fetuses with homozygous α-thalassemia, although there have been successful cases (12). This way, the fetus can be kept alive, but the child will need life-long transfusions and chelation as in β-thalassemia. There may be a role for gene therapy for α-thalassemia in the future.

In many cases of nonimmune hydrops, the diagnosis is not immediately clear. Using ultrasound and Doppler, it is often possible to distinguish between a likely anemic and nonanemic type of hydrops. In fetuses with ascites, edema, cardiomegaly, and high flow velocities in the middle cerebral artery, a diagnostic cordocentesis with full preparation for intrauterine transfusion seems a logical choice. If anemia is found, transfusion can buy time for the diagnostic work-up.

Platelet transfusion may be indicated in fetuses with severe thrombocytopenia, commonly defined as a platelet count $<50 \times 10^9/L$. Apart from the above-mentioned parvovirus infected fetuses, some fetuses with anemia due to red cell alloimmunization are found to be severely thrombocytopenic. This is thought to be due to decreased production from an overgrowth of erythropoetic precursor cells, but this has not been proven. It is more often found in hydropic fetuses, but as it seems hard to predict which fetus with Rh-disease is also thrombocytopenic, we do not routinely have platelets available for co-transfusion.

Another indication for fetal platelet transfusion is AITP. In Caucasians, the most common cause for this disease is the presence of human platelet antigen (HPA)-1a antibodies in maternal serum. The incidence of these antibodies in Europe and Canada is 0.1% to 0.2%. In 10% of pregnant women with these antibodies, fetal thrombocytopenia occurs. This may result in fetal intracranial hemorrhage (ICH) and intrauterine death. The highest risk for ICH in a thrombocytopenic fetus is in the third trimester and during delivery, but has been observed as early as 16 to 24 weeks' gestation. In the absence of a screening program, most AITP cases are detected after birth. In a subsequent pregnancy, prevention of ICH used to be done by serial (weekly) platelet transfusions. The cumulative risk of these procedures is now thought to be too high, and most centers have switched to a less invasive management protocol in which weekly administration of intravenous gammaglobulins is the cornerstone (66). Whether the hazards of diagnostic fetal blood sampling before or during IVIG treatment, or just before delivery outweigh the benefits is still under debate (67). Most clinicians who perform fetal blood samplings for AITP make sure they have platelets ready to transfuse immediately. However, rapid platelet transfusion in case of a bleeding from the puncture site unfortunately does not guarantee cessation of bleeding.

REFERENCES

1. Freda VJ. Antepartum management of the Rh problem. Prog Hematol 1966; 5:2 66–296.
2. Adamsons K Jr, Freda VJ, James LS, Towell ME. Prenatal treatment of erythroblastosis fetalis following hysterotomy. Pediatrics 1965; 35:848–855.
3. Liley AW. Intrauterine transfusion of foetus in haemolytic disease. Br Med J 1963; 5365:1107–1109.
4. Bennebroek Gravenhorst J, Kanhai HH, et al. Twenty-two years of intra-uterine intra-peritoneal transfusions. Eur J Obstet Gynecol Reprod Biol 1989; 33(1):71–77.
5. Rodeck CH, Kemp JR, Holman CA, Whitmore DN, Karnicki J, Austin MA. Direct intravascular fetal blood transfusion by fetoscopy in severe rhesus isoimmunisation. Lancet 1981; 1(8221):625–627.
6. Bang J, Bock JE, Trolle D. Ultrasound-guided fetal intravenous transfusion for severe rhesus haemolytic disease. Br Med J 1982; 284(6313):373–374.
7. Daffos F, Capella-Pavlovsky M, Forestier F. A new procedure for fetal blood sampling in utero: preliminary results of fifty-three cases. Am J Obstet Gynecol 1983; 146(8): 985–987.

8. Xu J, Raff TC, Muallem NS, Neubert AG. Hydrops fetalis secondary to parvovirus B19 infections. J Am Board Fam Pract 2003; 16(1):63–68.

9. Rodis JF, Borgida AF, Wilson M, et al. Management of parvovirus infection in pregnancy and outcomes of hydrops: a survey of members of the society of perinatal obstetricians. Am. J. Obstet. Gynecol 1998; 179(4):985–988.

10. Giacoia GP. Severe fetomaternal hemorrhage: a review. Obstet Gynecol Surv 1997; 52(6):372–380.

11. Haak MC, Oosterhof H, Mouw RJ, Oepkes D, Vandenbussche FP. Pathophysiology and treatment of fetal anemia due to placental chorioangioma. Ultrasound Obstet Gynecol 1999; 14(1):68–70.

12. Carr S, Rubin L, Dixon D, Star J, Dailey J. Intrauterine therapy for homozygous alpha-thalassemia. Obstet Gynecol 1995; 85(5, Pt 2):876–879.

13. Thornley I, Lehmann L, Ferguson WS, Davis I, Forman EN, Guinan EC. Homozygous alpha-thalassemia treated with intrauterine transfusions and postnatal hematopoietic stem cell transplantation. Bone Marrow Transplant 2003; 32(3):341–342.

14. van Kamp IL, Klumper FJ, Bakkum RS, et al. The severity of immune fetal hydrops is predictive of fetal outcome after intrauterine treatment. Am J Obstet Gynecol 2001; 185(3):668–673.

15. Radunovic N, Lockwood CJ, Alvarez M, Plecas D, Chitkara U, Berkowitz RL. The severely anemic and hydropic isoimmune fetus: changes in fetal hematocrit associated with intrauterine death. Obstet Gynecol 1992; 79(3):390–393.

16. Oepkes D, Brand R, Vandenbussche FP, Meerman RH, Kanhai HH. The use of ultrasonography and Doppler in the prediction of fetal haemolytic anaemia: a multivariate analysis. Br J Obstet Gynaecol 1994; 101(8):680–684.

17. Hecher K, Snijders R, Campbell S, Nicolaides K. Fetal venous, intracardiac, and arterial blood flow measurements in intrauterine growth retardation: relationship with fetal blood gases. Am J Obstet Gynecol 1995; 173(1):10–15.

18. Kirkinen P, Jouppila P, Eik-Nes S. Umbilical vein blood Flow in rhesus-isoimmunization. Br J Obstet Gynaecol 1983; 90(7):640–643.

19. Steiner H, Schaffer H, Spitzer D, Batka M, Graf AH, Staudach A. The relationship between peak velocity in the fetal descending aorta and hematocrit in rhesus isoimmunization. Obstet Gynecol 1995; 85(5, Pt 1):659–662.

20. Zimmerman R, Carpenter RJ Jr, Durig P, Mari G. Longitudinal measurement of peak systolic velocity in the fetal middle cerebral artery for monitoring pregnancies complicated by red cell alloimmunisation: a prospective multicentre trial with intention-to-treat. Br J Obstet Gynaecol 2002; 109(7):746–752.

21. Dukler D, Oepkes D, Seaward G, Windrim R, Ryan G. Noninvasive tests to predict fetal anemia: a study comparing Doppler and ultrasound parameters. Am J Obstet Gynecol 2003; 188(5):1310–1314.

22. van Dongen H, Klumper FJ, Sikkel E, Vandenbussche FP, Oepkes D. Noninvasive tests to predict fetal anemia in Kell alloimmunized pregnancies. Ultrasound Obstet Gynecol 2005; 25(4):341–345.

23. Bevis DC. The antenatal prediction of haemolytic disease of the newborn. Lancet 1952; 1(8):395–398.

24. Liley AW. Liquor amnii analysis in the management of the pregnancy complicated by rhesus sensitization. Am J Obstet Gynecol 1961; 82:1359–1370.

25. Queenan JT, Tomai TP, Ural SH, King JC. Deviation in amniotic fluid optical density at a wavelength of 450 nm in Rh-immunized pregnancies from 14 to 40 weeks' gestation: a proposal for clinical management. Am J Obstet Gynecol 1993; 168(5): 1370–1376.

26. Rodeck CH, Deans A. Red cell alloimmunisation. In: Rodeck CH, Whittle MJ, eds. Fetal Medicine, Basic Science and Clinical Practice. London: Churchill Livingstone, 1999:785–804.

27. Ryan G, Morrow RJ. Fetal blood transfusion. Clin Perinatol 1994; 21(3):573–589.

28. Weiner CP, Okamura K. Diagnostic fetal blood sampling-technique related losses. Fetal Diagn Ther 1996; 11(3):169–175.

29. Weiner CP. Fetal hemolytic disease. In: James DK, Steer PJ, Weiner CP, Gonik G, eds. High Risk Pregnancy; Management Options. 2nd. London: WB Saunders, 1999:343–362.

30. Fisk NM, Gitau R, Teixeira JM, Giannakoulopoulos X, Cameron AD, Glover VA. Effect of direct fetal opioid analgesia on fetal hormonal and hemodynamic stress response to intrauterine needling. Anesthesiology 2001; 95(4):828–835.

31. Moise KW Jr. The fetus with immune hydrops. In: Harrison MR, Evans MI, Adzick NS, Holzgreve W, eds. The Unborn Patient; the Art and Science of Fetal Therapy. Philadelphia: Saunders, 2001:513–523.

32. Anand KJ, Maze M. Fetuses, fentanyl, and the stress response: signals from the beginnings of pain? Anesthesiology 2001; 95(4):823–825.

33. van Kamp IL, Klumper FJ, Oepkes D, et al. Complications of intrauterine intravascular transfusion for fetal anemia due to maternal red-cell alloimmunization. Am J Obstet Gynecol 2005; 192(1):171–177.

34. Moise KW Jr. Hemolytic disease of the fetus and newborn. In: Creasy RK, Resnik R, eds. Maternal–fetal Medicine. Principle and Practice. 5th ed. Philadelphia: WB Saunders, 2004:537–561.

35. Giannakoulopoulos X, Sepulveda W, Kourtis P, Glover V, Fisk NM. Fetal plasma cortisol and beta-endorphin response to intrauterine needling. Lancet 1994; 344(8915):77–81.

36. Giannakoulopoulos X, Teixeira J, Fisk N, Glover V. Human fetal and maternal noradrenaline responses to invasive procedures. Pediatr Res 1999; 45(4, Pt 1):494–499.

37. Huang W, Deprest J, Missant C, van de Velde M. Management of fetal pain during invasive fetal procedures. A review. Acta Anesthesiol Belg 2004; 55(2):119–123.

38. Nicolini U, Nicolaidis P, Fisk NM, Tannirandorn Y, Rodeck CH. Fetal blood sampling from the intrahepatic vein: analysis of safety and clinical experience with 214 procedures. Obstet Gynecol 1990; 76(1):47–53.

39. Weiner CP, Wenstrom KD, Sipes SL, Williamson RA. Risk factors for cordocentesis and fetal intravascular transfusion. Am J Obstet Gynecol 1991; 165(4, Pt 1):1020–1025.

40. Westgren M, Selbing A, Stangenberg M. Fetal intracardiac transfusions in patients with severe rhesus isoimmunisation. Br Med J 1988; 296(6626):885–886.

41. Nicolaides KH, Soothill PW, Rodeck CH, Clewell W. Rh disease: intravascular fetal blood transfusion by cordocentesis. Fetal Ther 1986; 1(4):185–192.

42. Mandelbrot L, Daffos F, Forestier F, MacAleese J, Descombey D. Assessment of fetal blood volume for computer-assisted management of in utero transfusion. Fetal Ther 1988; 3(1–2):60–66.

43. Welch R, Rampling MW, Anwar A, Talbert DG, Rodeck CH. Changes in hemorheology with fetal intravascular transfusion. Am J Obstet Gynecol 1994; 170(3):726–732.

44. Harman CR, Bowman JM, Manning FA, Menticoglou SM. Intrauterine transfusion— intraperitoneal versus intravascular approach: a case–control comparison. Am J Obstet Gynecol 1990; 162(4):1053–1059.

45. Nicolini U, Kochenour NK, Greco P, Letsky E, Rodeck CH. When to perform the next intra-uterine transfusion in patients with Rh allo-immunization: combined intravascular and intraperitoneal transfusion allows longer intervals. Fetal Ther 1989; 4(1):14–20.

46. Moise, KJ Jr, Carpenter RJ Jr, Kirshon B, Deter RL, Sala JD, Cano LE. Comparison of four types of intrauterine transfusion: effect on fetal hematocrit. Fetal Ther 1989; 4(2–3): 126–137.

47. el Azeem SA, Samuels P, Rose RL, Kennedy M, O'Shaughnessy RW. The effect of the source of transfused blood on the rate of consumption of transfused red blood cells in pregnancies affected by red blood cell alloimmunization. Am J Obstet Gynecol 1997; 177(4):753–757.

48. Berkowitz RL, Chitkara U, Wilkins IA, Lynch L, Plosker H, Bernstein HH. Intravascular monitoring and management of erythroblastosis fetalis. Am J Obstet Gynecol 1988; 158(4):783–795.

49. Ronkin S, Chayen B, Wapner RJ, et al. Intravascular exchange and bolus transfusion in the severely isoimmunized fetus. Am J Obstet Gynecol 1989; 160(2):407–411.

50. Hallak M, Moise KJ Jr, Hesketh DE, Cano LE, Carpenter RJ Jr. Intravascular transfusion of fetuses with rhesus incompatibility: prediction of fetal outcome by changes in umbilical venous pressure. Obstet Gynecol 1992; 80(2):286–290.

51. Klumper FJ, van Kamp IL, Vandenbussche FP, et al. Benefits and risks of fetal red-cell transfusion after 32 weeks gestation. Eur J Obstet Gynecol Reprod Biol 2000; 92(1): 91–96.

52. Sampson AJ, Permezel M, Doyle LW, de Crespigny L, Ngu A, Robinson H. Ultrasound-guided fetal intravascular transfusions for severe erythroblastosis, 1984–1993. Aust N Z J Obstet Gynaecol 1994; 34(2):125–130.

53. Poissonnier MH, Brossard Y, Demedeiros N, et al. Two hundred intrauterine exchange transfusions in severe blood incompatibilities. Am J Obstet Gynecol 1989; 161(3):709–713.

54. Weiner CP, Williamson RA, Wenstrom KD, et al. Management of fetal hemolytic disease by cordocentesis. II. Outcome of treatment. Am J Obstet Gynecol 1991; 165(5, Pt 1):1302–1307.

55. van Kamp IL, Klumper FJ, Meerman RH, Oepkes D, Scherjon SA, Kanhai HH. Treatment of fetal anemia due to red-cell alloimmunization with intrauterine transfusions in the Netherlands, 1988–1999. Acta Obstet Gynecol Scand 2004; 83(8):731–737.

56. Janssens HM, de Haan MJ, van Kamp IL, Brand R, Kanhai HH, Veen S. Outcome for children treated with fetal intravascular transfusions because of severe blood group antagonism. J Pediatr 1997; 131(3):373–380.

57. Hudon L, Moise KJ Jr, Hegemier SE, et al. Long-term neurodevelopmental outcome after intrauterine transfusion for the treatment of fetal hemolytic disease. Am J Obstet Gynecol 1998; 179(4):858–863.

58. Newman TB, Maisels MJ. Evaluation and treatment of jaundice in the term newborn: a kinder, gentler approach. Pediatrics 1992; 89(5, Pt 1):809–818.

59. Valaes T, Kipouros K, Petmezaki S, Solman M, Doxiadis SA. Effectiveness and safety of prenatal phenobarbital for the prevention of neonatal jaundice. Pediatr Res 1980; 14(8):947–952.

60. von Kaisenberg CS, Jonat W. Fetal parvovirus B19 infection. Ultrasound Obstet Gynecol 2001; 18(3):280–288.

61. Peters MT, Nicolaides KH. Cordocentesis for the diagnosis and treatment of human fetal parvovirus infection. Obstet Gynecol 1990; 75(3, Pt 2):501–504.

62. de Jong EP, de Haan TR, Kroes AC, Beersma MF, Oepkes D, Walther FJ. Parvovirus B19 infection in pregnancy. J Clin Virol 2006. In press.

63. Sueters M, Arabin B, Oepkes D. Doppler sonography for predicting fetal anemia caused by massive fetomaternal hemorrhage. Ultrasound Obstet Gynecol 2003; 22(2):186–189.

64. Lam YH, Tang MH, Lee CP, Tse HY. Cardiac blood flow studies in fetuses with homozygous alpha-thalassemia-1 at 12–13 weeks of gestation. Ultrasound Obstet Gynecol 1999; 13(1):48–51.

65. Leung WC, Oepkes D, Seaward G, Ryan G. Serial sonographic findings of four fetuses with homozygous alpha-thalassemia-1 from 21 weeks onwards. Ultrasound Obstet Gynecol 2002; 19(1):56–59.

66. Radder CM, Brand A, Kanhai HH. A less invasive treatment strategy to prevent intracranial hemorrhage in fetal and neonatal alloimmune thrombocytopenia. Am J Obstet Gynecol 2001; 185(3):683–688.

67. Radder CM, Brand A, Kanhai HH. Will it ever be possible to balance the risk of intracranial haemorrhage in fetal or neonatal alloimmune thrombocytopenia against the risk of treatment strategies to prevent it? Vox Sang 2003; 84(4):318–325.

24
Gastroschisis

Julien Saada
Département de Périnatologie, Maternité de l'Hôpital Robert Debré (AP-HP), and Ecole de Chirurgie du Fer à Moulin (AP-HP), Paris, and Fédération de Gynécologie-Obstétrique, Secteur Échographie et Diagnostic Anténatal, Hôpital Paule de Viguier, Toulouse, France

Jean-François Oury
Département de Périnatologie, Maternité de l'Hôpital Robert Debré (AP-HP), and Université Paris VII (UFR Lariboisière Saint Louis), and Unité de Recherche EA3102, Paris, France

Edith Vuillard
Département de Périnatologie, Maternité de l'Hôpital Robert Debré (AP-HP), Paris, France

Pascal De Lagausie
Ecole de Chirurgie du Fer à Moulin (AP-HP), and Unité de Recherche EA3102, Paris, and Service de Chirurgie Pédiatrique, Hôpital la Timone, AP-HM, Marseille, France

Joe Bruner
Vanderbilt University Medical Center, Nashville, Tennessee, U.S.A.

Jean Guibourdenche
Biochimie-Hormonologie, Hôpital Robert Debré (AP-HP), Paris, France

Ghislaine Sterkers
Laboratoire d'Immunologie, Hôpital Robert Debré (AP-HP), Paris, France

Dominique Luton
Département de Périnatologie, Maternité de l'Hôpital Robert Debré (AP-HP), and Université Paris VII (UFR Lariboisière Saint Louis), and, Unité de Recherche EA3102, Ecole de Chirurgie du Fer à Moulin (AP-HP), Paris, France

GENERAL INTRODUCTION

Moore (1) first differentiated gastroschisis from omphalocele in 1953. It is defined as an abdominal wall defect that involves herniation of gut and occasionally spleen, liver, or genitourinary tract. It occurs mostly to the right side of the umbilicus and is characterized by the absence of membrane covering the prolapsed organs,

431

the loops of gut floating in the amniotic fluid. Thanks to sonographic scan, it is a common prenatally diagnosed condition, with a diagnostic rate about 95%.

Its overall prognosis is excellent with 90% survival rate (2,3) and its morbidity depends on prematurity, intrauterine growth restriction (IUGR), bowel atresia, and perivisceritis due to contact with the amniotic fluid.

First, perivisceritis was thought to be due to the presence of urine in the amniotic fluid, but, recently, digestive compounds in amniotic fluid have been established as the major responsible element. Besides the gold standard treatment of postnatal immediate surgery, recent advances in the understanding of the mechanisms responsible for the bowel damage may cause changes in therapeutic strategy. Prenatal treatment, using amnioexchange, may become an important step in the treatment of gastroschisis.

PREVALENCE AND EPIDEMIOLOGY

The total prevalence of gastroschisis, including live births, stillbirths, and terminations of pregnancy, is about 1–3 in 10,000 live births (2,3) with a sex ratio ~1. Although the total prevalence varies among geographic areas (3,4), several studies report a global increase of gastroschisis during recent years (2–5). Rankin et al. (3) have found a significant increase in the total prevalence from 1.48 per births in 1986 to 5.29 in 1996 in the north of England in patients who were identified from the Northern Cargenital Survey Abnormality.

The major epidemiological association with gastroschisis is young maternal age. It is more frequent in primiparas (3,6,7), and it is associated with low social economic status, poor maternal education, and drug abuse (cigarettes, alcohol, and cocaine) (8–10). Other teratogens have been implicated and are reported in Table 1. It has been suggested that these substances may have vasoreactive effects during embryo development.

Some isolated associations have been described with aneuploidy, trisomies 13, 18, 21, and monosomy 22 (11), and some familial cases have been reported (12–19). The role of genetic, epigenetic, and environmental factors is not yet clearly established (12).

EMBRYOLOGY AND PATHOGENESIS

While the fusion of the anterior abdominal wall muscles is complete by 8 weeks of gestation, the physiological umbilical herniation appears at the beginning of

Table 1 Teratogens Implicated in Gastroschisis and Epidemiological Associations

Teratogens	Cigarette smoking
	Alcohol
	Cocaine
	Aspirin
	Ibuprofen
	Pseudoephedrine
	Acetaminophen
	Phenylpropanolamine
Epidemiological associations	Young maternal age and short interval
	between menarche and first pregnancy
	Low social economic status
	Poor maternal education

the sixth week of gestation and ends by 10 weeks of gestation. The occurrence of the herniation is explained by the fact that, at this time, the liver and kidneys are proportionally bigger and occupy the majority of the abdomen. The herniation first tends to increase because of the rapid growth of the bowel, but then, as the embryo grows, the bowel loops return to the abdominal cavity. The reduction of the physiological herniation is accompanied by a 270° rotation of the bowel and the abdominal closure is complete by 10 weeks of gestation.

The pathogenesis of gastroschisis is not clearly understood; the most cited mechanism is the premature regression, by the fifth or sixth weeks of gestation, of the right omphalomesenteric artery or of the right umbilical vein (20,21). This premature regression leads to a mesodermal component failure of the abdominal wall, and intestinal malrotation is almost always associated with gastroschisis.

Others consider that it may be related to an early in utero rupture of an umbilical cord hernia (22).

BOWEL LESIONS, INFLAMMATORY PROCESS, AND AMNIOTIC DIGESTIVE COMPOUNDS IN GASTROSCHISIS

Bowel contact with the amniotic fluid is associated with a sterile inflammation of its wall resulting in a fibrous coat called perivisceritis (Fig. 1). Other bowel lesions of increasing gravity such as ischemia, perforation, stenosis, atresia, and partial or complete necrosis may be present and are implicated in morbidity, mortality, and in prognosis (23–27).

Two types of mechanism—a chemical and a constrictive one—are responsible for bowel lesions in gastroschisis (28–32).

Chemical Mechanism

Measurement of intra-amniotic values of tumor necrosis factor α (TNFα), interleukin 1β (IL1β), IL8, IL6, total protein, and ferritin levels displayed a chronic inflammatory profile in cases of gastroschisis. The levels of IL6, IL8, total protein, and ferritin are increased (33), where as the levels of TNFα and IL1β are not (Table 2). These

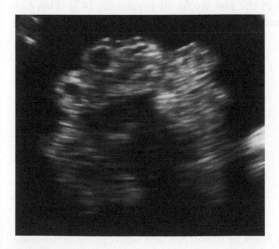

Figure 1 Ultrasonographic view of gastroschisis with matted and thickened bowel wall.

Table 2 Amniotic Fluid Concentrations of IL6, TNFα, IL1β, Ferritin, and Total Protein in
Gastroschisis Affected Fetuses, Expressed in MoM Relative to Normal Controls

	MoM	p
IL6	> 2,1	< 0,05
TNFα	1	NS
IL1β	1	NS
Ferritin	8.25	< 0,001
Total Protein	2.6	< 0,001

results suggest that a chronic in utero inflammatory reaction exists in gastroschisis
and that, because of the occurrence of meconium-stained amniotic fluid, gastrointestinal waste products are implicated in this reaction (33–35). The presence of
perivisceritis, which has the characteristics of an inflammatory reaction, also suggests
that a chronic inflammatory reaction exists. In 2000, Correira-Pinto (36) demonstrated
in a rat model of gastroschisis that perivisceritis was dependent on the presence of meconium. It has also been demonstrated in a chik model that exchanging amnioallantoic
fluid decreased bowel lesion intensity (37), and this result went along with a decrease
of gastrointestinal waste products, whereas urinary waste products did not vary.

Most histological studies have been conducted on resection samples of atretic
bowel from initial or iterative surgery or performed quickly after birth on necroti-
scopic samples. They revealed the presence of edema, fibrin deposits, fibrosis, capillary proliferation, cellular infiltration of epithelial cells, and macrophages in the
bowel wall (38,39). These results have also been described in animal models (40–43).
A few specimens of appendices retrieved at the time of initial surgery show a subser-
ous fibrosis with a polymorphic infiltrate of neutrophils, macrophages, and small
lymphocytes (personal data). Flow cytometry in the amniotic fluid of fetuses affected
by gastroschisis reveals the presence of inflammatory cells (neutrophils and monocytes) (personal data) (Fig. 2). In a rat model, Yu et al. (44) demonstrated that late
injection of dexamethasone in amniotic fluid of fetuses with gastroschisis had
beneficial effects on bowel wall thickening, normalized total DNA, induced cellular
proliferation, and decreased apoptosis.

Recently, it has been suggested that in utero defecation is a physiologic event
during normal fetal life and increases in the last weeks of pregnancy (45). This has
been supported by the presence of intestinal enzymes in the amniotic fluid of normal

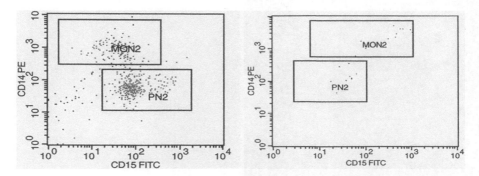

Figure 2 Flow cytometry showing high levels of monocytes and neutrophiles in amniotic
fluid of gastroschisis affected fetuses (*left*) compared to normal controls (*right*).

pregnancies (46,47). Meconium stain in amniotic fluid would not only be related to meconium passage but might be due to impaired clearance of amniotic fluid (45). Digestive compounds present in the amniotic fluid could be responsible for the chemical mechanism (41,48). They are associated with an inflammatory reaction in the bowel wall with aseptic peritonitis leading to edema, fibrin deposition, and cell infiltration, resulting in perivisceritis that may cover the whole bowel.

Constrictive Mechanism

The inextensible parietal defect, which can vary from 2 to 5 cm, is responsible for the constrictive mechanism. It may directly compress the superior mesenteric artery or vein and be responsible for ischemic complications or venous congestion. This may explain the frequency (10%) of bowel atresia in cases of gastroschisis.

Occlusive and subocclusive complications may also occur and be responsible for in utero vomiting, abnormal defecation (49), and decreased clearance of amniotic fluid together with bowel hypoperistaltism (45). Over-expression of nitrous oxide synthase (50–53) has been implicated in the occurrence of bowel hypoperistaltism (54,55).

These results show that chronic inflammatory reactions in the amniotic fluid, together with ischemia secondary to vascular compression (31,38,39), are implicated in the occurrence of the bowel wall abnormalities. The exact impact of amniotic fluid on the peritoneal surface of bowel wall is not yet completely known; however, exposure of a fetal pleural surface to the amniotic fluid induces similar changes as seen in the bowel wall in cases of gastroschisis (56).

Bowel lesions seem to be associated with downregulation of various genes involved in amino acid and glucose absorption (55,57–59) in experimental models of gastroschisis, and with fetal protein loss (60).

PRENATAL DIAGNOSIS

Gastroschisis used to be suspected in cases of elevated maternal α-fetoprotein, although this test was first designed for detection of neural tube defects (61–64).

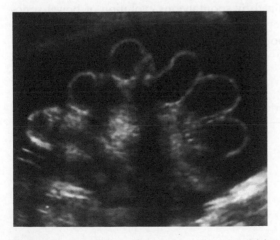

Figure 3 Ultrasonographic view of gastroschisis with a fine aspect of the bowel.

Table 3 Malformations Associated with Gastroschisis

Intrauterine growth restriction
Hydronephrosis
Arthrogryposis
Hypoplastic gallbladder
Meckel diverticulum
Oligoanhydramnios

Now, prenatal diagnosis relies on sonography with the typical feature of multiple bowel loops floating freely in the amniotic fluid as early as 10 weeks of gestation with no peritoneal membrane (Fig. 3). During the first trimester of pregnancy, bowel loops are collapsed and peristaltism may be seen. Later, meconium may appear as echogenic spots in the lumen of the hypoechoic bowel.

In contrast to omphalocele, gastroschisis is said not to be associated with an increased risk of chromosomal abnormality or of associated extragastrointestinal malformation. Some studies have yielded contradictory results; although Rankin et al. reported a malformation rate of 5.3% associated with gastroschisis and Roland et al. a rate of 5.5%, the EUROCAT study has reported a rate of 20.8% associated malformations. The most common extragastrointestinal malformations associated with gastroschisis are reported in Table 3 (2,3). Moreover, some of these gastroschisis cases associated with extragastrointestinal malformations may be, in fact, undiagnosed omphalocele with an early rupture and resorption of the sac.

A complete anatomical fetal examination has to be conducted to exclude these conditions and the common differential diagnosis of gastroschisis that are reported in Table 4.

IUGR and oligoanhydramnios are frequently associated with gastroschisis. IUGR may yet be overestimated because of the smaller abdominal circumference measurements (65,66).

MONITORING

The principle of follow-up is determined by spontaneous evolution of bowel sonographic aspect and the potential onset of complications.

The aspect of the free bowel loops floating in the amniotic fluid progressively changes in the course of pregnancy with the formation of a coat (perivisceritis)

Table 4 Differential Diagnosis of Anterior Abdominal Wall Defect

Omphalocele
Cystic cord lesion
Urachal cysts
Bladder extrophy
Cloacal extrophy
Amniotic band syndrome
Limb body wall complex
Pentalogy of Cantrell

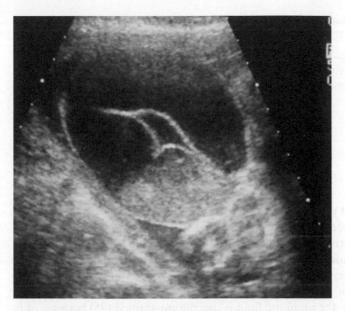

Figure 4 Ultrasonographic view of gastroschisis with an extra-abdominal bowel dilatation; a bowel atresia was discovered afterward.

covering the bowel loops. They then appear thicker and more echogenic. Sonography is not accurately able to identify partial necrosis (and secondary atresia), but a complete bowel necrosis may be associated with a sudden diminution of bowel size and has dramatic consequences.

Bowel dilatation and bowel wall thickening are often cited in studies as prognostic factors. Bowel dilatation would be, for some authors, a sign of occlusion and would reflect the bowel quality. Although data are not consistent, some authors have defined threshold values (11–18 mm) for prognosis and time of delivery. Others follow up bowel dilatation without recommending it as an appropriate indication for preterm delivery (24,67–79). Aina-Mumuney et al. found a significant correlation between gastric dilatation (Fig. 4) and length of stay in neonatal intensive care unit (NICU) and the occurrence of nonreactive nonstress test (80). The importance of bowel wall thickening is even more controversial and no consensus emerges from the different studies (67–78).

Mesenteric vascularization may be partially responsible for bowel abnormalities: Langer showed in a lamb model that a progressive constriction of bowel induced lesions independent of contact with amniotic fluid (28). Doppler measurement of the superior mesenteric artery may thus represent a potential tool for the follow-up in gastroschisis. Studies have contradictory results; Achiron (81) showed stability of vascular resistance from 29 weeks of gestation and Abuhaman (78) did not find any correlation between Doppler values in the extra-abdominal superior mesenteric artery and the outcome of gastroschisis. We found significant correlation between Doppler values and length of NICU stay and between maximal bowel dilatation and length of NICU stay. These results are yet to be confirmed by other studies and we do not use this parameter in our routine clinical practice (82).

The risk of in utero fetal death is higher in fetuses with gastroschisis (49,67,83,84). Fetal heart rate abnormalities are frequent during the third trimester of gestation (10%) and may prompt delivery (60,83,85–91). They consist of decreased

Table 5 Gastroschisis Monitoring

Sonography	Cardiotocography
Bowel dilatation and thickening	Decreased variability with or without
Bowel size sudden diminution	deceleration
Dilated stomach	
Oligohydramnios	
IUGR	

Abbreviation: IUGR, intrauterine growth retardation.

variability with or without decelerations. These abnormalities may partially be due to bowel torsion or subtorsion. They also may be due to IUGR and oligohydramnios that often complicate gastroschisis. Third trimester monitoring of fetal heart rate is thus a key tool in fetal surveillance for the diagnosis of fetal distress and may be repeated every day or every second day from 34 weeks of gestation (92). Table 5 reports the benchmarks of gastroschisis monitoring.

In most cases (79%), the amniotic fluid is meconium-stained (75) because of in utero vomiting, in utero defecation, meconium passage, or bowel perforation.

FETAL THERAPY: AMNIOEXCHANGE AND AMNIOINFUSION

Amnioinfusion and amnioexchange have been used to reduce gestational complications and to improve neonatal outcome.

Amnioinfusion

Amnioinfusion is an injection of warmed (37°C) physiologic saline. It is used in several situations: restoration of sufficient amniotic fluid volume in cases of abnormal fetal heart rate secondary to oligohydramnios, dilution of meconium-stained fluid to lower incidence of meconium aspiration syndrome, before morphologic sonographic scan in case of oligohydramnios, instillation of therapeutic drugs such as l-thyroxine, and in experimental protocols of endoscopic surgery.

Amnioinfusion must be done in surgical aseptic conditions to lower infectious complications. Other complications are rare but severe; cases of amniotic fluid embolism have been reported (93,94). Besides the occurrence of premature delivery, Dommergues (95) and Sapin (96) have reported cases of amnioinfusion in cases of oligohydramnios associated to gastroschisis with good outcomes.

Amnioexchange

Amnioexchange consists of the replacement of the amniotic fluid volume by volume with warm (37°C) saline and was first published in 1998 by Aktug (97) who performed four amnioexchanges with good outcome. In a lamb fetus model of gastroschisis (40,43), amnioexchange reduced inflammation in bowel wall. It induced a clearance of inflammatory compounds and gastrointestinal waste products and has a beneficial effect on amniotic fluid composition and bowel wall aspect. In humans, studies that evaluate the significance of amnioexchange are in progress.

DELIVERY

Delivery at a tertiary referral center is recommended as neonates have better outcomes because of a sharper coordination between obstetricians, neonatologists, and pediatric surgeons. The mean gestational age at spontaneous delivery is about 36–37 weeks (98), but the recommended mode (cesarean section vs. vaginal delivery) and timing of delivery is still debated as the hypothesis that labor is deleterious for the bowel has never been ascertained. Most authors have found no significant benefit to cesarean section (61,75,88,99–104). Moreover, it has been associated, in one study, with worse neonatal and infant outcomes (105). Others studies (106,107) suggest that cesarean section may benefit those fetuses.

As the available data do not provide evidence to support systematic cesarean section for fetuses with gastroschisis (108), we practice it only in cases of obstetrical indications.

IUGR is frequently associated with gastroschisis but does not constitute an indication of preterm delivery except in cases of abnormal middle cerebral artery Doppler and null or reversal diastolic flow of the umbilical artery (109).

POSTNATAL CARE

Immediately after delivery, the newborn trunk is wrapped in a sterile bag that covers the bowel loops, and appropriate care, which combines warmth and resuscitation, is given. The early complications are peritonitis and fluid, electrolyte, and caloric loss (Fig. 5). Adequate venous central lines and vesical and gastric tubes should be placed along with the administration of antibiotics and balanced electrolytes.

Surgery

The reference treatment is primary fascial closure but is only possible when the intraabdominal pressure (intravesical or intragastric pressure measurement) is <20 mmHg after the external bowel loops are returned to the abdominal cavity. It is associated with shorter interval of oral feeding, reduced hospital stay, and decreased surgery. Recently, studies have reported better outcomes for gastroschisis, particularly on the length of hospital stay, when a spring-loaded silo is used during the first 24 hours before fascial closure (110,111). In cases of increased abdominal pressure, fascial closure must be delayed using temporary coverage with intraabdominal pouch or mobilized lateral skin flaps (112).

Neonatal Intensive Care Unit

Most of the time, the increased intra-abdominal pressure necessitates first assisted ventilation, vasoactive and myorelaxant drugs, diuretics, and additional care that may be warranted because of the associated prematurity. Delayed total enteral nutrition requires the placement of a central venous line to provide appropriate caloric and hydroelectrolytic intake but is associated with septic complications (113,114).

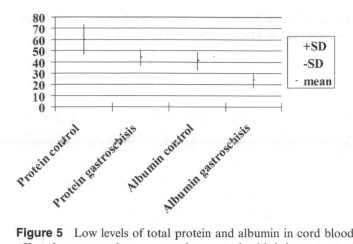

Figure 5 Low levels of total protein and albumin in cord blood at delivery in gastroschisis affected neonates when compared to controls; this is in contrast with the inflammatory profile observed in the amniotic fluid.

Parenteral nutrition is then replaced progressively by partial and complete enteral nutrition; the total duration of bowel rest will vary depending mostly on clinical evolution. The time of complete enteral nutrition is related to the length of hospital stay and duration of total parenteral nutrition (115). Infection and occlusive complications increase length of NICU stay and may jeopardize the outcome.

PROGNOSIS

The overall prognosis is good with mortality <10% (116,117). This result is first due to sonographic diagnosis that allows prenatal monitoring and delivery in a tertiary care center and then improvement in parenteral nutrition, surgery, and resuscitation techniques.

The first cause of mortality is sepsis (70%). Short-term and long-term outcomes (115,118) are related to the quality of the exteriorized bowel loops. Morbidity is still significant and mostly due to gastrointestinal complications; intestinal atresia is associated in 10% of cases and at least 25% of the newborns exhibit severe perivisceritis. As mentioned earlier, the time of total enteral nutrition is related to the length of hospital stay and duration of total parenteral nutrition (115).

Inguinal hernia is a frequent complication in infants with gastroschisis because of increased intra-abdominal pressure.

Long-term general and neurologic outcome is excellent in most cases (99,116,119).

REFERENCES

1. Moore TC, Stokes CE. Gastroschisis: report of two cases treated by a modification of the gross operation for omphalocele. Surgery 1953; 33:112–120.
2. Calzolari E, Bianchi F, Dolk H, Milan M. Omphalocele and gastroschisis in Europe: a survey of 3 million births 1980–1990. EUROCAT Working Group. Am J Med Genet 1995; 58:187–194.
3. Rankin J, Dillon E, Wright C. Congenital anterior abdominal wall defects in the North of England, 1986–1996: occurrence and outcome. Prenat Diagn 1999; 19:662–668.

4. Tan KH, Kilby MD, Whittle MJ, Beattie BR, Booth IW, Botting BJ. Congenital anterior abdominal wall defect in England and Wales 1987–1993: a retrospective analysis of OPCS data. Br Med J 1996; 313:903–906.

5. Barisic I, Clementi M, Hausler M, et al. Evaluation of prenatal ultrasound diagnosis of fetal abdominal wall defects by 19 European registries. Ultrasound Obstet Gynecol 2001; 18:309–316.

6. Roland A, Quijano F, Boos R, et al. Omphalocele and gastroschisis: prenatal diagnosis and perinatal management. A case analysis of the years 1989–1997 at the Department of Obstetrics and Gynecology, University of Homburg/Saar. Eur J Obstet Gynecol Reprod Biol 1999; 87:47–54.

7. Nichols CR, Dickinson JE, Pemberton PJ. Rising incidence of gastroschisis in teenage pregnancies. J Matern Fetal Med 1997; 6:225–229.

8. Torfs CP, Velie EM, Oechsli FW, Bateson TF, Curry CJ. A population-based study of gastroschisis: demographic, pregnancy and lifestyle factors. Teratology 1992; 50:44–53.

9. Werler MM, Mitchell AA, Shapiro S. First trimester maternal medication use in relation to gastroschisis. Teratology 1992; 45:361–367.

10. Werler MM, Mitchell AA, Shapiro S. Demographic, reproductive, medical, and environmental factors in relation to gastroschisis. Teratology 1992; 45:353–360.

11. Curry JI, McKinney P, Thornton JG, Stringer MD. The aetiology of gastroschisis. Br J Obstet Gynaecol 2000; 107:1339–1346.

12. Yang P, Beaty TH, Khoury MJ, Chee E, Stewart W, Gordis L. Genetic-epidemiologic study of omphalocele and gastroschisis: evidence of heterogeneity. Am J Med Genet 1992; 44:668–675.

13. Chun KH, Andrews G, White JJ. Gastroschisis in successive sibling: further evidence of acquired etiology. J Pediatr Surg 1993; 28:838–839.

14. Lowry RB, Baird PA. Familial gastroschisis and omphalocele. Am J Hum Genet 1982; 34:517–519.

15. Ventruto V, Stabile M, Lonardo F, et al. Gastroschisis in two sibs with abdominal hernia in maternal grandfather and great grandfather. Am J Med Genet 1985; 21:405–407.

16. Hershey DW, Haesslein HC, Mar CC, Adkins JC. Familial abdominal wall defect. Am J Med Genet 1989; 34:174–176.

17. Nelson TC, Toyama WM. Familial gastroschisis: a case of a mother and son occurrence. J Pediatr Surg 1995; 30:1706–1708.

18. Gorczyca DP, Lindfors KK, Giles KA, McGahan JP, Hanson FW, Tennant FP. Prenatally diagnosed gastroschisis in monozygotic twins. J Clin Ultrasound 1989; 17:216–218.

19. Bugge M, Petersen MB, Christensen MF. Monozygotic twins discordant for gastroschisis: case report and review of the literature of twins and familial occurrence of gastroschisis. Am J Med Genet 1994; 52:223–226.

20. Larsen WJ, ed. Development of gastrointestinal tract. In: Human Embryology. New York: Churchill Livingstone, 1993:224.

21. De Vries PA. The pathogenesis of gastroschisis and omphalocele. J Pediatr Surg 1980; 15:245–251.

22. Glick PL, Harrison MR, Adzick NS, Filly RA, deLorimier AA, Callen PW. The missing link in the pathogenesis of gastroschisis. J Pediatr Surg 1985; 20:406–409.

23. Moore TC. Gastroschisis and omphalocele: clinical differences. Surgery 1977; 82:561–568.

24. Louw JH. Jejunoileal atresia and stenosis. J Pediatr Surg 1996; 1:8–23.

25. Woodburne RT. Essentials of Human Anatomy. New York: Oxford University Press, 1961:418.

26. Colombani PM, Cunningham MD. Perinatal aspects of omphalocele and gastroschisis. Am J Dis Child 1977; 131:1386.

27. Bair JH, Russ PD, Pretorius DH, Manchester D, Manco-Johnson ML. Fetal omphalocele and gastroschisis: a review of 24 cases. Am J Radiol 1986; 147: 1047–1051.

28. Langer JC, Longaker MT, Crombleholme TM, et al. Etiology of intestinal damage in gastroschisis, I. Effect of amniotic fluid exposure and bowel constriction in a fetal lamb model. J Pediatr Surg 1989; 24:992–997.

29. Langer JC, Bell JG, Castillo RO, et al. Etiology of intestinal damage in gastroschisis, II. Timing and reversibility of histological changes, mucosal function, and contractility. J Pediatr Surg 1990; 25:1122–1126.

30. Albert A, Julia V, Morales SL, Parri FJ. Gastroschisis in the partially extraamniotic fetus: experimental study. J Pediatr Surg 1993; 28:656–659.

31. Kluck P, Tibboel D, van der Kamp AW, Molenaar JC. The effect of fetal urine on the development of the bowel in gastroschisis. J Pediatr Surg 1983; 18:47–50.

32. Aktug T, Erdag G, Kargi A, Akgur FM, Tibboel D. Amnio-allantoic fluid exchange for the prevention of intestinal damage in gastroschisis: an experimental study on chick embryos. J Pediatr Surg 1995; 30:384–387.

33. Burc L, Volumenie JL, de Lagausie P, et al. Amniotic fluid inflammatory proteins and digestive compounds profile in fetuses with gastroschisis undergoing amnioexchange. Br J Obstet Gynaecol 2004; 11:1–6.

34. Luton D, de Lagausie P, Guibourdenche J, et al. Effect of amnioinfusion on the outcome of prenatally diagnosed gastroschisis. Fetal Diagn Ther 1999; 14:152–155.

35. Morrison JJ, Klein N, Chitty LS, et al. Intra-amniotic inflammation in human gastroschisis: possible aetiology of postnatal bowel dysfunction. Br J Obstet Gynaecol 1998; 105:1200–1204.

36. Correia-Pinto J, Tavares M, Baptista M, Estevão-Costa J, Flake AW, Leite-Moreira AF. Meconium dependence of bowel damage in gastroschisis. In: Proceedings of A Journey from Gamete to Newborn, September 20–23, Leuven, Belgium, 2000:82.

37. Aktug T, Ucan B, Olguner M, et al. Amnio-allantoic fluid exchange for the prevention of intestinal damage in gastroschisis. III: Determination of the waste products removed by exchange. Eur J Pediatr Surg 1998; 8:326–328.

38. Tibboel D, Raine P, McNee M, et al. Developmental aspects of gastroschisis. J Pediatr Surg 1986; 21:865–869.

39. Tibboel D, Vermey-Keers C, Kluck P, Gaillard JL, Koppenberg J, Molenaar JC. The natural history of gastroschisis during fetal life: development of the fibrous coating on the bowel loops. Teratology 1986; 33:267–272.

40. Luton D, de Lagausie P, Guibourdenche J, et al. Influence of amnioinfusion in a model of in utero created gastroschisis in the pregnant ewe. Fetal Diagn Ther 2000; 15: 224–228.

41. Olguner M, Akgur FM, Api A, Ozer E, Aktug T. The effects of intraamniotic human neonatal urine and meconium on the intestines of the chick embryo with gastroschisis. J Pediatr Surg 2000; 35:458–461.

42. Albert A, Julia V, Morales L, Rovira J, Sancho A, Bombi JA. Role of the amniotic fluid in gastroschisis. An experimental study. Cir Pediatr 1992; 5:12–16.

43. de Lagausie P, Guibourdenche J, de Buis A, et al. Esophageal ligature in experimental gastroschisis. J Pediatr Surg 2002; 37:1160–1164.

44. Yu J, Gonzalez-Reyes S, Diez-Pardo JA, Tovar JA. Effects of prenatal dexamethasone on the intestine of rats with gastroschisis. J Pediatr Surg 2003; 38:1032–1035.

45. Ciftci AO, Tanyel FC, Bingol-Kologul M, Sahin S, Buyukpamukcu N. Fetal distress does not affect in utero defecation but does impair the clearance of amniotic fluid. J Pediatr Surg 1999; 34:246–250.

46. Morin PR, Potier M, Dallaire L, Melancon SB, Milunsky A. prenatal detection of intestinal obstruction: deficient amniotic fluid disaccharidases in affected fetuses. Clin Genet 1980; 18:217–222.

47. Kleijer WJ, Janse HC, Van Diggelen OP, Niermeijer MF. Intra-amniotic inflammation in human gastroschisis: possible aetiology of postnatal bowel dysfunction. Br J Obstet Gynaecol 1985; 105:1200–1204.
48. Ciftci AO, Tanyel FC, Ercan MT, Karnak I, Büyükpamukçu N, Hiçsönmez A. In utero defecation by the normal foetus: a radio nuclide study in the rabbit. J Pediatr Surg 1996; 31:1409–1412.
49. Adair CD, Rosnes J, Frye AH, Burrus DR, Nelson LH, Veille JC. The role of antepartum surveillance in the management of gastroschisis. Int J Gynaecol Obstet 1996; 52:141–144.
50. Bartho L, Koczan G, Petho G, Maggi CA. Blockade of nitric oxide synthase inhibits nerve mediated contraction in the rat small intestine. Neurosci Lett 1992; 145:43–46.
51. Sanders KM, Ward SM. Nitric oxide as a mediator of non adrenergic non cholinergic neurotransmission. Am J Physiol 1992; 262:379–392.
52. Bealer JF, Natuzzi ES, Buscher C, et al. Nitric oxide synthase is deficient in the aganglionic colon from patients with Hirschsprung's disease. Pediatrics 1994; 93:641–647.
53. Bealer JF, Graf J, Bruch SW, Adzick NS, Harrison MR. Gastroschisis increases small bowel nitric oxide synthase activity. J Pediatr Surg 1996; 31:1043–1046.
54. O'Neill JA, Grosfeld JL. Intestinal malfunction after antenatal exposure of viscera. Am J Surg 1974; 127:129–132.
55. Guo W, Swanicker F, Fonkalsrud EW, Vo K, Karamanoukian R. Effect of intraamniotic dexamethasone administration on intestinal absorption in a rabbit gastroschisis model. J Pediatr Surg 1996; 31:433–435.
56. Longaker MT, Whithy DJ, Jennings EW, et al. Fetal diaphragmatic wounds heal with scar formation. J Surg Res 1991; 50:375–385.
57. Lopez de Torre B, Tovar JA, Uriarte S, Aldazabal P. Transperitoneal exchange of water and solutes in the fetus with gastroschisis: experimental study in the chick embryo. Eur J Pediatr Surg 1991; 6:346–352.
58. Shaw K, Buchmiller TL, Curr M, et al. Impairment of nutrient uptake in a rabbit model of gastroschisis. J Pediatr Surg 1994; 29:376–378.
59. Srinathan SK, Langer JC, Wang JL, Rubin DC. Enterocyte gene expression is altered in experimental gastroschisis. J Surg Res 1997; 68:1–6.
60. Carroll SG, Kuo PY, Kyle PM, Soothill PW. Fetal protein loss in gastroschisis as an explanation of associated morbidity. Am J Obstet Gynecol 2001; 184:1297–1301.
61. Kirk EP, Wah RM. Obstetric management of the fetus with omphalocele or gastroschisis: a review and report of one hundred twelve cases. Am J Obstet Gynecol 1983; 146:512–518.
62. Milunsky A, Alpert E. Results and benefits of a maternal serum alpha fetoprotein screening program. J Am Med Assoc 1984; 252:1438–1442.
63. Simpson J, Baum L, Marder R, et al. Maternal serum afoetoprotein screening: low and high values for detection of genetic abnormalities. Am J Obstet Gynecol 1986; 155:593–597.
64. Burton B. Alpha foeto protein screening. Adv Pediatr 1986; 33:181–196.
65. Fries MH, Filly RA, Callen PW, Goldstein RB, Goldberg JD, Golbus MS. Growth retardation in prenatally diagnosed cases of gastroschisis. J Ultrasound Med 1993; 12:583–588.
66. Raynor BD, Richards D. Growth retardation in fetuses with gastroschisis. J Ultrasound Med 1997; 16:13–16.
67. Crawford RA, Ryan G, Wright VM, Rodeck CH. The importance of serial biophysical assessment of fetal wellbeing in gastroschisis. Br J Obstet Gynaecol 1992; 99:899–902.
68. Bond SJ, Harrison MR, Filly RA, Callen PW, Anderson RA, Golbus MS. Severity of intestinal damage in gastroschisis: correlation with prenatal sonographic findings. J Pediatr Surg 1988; 23:520–525.
69. Sipes SL, Weiner CP, Williamson RA, Pringle KC, Kimura K. Fetal gastroschisis complicated by bowel dilation: an indication for imminent delivery. Fetal Diagn Ther 1990; 5:100–103.

70. Lenke RR, Persutte WH, Nemes J. Ultrasonographic assessment of intestinal damage in fetuses with gastroschisis: is it of clinical value? Am J Obstet Gynecol 1990; 163:995–998.

71. Langer JC, Khanna J, Caco C, Dykes EH, Nicolaides KH. Prenatal diagnosis of gastroschisis: development of objective sonographic criteria for predicting outcome. Obstet Gynecol 1993; 81:53–56.

72. Pryde PG, Bardicef M, Treadwell MC, Klein M, Isada NB, Evans MI. Gastroschisis: can antenatal ultrasound predict infant outcomes? Obstet Gynecol 1994; 84:505–510.

73. Babcook CJ, Hedrick MH, Goldstein RB, et al. Gastroschisis: can sonography of the fetal bowel accurately predict postnatal outcome? J Ultrasound Med 1994; 13:701–706.

74. McMahon MJ, Kuller JA, Chescheir NC. Prenatal ultrasonographic findings associated with short bowel syndrome in two fetuses with gastroschisis. Obstet Gynecol 1996; 88:676–678.

75. Adra AM, Landy HJ, Nahmias J, Gomez-Marin O. The fetus with gastroschisis: impact of route of delivery and prenatal ultrasonography. Am J Obstet Gynecol 1996; 174:540–546.

76. Alsulyman OM, Monteiro H, Ouzounian JG, Barton L, Songster GS, Kovacs BW. Clinical significance of prenatal ultrasonographic intestinal dilatation in fetuses with gastroschisis. Am J Obstet Gynecol 1996; 175:982–984.

77. Brun M, Grignon A, Guibaud L, Garel L, Saint-Vil D. Gastroschisis: are prenatal ultrasonographic findings useful for assessing the prognosis? Pediatr Radiol 1996; 26:723–726.

78. Abuhamad AZ, Mari G, Cortina RM, Croitoru DP, Evans AT. Superior mesenteric artery Doppler velocimetry and ultrasonographic assessment of fetal bowel in gastroschisis: a prospective longitudinal study. Am J Obstet Gynecol 1997; 176:985–990.

79. Weitzman JJ, Vanderhoof RS. Jejunal atresia with agenesis of the dorsal mesentery with "christmas tree" deformity of the small intestine. Am J Surg 1966; 111:443–449.

80. Aina-Mumuney AJ, Fischer AC, Blackmore KJ, et al. A dilated fetal stomach predicts a complicated postnatal course in cases of prenatally diagnosed gastroschisis. Am J Obstet Gynecol 2004; 190:1326–1330.

81. Achiron R, Orvieto R, Lipitz S, Yagel S, Rotstein Z. Superior mesenteric artery blood flow velocimetry: cross-sectional Doppler sonographic study in normal fetuses. J Ultrasound Med 1998; 17:769–773.

82. Volumenic JL, de Lagausic P, Guibourdenche J, et al. Improvement of mesenteric superior artery Doppler velocimetry by amnio-infusion in fetal gastroschisis. Prenat Diagn 2001; 21:1171–1174.

83. Burge DM, Ade-Ajayi N. Adverse outcome after prenatal diagnosis of gastroschisis: the role of fetal monitoring. J Pediatr Surg 1997; 32:441–444.

84. Fisher R, Attah A, Partington A, Dykes E. Impact of antenatal diagnosis on incidence and prognosis in abdominal wall defects. J Pediatr Surg 1996; 31:538–541.

85. Poulain P, Milon J, Fremont B, et al. Remarks about the prognosis in case of antenatal diagnosis of gastroschisis. Eur J Obstet Gynecol Reprod Biol 1994; 54:185–190.

86. Haddock G, Davis CF, Raine PAM. Gastroschisis in the decade of prenatal diagnosis: 1983–1993. Eur J Pediatr Surg 1996; 6:18–22.

87. Dixon JC, Penman DM, Soothill PW. The influence of bowel atresia in gastroschisis on fetal growth, cardiotocograph abnormalities and amniotic fluid staining. Br J Obstet Gynaecol 2000; 107:472–475.

88. Moretti M, Khoury A, Rodriguez J, Lobe T, Shaver D, Sibai B. The effect of mode of delivery on the perinatal outcome in fetuses with abdominal wall defects. Am J Obstet Gynecol 1990; 163:833–838.

89. Stringer MD, Brereton RJ, Wright VM. Controversies in the management of gastroschisis: a study of 40 patients. Arch Dis Child 1991; 66:34–36.

90. Nihoul-Fekete C, Pellerin D. Manifestations digestives des coelosomies supérieures et moyennes (omphalocèles, laparoschisis). In: Navarro J, Schmitz J, eds. Gastroentérologie pédiatrique. 1st ed. Paris: Flammarion Med Science, 1987:397–398.

91. Ingamells S, Saunders NJ, Burge D. Gastroschisis and reduced fetal heart-rate variability. Lancet 1995; 345:1024–1025.
92. Brantberg A, Blaas HGK, Salvesen KA, Haugen SE, Eik-Nes SH. Surveillance and outcome in fetuses with gastroschisis. Ultrasound Obstet Gynecol 2004; 23:4–13.
93. Maher JE, Wenstrom KD, Hauth JC, Meis PJ. Amniotic fluid embolism after saline amnioinfusion: two cases and review of the literature. Obstet Gynecol 1994; 83:851–854.
94. Adair CD, Sanchez Ràmos L, Kaunitz AM, Briones D. A trial of labor complicated by uterine rupture following amnioinfusion. South Med J 1995; 88:847–848.
95. Dommergues M, Ansker Y, Aubry MC, et al. Serial transabdominal amnioinfusion in the management of gastroschisis with severe oligohydramnios. J Pediatr Surg 1996; 31:1297–1299.
96. Wenstrom K, Andrews WW, Maher JE. Amnioinfusion survey: prevalence, protocols, and complications. Obstet Gynecol 1995; 86:572–576.
97. Aktug T, Demir N, Akgur FM, Olguner M. Pretreatment of gastroschisis with transabdominal amniotic fluid exchanges. Obstet Gynecol 1998; 91:821–823.
98. Luton D, de Lagausie P, Guibourdenche J, et al. Prognostic factors of prenatally diagnosed gastroschisis. Fetal Diagn Ther 1997; 12:7–14.
99. Driver CP, Bruce J, Bianchi A, Doig CM, Dickson AP, Bowen J. The contemporary outcome of gastroschisis. J Pediatr Surg 2000; 35:1719–1723.
100. Lewis DF, Towers CV, Garite TJ, Jackson DN, Nageotte MP, Major CA. Fetal gastroschisis and omphalocele: is cesarean section the best mode of delivery? Am J Obstet Gynecol 1990; 163:773–775.
101. Rinehart BK, Terrone DA, Isler CM, Larmon JE, Perry KG Jr, Roberts WE. Modern obstetric management and outcome of infants with gastroschisis. Obstet Gynecol 1999; 94:112–116.
102. How HY, Harris BJ, Pietrantoni M, et al. Is vaginal delivery preferable to elective cesarean delivery in fetuses with a known ventral wall defect? Am J Obstet Gynecol 2000; 182:1527–1534.
103. Strauss RA, Balu R, Kuller JA, McMahon MJ. Gastroschisis: the effect of labor and ruptured membranes on neonatal outcome. Am J Obstet Gynecol 2003; 189:1672–1678.
104. Puligandla PS, Janvier A, Flageole H, Bouchard S, Laberge JM. Routine cesarean delivery does not improve outcome of infants with gastroschisis. J Pediatr Surg 2004; 39:742–745.
105. Quirk JG Jr, Fortney J, Collins HB II, West J, Hassad SJ, Wagner C. Outcomes of newborns with gastroschisis: the effects of mode of delivery, site of delivery, and interval from birth to surgery. Am J Obstet Gynecol 1996; 174:1134–1140.
106. Lenke PR, Hatch EI Jr. Fetal gastroschisis: a preliminary report advocating the use of cesarean section. Obstet Gynecol 1986; 67:395–398.
107. Sakala EP, Erhard LN, White JJ. Elective cesarean section improves outcomes of neonates with gastrischisis. Am J Obstet Gynecol 1993; 169:1050–1053.
108. Segel S, Marder S, Parry S, Macones G. Fetal abdominal wall defects and mode of delivery: a systematic review. Obstet Gynecol 2001; 98:867–873.
109. Puligandla PS, Janvier A, Flageole H, Bouchard S, Mok E, Laberge JM. The significance of intrauterine growth restriction is different from prematurity for the outcome of infants with gastroschisis. J Pediatr Surg 2004; 39:1200–1204.
110. Schlatter M, Norris K, Uitvlugt N, DeCou J, Connors R. Improved outcomes in the treatment of gastroschisis using a preformed silo and delayed repair approach. J Pediatr Surg 2003; 38:459–464.
111. Minkes RK, Langer JC, Mazziotti MV. Routine insertion of silastic spring-loaded silo for infants with gastroschisis. J Pediatr Surg 2000; 35:843–846.
112. Schuster SR. A new method for the staged repair of large omphalocele. Surg Gynecol Obstet 1967; 125:837–850.
113. Lefort J, Borde J, Mitrofanoff P, Ensel J. Laparoschisis: analyse d'une série de 19 cas. Chir Pédiatr 1978; 19:77–82.

114. Debeugny P, Jarde O, Herbaux B, et al. Le laparoschisis: problème thérapeutiques, à propos de 48 observations. Chir Pédiatr 1986; 27:41–49.
115. Sharp M, Bulsara M, Gollow, Pemberton P. Gastroschisis: early enteral feeds may improve outcome. J Pediatr Surg 2000; 36:472–476.
116. Snyder CL. Outcome analysis for gastroschisis. J Pediatr Surg 1999; 34:1253–1256.
117. Eurenius K, Axelsson O. Outcome for foetuses with abdominal wall defects detected by routine second trimester ultrasound. Acta Obstet Gynecol Scand 1994; 73:25–29.
118. Durfee SM, Downard CD, Benson CB, Wilson JM. Post-natal outcome of fetuses with prenatal diagnosis of gastroschisis. J Ultrasound Med 2002; 21:269–274.
119. Tarnowski KJ, King DR, Green L, Ginn-Pease ME. Congenital gastrointestinal anomalies: psychosocial functioning of children with imperforate anus, gastroschisis and omphalocele. J Consult Clin Psychol 1991; 59:587–590.

25

Twin-to-Twin Transfusion Syndrome

Liesbeth Lewi and Jan Deprest
*Department of Obstetrics and Gynaecology, University Hospitals Leuven,
Leuven, Belgium*

W. J. B. Dennes
*Centre for Fetal Care, Queen Charlotte's and Chelsea Hospital,
Hammersmith Campus, London, U.K.*

N. M. Fisk
*Institute of Reproductive and Developmental Biology, Imperial College London
and Queen Charlotte's and Chelsea Hospital, Hammersmith Campus, London, U.K.*

TWINS AND TWINS: DIFFERENT TYPES OF TWINNING

Twins can either be dizygotic (70%) or monozygotic (30%). Dizygotic twins result from the fertilization of two eggs, and there is a separate placenta and amniotic sac for each twin. Dizygotic twin pregnancies are, therefore, by definition dichorionic diamniotic and the few reported exceptions of dizygotic monochorionic twins due to fusion of two separate blastocysts only confirm this rule (1,2). In contrast, monozygotic twins arise from the fertilization of a single egg with subsequent splitting of the zygote. The longer the time period between fertilization and splitting, the more structures the twins have in common. In about 75% of monozygotic twins, splitting takes place after the third day postfertilization, resulting in a single placenta for both fetuses (monochorionic). The majority of monochorionic twins have separate amniotic sacs (diamniotic). Rarely, however, splitting occurs beyond the ninth day and these twins also share a single sac (monoamniotic), whereas splitting after the 12th day will result in conjoined twins. About 25% of monozygotic twins will be dichorionic diamniotic, when splitting occurs before the third day after fertilization.

Monochorionic twins not only share a single placenta, but vascular anastomoses also connect the blood circulation of both babies (Fig. 1). This shared fetal circulation means that the well-being of one fetus crucially depends on that of the other and accounts for the increased perinatal morbidity and mortality in monochorionic as compared to dichorionic twins (3). The vascular anastomoses are both unpredictable and randomly distributed and may account for some unique complications, such as twin-to-twin transfusion syndrome (TTTS), twin-reversed arterial perfusion, and in the event of single intrauterine fetal death (IUFD), acute exsanguination of the surviving twin into the fetoplacental circulation of the demised twin.

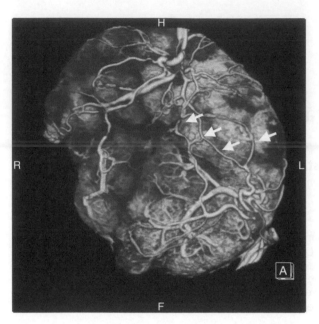

Figure 1 3D-reconstruction of a CT-angiogram of a monochorionic placenta demonstrating the vascular anastomoses connecting the two fetal circulations (*arrows*). *Source*: In collaboration with the Dept. of Radiology M. Cannie, UZ Leuven, Belgium.

Exact determination of chorionicity is, therefore, of utmost importance in the correct management of twin pregnancies and is reliably achieved on ultrasound scan prior to 14 weeks (4,5). At these early stages in pregnancy, the thin amniotic membrane is still separated from the thick intervening chorion and chorionicity determination is simply a matter of qualitative assessment or counting the layers that separate the twins (Fig. 2). Later on in pregnancy, it becomes far more difficult and often not possible to determine whether same sex twins do, or do not, share a single placenta. Whereas

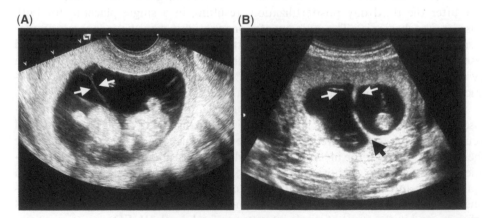

Figure 2 Chorionicity determination on the first trimester ultrasound scan (**A**) monochorionic diamniotic twins: only 2 thin amniotic membranes (*arrows*) separate the 2 fetuses; (**B**) dichorionic diamniotic twins: the fetuses are separated by 3 layers (amnion, chorion-chorion, amnion) (*arrows*).

chorionicity can be easily determined on early ultrasound, it is impossible to say whether dichorionic same-sex twins are dizygotic or monozygotic. All monochorionic twins are monozygotic and all dichorionic different-sex twins are dizygotic, but about 2 out of 10 dichorionic same-sex twins will still be monozygotic. In dichorionic same-sex twins, zygosity determination requires DNA fingerprinting, which prenatally would require an amniocentesis, chorionic villus sampling, or cordocentesis. Such an invasive procedure for zygosity determination is only rarely indicated, because in contrast to chorionicity, knowledge of zygosity is seldom crucial to obstetric management. However, zygosity remains of great interest to the parents. Now that these molecular techniques can be readily applied to accessible, postnatal tissue, such as hair and saliva, DNA fingerprinting on umbilical cord blood is less frequently offered after the birth of same-sex dichorionic twins.

TTTS: WHEN THE INTERTWIN TRANSFUSION BECOMES UNBALANCED

In monochorionic twins, intertwin transfusion is usually a constant, but balanced, phenomenon. However, in about 10% to 15%, a chronic imbalance in net flow occurs from one fetus (the donor) to the other (the recipient) resulting in TTTS, which typically occurs between 16 and 26 weeks of gestation. Hypovolemia, oliguria, and oligohydramnios develop in the donor, resulting in the "stuck twin" phenomenon, whereas hypervolemia, polyuria, and hydramnios evolve in the recipient, which may develop circulatory overload and hydrops. TTTS is a sonographic diagnosis usually based on the following criteria (6): hydramnios in the sac of the recipient twin (defined as deepest vertical pocket ≥ 8 cm before 20 weeks and ≥ 10 cm after 20 weeks) secondary to polyuria (distended bladder), combined with oligohydramnios in the donor's sac (deepest vertical pocket ≤ 2 cm) secondary to oliguria (collapsed or empty bladder) (Fig. 3). Although growth restriction is often present in the donor twin, it is not essential for the diagnosis. In severe cases of TTTS, Doppler investigation of the fetal circulation will show signs of congestive heart failure due to hypervolemia in the recipient (negative or reverse a-wave in the ductus venosus, pulsatile flow in the umbilical vein, tricuspid regurgitation) and signs of hypovolemia or increased vascular resistance in the donor (absent or reversed flow in the umbilical artery) (7,8). The mortality of untreated TTTS has traditionally been quoted as >80%; however, with advances in neonatal care it has decreased to 63% in the past decade (9).

The differential diagnosis includes monoamnionicity, discordant growth, and isolated hydramnios/oligohydramnios. In TTTS, the intertwin membrane may be difficult to see as it is wrapped tightly around the body of the donor twin. This may lead to an incorrect diagnosis of monoamnionicity. Although TTTS may occur in monoamniotic pregnancies (10), monoamniotic twins move freely in the amniotic cavity, whereas in diamniotic twins with TTTS, the donor twin remains fixed against the uterine wall. Discordant growth is also often confused with TTTS, as the growth-restricted twin may appear "stuck" due to oligohydramnios, but hydramnios is absent in the appropriately grown twin. The isolated presence of hydramnios or oligohydramnios in one sac with normal amniotic fluid in the other precludes the diagnosis of TTTS. Finally, a severe intertwin hemoglobin difference (with or without weight difference) diagnosed at birth should not be labeled TTTS (Fig. 4). Although, this reflects unbalanced intertwin transfusion, most cases of TTTS have an intertwin hemoglobin difference of <5 g/dL (11).

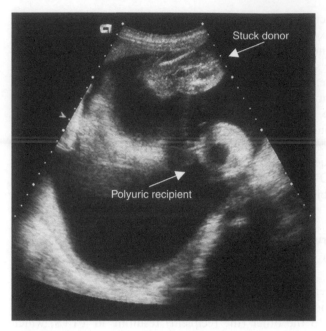

Figure 3 Ultrasound image of TTTS: the donor is stuck to the uterine wall without bladder filling; there is hydramnios in the sac of the recipient, who has a distended bladder. *Abbreviation*: TTTS, Twin-to-twin transfusion syndrome.

PATHOPHYSIOLOGY OF TTTS: VASCULAR ANASTOMOSES AND HEMODYNAMIC/HORMONAL FACTORS

The pathophysiology of TTTS has largely been explained on an angioarchitectural basis. Placental anastomoses are traditionally denoted as arterio-arterial (AA), veno-venous (VV), or arterio-venous (AV) (Fig. 5) (12). AA and VV anastomoses

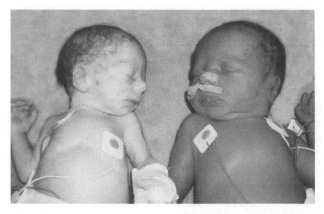

Figure 4 Macroscopic image of a monochorionic twin pair at 33 weeks with severe intertwin hemoglobin difference (5–20 g/dL) and 35% weight discrepancy. Prenatal ultrasound scan did not show discordant amniotic fluid volumes as required for the diagnosis of TTTS. *Abbreviation*: TTTS, twin-to-twin transfusion syndrome. *Source*: Courtesy of NICU, UZ Leuven, Belgium. (*See color insert.*)

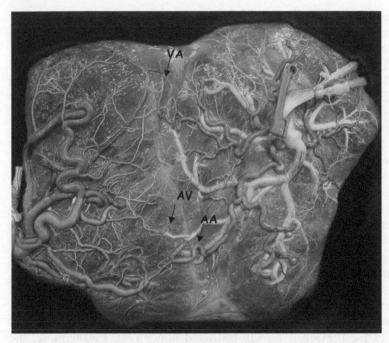

Figure 5 Macroscopic image after dye injection of a monochorionic placenta: superficial AA anastomosis, deep AV and oppositely directed VA anastomosis. *Abbreviations*: AA, arterio-arterial; AV arterio-venous; VV, veno-venous. (*See color insert.*)

are typically superficial, bidirectional anastomoses on the surface of the chorionic plate, forming direct communications between the arteries and veins of the two fetal circulations. The direction of flow depends on the relative interfetal vascular pressure gradients. AV anastomoses are usually considered "deep" anastomoses. They represent a shared cotyledon, receiving arterial supply from one twin and providing venous (well-oxygenated) drainage to the other twin. Thus, they are not strictly anastomoses as they do not bypass the capillary circulation. The supplying artery and draining vein of an AV anastomosis can be visualized on the placental surface as an unpaired artery and vein that pierce the chorionic plate at close proximity to each other (13). The AV anastomoses allow flow in one direction only, and hence may create imbalance in interfetal transfusion leading to TTTS, unless balanced by oppositely directed transfusion through other superficial or deep anastomoses.

Both postnatal injection studies (14) and in vivo fetoscopic observations (15,16) indicate the presence of at least one unidirectional AV anastomosis as an anatomical prerequisite for the development of TTTS. However, a case of TTTS has been reported with only superficial anastomoses (one AA and one VV) (16), but this seems an exception. Bidirectional AA anastomoses are believed to protect against the development of TTTS since most non-TTTS monochorionic placentas have AA anastomoses (84%) in contrast to TTTS placentas (20–30%) (14). AA, VV, and AV anastomoses have all been considered easily identifiable on inspecting the chorionic surface and were believed to be the only anastomoses present. However, recent data based on vascular casting and angiography suggest that placental angioarchitecture may actually be more complex than previously assumed with the existence of smaller anastomoses that are not visible from the chorionic surface (17,18).

Even if vascular anastomoses are an anatomical prerequisite for the development of TTTS, no specific pattern of anastomoses distinguishes monochorionic placentas that develop TTTS from those that do not. Other pathophysiologic mechanisms are likely to be involved, as simple transfusional blood volume effects cannot explain all the clinical manifestations. In the recipient, these include systemic hypertension (19,20) and hypertrophic outflow tract obstruction (19,21), and in the donor, increased placental vascular resistance in utero (22) and reduced arterial compliance in infancy (23). Further, there is little correlation between hemoglobin discordance and disease severity (11). The discordant long-term vascular programming demonstrated in genetically identical TTTS survivors appears preventable with timely intrauterine therapy (24), thus implicating deranged fetoplacental vascular function in utero.

It has been suggested that discordant placental function may offset TTTS. Placental dysfunction is associated with an increased fetoplacental resistance, which might promote transfusion from the growth-restricted donor to the recipient. Reduced insulin growth factor-II (25) and decreased leptin levels in donors, compared to recipients, reflects discordant placental development rather than transfusion as a cause of growth restriction (26). Notwithstanding this, twin transfusion must contribute to poor growth in some cases, as successful laser coagulation of the vascular anastomoses or selective termination of the recipient (27) often leads to a catch-up growth of the previously growth-restricted donor (28). Furthermore, the observation that end-diastolic frequencies, when absent in the umbilical artery of growth-restricted donors return acutely to normal following cord occlusion of the recipient is not in keeping with absent end-diastolic flow being a manifestation of the increased downstream placental resistance typical of IUGR, which is attributed to uteroplacental insufficiency.

Recent data implicate discordant hormonal vasodilatation in the donor and recipient in the phenotypic changes in TTTS. Raised endothelin-1 levels in recipients potentially contribute to increased peripheral vasoconstriction and hypertension. Recipients, as expected, have increased levels of atrial natriuretic peptide, but further, those with severe cardiac dysfunction have higher levels of brain natriuretic peptide, suggesting cardiac remodeling (29). Increased renin gene and protein expression are found in donor kidneys, whereas it is virtually absent in recipient kidneys, implicating discordant renin–angiotensin system activation in TTTS (30,31). Thus, the pathophysiology of TTTS is most likely multifactorial with vascular anastomoses providing the anatomical basis, and hemodynamic and hormonal factors then contributing in variable degrees to its clinical expression.

PREDICTION OF TTTS: IDENTIFICATION OF THE MONOCHORIONIC TWINS AT HIGHEST RISK

Identification of monochorionic twins at increased risk of TTTS would be helpful in patient counseling and planning of follow-up. Further, early diagnosis and treatment of TTTS may improve outcome, although the extent to which earlier treatment leads to a better outcome has yet to be determined. Nevertheless, undiagnosed TTTS may trigger cervical changes, which may increase the risk of preterm prelabor rupture of the membranes (PPROM) and preterm labor before or after therapy (32). As such, a short cervical length on transvaginal scan has been shown to be an important risk factor for delivery prior to 34 weeks after laser coagulation of vascular anastomoses

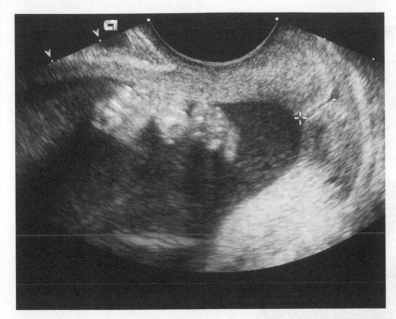

Figure 6 Preoperative ultrasound image of a short cervical length on transvaginal scan in a case of TTTS. *Abbreviation*: TTTS, twin-to-twin transfusion syndrome.

(Fig. 6) (33). Also, advanced disease with worsening hemodynamic dysfunction may increase the risk of long-term cardiac and neurological damage. Four markers have been proposed to predict TTTS: increased nuchal translucency (NT) in the first trimester, membrane folding, the absence of an AA anastomosis, and a velamentous cord insertion (Fig. 7).

On first-trimester scan, an increased NT (>95th centile) is a marker for chromosomal anomalies, cardiac defects, and a wide range of genetic syndromes. However, the frequency of increased NT is increased in monochorionic twins (13%), where it may reflect additionally early cardiac dysfunction due to hypervolemia in the recipient and thus predict the subsequent development of TTTS. As such, fetuses of monochorionic twin pregnancies with increased NT have a higher likelihood of developing TTTS [likelihood ratio: 3.5; 95% confidence interval (CI) 1.9–6.2] (34). However, the sensitivity of raised NT for TTTS is only 28% with a positive predictive value of 33%. As 72% of TTTS cases had NT measurements within the normal range, it does not perform well as a screening test. If TTTS truly results from a random, asymmetrical reduction in vascular anastomoses in the second trimester, then it may just not be possible to predict TTTS as early as the first trimester (35).

Folding of the intertwin membrane early in the second trimester may be a more promising sign for the prediction of TTTS. It is seen in 32% of monochorionic twin pregnancies and is believed to reflect oliguria and reduced amniotic fluid in one twin. It is associated with an increased likelihood for the development of TTTS (likelihood ratio: 4.2; 95% CI 3.0–6.0). As such, membrane folding identified 91% of TTTS cases with a positive predictive value of 43% (34).

Another marker for the prediction of TTTS is the absence of AA anastomoses. These anastomoses can be detected by color flow mapping and pulsed Doppler as early as 12 weeks, though the majority are detectable only after 18 weeks (36). When

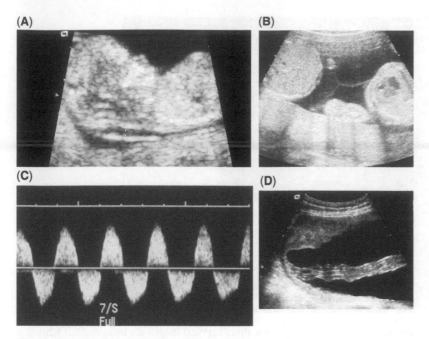

Figure 7 Ultrasound images of the 4 markers that may allow early identification of twin pregnancies at highest risk of TTTS: (**A**) increased NT in the first trimester, (**B**) membrane folding in the early second trimester, (**C**) the presence of an AA anastomosis with its typical bidirectional wave flow, and (**D**) a velamentous insertion in one of the twins. *Abbreviations*: TTTS, twin-to-twin transfusion syndrome; NT, nuchal translucency; AA, arterio-arterial.

an AA anastomosis is identified, only 15% of monochorionic twin pregnancies develop TTTS, compared to 61% where no AA anastomosis is detected (likelihood ratio 3.0, 95% CI 1.7–5.4) (36). Furthermore, in those that do develop TTTS, perinatal mortality is lower if an AA anastomoses is present. However, the clinical problem with using the absence of AA anastomoses as a prognostic sign is that it is not possible to ascertain whether they are truly absent or just undetected. Thus, its value lies principally in denoting a risk reduction in those in whom it is detected.

Finally, a velamentous cord insertion in one of the twins may increase the risk of TTTS, and this can be reliably detected by 18 weeks. Although this marker has not yet been evaluated in the antenatal period, postnatal studies demonstrate that 60% of monochorionic twins with a velamentous cord insertion were complicated by TTTS, while 65% of those pregnancies that developed TTTS had a velamentous cord (compared with 18.5% in those without) (37).

Although none of the proposed markers performs well for accurate and early prediction of TTTS, a combination of markers may improve risk stratification in the early second trimester. Such a risk assessment system is currently being assessed by a prospective multicenter study funded by the European Commission (Euro-Twin-2-Twin). In the absence of firm data on optimal follow-up schedule, all monochorionic twin pregnancies should be scanned every 2 weeks, especially between 16 and 26 weeks. If differences in amniotic fluid volume and bladder filling develop, weekly scans are recommended. Patients should also be warned to seek medical advice if symptoms of hydramnios develop, such as a rapid increase in uterine size, shortness of breath, or premature contractions.

STAGING OF TTTS: REFLECTION OF THE VARIABLE PRESENTATIONS OF TTTS AND OUTCOME

The natural history of TTTS is variable. It is not possible to say whether a patient will show stable rather than rapidly progressive disease, although the latter is more likely in the absence of an AA anastomosis. Quintero et al. suggested a formal sonographic staging system based on the presence or absence of bladder filling, Doppler changes, hydrops, and intrauterine death (Fig. 8) (38). The staging system probably does not reflect the chronologic time sequence of progressive disease, but rather defines the different disease manifestations. As such, IUFD of one or both twins may occur in stage I or II cases without passing through stage III or IV, while absent end-diastolic flow in the donor may precede differences in amniotic fluid volume. Nevertheless, the staging system appears broadly to predict outcome, with stages I and II (fluid balance changes only) having better outcomes than stages III and IV (circulatory compromise) with serial amnioreduction as well as with laser treatment (39,40). Recently, Tan et al. (41) showed that the presence of an AA anastomosis on Doppler predicted better perinatal survival independent of Quintero staging.

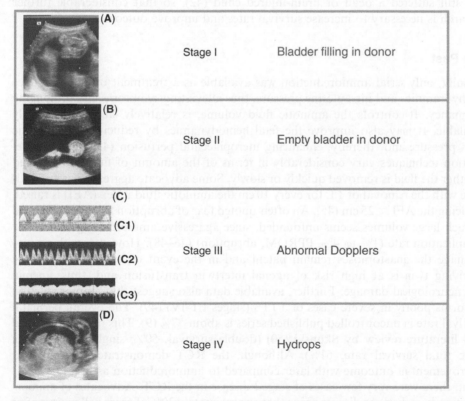

Figure 8 Sonographic staging system for TTTS. Deepest vertical pocket of ≥8 cm before 20 weeks and ≥10 cm after 20 weeks in the recipient and ≤2 cm in the donor (**A**) Stage I: bladder filling in the donor, (**B**) Stage II: no visible bladder in the donor, (**C**) Stage III: abnormal Dopplers (**C-1**) absent end-diastolic flow in the umbilical artery, (**C-2**) reversed a-wave in the ductus venosus, (**C-3**) pulsatile umbilical vein, (**D**) Stage IV: hydrops. *Source*: From Ref. 38.

TREATMENT OF TTTS: THE PAST, PRESENT, AND FUTURE

Untreated TTTS has a bleak prognosis. Hydramnios may lead to spontaneous abortion or extreme preterm delivery, and IUFD may result from cardiac failure in the recipient or poor perfusion in the donor. Moreover, there are substantial risks of cerebral and cardiac sequelae in survivors due to chronic hemodynamic imbalances. Both the donor and recipient are at risk of antenatally acquired brain injury. In donor twins, the mechanism presumably involves hypovolemia, hypotension, and anemia leading to cerebral hypoxia, whereas in the recipient, hyperviscosity and cardiac failure impairing cerebral perfusion are implicated. The risks of neurological damage are especially increased after single IUFD due to acute exsanguination of the survivor across the vascular anastomoses into the fetoplacental unit of the dead co-twin. In view of the poor outcome of untreated TTTS, there has been general consensus that therapy should be offered, although considerable controversy exists as to which treatment to offer. There are essentially four treatment options: serial amnioreduction, septostomy, selective feticide by cord occlusion, and fetoscopic laser coagulation of the vascular anastomoses. The recent randomized controlled trial (RCT) comparing serial amnioreduction and laser coagulation demonstrates that laser is currently the best overall treatment in terms of survival and neurological complications (39). However, this trial also showed that even with the better treatment, two-thirds of pregnancies still suffered a dead or brain-injured child (42), so that considerable further research is necessary to increase survival rates and improve outcome.

The Past

Initially, only serial amnioreduction was available as a treatment option to reduce the hydramnios and intrauterine pressure, thus alleviating symptoms and prolonging pregnancy. It controls the amniotic fluid volume, is relatively simple and widely available. It may also improve the fetal hemodynamics by reducing the amniotic fluid pressure and, thereby, enhancing uteroplacental perfusion (43,44). Amnioreduction techniques vary considerably in terms of the amount of fluid drained and whether the fluid is removed quickly or slowly. Some advocate aggressive amniodrainage with the removal of 1 L for every 10 cm the amniotic fluid index (AFI) is raised, reducing the AFI < 25 cm (45). An often-quoted fear of abruption following removal of such large volumes seems unfounded, since aggressive amniodrainage has a low complication rate (1% to 4%, PPROM, abruption) (46–48). However, with amniodrainage the anastomoses remain patent and in the event of a single IUFD, the surviving twin is at high risk of agonal intertwin transfusion and, thus, anemia and neurological damage. Further, available data also suggest that amnioreduction performs poorly in severe cases of TTTS (stages III–IV) (49). The overall perinatal survival rate in uncontrolled published series is about 57% (9). This rate is confirmed in a literature review by Skupski (50) (double survival, 50%; single survival rate, 20%; total survival rate, 61%). Although, the RCT demonstrated a significant improvement in outcome with laser compared to amnioreduction as first-line treatment, there were very few cases of stage I disease in the RCT. Advocates of amnioreduction in early stage disease argue that approximately 20% of cases will regress after a single amnioreduction without further treatment (40,51). A large comparative series suggested better results with amnioreduction compared to laser in early stage disease (49,52). This has led to the concept of a test amnioreduction in early stage disease (I and possibly II) with laser reserved for those that progress (53). However, one risk with this approach is that iatrogenic or intentional septostomy may substantially impair visualization at subsequent endoscopic laser use, and accordingly, this approach warrants testing in an RCT (54).

Intentional puncturing of the intertwin septum ("septostomy") with or without amnioreduction aims at normalizing the amniotic fluid of the donor and has been suggested as a treatment for TTTS largely based on the rarity of TTTS in monoamniotic twins. However, there is little evidence to support this as a primary, therapeutic technique. A small retrospective study comparing amnioreduction to septostomy ($n = 14$), did not show a survival benefit (55), and more recently an RCT comparing the two showed no improvement in survival, although there was a reduction in the frequency of repeat amnioreduction in those undergoing initial septostomy (56). Additionally, the pathophysiologic rationale remains unclear; although it increases the amniotic fluid volume in the donor's sac, allowing restoration of swallowing and intravascular volume in the donor, it does not address the underlying pathophysiology. There is also concern that it may create an iatrogenic monoamniotic state with possibility of cord entanglement (Fig. 9), although this has been borne out neither in the RCT nor in the series of single needle amniocenteses in twins (57).

Recently, selective feticide has been suggested as a treatment for stage III/IV TTTS (27). In monochorionic twins, selective feticide cannot be done by injection of KCl into the target fetus, as the co-twin is then exposed to a substantial risk of co-twin death or brain injury due to agonal intertwin transfusion. More elaborate techniques are necessary to isolate and permanently occlude the circulation in the target fetus. As such, bipolar umbilical cord coagulation has been shown to be an effective method with survival rates of ~80% (Fig. 10) (58). However, the use of selective feticide as a treatment for TTTS is certainly open to debate and may lead to some difficult decisions for both clinicians and the parents. This applies particularly because of the natural reluctance to terminate an otherwise healthy fetus, at

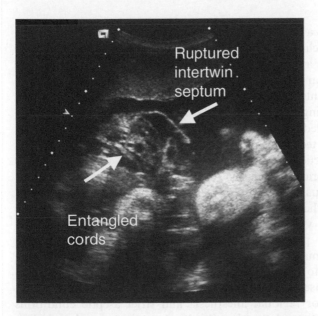

Figure 9 Sonographic image of cord entanglement after septostomy with iatrogenic monoamnionicity.

(A)   (B)

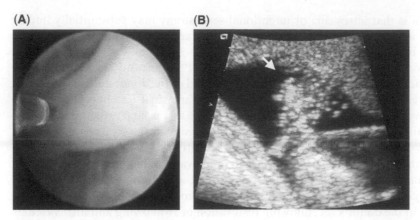

Figure 10 (A) Fetoscopic image of laser cord coagulation; (B) ultrasound image of bipolar cord coagulation, ascending steam bubbles (*arrow*) confirm adequate coagulation impact.

least with the potential to survive. An intrinsic limitation is that the maximum survival rate is only 50%. It is not always easy to determine which fetus has the worst prognosis. Initial preference for selective feticide of the donor, because of concerns about the poor outcome of a growth-restricted donor reaching viability, proved unfounded as absent end-diastolic flow may return and catch-up growth occurs following laser use (27). Current technical preference for the recipient allows the procedure usually to be done with concomitant amnioreduction. Selective feticide should, in our opinion, be reserved for cases with discordant anomaly, where imminent death of one twin is anticipated, or in stage III or IV cases where full inspection of the vascular equator is technically impossible.

The Present

Fetoscopic laser coagulation is a relatively new technique that is only available in a few specialized centers. The technique was first described by De Lia et al., in 1990 (59). Where amnioreduction is a palliative and often repetitive measure, fetoscopic laser coagulation of the vascular anastomoses aims to address the underlying cause of the disease through a single intervention. Most fetoscopic laser centers concur that coagulation of nonanastomosing vessels should be avoided, as this increases the number of nonfunctional cotyledons and may contribute to procedure-related loss. Consequently, the nonselective technique of coagulating all vessels crossing the inter-twin septum is no longer practiced (60) in most centers, as the vascular equator rarely coincides with the membranous equator. Accordingly, most groups selectively coagulate all anastomoses visualized. A "hyperselective" approach, proposed by Machin et al. (61) where only the causative AV anastomoses are coagulated, is only interesting from a theoretical viewpoint because it is impossible to identify the causative anastomoses in the presence of others. Furthermore, leaving certain anastomoses patent puts the remaining fetuses at risk for hypovolemic events in case of single IUFD and may lead to a reversal of transfusion (62,63).

In Europe and Canada, laser coagulation is performed percutaneously through a 3-mm incision under local or regional anesthesia and strict aseptic conditions (Fig. 11). Investing in good-quality video-endoscopic hardware is essential, including a high-quality light source, video camera, and monitor, and purpose-designed

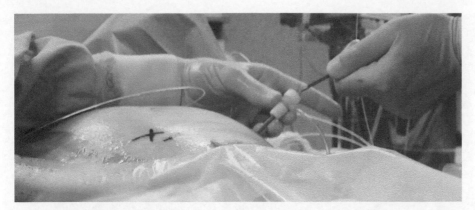

Figure 11 Image of the operative set-up and percutaneous access used for fetoscopic intervention.

fetoscopes. Further, appropriate energy sources are needed to coagulate the anastomosing vessels. For laser coagulation in TTTS, a Nd:YAG (minimal power requirements 60–100 W) or diode laser (30–60 W) with fibers of 400–600 µm are used.

Fetoscopic endoscopes differ from their hysteroscopic or laparoscopic counterparts, but are delivered by the same suppliers. At present, the experience gathered with any type of fetoscope is limited, and there is no indication that one particular brand performs better than another. Intuitively, one strives for a combination of minimal diameter, appropriate length, and maximal resolution. Personal preference, local factors such as after-sales service and compatibility with other operating room equipment will determine the choice of manufacturer. In Europe, considerable investment has been made by the European Commission in its "Biomed 2 Programme" for instrument development by a partner of the Eurofoetus research consortium (Karl Storz Endoskope). As a result of this project, a range of 20–30 cm fetoscopes with diameters of 1.0–2.3 mm is now available. The majority are semiflexible 0° fiber-optic scopes that can be curved, e.g., to direct the scope toward an anterior located placenta (64). More usual nonflexible rod lens telescopes have also been fabricated with angles of inclination up to 30° or with an associated deflecting mechanism for the laser fiber. Steerable fiber scopes have been used for an anterior placenta (65,66) but are limited by suboptimal image quality because of poor light transmission (unpublished observations). All scopes are used within a sheath, housing the endoscope and the laser fiber (Fig. 12). Fibers are usually inserted through an additional working channel, keeping the fiber in a stable position. Luer lock connections allow irrigation or drainage of fluid.

To gain entry, the sheath can either be introduced directly or through a cannula. For direct introduction, the sheath is loaded with its accompanying trocar. The sheath is inserted into the amniotic cavity under ultrasound guidance and once inside, the trocar is removed and replaced by the fetoscope. During the procedure, the sheath can be moved back and forward, but cannot be withdrawn without losing access to the amniotic cavity. The use of formal cannulas obviates this problem, as the port remains in situ during the entire procedure, through which different instruments and scopes can be introduced. In Leuven, thin-walled cannulas are used that are semiflexible, to accommodate curved instruments. These come in a variety of sizes with purpose-developed fitting trocars. There are currently no data to support either the direct or cannula access method. Further

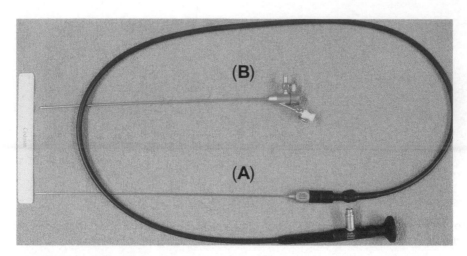

Figure 12 Example of fetoscopic instruments as used for laser coagulation of the vascular anastomoses in TTTS: (**A**) straightforward telescope, diameter 2 mm/length 30 cm with remote eyepiece, (**B**) fetoscopic sheath with channel for laser fibers up to 600 μm with 1 stopcock and 1 LUER-lock adaptor. *Source*: Karl Stroz, Tuttlingen, Germany.

technical details on endoscopes and ancillary equipment are available in more recent handbooks on fetal therapy (67).

Preoperatively, the position of the fetuses, umbilical cord insertions, and placenta are mapped by ultrasound. Under ultrasound guidance, the cannula or fetoscopic sheath is inserted into the hydramniotic sac. At all times, the placenta, fetal parts, maternal vessels, and bowel are avoided. In TTTS, fetoscopic detection of the anastomoses is improved by the presence of hydramnios, which flattens the placenta. Occasionally, vision may be hampered by blood or debris, for which amnioexchange with warmed Hartmann's solution heated by a blood warmer or a special amnioirrigator can improve visibility (68). Three fixed landmarks are available to identify any anastomosing vessels: the intertwin membrane, the recipient's and the donor's cord insertion. The intertwin septum and its placental insertion are easily identified as a thin white line on the chorionic surface. From there, blood vessels leaving the donor usually cross under the septum in the direction of the recipient. These blood vessels can be followed to identify any anastomosing vessels. Alternatively, anastomosing vessels can also be identified starting from the recipient's or donor's cord insertion. The purpose of the procedure is to visualize the entire vascular equator and to coagulate all visible anastomoses. Arteries are distinguishable from veins, as they have a darker color and cross over the veins.

Occasionally, it may be impossible to determine whether vessels anastomose or not, due to the position of the intertwin septum, placenta, fetus, or other physical limitations. In these instances, these vessels are coagulated as well. Also, with an anterior placenta, the amniotic sac as well as the vessels on the placenta may be more difficult to access. As mentioned above, instruments for anterior placentas have been developed, but it is yet unclear whether they improve performance. So far, similar outcomes have been reported for anteriorly and posteriorly located placentas (8,66). Coagulation is performed at a distance of ~1 cm and ideally at a 90° angle, using a nontouch technique (Fig. 13). Sections of ~1–2 cm are coagulated with shots of ~3–4 seconds, according to tissue response. Laser energy is adapted to the source

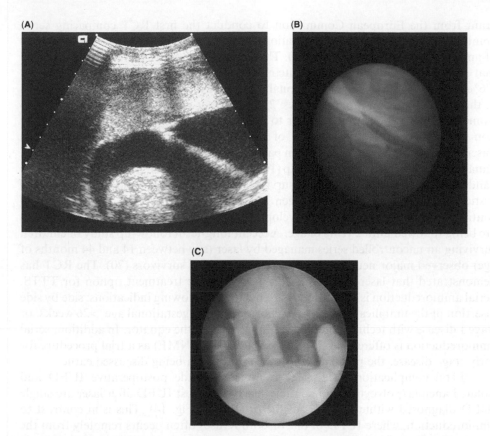

Figure 13 (A) Ultrasound image of laser coagulation of anastomoses on the chorionic plate in an anterior placenta; (B) fetoscopic image of a vessel crossing underneath the intertwin septum; (C) fetoscopic image of recipient's hand touching the face of the donor, who is stuck behind the intertwin septum.

used, the diameter of the vessels, and the tissue response. Typically, an Nd:YAG laser is set at 50–70 W and a diode laser at 30–40 W. The use of excessive laser power levels should be avoided, as this may cause vessel perforation and fetal hemorrhage. Large vessels can be coagulated from various angles to obtain progressive narrowing and eventual coagulation. Once all vessels are coagulated, the vascular equator is followed once more to ascertain that all anastomoses have indeed been fully coagulated and that flow has not resumed. The procedure is completed by amnioreduction until normal amniotic fluid volume is seen on ultrasound scan. The cannula or sheath is removed under ultrasound guidance to detect any significant bleeding from the uterine wall. Preoperatively, the patient receives prophylactic antibiotics (cefazolin, 2 g IV). Postoperatively, the patient remains as an in-patient for 1 to 2 days and ultrasound scans are repeated on these days to document fetal viability, amniotic fluid volume, and changes in the phenotypic features of TTTS, particularly bladder filling and Dopplers.

In uncontrolled series, the overall fetal survival has consistently been between 55% and 68%, with a risk of 2% to 11% for neurologic morbidity in survivors. Hecher et al. demonstrated a learning curve, arguing against scattering the experience over too many centers (69). The Eurofoetus research consortium received a grant from the European Commission to conduct the first RCT comparing serial amnioreduction versus laser coagulation as a primary therapy (i.e., no treatment of any form prior to enrollment) (39). This RCT was recently published and showed that laser had significantly better outcome in terms of survival of at least one twin (76% vs. 51%). Also, median gestational age at delivery was higher in the laser than in the amnioreduction group (33.3 vs. 29.0 weeks of gestation), with 42% and 69% women, respectively, delivering prior to 32 weeks. Also, infants in the amnioreduction group had a higher incidence of cystic periventricular leukomalacia (PVL) (laser: 6% vs. amniodrainage: 14%), in particular recipients. The high incidence of termination in the amnioreduction group (16% vs. 0% in the laser group) may on the one hand have contributed to the lower survival, but on the other hand the frequency of cystic PVL would arguably have been higher if severe cases had been allowed to continue (42). Longer-term neurodevelopmental results are awaited as these children are being followed until 2 years of age. A recent long-term follow-up study of children surviving an uncontrolled series managed by laser (age between 14 and 44 months of age) observed major neurological problems in 11% of survivors (70). The RCT has demonstrated that laser is currently the best first-line treatment option for TTTS. Serial amnioreduction is, therefore, restricted to the following indications: side by side insertion of the umbilical cords on the chorionic plate, gestational age >26 weeks, or stage I disease with technical limitations in visualizing the equator. In addition, serial amnioreduction is offered in one of our groups (WD, NMF) as a trial procedure for early stage disease, the pros and cons of this approach being discussed earlier.

Fetal complications after laser treatment include postoperative IUFD and isolated anemia/polycythemia in double survivors. Most IUFD after laser are single IUFD diagnosed within 48 hours of the procedure (Fig. 14). This is in contrast to amnioreduction, where IUFD of one or both fetuses often occurs remotely from the procedure. Also, the surviving twin after laser appears far less likely to be anemic (71) or to sustain neurological sequelae (72) compared to single IUFD survivors after amnioreduction (73), where the anastomoses remain patent. Another

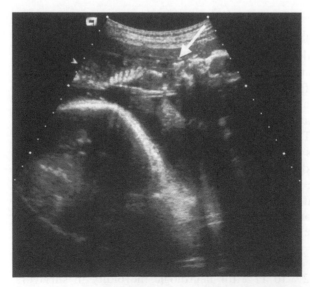

Figure 14 Ultrasound image after sIUFD with the head of the surviving twin and the macerated demised twin (*arrow*). *Abbreviation*: sIUFD, single intrauterine fetal death.

previously unrecognized fetal complication is the development of anemia/poly-cythemia without other signs of TTTS a few days or several weeks after laser treat-ment, which may complicate up to 10% of double survivors of laser (62,63). Doppler measurement of middle cerebral artery peak velocity (Fig. 15) helps iden-tify such cases, which can be treated by intrauterine transfusion/exchange transfu-sion, re-laser or cord occlusion. Consistently, it is the recipient that develops anemia, whereas the donor becomes polycythemic. The exact mechanism is not yet fully understood. The lack of preexisting intertwin differences in hemoglobin in most cases of TTTS argues against a downregulation of erythropoietin in the chronically transfused recipient and upregulation in the anemic donor. Also, the phenomenon is only seen in double survivors. Reverse transfusion through remain-ing anastomoses on the chorionic surface is an alternative explanation documented in one case in association with late phenotypic reversal of TTTS features 11 weeks after successful laser (62). In this light, one ex vivo study identified a mean of two anastomoses left patent after endoscopic laser (74). Further recent data (17) suggest that placental angioarchitecture is more complex than previously thought, with small, deep atypical AV anastomoses found in >50% of placentas. Consistent with this, detailed angiography in a recent study on 16 placentas of double survivors after laser, showed no remaining anastomoses indicating successful "bichorioniza-tion" (18). However, detailed angiography demonstrated remaining anastomoses not visible on the chorionic surface in nearly all placentas (Fig. 16). All these 16 cases had resolution of TTTS and a favorable outcome, although two cases devel-oped anemia/polycythemia without other signs of TTTS. These atypical anasto-moses may thus account for lesser degrees of intertwin transfusion, and close surveillance after laser is, therefore, recommended in double survivors with weekly middle cerebral artery Dopplers for the first month, then twice a week until deliv-ery. Other rare fetal complications after laser are congenital skin loss, gangrenous limb lesions, micropthalmia, and intestinal atresia (75,76). These anomalies have also been described in untreated TTTS and TTTS treated by other methods and, therefore, may originate from the disease process itself (77). Similarly, rare inci-dences of limb or umbilical cord constriction due to amniotic membrane disruption can occur as after any invasive intrauterine procedure (78).

(A)   **(B)**

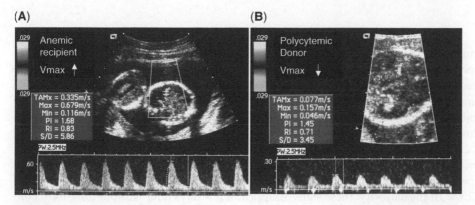

Figure 15 (A) Ultrasound image of discordant middle cerebral artery peak velocity (V max). (B) Doppler measurement in cases of anemia/polycytemia without other signs of TTTS 2 weeks after laser treatment. *Abbreviation*: TTTS, twin-to-twin transfusion syndrome.

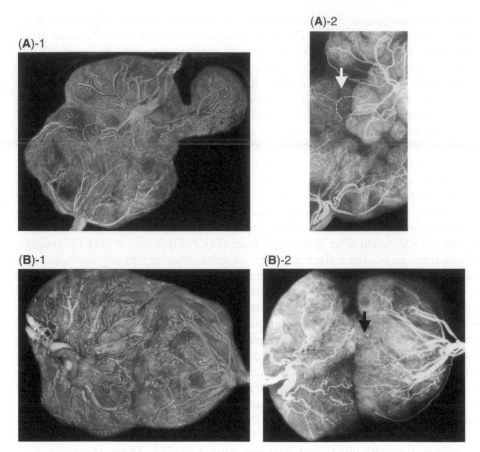

Figure 16 (**A-1**) and (**B-1**): macroscopic image of two placentas after laser. There are no visible anastomoses left on the chorionic surface. (**A-2**) and (**B-2**): Rx angiography shows remaining anastomoses not visible on the chorionic surface of 2 types. (**A-2**): vessels of 1 twin visible on the chorionic surface but dropping unexpectedly into the cotyledon of the other (*arrow*). (**B-2**): capillary connections in between cotyledons not visible on the chorionic surface. *Source*: In collaboration with the Dept. of Radiology M. Cannie, UZ Leuven, Belgium. (*See color insert.*)

Although laser appears to prevent the increased arterial stiffness seen in long-term donor vessels after amnioreduction (24), it remains to be demonstrated whether laser also reduces the incidence of cardiac sequelae in recipients. Our groups have separately reported a 7% prevalence of pulmonary valve stenosis in recipients managed primarily by amnioreduction (21), and a 7% incidence of pulmonary valve stenosis in recipients managed by laser (79). At present, all our cases undergo echocardiography before and after laser to document the influence of laser treatment on cardiac function. It is clear that laser coagulation has a profound effect on fetal hemodynamics. Immediately after laser, the donor develops a state of relative hypervolemia, which accounts for the development of one or more hydropic signs in 25%. In the majority, these signs disappear a few days later without long-term consequences (80). Similarly, 27% of donors demonstrate absent or reversed a-wave in the ductus venosus on the first postoperative day. Also, if absent end-diastolic flow was present in the donor before laser, reappearance of positive end-diastolic flow is observed in 53% (8). Finally, laser coagulation may equalize previously discordant umbilical venous blood flow between donor and recipient (81).

Maternal safety of fetoscopic interventions must remain a priority, and serious maternal complications should be registered, such as in the registry set up by Eurofoetus (82). Cases of transient maternal mirror syndrome, placental abruption, chorioamnionitis, and bleeding requiring transfusion have been registered, but no maternal deaths. In the Eurofoetus RCT, there was no severe maternal morbidity (no woman required ICU admission or blood transfusion), although three placental abruptions occurred at the end of the amnioreduction (two in the drainage and one in the laser group); all requiring immediate delivery (39). Infection is another potential problem. In our study on fertility and pregnancy outcome in a consecutive series of 100 patients, fetoscopic interventions did not influence future fertility and pregnancy outcome, although the experience of a complicated pregnancy may influence parental decisions regarding further pregnancies (83).

The Future

At least two issues need to be addressed in the future to reduce fetal loss rates after laser: the high incidence of single postoperative IUFD and early PPROM. In our experience, single IUFD within 48 hours occurs in 18% of cases and affects the donor as often as the recipient. The cause of these deaths remains largely unexplained, and it is not possible to predict which cases will be complicated by single IUFD (84). It is generally assumed that with unequal placental sharing, too little placental mass may remain after laser for the fetus with the smallest placental portion (85). However, preoperative MRI appears to reflect placental distribution (Fig. 17) and postoperative IUFD was not restricted to the fetus with the smallest placental share (86). Prevention of such losses will require further research to identify their exact cause.

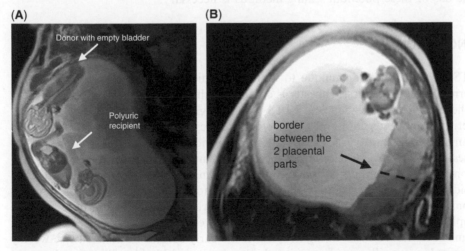

Figure 17 (A) MRI image of TTTS stage II prior to laser with the stuck donor and polyuric recipient in the hydramniotic sac; (B) preoperative MRI image of the placenta in TTTS demonstrating the intensity difference between the donor's and recipient's part, which allows calculation of placental distribution. *Abbreviations*: MRI, Magnetic Resonance Imaging; TTTS, twin-to-twin transfusion syndrome. *Source*: Dept. of Radiology M. Cannie, UZ Leuven, Belgium.

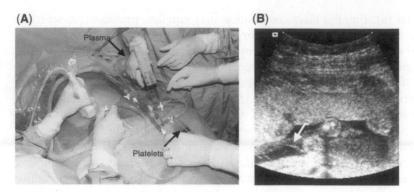

Figure 18 (**A**) Image of the set-up for an amniopatch procedure; platelets and plasma are injected through a 20 G needle into the amniotic cavity; (**B**) ultrasound image after the procedure: fibrin threads are visible (*arrow*) around the fetal limbs.

PPROM remains a major complication of invasive antenatal procedures, accounting for high morbidity and mortality if the membranes rupture prior to viability. In Leuven, PPROM within 5 weeks of the procedure occurs in 16%. The overall incidence of PPROM before 37 weeks is 45% with a median gestational age at delivery of 30 weeks in cases with PPROM, compared to 35 weeks in those without PPROM. At birth, fetoscopic membrane defects are easily identifiable in the gestational sac and histology shows little or no signs of spontaneous wound healing (87). Intra-amniotic injection of platelets and clotting factors may be a successful technique to treat early postoperative PPROM (Fig. 18) (88,89). In vitro research has demonstrated that a platelet plug adheres to the exposed extracellular matrix between amnion and chorion (90) and can seal a fetoscopic membrane defect. Platelets and clotting factors may stimulate membrane repair by releasing growth factors and by providing a scaffold for cell invasion (91). Further research into the prophylactic use of these potential sealing methods is necessary.

CONCLUSION

TTTS is a complication unique to monochorionic twins and correct chorionicity determination in the first trimester is crucial for the identification and management of these high-risk pregnancies. TTTS is a sonographic diagnosis based on strict criteria of amniotic fluid and bladder discordancy. TTTS is usually explained on an angioarchitectural basis. Nearly all monochorionic twins have placental anastomoses, but only 10% develop unbalanced intertwin transfusion mediated by unidirectional AV anastomoses with inadequate compensation by oppositely directed VA or bidirectional superficial anastomoses. Yet, hemodynamic factors, discordant hormonal control of vasculature, and placental chorioangioarchitecture may be more complex than previously thought. Because it is currently not possible to identify the monochorionic twins at highest risk in the early second trimester, twice-weekly sonographic surveillance of amniotic fluid volume and bladder filling is advocated for all monochorionic twins, from 16 weeks. The Eurofetus RCT shows that laser coagulation is currently the best first-line treatment for TTTS, although considerable further research is needed to improve survival rates and prevent single IUFD and early PPROM.

ACKNOWLEDGMENTS

Dr. L. Lewi is beneficiary of a grant of the European Commission in its 5th Framework Programme (#QLG1-CT-2002-01632 EuroTwin2Twin). Work in Leuven is supported by the Euro Twin2Twin consortium, the members of which include Y. Ville (Poissy), K. Hecher (Hamburg), E. Gratacos (Barcelona), R. Vlietinck (Leuven), M. van Gemert (Amsterdam), G. Barki (Tuttlingen), K. Nicolaides (London), R. Denk (Munchen), and C. Jackson (London). Work in London is supported by The Richard and Jack Wiseman Trust.

REFERENCES

1. Souter VL, Kapur RP, Nyholt DR, et al. A report of dizygous monochorionic twins. N Engl J Med 2003; 349(2):154–158.
2. Quintero RA, Mueller OT, Martinez JM, et al. Twin–twin transfusion syndrome in a dizygotic monochorionic–diamniotic twin pregnancy. J Matern Fetal Neonatal Med 2003; 14(4):279–281.
3. Sebire NJ, Snijders RJ, Hughes K, Sepulveda W, Nicolaides KH. The hidden mortality of monochorionic twin pregnancies. Br J Obstet Gynaecol 1997; 104(10):1203–1207.
4. Stenhouse E, Hardwick C, Maharaj S, Webb J, Kelly T, Mackenzie FM. Chorionicity determination in twin pregnancies: how accurate are we? Ultrasound Obstet Gynecol 2002; 19(4):350–352.
5. Carroll SG, Soothill PW, Abdel-Fattah SA, Porter H, Montague I, Kyle PM. Prediction of chorionicity in twin pregnancies at 10–14 weeks of gestation. Br J Obstet Gynaecol 2002; 109(2):182–186.
6. www.eurofoetus@eurofoetus.org.
7. Hecher K, Ville Y, Nicolaides KH. Fetal arterial Doppler studies in twin–twin transfusion syndrome. J Ultrasound Med 1995; 14(2):101–108.
8. Zikulnig L, Hecher K, Bregenzer T, Baz E, Hackeloer BJ. Prognostic factors in severe twin–twin transfusion syndrome treated by endoscopic laser surgery. Ultrasound Obstet Gynecol 1999; 14(6):380–387.
9. van Gemert MJ, Umur A, Tijssen JG, Ross MG. Twin–twin transfusion syndrome: etiology, severity and rational management. Curr Opin Obstet Gynecol 2001; 13(2): 193–206.
10. Rodis JF, McIlveen PF, Egan JF, Borgida AF, Turner GW, Campbell WA. Monoamniotic twins: improved perinatal survival with accurate prenatal diagnosis and antenatal fetal surveillance. Am J Obstet Gynecol 1997; 177(5):1046–1049.
11. Denbow M, Fogliani R, Kyle P, Letsky E, Nicolini U, Fisk N. Haematological indices at fetal blood sampling in monochorionic pregnancies complicated by feto-fetal transfusion syndrome. Prenat Diagn 1998; 18(9):941–946.
12. De Lia J, Fisk N, Hecher K, et al. Twin-to-twin transfusion syndrome—debates on the etiology, natural history and management. Ultrasound Obstet Gynecol 2000; 16(3):210–213.
13. Taylor MJ, Farquharson D, Cox PM, Fisk NM. Identification of arterio-venous anastomoses in vivo in monochorionic twin pregnancies: preliminary report. Ultrasound Obstet Gynecol 2000; 16(3):218–222.
14. Denbow ML, Cox P, Taylor M, Hammal DM, Fisk NM. Placental angioarchitecture in monochorionic twin pregnancies: relationship to fetal growth, fetofetal transfusion syndrome, and pregnancy outcome. Am J Obstet Gynecol 2000; 182(2):417–426.
15. Diehl W, Hecher K, Zikulnig L, Vetter M, Hackeloer BJ. Placental vascular anastomoses visualized during fetoscopic laser surgery in severe mid-trimester twin–twin transfusion syndrome. Placenta 2001; 22(10):876–881.
16. Bermudez C, Becerra CH, Bornick PW, Allen MH, Arroyo J, Quintero RA. Placental types and twin–twin transfusion syndrome. Am J Obstet Gynecol 2002; 187(2):489–494.

17. Wee LY, Taylor M, Watkins N, Franke V, Parker K, Fisk NM. Characterisation of deep arterio-venous anastomoses within monochorionic placentae by vascular casting. Placenta 2005; 26(1):19–24.

18. Lewi L, Cannie M, Jani J, et al. Placental angiography of double survivors and double fetal deaths after laser for twin–twin transfusion syndrome (TTTS). Am J Obstet Gynecol 2004; 191(Suppl 6):S162.

19. Zosmer N, Bajoria R, Weiner E, Rigby M, Vaughan J, Fisk N. Clinical and echographic features of in utero cardiac dysfunction in the recipient twin in twin–twin transfusion syndrome. Br Heart J 1994; 72:74–79.

20. Mahieu-Caputo D, Salomon LJ, Le Bidois J, et al. Fetal hypertension: an insight into the pathogenesis of the twin–twin transfusion syndrome. Prenat Diagn 2003; 23(8): 640–645.

21. Karatza AA, Wolfenden JL, Taylor MJ, Wee L, Fisk NM, Gardiner HM. Influence of twin–twin transfusion syndrome on fetal cardiovascular structure and function: prospective case–control study of 136 monochorionic twin pregnancies. Heart 2002; 88(3):271–277.

22. Wee LY, Taylor MJ, Vanderheyden T, Talbert D, Fisk NM. Transmitted arterio-arterial anastomosis waveforms causing cyclically intermittent absent/reversed end-diastolic umbilical artery flow in monochorionic twins. Placenta 2003; 24(7):772–778.

23. Cheung YF, Taylor MJ, Fisk NM, Redington AN, Gardiner HM. Fetal origins of reduced arterial distensibility in the donor twin in twin–twin transfusion syndrome. Lancet 2000; 355(9210):1157–1158.

24. Gardiner HM, Taylor MJ, Karatza A, et al. Twin–twin transfusion syndrome: the influence of intrauterine laser photocoagulation on arterial distensibility in childhood. Circulation 2003; 107(14):1906–1911.

25. Bajoria R, Gibson MJ, Ward S, Sooranna SR, Neilson JP, Westwood, M. Placental regulation of insulin-like growth factor axis in monochorionic twins with chronic twin–twin transfusion syndrome. J Clin Endocrinol Metab 2001; 86(7):3150–3156.

26. Sooranna SR, Ward S, Bajoria R. Discordant fetal leptin levels in monochorionic twins with chronic midtrimester twin–twin transfusion syndrome. Placenta 2001; 22(5): 392–398.

27. Taylor MJ, Shalev E, Tanawattanacharoen S, et al. Ultrasound-guided umbilical cord occlusion using bipolar diathermy for stage III/IV twin twin transfusion syndrome. Prenat Diagn 2002; 22(1):70–76.

28. van Gemert MJ, Vandenbussche FP, Schaap AH, et al. Classification of discordant fetal growth may contribute to risk stratification in monochorionic twin pregnancies. Ultrasound Obstet Gynecol 2000; 16(3):237–244.

29. Bajoria R, Ward S, Chatterjee R. Natriuretic peptides in the pathogenesis of cardiac dysfunction in the recipient fetus of twin–twin transfusion syndrome. Am J Obstet Gynecol 2002; 186(1):121–127.

30. Mahieu-Caputo D, Dommergues M, Delezoide AL, et al. Twin-to-twin transfusion syndrome. Role of the fetal renin–angiotensin system. Am J Pathol 2000; 156(2): 629–636.

31. Kilby MD, Platt C, Whittle MJ, Oxley J, Lindop GB. Renin gene expression in fetal kidneys of pregnancies complicated by twin–twin transfusion syndrome. Pediatr Dev Pathol 2001; 4(2):175–179.

32. De Lia JE, Carr MH. Pregnancy loss after successful laser surgery for previable twin–twin transfusion syndrome. Am J Obstet Gynecol 2002; 187(2):517–518, author reply 518.

33. Robyr R, Boulvain M, Ortqvist L, et al. OC119: prognostic factors for preterm delivery in twin-to-twin transfusion syndrome (TTTS) treated by laser coagulation. Ultrasound Obstet Gynecol 2004; 24(3):249–250.

34. Sebire NJ, Souka A, Skentou H, Geerts L, Nicolaides KH. Early prediction of severe twin-to-twin transfusion syndrome. Hum Reprod 2000; 15(9):2008–2010.

35. Sebire NJ, Talbert D, Fisk NM. Twin-to-twin transfusion syndrome results from dynamic asymmetrical reduction in placental anastomoses: a hypothesis. Placenta 2001; 22(5):383–391.

36. Taylor MJ, Denbow ML, Tanawattanacharoen S, Gannon C, Cox PM, Fisk, NM. Doppler detection of arterio-arterial anastomoses in monochorionic twins: feasibility and clinical application. Hum Reprod 2000; 15(7):1632–1636.

37. Fries MH, Goldstein RB, Kilpatrick SJ, Golbus MS, Callen PW, Filly RA. The role of velamentous cord insertion in the etiology of twin–twin transfusion syndrome. Obstet Gynecol 1993; 81(4):569–574.

38. Quintero RA, Morales WJ, Allen MH, Bornick PW, Johnson PK, Kruger M. Staging of twin–twin transfusion syndrome. J Perinatol 1999; 19(8, Pt 1):550–555.

39. Senat MV, Deprest J, Boulvain M, Paupe A, Winer N, Ville Y. Endoscopic laser surgery versus serial amnioreduction for severe twin-to-twin transfusion syndrome. N Engl J Med 2004; 351(2):136–144.

40. Taylor MJ, Govender L, Jolly M, Wee L, Fisk NM. Validation of the Quintero staging system for twin–twin transfusion syndrome. Obstet Gynecol 2002; 100(6):1257–1265.

41. Tan TY, Taylor MJ, Wee LY, Vanderheyden T, Wimalasundera R, Fisk NM. Doppler for artery–artery anastomosis and stage-independent survival in twin–twin transfusion. Obstet Gynecol 2004; 103(6):1174–1180.

42. Fisk NM, Galea P. Twin–twin transfusion—as good as it gets? N Engl J Med 2004; 351(2):182–184.

43. Fisk NM, Vaughan J, Talbert D. Impaired fetal blood gas status in polyhydramnios and its relation to raised amniotic pressure. Fetal Diagn Ther 1994; 9(1):7–13.

44. Bower SJ, Flack NJ, Sepulveda W, Talbert DG, Fisk NM. Uterine artery blood flow response to correction of amniotic fluid volume. Am J Obstet Gynecol 1995; 173(2):502–507.

45. Denbow ML, Sepulveda W, Ridout D, Fisk NM. Relationship between change in amniotic fluid index and volume of fluid removed at amnioreduction. Obstet Gynecol 1997; 90(4, Pt 1):529–532.

46. Elliott JP, Sawyer AT, Radin TG, Strong RE. Large-volume therapeutic amniocentesis in the treatment of hydramnios. Obstet Gynecol 1994; 84(6):1025–1027.

47. Mari G, Roberts A, Detti L, et al. Perinatal morbidity and mortality rates in severe twin–twin transfusion syndrome: results of the International Amnioreduction Registry. Am J Obstet Gynecol 2001; 185(3):708–715.

48. Leung WC, Jouannic JM, Hyett J, Rodeck C, Jauniaux E. Procedure-related complications of rapid amniodrainage in the treatment of polyhydramnios. Ultrasound Obstet Gynecol 2004; 23(2):154–158.

49. Quintero RA, Dickinson JE, Morales WJ, et al. Stage-based treatment of twin–twin transfusion syndrome. Am J Obstet Gynecol 2003; 188(5):1333–1340.

50. Skupski DW, Gurushanthaiah K, Chasen S. The effect of treatment of twin–twin transfusion syndrome on the diagnosis-to-delivery interval. Twin Res 2002; 5(1):1–4.

51. Dickinson JE, Evans SF. The progression of disease stage in twin–twin transfusion syndrome. J Matern Fetal Neonatal Med 2004; 16(2):95–101.

52. Fisk NM, Tan TY, Taylor MJ. Re: Stage-based treatment of twin–twin transfusion syndrome. Am J Obstet Gynecol 2004; 190(6):1809–1810. (author reply pp. 1810–1811).

53. Fisk NM, Tan TY, Taylor MJ. Stage-based treatment of twin–twin transfusion syndrome. Am J Obstet Gynecol 2004; 190(5):1491–1492.

54. Huber A, Hecher K. How can we diagnose and manage twin–twin transfusion syndrome? Best Pract Res Clin Obstet Gynaecol 2004; 18(4):543–556.

55. Johnson JR, Rossi KQ, O'Shaughnessy RW. Amnioreduction versus septostomy in twin–twin transfusion syndrome. Am J Obstet Gynecol 2001; 185(5):1044–1047.

56. Moise KJ, Dorman K, Lamvu G, et al. A randomized trial of amnioreduction versus septostomy in the treatment of twin–twin transfusion syndrome. Am J Obstet Gynecol 2005; 193(3 Pt 1):701–707.

57. Sebire NJ, Noble PL, Odibo A, Malligiannis P, Nicolaides KH. Single uterine entry for genetic amniocentesis in twin pregnancies. Ultrasound Obstet Gynecol 1996; 7(1):26–31.

58. Deprest J, Van Schoubroeck D, Senat MV, et al. Cord coagulation in monochorionic multiplets late in gestation. Am J Obstet Gynecol 2003; 189(6 Suppl 1):S226.

59. De Lia JE, Cruikshank DP, Keye WR Jr. Fetoscopic neodymium:YAG laser occlusion of placental vessels in severe twin–twin transfusion syndrome. Obstet Gynecol 1990; 75(6):1046–1053.

60. Ville Y, Hyett J, Hecher K, Nicolaides K. Preliminary experience with endoscopic laser surgery for severe twin–twin transfusion syndrome. N Engl J Med 1995; 332(4): 224–227.

61. Feldstein VA, Machin GA, Albanese CT, et al. Twin–twin transfusion syndrome: the 'Select' procedure. Fetal Diagn Ther 2000; 15(5):257–261.

62. Wee LY, Taylor MJ, Vanderheyden T, Wimalasundera R, Gardiner HM, Fisk NM. Reversal of twin–twin transfusion syndrome: frequency, vascular anatomy, associated anomalies and outcome. Prenat Diagn 2004; 24(2):104–110.

63. Robyr R, Lewi L, Yamamoto M, Ortqvist L, Deprest J, Ville Y. Permanent feto-fetal transfusion from the recipient to the donor twin. A complication of laser surgery in twin-to-twin transfusion syndrome (TTTS). Ultrasound Obstet Gynecol 2004; 24(3):339.

64. Deprest JA, Van Schoubroeck D, Van Ballaer PP, Flageole H, Van Assche FA, Vandenberghe K. Alternative technique for Nd:YAG laser coagulation in twin-to-twin transfusion syndrome with anterior placenta. Ultrasound Obstet Gynecol 1998; 11(5):347–352.

65. Luks FI, Deprest JA, Vandenberghe K, et al. Fetoscopy-guided fetal endoscopy in a sheep model. J Am Coll Surg 1994; 178(6):609–612.

66. Quintero RA, Bornick PW, Allen MH, Johson PK. Selective laser photocoagulation of communicating vessels in severe twin–twin transfusion syndrome in women with an anterior placenta. Obstet Gynecol 2001; 97(3):477–481.

67. Deprest J, Ville Y. Obstetric endoscopy. In: Harrison MR, Evan MI, Adzick NS, Holzgreve W, eds. The Unborn Patient: The Art and Science of Fetal Therapy. Philadelphia: W.B Saunders, 2000:213–232.

68. Bonati F, Perales A, Novak P, et al. Ex vivo testing of a temperature- and pressure-controlled amnio-irrigator for fetoscopic surgery. J Pediatr Surg 2002; 37(1):18–24.

69. Hecher K, Diehl W, Zikulnig L, Vetter M, Hackeloer BJ. Endoscopic laser coagulation of placental anastomoses in 200 pregnancies with severe mid-trimester twin-to-twin transfusion syndrome. Eur J Obstet Gynecol Reprod Biol 2000; 92(1):135–139.

70. Banek CS, Hecher K, Hackeloer BJ, Bartmann P. Long-term neurodevelopmental outcome after intrauterine laser treatment for severe twin–twin transfusion syndrome. Am J Obstet Gynecol 2003; 188(4):876–880.

71. Senat MV, Loizeau S, Couderc S, Bernard JP, Ville Y. The value of middle cerebral artery peak systolic velocity in the diagnosis of fetal anemia after intrauterine death of one monochorionic twin. Am J Obstet Gynecol 2003; 189(5):1320–1324.

72. Sutcliffe AG, Sebire NJ, Pigott AJ, Taylor B, Edwards PR, Nicolaides KH. Outcome for children born after in utero laser ablation therapy for severe twin-to-twin transfusion syndrome. Br J Obstet Gynaecol 2001; 108(12):1246–1250.

73. Lopriore E, Nagel HT, Vandenbussche FP, Walther FJ. Long-term neurodevelopmental outcome in twin-to-twin transfusion syndrome. Am J Obstet Gynecol 2003; 189(5): 1314–1319.

74. De Paepe ME, Friedman RM, Poch M, Hansen K, Carr SR, Luks FI. Placental findings after laser ablation of communicating vessels in twin-to-twin transfusion syndrome. Pediatr Dev Pathol 2004; 7(2):159–165.

75. Stone CA, Quinn MW, Saxby PJ. Congenital skin loss following Nd:YAG placental photocoagulation. Burns 1998; 24(3):275–277.

76. Luks FI, Carr SR, Tracy TF Jr. Intestinal atresia associated with twin–twin transfusion syndrome. J Pediatr Surg 2001; 36(7):1105–1106.

77. Carr SR, Luks F, Tracy T, Plevyak M. Antenatal necrotic injury in severe twin-to-twin transfusion syndrome. A case and review. Fetal Diagn Ther 2004; 19(4):370–372.

78. Lewi L, Hanssens M, Spitz B, Deprest J. Complete chorioamniotic membrane separation. Case report and review of the literature. Fetal Diagn Ther 2004; 19(1):78–82.

79. Witters I, Gewillig M, Lewi L, et al. OC123: prevalence of congenital heart disease in the neonatal period in TTTS treated by laserphotocoagulation. Ultrasound Obstet Gynecol 2004; 24(3):249–250.

80. Gratacos E, Van Schoubroeck D, Carreras E, et al. Transient hydropic signs in the donor fetus after fetoscopic laser coagulation in severe twin–twin transfusion syndrome: incidence and clinical relevance. Ultrasound Obstet Gynecol 2002; 19(5):449–453.

81. Ishii K, Chmait RH, Martinez JM, Nakata M, Quintero RA. Ultrasound assessment of venous blood flow before and after laser therapy: approach to understanding the pathophysiology of twin–twin transfusion syndrome. Ultrasound Obstet Gynecol 2004; 24(2):164–168.

82. Gratacos E, Deprest J. Current experience with fetoscopy and the Eurofoetus registry for fetoscopic procedures. Eur J Obstet Gynecol Reprod Biol 2000; 92(1):151–159.

83. Lewi L, Vandenberghe G, Deprest J. Fertility and pregnancy outcome after fetoscopic surgery. Am J Obstet Gynecol 2003; 189(6 Suppl 1):S222.

84. Martinez JM, Bermudez C, Becerra C, Lopez J, Morales WJ, Quintero RA. The role of Doppler studies in predicting individual intrauterine fetal demise after laser therapy for twin–twin transfusion syndrome. Ultrasound Obstet Gynecol 2003; 22(3):246–251.

85. Quintero RA, Comas C, Bornick PW, Allen MH, Kruger M. Selective versus non-selective laser photocoagulation of placental vessels in twin-to-twin transfusion syndrome. Ultrasound Obstet Gynecol 2000; 16(3):230–226.

86. Lewi L, Cannie M, Vandecaveye V, Jani J, Dymarkowski S, Deprest J. OC118: a pilot study to assess the role of placental MR imaging to predict placental distribution and the position of the vascular equator in twin-to-twin transfusion syndrome. Ultrasound Obstet Gynecol 2004; 24(3):248.

87. Gratacós E, Sanin-Blair J, Lewi L, Toran N, Cabero L, Deprest J. A histological study of fetoscopic membrane defects to document membrane healing. In press in Placenta.

88. Quintero RA, Morales WJ, Allen M, Bornick PW, Arroyo J, LeParc G. Treatment of iatrogenic previable premature rupture of membranes with intra-amniotic injection of platelets and cryoprecipitate (amniopatch): preliminary experience. Am J Obstet Gynecol 1999; 181(3):744–749.

89. Lewi L, Van Schoubroeck D, Van Ranst M, et al. Successful patching of iatrogenic rupture of the fetal membranes. Placenta 2004; 25(4):352–356.

90. Lewi L, Hoylaerts M, Verbist L, Beutels E, Deprest J. Platelet-rich plasma to prevent amniotic fluid leakage following fetoscopic interventions: an in vitro study. Am J Obstet Gynecol 2003; 189(6, Suppl 1):S222.

91. Lewi L, Poliard E, Verbist L, et al. Platelet rich plasma (PRP) to prevent amniotic fluid leakage after fetoscopic interventions: an in vitro study in a human amniochorion explant culture on a PRP matrix. J Soc Gynecol Investig 2004; 11:115.

26
Fetoscopic Instrumentation and Techniques

Jan Deprest, Liesbeth Lewi, Jacques Jani, Dominique van Schoubroeck,
Denis Gallot, Federico Spelzini, Marc Vandevelde, and Roland Devlieger
*Department of Obstetrics and Gynaecology, University Hospitals Leuven,
Leuven, Belgium*

Gerard Barki and Sabine Bueschle
Karl Storz Endoskope, Tuttlingen, Germany

Eduardo Gratacos
Hospital Clinic, Barcelona, Spain

INTRODUCTION

In the 1970s, direct fetal visualization through endoscopy was introduced into obstetrics. Various names were given to this technique: amnioscopy, fetoscopy, or embryoscopy, the latter referring to its application in the first trimester. Fetoscopy was performed for diagnostic purposes, e.g., to obtain fetal blood in the diagnosis of hemoglobinopathies, to demonstrate pathognomic malformations or to biopsy fetal skin or liver under direct vision. Fetoscopy was also used for therapeutic purposes, such as intravascular transfusion under direct visual control. The technique never became widely implemented because of its required skills, instruments, and invasiveness. The overall abortion rate, defined as any fetal loss prior to 28 weeks, was 4%. Abortions were more frequent following skin biopsy (16%) and fetal visualization (7.9%). The relatively large diameter of the instruments used may have played a role: rod lens telescopes of 3 mm were the minimum for sufficient illumination and appropriate image resolution. As a consequence, instruments were also much shorter than what is used today. Some complications were also attributed to the "blind" introduction technique, i.e., without ultrasound (US) guidance. Anyway, fetoscopy soon was nearly completely abandoned because of advances in high-resolution US, used for diagnostic purposes or to guide invasive procedures.

Rapid advances of video-endoscopic technology and miniaturization of lightweight cameras boosted laparoscopy and hysteroscopy in the 1980s. Simultaneously, diameters of the endoscopes decreased dramatically, particularly, fiber endoscopes with a high number of pixels offered better image quality at a very small diameter. This renewed the interest in direct visual access to the fetus, both for diagnostic and

473

therapeutic procedures: the "new" fetoscopy returned to fetal medicine (1,2). Fetoscopy has meanwhile gained again its place in modern fetal medicine, where it is mainly used to operate on the placenta, cord, membranes, and even the fetus (3). Obstetricians may be not familiar with current video-endoscopy. We, therefore, first introduce the reader to instrumental requirements for and surgical or technical aspects of fetoscopy. Subsequently, we describe how fetoscopy is now being used to guide in utero operations on the placenta, umbilical cord, fetal membranes, and also the fetus. The potential and the place of these operations for given conditions are described elsewhere in this book. To distinguish between types of fetoscopic interventions of the fetus, fetoscopic manipulations on the fetal adnexae are usually called "obstetrical endoscopy." In contrast, manipulations on the fetus itself can be called endoscopic *fetal* surgery (3). In addition, it must be remembered that any fetoscopy is a surgical intervention, subject to complications. This aspect will be dealt with in the last paragraph.

INSTRUMENTATION AND TECHNIQUE FOR OPERATIVE FETOSCOPY

Fetoscopes and Image Display

Modern fetoscopes are quite different from their hysteroscopic or laparoscopic counterparts. In Europe, the European Commission made considerable investments in its "Biomed 2 Programme" to allow instrument development in fetal medicine, and granted Karl Storz Endoskope (Tuttlingen, Germany) permission and resources to form a partnership with clinicians in the Eurofoetus research consortium (1997) (4). A range of 20 to 30 cm fetoscopes with diameters of 1.0 to 2.3 mm are now available, thanks to this project. Typically, modern fetoscopes have a *deported* eyepiece. The typical fixed eyepiece at the back of the scope, with the camera connected to it, increases weight and prevents the fetal medicine specialist from manipulating the instrument as easily as s when using a needle steered under US guidance. Today, most clinicians use endoscopes of diameters of 2.0 mm or less. Key elements of the scope are the diameter, length, field, and angle of vision, as well as the technology of the image and light transmission within the scope, which determines the depth of vision. Image and light transmission can be either through fiber-optic bundles or through a conventional rod lens system. In general, the diameter of fiber-optic scopes determines the number of individual fibers of the scope, although the newer generation accommodates more fibers for the same diameter, providing a clearer image and better resolution for the same diameter. Fiberscopes have in theory a larger opening angle, and, therefore, a panoramic view, in spite of having no real lens at their tip. Current technology does not offer the possibility yet to look through the scope at a certain angle, as for instance standard (rod lens) hysteroscopes do, where a 12° or 30° angle is typical.

In our current clinical practice, we mostly use fiber-endoscopes with diameters ranging from 1.0 to 2.3 mm (Karl Storz, Fig 1). These continue to improve in resolution, having up to 50,000 pixels at the time of writing this chapter, and there is more to come. The fibers in the scope are flexible and these optics can, therefore, be curved to a certain degree, which helps to overcome the current limitation of a 0° angle of view. This may be particularly helpful for operating on the anterior side of the uterus, without the need to enter the uterus posteriorly. We have also used steerable endoscopes in experimentation, as well as in cases of laser coagulation on an anteriorly located placenta (5–7). However, we were not impressed with image quality; particularly, light transmission was very poor (unpublished observations).

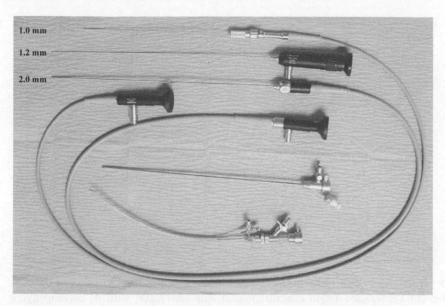

Figure 1 Overview of our fiber-optic endoscopes. From top to bottom: 1.0 mm embryoscope, 1.2 and 2.0 mm 0° fiber fetoscopes with deported eyepieces, except for 1.2 mm endoscope with conventional eyepiece. A straight sheath and curved sheath are shown at the bottom of the image. These exist in diameters and lengths adapted to the type of scope used.

Rod lens endoscopes also contain fibers for illuminational light transmission, but the image itself is focused by a lens system. Rod lens scopes usually have a relatively large opening angle and offer a panoramic view, thanks to their lens design. However, these features may be limited by the diameter of the scope. With current technology, there is a critical level of ~2 mm diameter, under which it is difficult to obtain enough light to work clinically, at least for longer fetoscopes. The smallest rod lens fetoscope we have been using is a pediatric cystoscope with a diameter of 1.9 mm (Olympus, Hamburg, Germany). This scope is, however, very short; a 25 cm or longer fetoscope seems more appropriate to meet the depth of a polyhydramniotic cavity or to bridge maternal adiposity in some cases. These instruments are also very frail. A special operative fetoscope, comparable to an operative hysteroscope has been developed for this indication. It consists of a 2.0 mm rod lens fetoscope with a 12° or 30° direction of view. Its length is limited to 26 cm. It comes with a double sheath. The inner sheath has a working channel for the fiber. At its tip an Alberran deflecting mechanism is installed to help guide the fiber to the target. The outer sheath can be used for exchange of fluid (4).

Embryoscopes have a smaller diameter, but light instillation requirements are obviously much lower. Dumez initially used rod lens equipment of 1.7 mm, but smaller fiber optics of 0.5–1.0 mm are available today. These semiflexible optics contain 10,000 pixels or more, and have a 70° field of vision (8). Introduction is done through a single 18 gauge, or a larger and double needle for operative manipulations. The second needle lumen acts as a side port for the introduction of an aspiration needle (24 gauge) or instruments to be used during the procedure (Fig 2). Because of the limited view, the endoscope must be directed to the area to be visualized under US guidance.

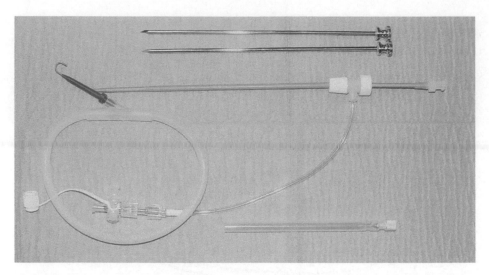

Figure 2   A set of a 9- and 10-Fr trocar (*top*) for sharp and direct introduction of the cannula. (*Bottom*) Thin-walled teflon cannula, loaded with obturator, with its accompanying guide wire. These cannualas as well as the trocars exist in any size between 6 and 15 Fr. The cannula can be connected to infusion or drainage systems via the luer lock connections. The needle and the guide wire can be used for introduction with the Seldinger technique.

Additional Hardware

The fetoscope is connected to a good quality light fountain and a videocamera. We use a Xenon light source, and a one or three-chip digital image processing camera, as used in conventional laparoscopy. The camera projects the fetoscopic images on a videoscreen, but as US backup is crucial, both images should be available to the operator. We, therefore, use a so-called "twin"-video system (Karl Storz) to project both endoscopic and US images simultaneously; the relative size of each of those images on the screen can be decided upon by the operator. In very complex interventions, several monitors can be used. The monitor(s) is (are) set according to the rules applying in any endoscopic procedure: the operator, the target area, and the screen should be in one line, to allow comfortable manipulation of instruments by both the surgeon and the assistants. Appropriate documentation systems such as a digital videorecorder, printer, or writer may be useful.

Although fetoscopy can be performed in a natural amniotic fluid environment, the use of a distension medium can improve visualization or create more working space. We always have Hartmann's solution available, warmed to body temperature and infused by either a blood warmer or a special amnio-irrigator (9). Care should be taken to avoid a rise in intra-amniotic pressure, and intermittent drainage may be needed. So far, its clinical use has been safe in normal working conditions, as was reported earlier in experimental conditions (10). In one report on fetoscopic covering of a myelomeningocele, uterine distention was achieved with CO_2. No experience with this medium for "obstetrical" interventions has been reported so far. The use of a gas distention medium probably facilitates complex endoscopic procedures, because of a better depth of vision, allowing more working space and the ability to work in conditions with limited bleeding (11). We have been hesitant to use CO_2, as it causes fetal acidosis (12). However, other investigators have demonstrated in sheep that maternal hyperventilation could correct for this, an observation which we could not confirm in physiologic conditions (13,14). In theory, inert gases such as helium could also be used. However, none of these distention techniques have been tested more formally in experimental conditions nor widely used clinically to date.

Energy sources are needed to coagulate the vessels of interest. When using a laser, a machine with appropriate coagulation capabilities is needed. We use either a Nd:YAG laser (minimal power requirements 60–100 W) or diode laser (30–60 W) (Dornier Medilas, Germany) with fibers of 400–600 μm. Quintero described the use of larger fibers with side-firing capabilities, which are used to coagulate anteriorly located placentas. This requires, however, a second introduction port as they are too large to work through the working channel (15). Interstitial laser has been described by Soothill et al. (16). Electrosurgery is obviously a more widely available tool. In 2000, we described the use of bipolar forceps to coagulate the umbilical cord, a procedure that can be done entirely under US guidance (17). Forceps of 5, 3, and more recently 2.3 mm have been marketed. Monopolar energy was first described by Rodeck (18): a needle is inserted in or around the aorta or cord of the target acardiac fetus, through which an isolated electrode is advanced.

Techniques to Access the Pregnant Uterus

Sheaths and Cannulas

The endoscope is housed within a sheath, its diameter and shape being dependent on the purpose of the endoscopic procedure. The sheath can be used for irrigation of the operative field and/or instrument insertion. Some sheaths have separate openings for instrument insertion. For instance, in laser surgery, fibers are stabilized by insertion in an instrument channel. Alternatively, the sheath can be oval-shaped with the fiber located in the narrowest part. To penetrate the abdominal and uterine wall directly with this sheath, the latter is first loaded with a sharp trocar. After introduction under US guidance, the trocar is withdrawn and the sheath accommodates the scope, and eventually a laser fiber, forceps, scissors, catheters, and irrigation as required.

During the procedure, the sheath will inevitably be advanced or withdrawn to some extent, which causes some friction and possibly membrane disruption. In lengthy or complex procedures, so many manipulations or reinsertions of instruments are needed, that a real endoscopic port or cannula is preferable, just as in laparoscopy. The diameter of the cannula is chosen according to the largest instrument to be used through the port. At this moment, we are working on a system to exchange cannulas of different diameters. So far, we ourselves have been using cannulas designed for vascular access, which come in any diameter between 4 and 15 Fr (1.6–5.0 mm—Performa, Cook, Belgium; Fig. 2). They are inserted either with the Seldinger technique (7), which gradually expands the myometrial and membrane stab wound up to the desired diameter, or directly with purpose-designed pyramidal trocars (Karl Storz). The cannulas offer a leakproof seal and a side channel for infusion or removal of fluid; they are made of flexible material allowing for the use of curved instruments. Others have used different types of cannulas, particularly during experimental fetal surgical procedures (19). Completely reusable cannulas are also marketed; but they are usually larger in diameter for the same inner diameter (4).

Uterine Entry Point

The exact point of entry into the amniotic cavity is a compromise between the theoretical optimal cannula position toward the target area and the limitations imposed by the actual position of the fetus and placenta. The majority of fetoscopic procedures are performed percutaneously with local anesthesia of the abdominal wall down to the myometrium, as earlier mentioned, or under loco-regional anesthesia. The sheath can be easily inserted through an area free of placenta (Fig. 3). When an anterior placenta hampers entry through the anterior uterine wall, we earlier suggested a transfundal insertion and the use of a flexible cannula and curved instruments. To do this safely, we made a 2–3 cm mini-laparotomy to avoid bowel injury (Fig. 4). However, this approach requires loco-regional or general anesthesia, and is certainly more invasive than the percutaneous approach. As an alternative in a case of an anteriorly located placenta, a very lateral uterine insertion with previous identification of uterine vessels using Doppler and a steerable or slightly bent endoscope can be used (Fig. 5). So far, it has not been shown that results for twin-to-twin transfusion syndrome (TTTS) cases with an anterior placenta are worse, and would require more invasiveness.

However, in complex operative procedures, such as two-port fetoscopic cord ligation or fetal surgery, multiple cannulas are simply a necessity, and varying degrees of uterine distention may occur during the operation. Such operations are usually carried out through (a) formal abdominal incision(s) so that the uterine cannulas can move freely in relation to the maternal wall, and uterine tearing is thus prevented. Although many obstetricians would try to perform all interventions percutaneously at all costs, we feel that the maternal incision and morbidity should

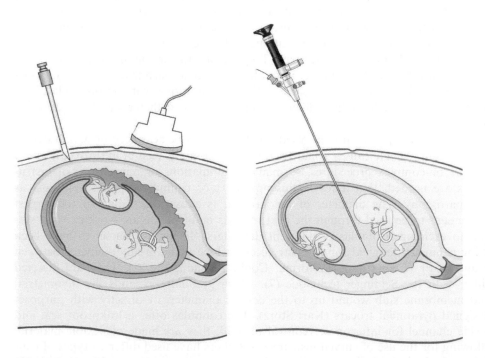

Figure 3 Schematic drawing of fetoscopic laser coagulation of chorionic plate vessels, in a case of a posterior placenta. The trocar is first inserted percutaneously, and later a straight endoscope is inserted through the cannula. *Drawing*: Katja Dalkowski.

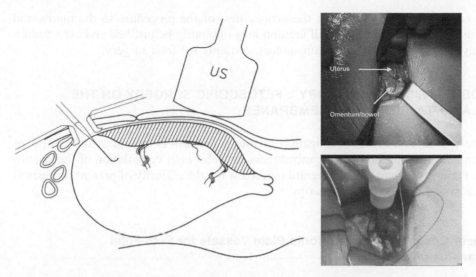

Figure 4 In exceptional situations, a mini-laparotomy may be preferred to introduce the trocar safely through the fundus or toward the posterior side of the uterus. *Inset*: Outside view of mini-laparotomy and trocar inserted. *Source*: From Ref. 7.

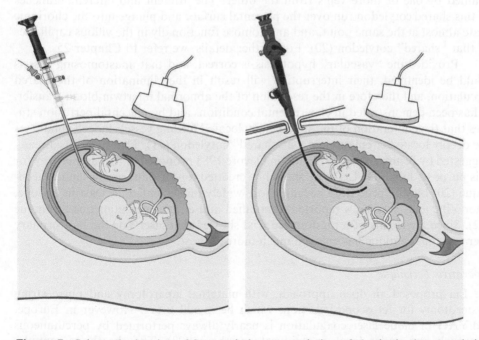

Figure 5 Schematic drawing of fetoscopic laser coagulation of chorionic plate vessels in a case of an anterior placenta. A percutaneous trocar insertion has been used and the curved endoscope allows a more appropriate inclination toward the placenta. We have used a steerable endoscope, but the image quality so far remains poor. *Drawing*: Katja Dalkowski.

be considered separately from the invasiveness of the procedure to the uterus and fetus. Maternal abdominal wall incision may obviously be justified and even technically necessary in selected circumstances, certainly for fetal surgery.

"OBSTETRICAL ENDOSCOPY": FETOSCOPIC SURGERY ON THE PLACENTA, CORD, AND MEMBRANES

Apart from case reports on ligation of the major vessels in a placental chorioangioma and section of amniotic membranes or webs, laser coagulation of the chorionic plate vessels and cord obliteration account for the majority of present obstetrical indications for operative fetoscopy.

Laser Coagulation of Chorionic Plate Vessels for Feto-Fetal Transfusion Syndrome

Pathophysiology

Laser coagulation of chorionic plate vessels has been introduced as a more cause-oriented approach than, for instance, amniodrainage. Feto-fetal transfusion syndrome (FFTS) is related to the presence of arterio-venous (AV) anastomoses in combination with a paucity (or absence) of arterio-arterial (AA) or veno-venous (VV) anastomoses, which normally compensate for the hemodynamic effects of AV communications. For clarity, an AV anastomosis is not a real "anatomical" anastomosis, but a cotyledon that is fed by at least one artery from one fetus, and drained by one or more veins from the other. The afferent and efferent branches of this shared cotyledon run over the placental surface and plunge into the chorionic plate almost at the same point, and anastomose functionally in the villous capillaries of that "shared" cotyledon (20). For further details, we refer to Chapter 25.

Provided the "vascular" hypothesis is correct, and that anastomosing vessels could be identified, their interruption will result in the elimination of the shared circulation, and therefore in the resolution of the abnormal intertwin blood transfer. It has been demonstrated in experimental conditions and by placental perfusion studies that the obliteration of the superficially located feeding vessels indeed eliminates the deeply located circulation or the "shared" cotyledon (21). That idea was already suggested by Benirschke in 1973, and in Devore 1983 proposed to use laser energy for this purpose. Julian De Lia et al. should be credited for introducing the clinical technique (20) but the procedure became more widely implemented, at least in Europe, after Ville and Nicolaides reported a modified and elegant percutaneous technique (22). Since the results of a randomized trial showed that laser was the best primary therapy, the technique has enjoyed much more interest.

Operative Technique

De Lia proposed an open approach, with maternal laparotomy and purse string hysterotomy for fetoscope insertion, which he is still using. However in Europe, Nd:YAG or diode laser coagulation is nearly always performed by percutaneous approach and under local or epidural anesthesia (23). The sheath or cannula, loaded with a trocar, is inserted under US guidance into the polyhydramniotic sac (Figs. 3–6). The surgeon has, at least in planning, to map ahead of time the target, which is the (externally invisible) vascular equator. For this purpose, the

(A)   (B)

(C)   (D)

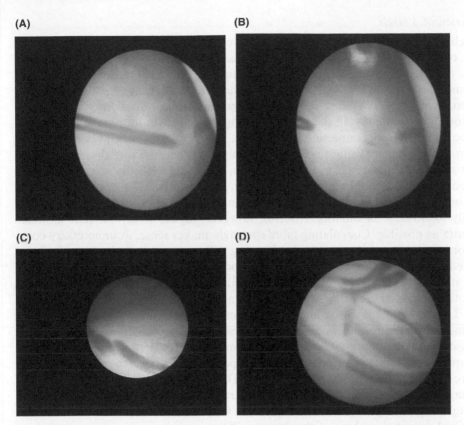

Figure 6 Fetoscopic appearance of anastomosing vessels on a monochorionic placenta. Artery-to-vein anastomosis prior to (**A**) and after (**B**) coagulation. (**C**) Artery-to-artery anastomosis. (**D**) Superficial chorionic plate vessels crossing the intertwin membrane.

insertion of the two cords with color Doppler can be of much help, and potentially ultrasound can reveal some difference in echogenicity between the two parts of the placenta. Without this, directing the scope at a perpendicular angle to the donor may also work, which will allow the easy identification of the intertwin membrane and the vessels crossing under it. The placenta is avoided, but due to flattening and the inability to determine the lateral borders, occasionally one may partly hit it. The anticipated tract of the cannula is infiltrated with xylocain 1% (up 20 mL) down to the myometrium, for local anesthesia. We frequently use combined spinal–epidural anesthesia, with hyperbaric bupivacaine (8 mg) injected into the spinal space at the L3–L4 or L4–L5 interspace (23). The trocar and cannula are advanced stepwise through the different layers, monitored under US guidance. The trocar is then removed and a fetoscope and 400–600 μm Nd:YAG or diode laser fiber are inserted into the sheath. The laser tip is directed as close as possible to a 90° angle toward the target vessels. Coagulation is done using a no touch technique with power settings of 40–100 W (Nd:YAG) at about 1 cm distance or less. Selection of the vessels to be targeted will be discussed subsequently. Sections of ~1 cm are coagulated. Amnio-infusion may be needed to improve visualization or to clear the operative field in case of stained fluid, or to prevent suspended amniotic debris to become stuck to the tip of the fiber, making laser energy inefficacious and finally burn the fiber tip.

Selection of Vessels

The chorionic plate is inspected and the course of the vessels determined. Fetoscopic laser occlusion of the chorioangiopagus vessels (FLOC), as proposed by De Lia et al. (20), is the identification and coagulation of all anastomosing vessels along the vascular equator (Fig. 4). It is not clear whether this is always possible. In a more pragmatic approach, Ville et al. (22) described the surgical division of the vascular territory by coagulating all the vessels crossing the intertwin membrane, which cannot be excluded from connecting both fetuses. In other words, when vessels originating from the recipient cannot be followed completely, because they disappear on the other side of the membrane or under the fetus, and could in theory anastomose, they will be coagulated, too. In an unselective way, lasering all vessels along the intertwin membrane is probably much easier, faster, and readily reproducible, because of its readily identifiable landmarks. It seems, however, logical to try to spare as much placenta as possible. Coagulating more sparingly makes sense, as unnecessary coagulation of vessels not involved in the shunting will lead to the elimination of normal cotyledons and may impair fetomaternal blood–gas interchange for an already critically distressed fetus. Meanwhile, several teams have shown the feasibility of this operation in higher-order multiplets with comparable results (24).

Large vessels may need higher power settings, and initial tissue effect may be obtained by lasering first laterally at the vessels. Progressively, they will narrow and get coagulated. Larger vessels may be at more risk for perforation. Once all vessels are coagulated, and prior to drainage, operative sites need to be reinspected to ensure that coagulation has been effective. The procedure is completed by amniodrainage till normal amniotic fluid pockets are seen on US. We use rapid drainage through the fetoscopic cannula with as well as without aspiration. Abruptio has been described during this phase of the therapy (25).

FETOSCOPIC CORD OBLITERATION

Next to FFTS, monochorionic (MC) twinning may be complicated by a number of rare conditions, such as twin reversed arterial perfusion sequence (TRAP), or twins may be discordant for structural or genetic anomalies, for which they are at higher risk than singletons. In all these circumstances, selective feticide may be contemplated for selected cases. In *dichorionic* multiple pregnancies, selective feticide with intracardiac or intrathoracic injection of potassium chloride is a well-established modality. The loss rate for the other twin is ~7% and may be independent of gestation. The cause of this remains unknown. In *monochorionic* twins, vascular communications between the two fetuses are virtually always present and feticide by intracardiac KCl is not suitable, as the product may embolize to the other fetus. Also, following intrauterine fetal death (IUFD), blood may be "dumped" from the surviving twin into the dead fetus, since intertwin vessels remain patent. Such acute, agonal feto-fetal transfusion may lead to hypovolemic shock in the survivor, causing either central nervous system damage or IUFD of the survivor. Umbilical cord embolization is also discouraged as any embolic agent can embolize to the other fetus. Denbow et al. reported 12 attempts of umbilical vessel occlusion with absolute alcohol or enbucrilate gel and observed an overall success rate of 33% in six MC twins (26). Accordingly, techniques for selective feticide in MC twins must include a method for arresting flow in the cord of the target fetus completely and permanently (27).

Techniques for Cord Occlusion in Monochorionic Twins

Surgical ligation of the umbilical cord causes immediate, complete, and permanent interruption of both arterial and venous flow in the umbilical cord, irrespective of its diameter. Fetoscopic cord ligation was the first clinical procedure to become clinically acceptable but lost favor because of alternative cord occlusion techniques that are easier (28).

Early in gestation one can use fetoscopic laser coagulation, as described before, but targeted to the cord or cord root vessels. This has been described as early as 16 weeks. A double lumen needle can be used, accommodating a 1.0-mm fetoscope and a 400-µm laser fiber (Figs. 1 and 7) (29). Coagulation of the umbilical cord is a fairly easy and straightforward procedure; the cord root of the target fetus is visualized, and the vessels are then coagulated using a "no touch" technique. The successful use of laser cord coagulation has been reported for an acardiac twin as late as 24 weeks, but overall it has a high failure rate beyond 20 to 22 weeks of gestation. In a large follow-up study, there was a higher risk for postoperative IUFD, which occurred within 48 hours, and it was believed that incomplete coagulation might be the cause of postmortem feto-fetal hemorrhage, with subsequent double IUFD as a consequence (30).

We later described the use of bipolar energy to occlude the cord. This has a number of theoretical and practical advantages (31). First, it obliterates simultaneously both the umbilical arteries and vein, causing immediate cessation of flow, thus preventing agonal interfetal hemorrhage when a vessel would remain or become patent (again). Second, the procedure can be performed through a single port. Moreover, the technique relies on existing standard and relatively inexpensive

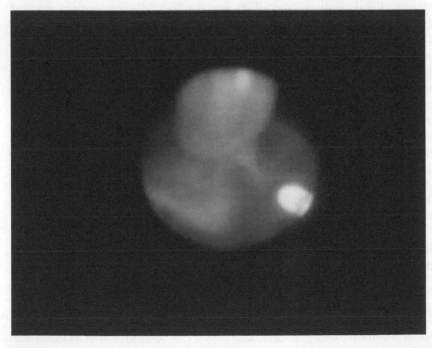

Figure 7 Laser coagulation of cord vessels. A 1.0 mm embryoscope and a 400 µm fiber are used here.

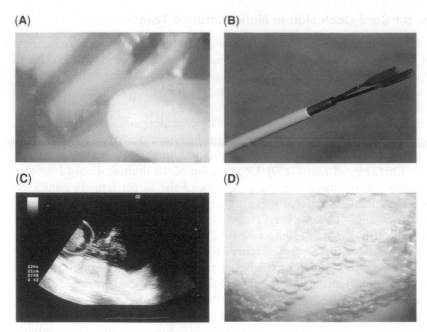

Figure 8 (**A**) Technique of fetoscopic cord coagulation, using a 3-mm bipolar forceps. (**B**) Smaller instruments are now available, like this 7.0 Fr (2.3 mm) bipolar forceps, which can be manipulated under ultrasound control. (**C**) Ultrasound image: local heat production is visible as turbulences and/or steam bubbles. (**D**) Fetoscopic image of the local effect of coagulation.

instrumentation. Fetal medicine specialists are familiar with performing invasive procedures under real-time US guidance. If the cannula cannot be directly inserted into the target amniotic sac, the cord can even be grasped through the intertwin membranes. The latter, however, may create iatrogenic monoamniotic twin pregnancy, and as a consequence cord accidents, as described in (30). The key instrument in the procedure is a small diameter bipolar coagulation forceps. Over time, we have used different commercially available instruments, such as a disposable 3.0-mm forceps (Everest Medical, Minneapolis, Minnesota, U.S.A.), or more recently a 3.0-mm and 2.7 mm reusable instrument (Fig. 8). Applying too high energy may lead to cord transection; insufficient coagulation may cause interfetal transfusion after the fetus dies. The current instrumentation allows for cord coagulation even in the third trimester (32). Additional improvement might be the currently tested bipolar forceps, with a built in scope, as to facilitate identification and grasping of the cord becomes easier and faster.

Monopolar or Intestitial Laser Coagulation of the Cord and Other Fetal Vessels

Rodeck et al. described the use of monopolar thermocoagulation to arrest blood flow using conventional US-guided needling techniques (18). This elegant needle-based US-guided technique is certainly less complex and invasive than fetoscopic ligation. As an alternative energy source, again laser can be used, but in its interstitial mode (33). However, it remains to be demonstrated whether (i) arresting flow in the aorta precludes internal fetal hemorrhage or (ii) feto-fetal hemorrhage, and (iii) if the technique would also work in other hemodynamic conditions and/or at a later gestational age. In their first report, the procedure actually failed occasionally and in later reports this was confirmed (34). In personal communications, the group confirmed that the procedure does not work in FFTS. It is likely that the hemodynamic conditions, which are clearly different for TRAP as compared to FFTS and/or discordant MC twins, in a normal pumping heart, play a role in this. A marketed monopolar electrode is now available, purpose-designed, within the Eurofoetus project (4).

Currently, it is not possible to say what the single best method is for selective feticide in MC pregnancies. The surgeon should be familiar with several techniques in order to tailor therapy to the individual requirements of each case. Initially, we recommended laser coagulation of the cord as a primary technique, with bipolar coagulation to be used beyond 22 weeks or when laser fails (28). However, in our total experience, laser coagulation has a higher risk of postoperative IUFD, and perhaps bipolar should be used more liberally. In addition, and somewhat surprising, there was also a clear learning curve effect with a dramatic fall in complications after 40 procedures (30). Therefore, even if the hardware is available, these procedures should be performed in experienced tertiary referral centers, and by the same operators to ensure adequate experience.

AMNIOTIC BAND SYNDROME

To date, the pathogenesis of amniotic bands and even their existence as a cause for some congenital anomalies are still controversial. Amniotic band syndrome (ABSd) refers to amputation of fingers and/or limbs, and a wide spectrum of associated anomalies involving trunk and craniofacial anomalies. Two theories have been proposed to explain the pathogenesis. Streeter's theory is based on a developmental anomaly of the embryonic germinal disc, and the amniotic band would be a byproduct rather than the cause of fetal anomalies. Torpin's theory claims that the primary problem is rupture of the amniotic membrane, and its detachment from the chorion. In that scenario, the fetus would exit the amniotic cavity, and the outer amnion and naked chorion produce mesodermic fibrous strings that entangle and entrap different fetal organs like a "guillotine," leading to constriction and amputation. This theory became widely accepted, despite the small number of cases and inconsistent findings (35).

It has so far been difficult to visualize an amnion at the precise place of amputation, or in most instances no amniotic sheet at all. The full sequence of a normal fetus, followed by the occurrence of amniotic rupture, then by adhesion to the limbs, and finally by amputation has not been described. Bronshtein, therefore, doubts this etiology. It is, for instance, difficult to explain why bands always cause transverse amputations and not diagonal constriction rings. The adhesion and constriction theory of Torpin does, for instance, explain neither the associated anomalies nor the damage to internal organs. Brohnstein concludes, therefore, that the underlying reason must be an embryonic or teratogenic factor.

Moerman et al. have reconciled both theories, and accept that both entities exist, and are just of different origin (36). Schwartzler and Ville recently investigated a case of ABSd at 12 weeks of gestation in which the fetus appeared to be trapped in a "cob web" of bands (37). These bands were examined by transmission electron microscopy, and appeared to be cell-free tubules, carrying hooks acting like a "velcro" and constricting fetal elements. The case demonstrates early and increasing constriction as the fetus grows and moves. In addition, this fetus had grade 3 intra-ventricular hemorrhage, suggesting that bands could cause internal damage by redis-tributing blood flow under external pressure. Also at later gestational age, US allows detection of limb or finger amputations. In a recent report, Tadmor et al. observed the progressive constriction of the lower limbs from 21 weeks onward (38).

Though the consequences of ABSd are dramatic, they are not life-threatening. Despite that, it would seem logical to try to arrest this process, particularly when the diagnosis of bands is made early and the amputation process has just started. A causal relationship between the bands and the amputation is plausible. The in utero release of amniotic bands in humans was, therefore, only a logical step pioneered by Quintero et al. (39). His group treated two cases of ABSd in animals, at 22 and 23 weeks, lysing the band under sono-endoscopic control. The procedure restored adequate blood flow distal to the obstruction and the limb could be pre-served. In both cases, only mild or minimal limb dysfunction was present at birth. The assumption that human amniotic bands are amenable to a similar form of sur-gical release as in the animal model, remains indeed speculative, and the success of surgery is based on the mechanistic etiologic mechanism.

FETOSCOPIC SURGERY FOR CONGENITAL DIAPHRAGMATIC HERNIA

Congenital diaphragmatic hernia (CDH) is a sporadic condition, affecting 1or 2 in 5000 live births (40). In just over half of the cases, the condition will be isolated, while the rest may have associated chromosomal, syndromal, or structural anomalies, being independent determinants of survival. Although in essence only an anatomical defect, the leading problem of these infants is pulmonary hypoplasia and pulmonary hyper-tension (41,42). Today, screening programs usually allow for early diagnosis of CDH and such patients ought to be referred to tertiary units for (i) further structural and genetic work up; (ii) prenatal prognostication; (iii) multidisciplinary counseling and (iv) further in utero management and/or timed term delivery, neonatal resuscitation, and delayed repair. Today, still only 64% of antenatal diagnosed and live born cases survive the neonatal period, and for isolated cases this is 70% (43).

Given the potential impact of the diagnosis of CDH, the fetal medicine specia-list logically will be expected to predict outcome of the individual case and to assist in choosing between available options, including for severe cases prenatal therapy or termination. It has been shown that *lethal* pulmonary hypoplasia may be predicted on the basis of indirect assessment of lung development. Several imaging techniques to quantitate lung development are currently evaluated (44). For left-sided CDH, the presence of herniation of the left liver lobe into the thorax (45) and a low lung-to-head ratio (LHR) during midgestation can predict neonatal mortality reasonably well (46,49).

Concept and Technique of Antenatal Intervention

Current postnatal care does not solve the underlying pulmonary hypoplasia. Prena-tal measures that would improve lung development to viable levels are, therefore, a logical next step. Congenital laryngeal atresia is an experiment of nature, where congenital tracheal occlusion (TO) leads to triggered lung growth (50). Experimental TO also prevents egress of lung liquid, leading to increased levels of lung tissue stretch and has been extensively studied by many groups in different in vitro and

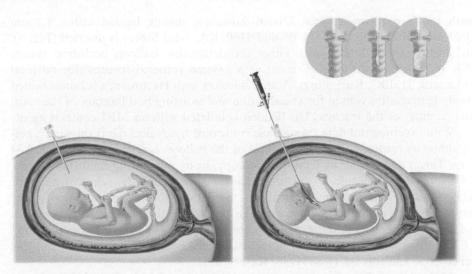

Figure 9 The cannula has been inserted in the direction of the fetal mouth. The endoscope is then advanced into the fetal pharynx and trachea. Inset: Balloon deposition. *Source*: From ISUOG and John Wiley & Sons, Ltd.

animal models (51,52). Our group showed that for pulmonary response timing and duration of the occlusion period are crucial for the nature of the response of airways and pulmonary vessels (52). This led us to the concept of temporary TO in the late canalicular phase with prenatal reversal [plug–unplug sequence (53)], which yields in animal models optimal response of airways and vessels (52). To make this clinically acceptable, we developed a percutaneous, fetoscopic endoluminal technique of (reversible) balloon occlusion (FETO) (54). It avoids laparotomy, hysterotomy, and fetal neck dissection, and does not require the restoration of airways by a so-called ex utero intrapartum therapy (EXIT) procedure (55). Feasibility of the procedure was demonstrated and we were the first to report survivors after a percutaneous balloon occlusion (56,57).

Clinical Fetoscopic Program and Instrumentation

Selection criteria are (i) singleton pregnancy with severe CDH in an anatomically and chromosomally normal fetus diagnosed prior to 28 weeks, (ii) Irrespective of the side of the herniation, the liver should be herniated into the thorax and the LHR <1.0, as measured between 26 and 28 weeks. For consistency, all ultrasound examinations are performed by the same specialists in each of the participating institutions. (iii) Following FETO and unless the balloon could be removed prior to birth, patients should have their delivery at an institution with facilities for neonatal balloon removal by EXIT procedure, to permit tracheoscopic retrieval of the balloon.

Typically FETO (at 26–28 weeks), as well as fetoscopic retrieval of the balloon (at 34 weeks), is performed under loco-regional anesthesia, perioperative prophylactic tocolysis, and antibiotics. Fetal medication consists of fentanyl and pancuronium for analgesia and immobilization by intramuscular injection. A 10 Fr cannula similar to the one for laser coagulation in twins is inserted toward the fetal mouth, and a purpose-designed 3.0 mm fetoscopic sheath, loaded with a 1.2-mm 10,000 pixel fiber-endoscope (11505 and 11605KA, Karl Storz) is inserted (Fig. 9). This sheath can be loaded with either the detachable balloon occlusion system (GVB 16, MicroVasys, Paris, France) or a 1.0-mm retrieval forceps (for retrieval at 34 weeks; 11510C, Karl Storz). Amnio-infusion with Hartmann's solution heated to body temperature is used for visualization and assisting in dilatation of the vocal cords on entry of the trachea. The balloon is inflated with an MRI contrast agent.

With experimental data (meanwhile confirmed by clinical data) showing a better pulmonary response, prenatal retrieval of the balloon is scheduled, at around 34 weeks. This is done either by fetal tracheoscopy, or by puncturing the balloon using an US-guided 20G needle. Prepartum removal also avoids the inherent need for EXIT-associated hysterotomy, and allows the patient to return home for further postnatal management, certainly posing less burden on the patient. In case of preterm delivery, or earlier in our experience, the balloon might also be retrieved during an EXIT procedure, using another purpose-designed blunt tip, double flow rod lens tracheoscope and forceps (KST 1138, Karl Storz).

The results of this operation are beyond the scope of this technical chapter, and we refer to the current literature (49,57). On US lungs showed increasing echogenicity and LHR from a median 0.7 before FETO to 1.8 within 2 weeks after surgery. Overall, early neonatal survival increase is >60%; survival till discharge is >50% for severe cases managed postnatally. Survivors do not seem to be neurologically impaired. This procedure remains invasive with its well-identified problems. Membranes ruptured <32 weeks in 35%, however, not necessarily leading to preterm delivery (30%). There was a decreasing trend for these complications as experience increased. It seems that severe CDH may be successfully treated with temporary TO, which can be achieved by minimally invasive techniques (58).

ACKNOWLEDGMENTS

Drs L. Lewi and J. Jani are beneficiaries of a grant of the European Commission in its 5th Framework Programme (#QLG1-CT-2002–01632 EuroTwin2Twin). The Eurofoetus project (BMH4 CT 97 23 83) was funded in the Biomed 2 Programme of the E.C. Other members of these projects are thanked: Y. Ville (Poissy), K. Hecher (Hamburg), T. H. Bui (Stockholm), R. Vlietinck (Leuven), M. van Gemert (Amsterdam), U. Nicolini (Milan), K. Nicolaides (London), R. Denk (Munchen), and C. Jackson (London).

REFERENCES

1. Quintero RA, Abuhamad A, Hobbins JC, Mahoney MJ. Transabdominal thin gauge embryofetoscopy: a technique for early prenatal diagnosis and its use in the diagnosis of a case of Meckel Gruber Syndrome. Am J Obstet Gynecol 1993; 168:1552–1557.
2. Luks FI, Deprest JA. Endoscopic fetal surgery: a new alternative? (editorial). Eur J Obstet Gynecol Reprod Biol 1993; 52:1–3.
3. Gratacós E, Deprest J. Current experience with fetoscopy and the Eurofoetus registry for fetoscopic procedures. Eur J Obstet Gynecol Reprod Biol 2000; 92:151–160.
4. Deprest J, Ville Y, Bui TH, Hecher K, Dumez Y, Nicolini U. Eurofoetus. Endoscopic fetoplacental surgery: from animal experimentation to early human experimentation.

Programme funded by the European Commision, within the Biomed 2 Programme, BMH4 CT97 2383. Endreport ISBN 23–89756–427–0. Tuttlingen, Germany:Endo-Press, 2004:1–56.

5. Luks FI, Deprest JA, Vandenberghe K, et al. Fetoscopy-guided fetal endoscopy in a sheep model. J Am Coll Surg 1994; 178:609–612.

6. Ville Y, Van Peborgh P, Gagnon A, Frydman R, Fernandez H. Traitement chirurgical du syndrome transfuseur-transfusé: coagulation des anastomoses par un laser Nd:YAG sous contrôle écho-endoscopique. J Gynecol Obstet Biol Reprod 1997; 26:175–181.

7. Deprest J, Van Schoubroeck D, Van Ballaer P, Flageole H, Van Assche FA, Vandenberghe K. Alternative access for fetoscopic Nd: YAG laser in TTS with anterior placenta. Ultrasound Obstet Gynecol 1998; 12:347–352.

8. Deprest J, Ville Y. Obstetric endoscopy. In: Harrison M, Evans M, Adzick NS, Holzgreve W, eds. The Unborn Patient: The Art and Science of Fetal Therapy. Chap 15. Philadelphia: W.B. Saunders, 2000:213–232.

9. Bonati F, Perales A, Novak P. Ex vivo testing of a temperature and pressure controlled amnio-irrigator for fetoscopic surgery. J Pediatr Surg 2002; 37:18–24.

10. Evrard V, Deprest J, Luks F, et al. (1997). Amnio-infusion with Hartmann's solution: a safe distension medium for endoscopic fetal surgery in the ovine model. Fetal Diagn Ther 1997; 12:188–192.

11. Bruner JP, Richards WO, Tulipan NB, Arney TL. Endoscopic coverage of fetal myelomeningocele in utero. Am J Obstet Gynecol 1999; 180:153–158.

12. Luks FI, Deprest JA, Marcus M, et al. Carbon dioxide pneumamnios causes acidosis in the fetal lamb. Fetal Diagn Ther 1994; 9:101–104.

13. Saiki Y, Litwin DEM, Bigras JL, et al. Reducing the deleterious effects of intrauterine CO_2 during fetoscopic surgery. J Surg Res 1997; 69:51–54.

14. Gratacos E, Wu J, Devlieger R, Vandevelde M, Deprest J. Effects of amniodistention with carbon dioxide on fetal acid-base status during fetoscopic surgery in a sheep model. Surg Endosc 2001; 15:368–372.

15. Quintero RA, Bornick PW, Allen MH, Johnson PK. Selective photocoagulation of communicating vessels in severe twin–twin transfusion syndrome in women with an anterior placenta. Obstet Gynecol 2001; 97:477–481.

16. Soothill P, Sohan K Carroll S, Kyle P. Ultrasound-guided, intra-abdominal laser to treat acardiac pregnancies. Br J Obstet Gynaecol 2002; 109(3):352–354.

17. Deprest J, Audibert F, Van Schoubroeck D, Hecher K, Mahieu-Caputo D. Bipolar cord coagulation of the umbilical cord in complicated monochorionic twin pregnancy. Am J Obstet Gynecol 2000; 182:340–345.

18. Rodeck C, Deans A, Jauniaux E. Thermocoagulation for the early treatment of pregnancy with an acardiac twin. N Engl J Med 1998; 339:1293–1294.

19. Luks FI, Deprest JA, Gilchrist BF, et al. Access techniques in endoscopic fetal surgery. Eur J Pediatr Surg 1997; 7:131–134.

20. De Lia JE, Cruikshank DP, Keye WR. Fetoscopic neodymium: YAG laser occlusion of placental vessels in severe twin–twin transfusion syndrome. Obstet Gynecol 1990; 75:1046–1053.

21. Dumitrascu-Branisteanu I, Deprest J, Evrard V, et al. Time-related cotyledonary effects of laser coagulation of superficial chorionic vessels in an ovine model. Prenat Diagn 1999; 19:205–210.

22. Ville Y, Hyett J, Hecher K, Nicolaides K. Preliminary experience with endoscopic laser surgery for severe twin–twin transfusion syndrome. N Engl J Med 1995; 332: 224–227.

23. Vandevelde M, Van Schoubroeck D, Lewi L, et al. Randomized double-blind comparison of remifentanil and diazepam for fetal immobilization and maternal sedation during fetoscopic surgery. Anesth and Analg 2005; 101(1):251–258.

24. Van Schoubroeck D, Lewi L, Ryan G, et al. Fetoscopic surgery in triplet pregnancies–a multicenter case series. Am J Obstet Gynecol 2004; 191:1529–1532.

25. Senat MV, Deprest J, Boulvain M, Paupe A, Winer N, Ville Y. A randomized trial of endoscopic laser surgery versus serial amnioreduction for severe twin-to-twin transfusion syndrome at midgestation. N Engl J Med 2004; 351:136–144.

26. Denbow ML, Overton TG, Duncan KR, Cox PM, Fisk NM. High failure rate of umbilical vessel occlusion by ultrasound-guided injection of absolute alcohol or enbucrilate gel. Prenat Diagn 1999; 19:527–532.

27. Deprest JA, Evrard VA, Van Ballaer PP, et al. Experience with fetoscopic cord ligation. Eur J Obstet Gynecol Reprod Biol 1998; 81:157–164.

28. Challis D, Gratacós E, Deprest J. Selective termination in monochorionic twins. J Perinat Med 1999; 27:327–338.

29. Hecher K, Hackeloër BJ, Ville Y. Umbilical cord coagulation by operative microendoscopy at 16 weeks gestation in an acardiac twin. Ultrasound Obstet Gynecol 1997; 10:130.

30. Lewi L, Gratacos E, Ortibus E, et al. Pregnancy and infant outcome of 80 consecutive cord coagulations in complicated monochorionic multiple pregnancies. Am J Obstet Gynecol 2006; 194:782–789.

31. Deprest J, Audibert F, Van Schoubroeck D, Hecher K, Mahieu-Caputo D. Bipolar cord coagulation of the umbilical cord in complicated monochorionic twin pregnancy. Am J Obstet Gynecol 2000; 182:340–345.

32. Deprest J, Van Schoubroeck D, Senat MV, et al. Cord coagulation in monochorionic multiplets late in gestation (abstract 612). Am J Obstet Gynecol 2003; 189:S226.

33. Soothill P, Sohan K, Carroll S, Kyle P. Ultrasound-guided, intra-abdominal laser to treat acardiac pregnancies. Br J Obstet Gynaecol 2002; 109(3):352–354.

34. Holmes A, Jauniaux E, Rodeck C. Monopolar thermocoagulation in acardiac twinning. Br J Obstet Gynecol 2001; 108:1000–1002.

35. Bronshtein M, Zimmer EZ. Do amniotic bands amputate fetal organs? Ultrasound Obstet Gynecol 1997; 10:309–311.

36. Moerman P, Fryns JP, Vandenberghe K, Lauweryns JM. Constrictive amniotic bands, amniotic adhesions, and limb–body wall complex: discrete disruption sequences with pathogenetic overlap. Am J Med Genet 1992; 42:470–479.

37. Schwartzler P, Moscoso G, Senat M, Ville Y. The cobweb syndrome: 1st trimester sonographic diagnosis of multiple amniotic bands confirmed by fetoscopy and pathological examination. Hum Reprod 1998; 13:2966–2969.

38. Tadmor O, Kreisberg G, Achiron R, Porat S, Yagel S. Limb amputation in amniotic band syndrome: serial ultrasonographic and Doppler observations. Ultrasound Obstet Gynecol 1997; 10:312–315.

39. Quintero R, Morales WJ, Kalter CS, Angel JL. In utero lysis of amniotic bands. Ultrasound Obstet Gynecol 1997; 10:316–320.

40. Torfs CD, Curry CJR, Bateson TF, et al. A population-based study of congenital diaphragmatic hernia. Teratology 1992; 46:355.

41. Jesudason EC, Connell MG, Fernig DG, et al. Early lung malformations in congenital diaphragmatic hernia. J Pediatr Surg 2000; 35:124–128.

42. Ijsselstein H, Tibboel D. The lungs in congenital diaphragmatic hernia: do we understand? Pediatr Surg 2000; 35:124–128.

43. Stege G, Fenton A, Jaffray B. Nihilism in the 1990s. The true mortality of CDH. Pediatrics 2003; 112:532–535.

44. Deprest J, Jani J, Cannie M, et al. Progress in intra-uterine assessment of the fetal lung and prediction of neonatal function. Ultrasound Obstet Gynaecol 2005; 25(2): 108–111.

45. Albanese CT, Lopoo DV, Paek BW, et al. Fetal liver position and perinatal outcome for congential diaphragmatic hernia. Prenat Diagn 1998; 18:1138–1842.

46. Metkus AP, Filly RA, Stringer MD, et al. Sonographic predictors of survival in fetal diaphragmatic hernia. J Pediatr Surg 1996; 31:148–152.

47. Flake A, Crombleholme T, Johnson M, et al. Treatment of severe congenital diaphragmatic hernia by fetal tracheal occlusion: clinical experience with fifteen cases. Am J Obstet Gynecol 2000; 183:1059–1066.

48. Laudy JAM, Van Gucht M, Van Dooren MF, et al. Congenital diaphragmatic hernia: an evaluation of the prognostic value of the lung-to-head ratio and other prenatal parameters. Prenat Diagn 2003; 23:634–639.

49. Deprest J, Jani J, Gratacos E, et al. Fetal intervention for congenital diaphragmatic hernia. Semin Perinatol 2005; 29(2):94–103.

50. Oepkes D, Teunissen AK, Van de Velde M, Devlieger H, Delaere P, Deprest J. Congenital high airway obstruction syndrome successfully treated with ex utero intrapartum treatment. Ultrasound Obstet Gynaecol 2003; 22:437–439.

51. Di Fiore JW, Fauza DO, Slavin R, et al. Experimental fetal tracheal ligation reverses the structural and physiological effects of pulmonary hypoplasia in CDH. J Pediatr Surg 1997; 29:248–256.

52. Deprest J. Towards an endoscopic intra-uterine treatment for congenital diaphragmatic hernia. Verh K Acad Geneesk Belg 2002; 49:55–70.

53. Flageole H, Evrard V, Piedboeuf B, et al. The plug-unplug sequence: an important step to achieve type II pneumocyte maturation in the fetal lamb model. J Pediatr Surg 1998; 33:299–303.

54. Deprest JA, Evrard VA, Van Ballaer PP, et al. Tracheoscopic endoluminal plugging using an inflatable device in the fetal lamb model. Eur J Obstet Gynaecol Reprod Biol 1998; 81:165–169.

55. Bouchard S, Johnson P, Flake A, et al. The EXIT procedure: experience and outcome in 31 cases. J Pediatr Surg 2002; 37:418–426.

56. Quintero RA, Morales WJ, Bornick PW, Allen MH, Johnson PK. Minimally invasive intraluminal tracheal occlusion in a human fetus with left congenital diaphragmatic hernia at 27 weeks gestation via direct fetal laryngoscopy. Prenat Neonat Med 2000; 5:134–140.

57. Deprest J, Gratacos E, Nicolaides KH, et al. Fetoscopic tracheal occlusion (FETO) for severe congenital diaphragmatic hernia: evolution of a technique. Ultrasound Obstet Gynaecol 2004; 24:121–126.

58. Deprest J, Jani J, van Schoubroeck D, et al. Current consequences of prenatal diagnosis of congenital diaphragmatic hernia. J Ped Surg 2006; 41:423–430.

27

Open Fetal Surgery

Michael W. Bebbington, Mark P. Johnson, R. Douglas Wilson, and N. Scott Adzick
*The Center for Fetal Diagnosis and Treatment, The Children's Hospital of Philadelphia,
The University of Pennsylvania School of Medicine, Philadelphia, Pennsylvania, U.S.A.*

INTRODUCTION

With the widespread acceptance of prenatal diagnosis, new arrays of challenges present themselves for the management of the fetus with congenital anomalies. Despite advances in prenatal care, planned delivery and neonatal care at a tertiary care center, improvements in mortality and morbidity for some fetuses have been elusive. By the time they are delivered, the disease process has progressed to the point that they are too ill to be successfully treated postnatally. It is this group of fetuses that may benefit from fetal surgical intervention.

As with any invasive procedure, the risks and benefits must be weighed for each case. For a fetus with a life-threatening condition, the risks may be small compared with the potential benefits. However, the maternal risks and benefits must also be weighed as the mother assumes a significant pregnancy risk associated with fetal surgical procedures as well as the risk to future pregnancies of the prior hysterotomy. Until recently, open fetal surgery has been reserved for cases where expectant management had a lethal outcome. The goal is to prevent mortality where anomalies are potentially correctable. This requires knowledge of the natural history and pathophysiology of the abnormality, the availability of accurate prenatal diagnosis, a surgical procedure to alter the natural history of the anomaly, and the ability to allow the pregnancy to continue to minimize the risks of premature delivery. Recently, these same principles have been applied to a nonlethal anomaly in an attempt to prevent life-long morbidity.

Despite progress, fetal surgery remains controversial. The controversy arises around the issues of the natural history of a specific anomaly and whether this is improved by the fetal surgical intervention. In the short term, the most important consideration that needs to be met before open fetal surgery becomes an accepted option is for the benefits to be clearly demonstrated through studies in animal models, careful case studies, then randomized clinical trials. Already several potential interventions have been discontinued when they failed to show a demonstrable improvement when compared to standard therapy. This chapter will summarize the current status of open maternal–fetal surgery for fetuses with life-threatening anomalies related to congenital cystic adenomatoid malformation (CCAM), bronchopulmonary sequestration (BPS), sacrococcygeal teratoma (SCT), and congenital

493

diaphragmatic hernia (CDH), as well as the prevention of long-term morbidity from midgestation repair of myelomeningocele (MMC).

PERIOPERATIVE MANAGEMENT OF FETAL SURGICAL PATIENTS

Preoperative Management

Patients referred to a fetal treatment center for possible fetal surgical intervention undergo an extensive evaluation. This evaluation includes: (i) detailed ultrasonography to confirm the diagnosis and exclude any additional abnormalities that might impact clinical outcome, (ii) ultrafast fetal magnetic resonance imaging (MRI) for additional anatomic information, (iii) fetal echocardiography to rule out congenital heart defects and to provide a functional assessment of fetal cardiac function, and (iv) fetal karyotype to exclude a cytogenetic or possibly molecular chromosomal anomaly as the basis for the anomaly. In general, chromosomal or other genetic anomalies, multiple gestations, additional major anomalies, and maternal medical, obstetrical, social, or psychological risk factors are contraindications for open fetal surgery.

Following completion of their evaluation, families meet with both the maternal–fetal medicine/obstetrical and pediatric surgery physicians to discuss the nature of the anomaly, its natural history, prognosis, and therapeutic options. If open maternal–fetal surgery is considered, a psychological evaluation is also performed by the team's social worker. A team meeting that includes all members of the fetal surgery team along with the family is held to discuss each step of the proposed surgery and postoperative care, the risk and benefits of the intervention, and the potential alternatives to fetal therapy. Members of the team include the fetal/pediatric surgeon, maternal–fetal medicine/obstetrical/genetics specialist, anesthesiologist, perinatal advanced practice nurse, nurse sonographer, operating room nurses, and social worker. Potential risks include operative complications, preterm labor, preterm rupture of the membranes, chorioamnionitis, fetal demise, uterine rupture, complications of postoperative tocolytic therapy, and the need for cesarean delivery in all future pregnancies. These risks are clearly outlined and discussed before consent is obtained. This meeting allows the family the opportunity to ask more questions and make decisions with the most complete information available.

Operative Management

Patients are admitted the morning of surgery for preoperative obstetrical monitoring. Prophylactic tocolysis with a 50 mg oral dose of indomethacin is started preoperatively. Large bore venous access is obtained and both epidural anesthesia and general anesthesia are used to provide pain relief to the mother and fetus and to provide maximal uterine relaxation. The mother is positioned to ensure sufficient lateral tilt to prevent compression of the vena cava by the gravid uterus that can impair venous return. Perioperative monitoring via an arterial line, a bladder catheter, electrocardiogram leads, and a transcutaneous pulse oximeter is undertaken. Maternal intraoperative fluid administration is conservatively managed to minimize the risk of postoperative pulmonary edema. Pneumatic compression boots are used to reduce the risk of venous thrombosis. After the laparotomy incision, sterile intraoperative ultrasound is used to confirm fetal position and placental location. Placental margins are localized and marked on the uterine surface using electrocautery. The uterine incision is planned so that the incision is at least 6 cm away from the placental edge but still allows exposure of the appropriate fetal anatomy. Manipulation of the fetal position is sometimes required prior to the hysterotomy in order to optimize fetal operative exposure.

Under sonographic guidance, two PDS (polydioxanone) stay sutures (Ethicon, New Brunswick, NJ) are placed parallel to the intended hysterotomy site and through the full thickness of the uterine wall to secure the membranes. Electrocautery is used to incise the myometrium between the stay sutures, through the full-thickness of the uterine wall and membranes. A uterine stapling device with absorbable Lactomer staples (US Surgical, Norwalk, CT) is then introduced under ultrasound guidance, using a piercing attachment that locks onto the lower limb of the stapler. Once the stapler is appropriately placed, it is deployed, anchoring the fetal membranes to the uterine wall, creating a hemostatic hysterotomy, and minimizing the risk of chorioamniotic separation. A second stapler is introduced to extend the incision in the opposite direction and care is taken to ensure hemostasis where the two staple lines overlap. The fetus is positioned with the appropriate portion of fetal anatomy visible through the incision. Only a minimal amount of the fetus is allowed to extrude through the incision. For surgery involving removal of fetal lung lesions or SCTs, intraoperative fetal monitoring is provided by the use of a miniaturized pulse oximeter wrapped around the fetal palm or foot and protected by aluminum foil and tegaderm to minimize light exposure and moisture. Continuous intraoperative fetal echocardiography is performed in all open fetal surgical procedures to monitor the fetal heart rate and ventricular function. The fetus receives an injection of a combination of fentanyl 20 mcg/kg, atropine 20 mcg/kg, and vecuronium 20 mcg/kg. The fentanyl provides intraoperative and postoperative fetal analgesia, atropine ablates the bradycardic response with fetal surgical manipulation, and vecuronium ensures that the fetus does not move during the surgical procedure. The fetus is kept warm and buoyant within the uterus through the use of a continuous intrauterine infusion of Ringer's Lactate warmed to between 37°C and 39°C and infused through a level I rapid infusion device. This maintains uterine volume and temperature and prevents compression of the umbilical cord and the placenta during the procedure. Care must be taken not to overfill the uterus as this can result in altered placental perfusion, risk of cervical change, and a higher risk for postoperative preterm labor.

After completion of the fetal surgery, a watertight two-layer uterine closure is performed with double-armed, full-thickness 0 PDS interrupted stay sutures followed by a running 0 PDS suture. Before completing the running layer, the amniotic fluid is reconstituted by infusing warmed Ringers Lactate through the level 1 pump catheter until ultrasound demonstrates a subjectively normal amniotic fluid volume. Near the end of the infusion, 500 mg of oxycillin or 900 mg of clindamycin is instilled into the amniotic cavity. The catheter is then withdrawn and the uterine closure is completed. An omental flap is mobilized and secured over the hysterotomy site. During closure of the hysterotomy, a 6-g intravenous loading dose of magnesium sulfate is administered to the mother over 20 minutes. The maternal abdomen is closed in anatomic layers. The skin is closed with a subcuticular suture and a transparent dressing applied so that postoperative monitoring can be performed.

Postoperative Management

Patients are transferred to the labor and delivery unit for the first 24–48 hours of postoperative care. Depending on the degree of uterine irritability, a continuous infusion of magnesium sulfate is maintained between 3 and 4 g/hr. This infusion is continued for 24 to 48 hours postoperatively while serum magnesium levels are monitored as needed, along with clinical evaluation for signs of magnesium toxicity. Indomethacin is administered postoperatively at a dose of 50 mg PR every six hours for the first 24 hours. This is decreased to 25 mg orally every six hours for another 24 hours if the patient remains free of contractions. Daily fetal echocardiography is performed during this time to monitor for signs of constriction of the ductus arteriosus, tricuspid regurgitation, or other signs of cardiac dysfunction. Pain relief is obtained by means of patient controlled epidural anesthesia. Patients are converted to a tocolytic regimen of nifedipine 10 to 20 mg every six hours by postoperative day 2. This is continued after discharge until delivery. Prophylactic intravenous antibiotics are continued for 24 hours postoperatively.

Uterine activity is monitored using an external tocodynamometer for the first 48 hours postoperatively. For previable fetuses, the fetal heart is auscultated on an every 4-hour basis. For viable fetuses, continuous external monitoring is performed. An ultrasound evaluation of the hysterotomy site, amniotic fluid volume, and Doppler studies of the umbilical vessels is undertaken daily while the patient remains hospitalized. Patients are gradually ambulated and discharge is arranged on the fourth postoperative day if they are stable and contraction free. Following discharge, management consists of bed rest and weekly assessment of both the mother and fetus. After two weeks, the maternal activity level is slowly increased but remains limited for the duration of the pregnancy. Since the midgestation hysterotomy is not located in a well-developed lower uterine segment, all pregnancies must be delivered by cesarean section to avoid the risk of uterine rupture. At 36 weeks, prior to undertaking delivery, an amniocentesis is performed to confirm lung maturity.

Complications to Open Fetal Surgery

Preterm labor and delivery remains the single most significant risk of fetal surgery and can minimize any benefits because of the complications of prematurity. The risks of premature labor appear to correlate with the degree of physiologic distress of the fetus undergoing surgery. Those fetuses undergoing an elective repair of a MMC have fewer complications than a hydropic fetus undergoing a resection of an intrathoracic lung mass.

Prior to instituting careful regulation of intraoperative fluids, noncardiogenic pulmonary edema was a frequent and serious complication in as many as 25% of cases. The combination of tocolytic therapy, generous intravenous hydration, and the release of vasoactive substances at the time of surgery resulted in increased maternal vascular permeability and pulmonary capillary leak. This risk peaks early on postoperative day 2. The use of careful restriction of intravenous fluids both intraoperatively and postoperatively has dramatically reduced the incidence of this complication.

Amniotic fluid leak can occur either into the abdomen, from the site of the hysterotomy or from the vagina as a result of membrane separation at the hysterotomy site. Chorioamniotic separation is a recognized complication that increases the risks of membrane rupture (1). Evaluation of the hysterotomy site for signs of membrane separation is a recommended part of the routine weekly assessment because of the increased risk of premature preterm rupture of the membranes (PPROM) with large membrane separations and potential need for urgent delivery should the membrane separation extend to involve the umbilical cord.

Indications for Open Fetal Surgery

At the present time only two anomalies can be considered to have been shown to have unequivocal, life-saving benefit from open fetal intervention: CCAM and fetal SCT. Each of these has a well-defined pathophysiology and a clear-cut natural history. Progressive enlargement of the lesion can lead to the development of hydrops that is associated with fetal death. A number of other anomalies, including CDH and obstructive uropathy have been investigated to determine if fetal intervention is beneficial. Significant questions remain to determine if we can accurately select those fetuses that may benefit from intervention and whether fetal intervention can alter and improve the natural history of the disease. Recently, the traditional rationale for fetal surgery has been challenged by the application of open maternal–fetal surgery to the repair of fetal MMC. As this is a nonlethal anomaly, the rationale for surgery is not to prevent fetal or neonatal death, but to prevent or reduce life-long disability. It remains to be demonstrated whether fetal surgery will reduce long-term disability that is associated with MMC. This is the subject of an ongoing multicenter randomized trial currently being supported by the National Institutes of Health (NICHD).

Fetal Lung Lesions

CCAM is a benign cystic lung mass that is usually lobar in distribution. It is characterized histologically by an overgrowth of terminal respiratory bronchioles that form cysts of various sizes and by a lack of normal alveolar development. Many consider CCAM to be a hamartoma. This is a developmental abnormality with an excess of one or several tissue components. Most CCAM lesions communicate with the bronchial tree and derive their blood supply from the pulmonary circulation (Fig. 1).

BPS is a nonfunctioning lung mass that arises as an aberrant out-pouching from the developing foregut and has a systemic blood supply. BPS can be intralobar or extralobar. An extralobar sequestration consists of pulmonary tissue that is enveloped in its own pleura and does not communicate with the tracheobronchial tree. It may occur above or below the diaphragm. The intralobar form is found within the normal lung tissue, with or without communication with the normal bronchial tree (Fig. 2).

Some lesions appear to contain elements of both lung lesions; they can be both cystic and solid and can demonstrate both pulmonary and systemic vascular supplies. We have classified these as hybrid lesions.

Congenital lobar emphysema is a lobar overinflation without destruction of alveolar septa and is more common in the upper or middle lobes. It may develop secondary to anomalous development of a lobar or segmental bronchus or from intrinsic/extrinsic bronchial compression. It can be difficult to distinguish from the other lung lesions antenatally.

Each of these lung lesions can present with varying clinical features and the natural history can follow quite a variable course depending on their size, rate of growth, and the relative amounts of cystic or solid components. A large lung mass with mediastinal shift that is diagnosed early in pregnancy can initially appear to carry a poor prognosis. These lesions can enlarge until the third trimester when they stabilize and start to regress with a decrease in size and secondary mass effects. The echo texture on ultrasound can also change, with the lesions becoming isoechoic with the surrounding lung, making them effectively disappear (2). Postnatal CT imaging,

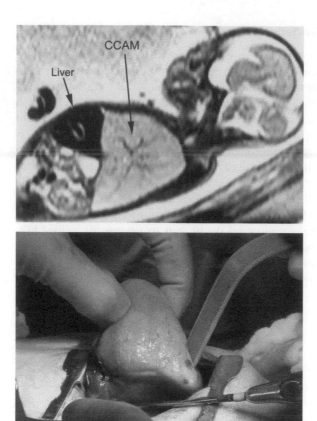

Figure 1 Fetal congenital cystic adenomatoid malformation. *Top panel*: Ultrafast fetal MRI image of very large microcystic CCAM filling the majority of the fetal chest, displacing the posterior diaphragm into the renal fossa and the kidney downward into the pelvis, and the heart and contralateral normal left lung against the left chest wall. *Lower panel*: Fetal mass resection following onset of hydrops. *Abbreviations*: MRI, magnetic resonance imaging; CCAM, congenital cystic adenomatoid malformation. (*See color insert.*)

however, will still reveal the presence of the lesion, thus, emphasizing the need for postnatal follow-up in all patients. Given the variable natural history and unpredictable growth potential, selection of fetuses that will need to undergo open excision can only be determined by close serial ultrasound observation to follow the rate of growth using the CCAM volume ratio (CVR) and screening for the onset of secondary complications such as hydrops or polyhydramnios. At each visit, the lesion is measured in three dimensions and the volume calculated using the formula for the volume of an ellipse (length × width × depth × 0.523). The CVR is determined by dividing this value by the head circumference to correct for increasing fetal size and gestational age (3).

The development of hydrops before 32 weeks' gestation is currently the only consistent indication for open surgery. In fetuses with large lesions (CVR >1.6), serial measurements of the CVR are made two to three times a week. Ascites is typically the first sign of hydropic change. The ascites does not seem to be related to cardiac dysfunction created by the shift of the heart, but rather to impaired venous return. Cardiac compression or obstruction of the great vessels by the expanding mass can contribute to the progression of hydropic changes by impairing cardiac

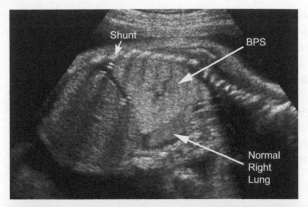

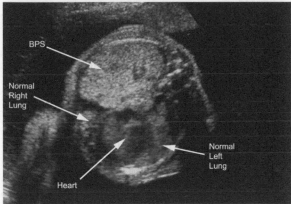

Figure 2 Fetal extralobar bronchopulmonary sequestration. *Top panel*: Sagittal view of the right chest with the large homogenous BPS mass, normal right lung compressed anterior, and residual effusion following placement of a thoracoamniotic shunt for a prior severe effusion. *Lower panel*: Transverse view, again showing large BPS, small effusion, displaced and compressed right lung, and mild mediastinal and cardiac shift to the left. *Abbreviation*: BPS, bronchopulmonary sequestration.

output and causing congestion in the liver. It is not until the fetus demonstrates further changes in terms of the development of pleural or pericardial effusions, skin or scalp edema, or placentomegally that open resection is indicated. Fetuses with solid, nonmacrocystic lesions and a CVR of ≤1.2 have not been shown to go on to develop hydrops. The same is not true for macrocystic lesions where rapid cyst expansion is possible.

If the fetus develops hydrops and the CCAM is of the macrocystic type, aspiration of the cyst(s) under ultrasound guidance can be a useful initial treatment. While many of the cysts will recur, drainage can provide a temporary decrease in size or volume of the lesion. This may slow or even halt the progression of hydrops. Reevaluation of the mass size and position following drainage can help to determine whether chronic drainage may be helpful and may help in planning the best position for placement of a thoracoamniotic shunt.

At the Children's Hospital of Philadelphia, open resection has been performed for lung lesions on 15 hydropic fetuses with eight survivors. In the earliest cases, it was observed that several fetuses exhibited a profound bradycardia following removal of the mass from the fetal chest. We postulated that the removal of cardiac compression resulted in pathophysiology similar to the abrupt relief of a pericardial tamponade with fetal hemodynamic collapse and bradycardia. These fetuses were also among the most physiologically compromised since advanced hydrops was present before open resection was considered. In the cases that have undergone open resection since 2000, intravenous access was established in the fetus prior to commencing the thoracotomy (4). Continuous fetal echocardiography is used to monitor cardiac function during thoracotomy and lobectomy. Appropriate fluid resuscitation is administered to the fetus during the surgery if there is any evidence of altered cardiac contractility as the lung mass is removed. The survival rate has improved since this change in procedure was initiated.

Sacrococcygeal Teratoma

SCT is the most common tumor in newborns. These are rarely associated with other congenital malformations or chromosomal anomalies. The tumors uniformly arise from the coccyx and are classified by the relative amounts of intrapelvic and external tumor. Type 1 is almost completely external, Type 2 is predominantly external but has a significant internal component, Type 3 is partially external but is predominantly internal with intra-abdominal extension, and Type 4 is located entirely within the pelvis and abdomen. This classification predicts the likelihood of prenatal detection, ease of resection, and likelihood of malignancy. Type 1 is easier to resect with a low incidence of malignancy while Type 4 is not amenable to fetal resection and is more likely to be malignant at the time of diagnosis when first diagnosed postnatally. An SCT diagnosed before birth carries a mortality rate of between 30% and 50%. A rapid phase of tumor growth in a predominantly solid, vascular tumor usually precedes the development of hydropic changes and impending fetal demise. Some lesions are unusually vascular resulting in shunting of large volumes of blood to the tumor (Fig. 3). This can create a state of high-output physiology that can lead to fetal cardiac failure.

Pregnancies complicated by the diagnosis of an SCT require intensive surveillance. Serial ultrasounds are required to assess fetal growth as well as the growth and echotexture of the mass. Frequent determinations of the combined cardiac output allow for assessment of the increased workload placed on the heart by the expanding mass. Measuring the diameter of the inferior vena cava can be used to reflect the degree of increased venous return that results from the perfusion of the mass. Doppler studies can demonstrate reversal of diastolic flow in the umbilical arteries as the lower resistance to flow in the tumor effectively "steals" blood from the fetus and placenta. The high output state can contribute to the development of polyhydramnios and premature rupture of the membranes resulting in premature delivery. There is also the possibility for spontaneous or traumatic tumor rupture and subsequent hemorrhage.

The fetus can be followed closely if no signs of high-output cardiac failure are observed. Serial amnioreductions can be used to manage the polyhydramnios for maternal discomfort, evidence of cervical change, or if preterm labor develops. If the lesion contains a significant cystic component, and if increasing size of the lesion places the pregnancy at risk for preterm labor, aspiration of the cyst can be considered to reduce the overall volume of the SCT. Cyst aspiration can also be considered prior to delivery to minimize mass size and the risk of rupture of the SCT. If hydropic changes develop after 30 weeks, delivery is indicated. Fetal surgery to resect an SCT can be considered if hydrops or placentomegally develop before that gestational age.

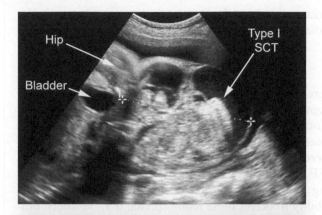

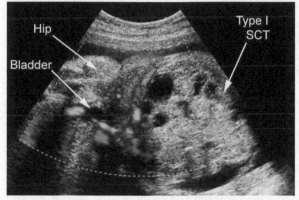

Figure 3 Fetal sacrococcygeal teratoma. *Top panel*: The predominately external SCT mass arising from the distal coccyx, containing both solid and cystic components. There is a small internal component that is not displacing the bladder or obstructing the ureters. *Lower panel*: Power Doppler image showing the rich blood supply to this tumor arising from the iliac vessels. *Abbreviation*: SCT, sacrococcygeal teratoma. (*See color insert.*)

Criteria for consideration of fetal surgery would include no maternal risk factors for anesthesia or surgery, a singleton pregnancy with a normal karyotype, no significant associated anomalies, and evidence of impending cardiac failure and favorable anatomy (Type 1 or 2). The development of Maternal Mirror Syndrome is a contraindication for fetal surgery and should be treated by immediate delivery. We reported on 30 SCT cases referred since 1995. Of these, four patients elected pregnancy termination, five had an intrauterine fetal demise, seven resulted in neonatal deaths, and 14 were survivors (5). Only four patients required open surgical resection because of hydropic changes with three of those having long-term survival. In the open surgery group, postsurgical preterm labor occurred in each case with the mean gestational age at delivery of 29 weeks (range 27.6–31.7 weeks) representing an average of five weeks from the time of fetal surgery to delivery (range 2.5–10.7 weeks). Postnatal hospital stay ranged from 16 to 34 weeks in the survivors. The one infant that did not survive was delivered for suspected chorioamnionitis four weeks postoperatively at 27.9 weeks. The fetus was severely depressed at birth with Apgar scores of 0^1, 0^5, and 4^{10}. This newborn died at six hours of age. On autopsy, there was evidence of significant cardiomegaly, a small pericardial effusion, and constriction of the ductus arteriosus. A second course of indomethacin had been administered for premature labor likely resulting in closure of the ductus arteriosus resulting in the development of biventricular hypertrophy and the newborn died from cardiac failure.

Myelomeningocele

The most recent condition where open maternal–fetal surgery has been applied is in selected cases of prenatally diagnosed MMC. MMC represent a failure of the distal neural tube to close during the fourth week of gestation. The lesion protrudes dorsally, is not covered by skin, and is usually associated with spinal-nerve paralysis. Leakage of α-fetoprotein (AFP) from the cerebrospinal fluid (CSF) into the amniotic fluid results in an increased transport of AFP into the maternal circulation. The use of second trimester maternal serum screening and the more routine use of midtrimester ultrasound have resulted in an increased ability to detect these lesions prenatally. Newborn outcome and disability vary greatly depending on the upper most level of the bony spinal defect. The ability to walk, control of bowel and bladder function, reproductive consequences in males, and degree of intracranial consequences of ventriculomegaly, the Chiari II malformation, and tethering of the spinal cord all contribute to determining the functional and neurodevelopmental disabilities these children face.

The exact etiology of MMC is poorly understood but is likely multifactorial. It was initially hypothesized that it is a disorder of neurulation during the embryonic development of the spinal cord. It is now thought that the primary disorder with MMC may not be neural but rather a mesoderm-related malformation of the posterior spine, meninges, and soft tissues leading to spina bifida, dorsally nonclosed dura and pia mater, and thus exposure of the spinal cord. Experimental work has shown that the unprotected but otherwise normal neural tissue is progressively damaged by exposure to the amniotic fluid and by direct trauma as a result of fetal movement and contact with the uterine wall resulting in mechanical trauma (Fig. 4).

Unlike other conditions where maternal–fetal surgery has been successfully applied, spina bifida is not a lethal anomaly. Thus, prior to the application of in utero closure in human fetuses, considerable animal experimentation has taken place to demonstrate the potential for long-term benefits in reducing chronic morbidity. Meuli et al. demonstrated that lesions, remarkably similar to human MMC, could be produced experimentally in fetal sheep by exposing the lumbar spinal cord to amniotic fluid by performing a dorsal laminectomy. This involved resecting the overlying skin, soft tissue, and posterior bony spinal elements (6). The same authors showed that subsequent delayed in utero closure of the muscle and skin layers over these created lesions decreased the expected spinal cord damage and preserved neurologic function (7,8). These studies demonstrated not only the technical feasibility of open fetal repair of spina bifida but also that in utero repair may prevent or diminish the ongoing neurological injury in human fetuses that contributes to the chronic disability experienced by children with open neural tube defects.

It is recognized that fetuses with thoracolumbar lesions have the poorest functional outcomes, while those with lower lesions tend to have better outcomes (9). With the significant risks associated with fetal surgery, fetal repair was initially only offered to patients carrying a fetus with a large lower thoracic or lumbar level defect, an Arnold–Chiari malformation, mild to moderate ventriculomegaly, normal leg movements, no apparent talipes deformity of the foot, a normal karyotype, and no other structural anomalies.

An initial review of the first 10 patients undergoing open fetal closure of MMC between 22 and 25 weeks at The Children's Hospital of Philadelphia demonstrated

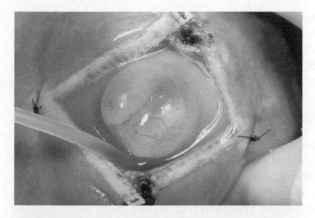

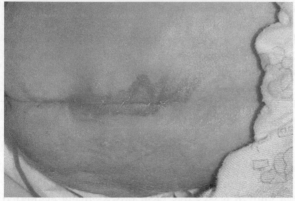

Figure 4 Fetal myelomeningocele. *Top panel*: Characteristic lower lumbosacral myelomeningocele at the time of fetal neurosurgical closure. *Lower panel*: Fetal repair site in the same infant after birth in the newborn nursery. (*See color insert.*)

improvement in hindbrain herniation on serial MRI scans (10). While one fetus delivered prematurely at 25 weeks and died from complications of prematurity, the remaining nine showed ascent of the hindbrain and increased CSF around the posterior fossa while still in utero. Bruner et al. reported similar findings after MMC repair performed between 24 and 30 weeks gestation (11). In addition, the need for ventriculoperitoneal shunting was less in the prenatal repair group compared to a historical control group of newborns undergoing postnatal repair. A retrospective review of 50 fetuses that underwent open fetal MMC closure at the Children's Hospital of Philadelphia demonstrated consistent in utero resolution of the hindbrain herniation and a slowing of the progress of ventriculomegaly (12). Reversal of hindbrain herniation and restoration of the extra-axial CSF spaces may slow progressive ventriculomegaly and the need for postnatal shunting. Perinatal survival in this study was 94% with only 43% of the fetuses requiring ventriculoperitoneal shunting compared to 85% in a group of historical controls (13).

Maternal–fetal surgery for MMC represents a departure from previous situations where the conditions treated were potentially lethal. Since the goal of MMC repair is to prevent or reduce lifelong morbidity, there is an increased need for more rigorous evaluation before this therapy is widely adopted. The NIH is currently supporting the Management of Myelomeningocele Study, a prospective, randomized controlled trial to compare standard postnatal repair with prenatal fetal repair between 20 and 26 weeks gestation. Multiple short-term and long-term outcomes are being assessed including survival, need for ventriculo-peritoneal shunting, bowel and bladder function, neurodevelopmental, functional, and psychosocial outcomes in these two groups of children.

Congenital Diaphragmatic Hernia

CDH represents a simple anatomic defect with profound physiologic consequences. It is thought to result from a failure of the pleuroperitoneal canal to close between 9 and 10 weeks' gestation. This allows herniation of abdominal viscera into the thoracic cavity. The herniation typically occurs during the pseudoglandular stage of lung development. This means that the major bronchial buds have formed but branching of the bronchial tree may be limited by the mass effect of the herniated viscera. The number of alveoli that develop is also limited. The pulmonary vascular bed is abnormal with fewer vessels present. Those that develop are smaller in caliber with muscular hyperplasia of the medial layer. Pulmonary hypoplasia and pulmonary hypertension are the primary postnatal sequellae that limit survival. Eighty-nine percent of CDH cases are left-sided, 9% are right-sided, and in 2% the defect is bilateral.

Previously, the presence of liver herniation (Fig. 5) was used to differentiate between good prognosis and poor prognosis cases (14,15). When the liver is not herniated into the fetal chest, survival is >90%. When the liver is herniated into the chest, survival falls dramatically to as low as 43%. The lung-to-head circumference ratio (LHR) is a two-dimensional measurement of the cross-sectional area of the right lung performed at the level of the four-chamber cardiac view. This measurement, when performed between 24 and 26 weeks has been prospectively evaluated as a predictor of outcome. In a review of patients at our institution from 1995 to 1999, survival was 85% with an LHR of >1.4. For an LHR between 1 and 1.4, survival dropped to 56% while for an LHR <1, no infants survived. A more recent review encompassing data from 1999 to 2004 has shown that with an LHR >1.4, survival is >90%. With an LHR between 1 and 1.4, survival dropped slightly to 85%. For the group with an LHR <1, survival was 60%. These figures likely reflect significant improvements in the postnatal management of newborns with CDH. Still, the combination of liver herniation and an LHR <1 identifies a group of fetuses with the poorest prognosis when managed with conventional postnatal treatment. This extremely at-risk group of fetuses would be the most appropriate group to evaluate the benefits, if any, of maternal–fetal surgery for CDH.

Initial attempts to complete an in utero open CDH repair were technically impossible when liver herniation was present. Fetal demise was related to an inability to completely reduce the liver and obtain an adequate repair and because acute reduction compromised umbilical venous and ductus venosus flow, resulting in fetal bradycardia and cardiac arrest (16). Attempts at open hysterotomy and repair of the diaphragmatic defect did not improve outcomes in prospective controlled and retrospective studies (17). More recent efforts at in utero treatment of CDH have utilized tracheal occlusion. In animal models, occlusion has been demonstrated to prevent the normal egress of lung fluid and promote lung growth. Initially, hemoclips were applied to the external surface of the fetal trachea under direct visualization. Subsequently, a video-endoscopic technique was developed (Fetendo Clip) where hysterotomy was not required (18). Complications related to uniform premature delivery, recurrent laryngeal nerve injury related to the tracheal dissection, and to long-term

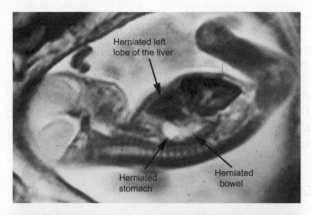

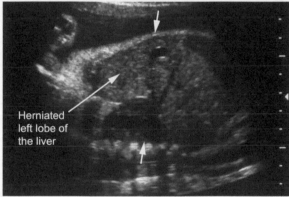

Figure 5 Fetal congenital diaphragmatic hernia. *Top panel*: Ultrafast fetal MRI image of a left-sided CDH showing the presence of bowel, stomach, and the left lobe of the fetal liver in the chest. *Lower panel*: Sonographic image of another fetus with a left-sided CDH showing herniation of a large portion of the left lobe of the liver into the chest. The *white arrows* show the level of the defect in the diaphragm. *Abbreviations*: MRI, magnetic resonance imaging; CDH, congenital diaphragmatic hernia.

morbidity in those newborns that survived. Maternal morbidity was also significant as reflected in the high incidence of chorioamniotic membrane separation, PPROM, pulmonary edema, and preterm delivery.

More recently, tracheal occlusion has been achieved through the endoscopic placement of a detachable balloon device in the fetal trachea midway between the vocal cords and the carina. As with other methods of tracheal occlusion, delivery by an EXIT (Ex-Utero Intrapartum Treatment) procedure is required in order for the occlusion to be removed before the fetus is separated from the placental circulation. A randomized controlled trial was performed comparing endoscopic tracheal occlusion using a detachable silicone balloon with standard postnatal care in fetuses with a severe left-sided CDH (19). The primary outcome was survival to 90 days of age. The study was discontinued after 24 of 40 patients were randomized because the survival in the two groups was similar. In the group randomized to standard care, 73% survived; while in the group that underwent in utero occlusion, survival was 77%. The group that underwent tracheal occlusion experienced significantly more postnatal morbidity. As a result of this study, in utero surgery for CDH continues to be studied in the laboratory but is no longer offered as a clinical treatment in North America. A recent case series of endoscopic tracheal occlusion has been reported by the FETO Task group in Europe (20). Their technique is similar to that reported on by Harrison et al. except that the procedure was performed without maternal laparotomy and many of the cases were performed under a combination of regional and local anesthesia instead of general anesthesia. As the survival rate from postnatal management of CHD varies from center to center, and as continued improvements occur in postnatal care, the decision on whether to adopt this technique outside of North America remains to be made.

MATERNAL RISKS OF MATERNAL–FETAL SURGERY

Any open maternal–fetal surgery includes risks to the mother, not only related to the primary surgery but also associated with the eventual surgical delivery and to all subsequent pregnancies. Morbidity related to the initial surgery can be associated with surgical bleeding or infection. Anesthesia complications can occur related to either the use of regional or general anesthesia. Side effects can occur from the medications used to prevent preterm labor in the perioperative period. Preterm PROM and preterm labor can result in prolonged hospitalization and the use of additional tocolytic therapy. Since the hysterotomy performed at the time of fetal surgery is usually located in the fundus of the uterus, there is a risk for uterine rupture as the pregnancy progresses regardless of any preterm labor that may ensue. Additional surgical risks, typical for any repeat surgery, are associated with the need for cesarean section for delivery in these cases.

Future pregnancies are also at increased risk related to weakness created by the initial surgical hysterotomy. A recent retrospective survey of 55 former fetal surgery patients assessed outcomes in 34 pregnancies occurring in 29 patients (21). There were greater than expected risks of spontaneous loss (18%) and preterm delivery (24%). Only 58% of the pregnancies resulted in a term delivery. Uterine dehiscence (four cases) or rupture (two cases) occurred in 18% of the study group. Cesarean hysterectomy was required in one case related to hemorrhage. The interpregnancy interval did appear to affect the rate of complications. This study was limited by its small numbers and retrospective nature but does indicate that there are increased risks that extend beyond the index pregnancy.

THE FUTURE

The field of maternal–fetal surgery continues to be an important area for research and development of new techniques and technology in conditions with a poor prognosis for the neonate. Many of the advances will likely utilize less invasive procedures as evidenced by the evolution of the techniques for CDH repair. Any advances, however, must be subjected to rigorous evaluation to determine whether treatments are effective. These evaluations must include long-term evaluation of outcomes including neurodevelopmental, cognitive, and quality of life indices for the newborn. Management of preterm labor and prevention of membrane separation leading to PPROM remain the primary challenges in fetal surgery. Consideration must always be given to the maternal risks in the index as well as future pregnancies when counseling these patients.

REFERENCES

1. Wilson RD, Johnson MP, Flake AW, et al. Chorioamniotic membrane separation following open fetal surgery: Pregnancy outcome. Fetal Diagn Ther 2003; 18:314–320.
2. Winters WD, Effman EL, Nghiem HV, Nyberg DA. Disappearing fetal lung masses: importance of postnatal imaging studies. Pediatr Radiol 1997; 27:535–539.
3. Crombleholme TM, Coleman B, Hedrick H, et al. Cystic adenomatoid malformation volume ratio predicts outcome in prenatally diagnosed cystic adenomatoid malformation of the lung. J Pediatr Surg 2002; 37:331–338.
4. Keswani SG, Crombleholme TM, Rychik J, et al. Impact of continuous intraoperative monitoring on outcomes in open fetal surgery. Fetal Diagn Ther 2005; 20(4):316–320.
5. Hedrick HL, Flake AW, Crombleholme TM, et al. Sacrococcygeal teratoma: prenatal assessment, fetal intervention and outcome. J Pediatr Surg 2004; 39:430–438.
6. Meuli M, Meuli-Simmon C, Yingling CD, et al. Creation of myelomeningocele in utero: a model of functional damage from spinal cord exposure in fetal sheep. J Pediatr Surg 1995; 30:1028–1033.
7. Meuli M, Meuli-Simmon C, Hutchins GM, et al. In utero surgery rescues neurological function at birth in sheep with spina bifida. Nat Med 1995; 1:342–347.
8. Meuli M, Meuli-Simmon C, Yingling CD, et al. In utero repair of experimental myelomeningocele saves neurologic function at birth. J Pediatr Surg 1996; 31:397–402.
9. Cochrane DD, Wilson RD, Stienbok P, et al. Prenatal spinal evaluation and functional outcome of patients born with melomeningocele: information for improved prenatal counselling and outcome prediction. Fetal Diagn Ther 1996; 11:159–168.
10. Sutton LN, Adzick NS, Bilaniuk LT, Johnson MP, Crombleholme TM, Flake AW. Improvement in hindbrain herniation demonstrated by serial fetal magnetic resonance imaging following fetal surgery for myelomeningocele. J Am Med Assoc 1999; 282: 1826–1831.
11. Bruner JP, Tulipan NB, Paschall RL, et al. Fetal surgery for myelomeningocele, and the incidence of shunt-dependant hydrocephalus. J Am Med Assoc 1999; 282:1819–1825.
12. Johnson MP, Sutton LN, Rintoul N, et al. Fetal myelomeningocele repair: short-term clinical outcomes. Am J Obstet Gynecol 2003; 189:482–487.
13. Rintoul NE, Sutton LN, Hubbard AM, et al. A new look at myelomeningoceles: functional level, vertebral level, shunting and the implications for fetal intervention. Pediatrics 2002; 109:1–5.
14. Metkus AP, Filly RA, Stringer MD, Harrison MR, Adzick NS. Sonographic predictors of survival in fetal diaphragmatic hernia. J Pediatr Surg 1996; 31:148–152.
15. Albanese CT, Lopoo J, Goldstein RB, et al. Fetal liver position and perinatal outcome for congenital diaphragmatic hernia. Prenat Diagn 1998; 18:1138–1142.
16. Flake A. Fetal surgery for congenital diaphragmatic hernia. Semin Pediatr Surg 1996; 5:266–274.
17. Harrison MR, Adzick NS, Bullard KM, et al. Correction of congenital diaphragmatic hernia in utero. VII. A prospective trial. J Pediatr Surg 1997; 32:1637–1642.
18. Harrison MR, Sydorak RM, Farrell JA, Kitterman JA, Filly RA, Albanese CT. Fetoscopic temporary tracheal occlusion for congenital diaphragmatic hernia: prelude to a randomized controlled trial. J Pediatr Surg 2003; 38:1012–1020.
19. Harrison MR, Keller RL, Hawgood SB, et al. A randomized trial of fetal endoscopic tracheal occlusion for severe fetal congenital diaphragmatic hernia. N Engl J Med 2003; 349:1916–1924.
20. Deprest J, Gratacos E, Nicolaides KH. Fetoscopic tracheal occlusion (FETO) for severe congenital diaphragmatic hernia: evolution of a technique and preliminary results. Ultrasound Obstet Gynecol 2004; 24:121–126.
21. Wilson RD, Johnson MP, Flake AW, et al. Reproductive outcomes after pregnancy complicated by maternal-fetal surgery. Am J Obstet Gynecol 2004; 191:1430–1436.

28
Termination of Pregnancy

Oi Shan Tang and Pak Chung Ho
Department of Obstetrics and Gynecology, Queen Mary Hospital,
Pokfulam, Hong Kong, Special Administrative Region, China

INTRODUCTION

The advances in the technology of prenatal diagnosis have made great changes in the management of fetal abnormality. The pregnant woman expects a normal and healthy baby. In the past, only the high-risk women were offered prenatal diagnostic tests or ultrasound examination to detect fetal abnormalities. Now, various screening tests and ultrasound examinations are available to exclude fetal abnormalities even in low-risk women. Screening tests using serum markers and nuchal thickness are commonly performed in many parts of the world to screen for Down syndrome. Routine ultrasound examination has been incorporated in many antenatal care programs to look for fetal structural abnormalities. As a result, more and more abnormal fetuses can be detected before viability. In the past, most of the fetal abnormalities were diagnosed in the second trimester. Now, the availability of first trimester serum screening and late first trimester ultrasound screening has made the detection of many fetal abnormalities possible at the late first trimester. While some of the fetal abnormalities may be amenable to prenatal therapy, most of the others will either be fatal or result in the delivery of babies with severe handicaps. Therefore, the majority of these women may have to make a decision on termination of pregnancy when they face the diagnosis of fetal anomaly.

It is always a difficult and emotionally stressful situation for a mother to terminate a wanted pregnancy. As soon as the diagnosis is made, the mother has to cope with it and make the decision to terminate the pregnancy. Subsequently, she has to go through the abortion process, which is sometimes painful and distressing, not to mention the possible risks associated with the procedures.

Most of the terminations of pregnancies for fetal anomaly are performed in the second trimester. In the past, before the availability of prostaglandin analogues, dilatation and evacuation (D&E), oxytocin infusion, and amniofusion of hypertonic saline or urea were the commonest methods for termination of pregnancy in the second trimester. Hypertonic saline instillation is associated with maternal hypernatrinemia and coagulation defects. Oxytocin infusion is not an effective method of abortion in the second trimester and is associated with complications, such as water intoxification.

509

These two methods are seldom used these days. D&E remains the commonest surgical method for second-trimester abortion.

If the diagnosis of fetal anomaly can be made in the first trimester, termination of pregnancy is usually performed by vacuum aspiration. Recently, the use of the combination of mifepristone and a prostaglandin analogue has been explored for medical abortion in the late first trimester.

METHODS OF ABORTION IN THE FIRST TRIMESTER

Vacuum Aspiration

Vacuum aspiration is commonly performed for termination of pregnancy at gestational age <12 weeks, and some experienced operators use vacuum aspiration for up to 14 weeks. Vacuum aspiration is currently the standard management for termination of pregnancy in the first trimester in many parts of the world. It is considered to be safe and effective with a success rate >95% (1). The procedure usually takes about 5–10 minutes. It can be done under local or general anesthesia depending on the needs of the women undergoing abortion. The cervix is gradually dilated to the necessary dilatation, depending on the gestational age, using dilators with increasing diameters. This is followed by the use of a plastic or metal cannula to evacuate the uterine contents by vacuum force. An electrical vacuum pump is more commonly used but manual vacuum aspiration may also be used in early gestations.

Vacuum aspiration is a very safe procedure although complications such as excessive hemorrhage, incomplete abortion, cervical tear, and uterine perforation may occur. It is associated with major morbidity in up to 1% of women and minor morbidity in 10% (2). In a more recent study of 170,000 first-trimester abortions carried out in New York City, only <0.1% of the women experienced serious complications requiring hospitalization (3). It appears that the incidence of severe morbidity associated with abortion has decreased recently in some of the developed countries. The seniority of the surgeon performing the procedure was found to affect the outcome of the surgical evacuation (4). The risk is also increased when difficulty is encountered during cervical dilatation, especially in nulliparous women. Various methods have been used for cervical priming before vacuum aspiration including osmotic dilators, mifepristone, and prostaglandin analogues. These days, vacuum aspiration is usually performed as a day-patient procedure. Osmotic dilators have to be inserted 12 hours before and mifepristone has to be taken 36–48 hours before the operation to produce adequate cervical priming effect. Therefore, they are less suitable for day-patients. Prostaglandin analogues are the cervical priming agents of choice, and misoprostol has been widely studied for this purpose (5). A single dose of 400 μg misoprostol given orally, vaginally, or sublingually three hours before the scheduled operation was found to be effective as a cervical priming agent (6,7). Misoprostol is also cheap and the incidence of side effects is low.

Dilatation and Curettage

Dilatation and curettage is different from vacuum aspiration. It involves the dilatation of the cervix followed by the use of sharp curettage to scrape the wall of the uterus. This procedure is not as safe as vacuum aspiration and is associated with more blood loss and major complications (8). A recent Cochrane review on the surgical methods for first-trimester abortion did not show any significant difference in the incidence of major complications, including excessive blood loss, blood transfusion, febrile morbidity, incomplete or repeat uterine evacuation procedure, rehospitalization, post-operative abdominal pain, or therapeutic antibiotic use, between dilatation and curettage and vacuum aspiration; however, the studies involved were small and lacked power to show any meaningful difference between the two methods (9). The only significant finding was the duration of operation, which was significantly shorter with vacuum aspiration when compared to dilatation and curettage. However, vacuum aspiration has replaced dilatation and curettage as the main surgical method of abortion in the first trimester.

Medical Abortion

Prostaglandins were known to terminate early pregnancies by the 1960s. However, prostaglandins and their analogues that were used in the 1960s and 1970s were associated with a high incidence of side effects like vomiting, diarrhea, and fever. Besides, repeated doses were required if prostaglandins were used alone. The introduction of the antiprogestogen mifepristone in the late 1980s led to extensive studies of medical abortion using mifepristone in combination with various prostaglandin analogues.

Progesterone maintains the uterus in a quiescent state by inducing hyperpolarization of the membrane of the myometrial cells, and a greater change in electric potential is necessary before contractions can occur (10). Progesterone antagonists are synthetic steroids that bind to the progesterone receptors and prevent endogenous progesterone from exerting its effects (11). Mifepristone is the antiprogesterone that is approved for use clinically for induction of abortion. It can increase the sensitivity of the uterus to prostaglandins. However, the complete abortion rate of using mifepristone alone was only 60–80% for termination of early pregnancy <6 weeks of gestation (12). This complete abortion rate is obviously not acceptable compared to surgical abortion, which has a complete abortion rate of >95%. It was then recognized that the complete abortion rate could be increased to 95% when mifepristone was combined with a suitable prostaglandin analogue (13,14). This regimen, consisting of a single dose of 600 mg mifepristone followed 48 hours later by either injection of sulprostone 0.25 mg or gemeprost 1 mg vaginal pessary, was tested extensively in large clinical trials (15,16). However, the use of sulprostone for the purpose of medical abortion was withdrawn following the report of a death due to myocardial infarction in association with its use (17).

Misoprostol is currently the commonest prostaglandin analogue used for the purpose of medical abortion in the first trimester. It has the advantages of being cheap and stable at room temperature when compared to gemeprost. Misoprostol is manufactured and licensed for oral use. The complete abortion rate with oral misoprostol, when combined with mifepristone, declines with increase in gestational age. The complete abortion rates were 92%, 83%, and 77% for gestational age of <49 days, 50–56 days, and 57–63 days, respectively (18). Subsequently, it was found that misoprostol could be administered vaginally. This route of administration was more potent when compared to the oral route in medical abortion (18). The complete abortion rate achieved by using mifepristone followed 48 hours later by 800 μg of vaginal misoprostol was 95–98% for up to 63 days of gestation (19–21). A randomized trial comparing 0.5 mg vaginal gemeprost with 800 μg vaginal misoprostol, after pretreatment with 200 mg mifepristone, showed that vaginal misoprostol was superior to gemeprost with a higher complete abortion rate, and fewer incomplete abortions and ongoing pregnancies. The incidences of side effects were similar. Therefore, vaginal misoprostol is currently the prostaglandin analogue of choice for medical abortion in the first trimester (21). The regimens mentioned above involve the use of mifepristone 200–600 mg given 48 hours before the administration of a prostaglandin analogue. The registered dose of mifepristone used for medical abortion in the first trimester is 600 mg. However, it has been shown in several studies that 200 mg was as effective as 600 mg for this purpose (22,23).

Complications with mifepristone and misoprostol for medical abortion are rare. Gastrointestinal symptoms, like diarrhea, vomiting, and fever are common with the use of misoprostol, but they are usually self-limiting. Other possible complications associated with medical abortion are hemorrhage, infection, and allergic reaction to the drugs.

Many of the prenatal diagnostic tests available currently cannot establish a definite diagnosis earlier than 63 days of gestation. The complete abortion rate of the regimen mentioned above, using a combination of mifepristone and a single dose of prostaglandin analogue is <90% when used beyond nine weeks of gestation. Additional doses of prostaglandin analogues are required to achieve a complete abortion rate of over 90% (24). However, the induction to abortion interval is increased when repeated doses of prostaglandin analogues are required. Therefore, vacuum aspiration may still be the preferred method of first-trimester abortion beyond nine weeks of gestation.

METHODS OF ABORTION IN THE SECOND TRIMESTER

Abortion in the second trimester can be performed either medically with mifepristone and prostaglandin analogues or surgically by D&E. The choice of the method used is sometimes a matter of preference of the gynecologists or the women undergoing abortion. As a matter of fact, D&E is more commonly used in the United States for abortion in the second trimester, whereas medical abortion is the preferred method in the United Kingdom.

Dilatation and Evacuation

D&E is the surgical method of choice for termination of pregnancy beyond 12 weeks of gestation. It is a quick procedure and can be performed as a day-patient procedure under local or general anesthesia. In order to remove the relatively large fetal parts, especially the fetal head, cervical dilatation to 14–16 mm is required. The membrane is ruptured, and the amniotic fluid is aspirated with suction cannula. The fetal parts and the placenta are then removed by the use of forceps (Sofer or Bierer). To minimize the risk of perforation and incomplete evacuation, the procedure is now commonly performed under ultrasound guidance. The fetal parts and the placenta should be examined carefully at the end of the procedure to ensure that the abortion is complete. Cervical priming is an essential part of this procedure. It has been shown that preoperative cervical priming can increase the safety of the procedure (25). It is actually the recommendation of the World Health Organization that cervical preparation should precede all abortions induced after 14 weeks of gestation (26). Adequate cervical priming can decrease the risk of cervical tears, uterine perforation, and incomplete evacuation of the uterus. Cervical priming can be performed by intracervical tents, mifepristone, or prostaglandin analogues. Laminaria tents, Lamicel, and Dilapan are the intracervical tents that can be used for this purpose.

Laminaria tents (*Laminaria japonica* or *digitata*) are derived from seaweed, which is dried and compressed into rods of about 5-cm long with variable widths. A thread is present at one end to aid extraction. The tents swell up slowly in the presence of moisture (hygroscopic), and increase to a size of about three to five times the original diameter within 4–12 hours. This also enhances the softening of the cervix. Lamicel and Dilapan are synthetic slow dilators. Lamicel is made of polyvinyl alcohol polymer sponge impregnated with approximately 450 mg of magnesium sulfate to form a cylindrical tent with a diameter of 3–5 mm and a length of 75 mm. This dilator swells up to about four times its dry size by absorption of water from neighboring cervical tissues. Dilapan is a hydrophilic polymer made of polyacrylonitrile. It swells up more rapidly and dilates more effectively than other slow dilators as it opens the cervix from 5 to 12 mm within 2–4 hours. It acts mainly via mechanical forces, although enzymatic and local humoral factors inducing cervical softening appear to be involved to a lesser extent. Its removal is more difficult due to the impaction in the cervix particularly if it is left inside the cervix for >4 hours. Pharmacological means of cervical priming such as misoprostol and mifepristone have been found to be as effective as intracervical tents (27,28). Misoprostol has advantages over the other agents since it is cheap and easily available. It can be given orally, vaginally, and sublingually, and it takes only 3 hours to achieve the cervical priming effect when compared to the other agents, which may take a day to work. Thus, misoprostol is considered to be more convenient especially for day-surgery procedures.

Apart from ultrasound guidance and cervical priming, the safety of D&E depends very much on the skill and experience of the operator. Second-trimester abortion by D&E, preceded by cervical preparation, is a safe and effective method when undertaken by specialist practitioners with access to the necessary instruments and who also have a sufficiently large case-load to maintain their skills (29).

The possible complications of D&E are cervical damage, uterine perforation, incomplete abortion, and infection. The risks of these complications increase with the gestational age when the procedure is performed (8). Although these complications are rare in expert hands, they may result in serious consequences which may jeopardize the future fertility potential of the women.

D&E is the method of choice for abortion in the second trimester in many parts of the world. This is a quick surgical procedure, which can be done under adequate anesthesia, and the woman does not have to go through a painful abortion procedure.

Medical Abortion

Before the availability of prostaglandin (PG) analogues, oxytocin infusion, and amniofusion of hypertonic saline or urea were the commonest medical methods used for termination of pregnancy in the second trimester. Hypertonic saline instillation may be associated with maternal hypernatrinemia and coagulation defects. Oxytocin infusion is not an effective method of abortion in the second trimester and is associated with complications like water intoxication. These two methods are seldom used anymore. The introduction of prostaglandin analogues in the late 1970s changed the management of medical termination of pregnancy in the second trimester. With the use of the antiprogestogen, mifepristone, the induction to abortion interval is shortened, and the dosage of prostaglandin analogue required is reduced. Currently, medical abortion is the method of choice in many centers that perform second trimester termination of pregnancy.

Prostaglandins can stimulate myometrial contraction and cause cervical ripening and dilatation. Their receptors exist throughout all stages of pregnancy and thus, prostaglandins and their analogues are effective in termination of first- and second-trimester pregnancy. The natural prostaglandins, $PGF_{2\alpha}$ and PGE_2 were first tested clinically for second trimester medical abortion but they were soon replaced by prostaglandin analogues because of their high incidence of gastrointestinal side effects when given parenterally or vaginally, especially with repeated administration. Prostaglandin analogues are relatively resistant to metabolism and, therefore, have prolonged action (10). The PGE analogue is preferable as it has more selective action on the myometrium and causes less gastrointestinal side effects (30). The three most extensively studied PGE analogues are sulprostone, gemeprost, and misoprostol.

Prostaglandin-Alone Regimens

Sulprostone (16-phenoxy-ω-17,18,19,20-tetranor PGE_2 methyl sulphonylamide) was studied in the early 1980s for medical abortion in the second trimester (30). It is usually given intramuscularly at a dose of 0.5 mg every four hours. It is more convenient than intra- or extra-amniotic administration. However, intramuscular sulprostone is no longer used clinically for medical abortion because of its association with myocardial infarction (17). Therefore, the two remaining PGE analogues, gemeprost and misoprostol, are the principal drugs used for second trimester medical abortion now.

Gemeprost (16,16-dimethyl trans-Δ^2 PGE_1 methyl ester) is a PGE_1 analogue. It is given in the form of a vaginal pessary. The studies using a vaginal gemeprost only regimen gave a complete abortion rate of 88–96.5% in 48 hours (31–33). The commonest regimen is 1 mg every three hours for five doses in the first 24 hours. The regimen is repeated if abortion does not occur in 24 hours. The induction to abortion interval ranged from 14 to 18 hours. The commonest side effects were vomiting, diarrhea, and fever. It was shown in one study that increasing the dosing interval to every six hours did not compromise the abortion rate or the induction to abortion interval for 12 to 18 weeks of gestation (34). It had the advantages of using fewer pessaries and caused fewer side effects. Cost and the need for storage in a refrigerator are the drawbacks of gemeprost. These make its use only practicable in prosperous countries.

Misoprostol (15-deoxy-16-hydroxy-16-methyl PGE_1), a synthetic PGE_1 analogue, was initially developed orally for the prevention and treatment of peptic ulcer. Later on, it was discovered that it could be used off-label as an abortifacient. It is cheap, stable at room temperature and is easily available in many developing countries. Most of the misoprostol only regimens that were studied in the second trimester involved the use of the vaginal route. It had been demonstrated by a pharmacokinetic study that the systemic bioavailability of vaginally administered misoprostol was three times higher than that of orally administered misoprostol. With vaginal administration, peak plasma levels were reached more slowly and slightly lower but were sustained for up to four hours (35). The studies comparing oral with vaginal administration of misoprostol in second-trimester abortion showed that the vaginal route was more effective (36). In the literature, the dosage of misoprostol used in the studies involving misoprostol alone regimen varied from 100 to 600 μg, and the dosing interval ranged from 3 to 12 hours. A randomized study demonstrated that misoprostol 400 μg given vaginally every three hours was the optimal regimen for second-trimester abortion, and the complete abortion rate and induction to abortion interval was compromised by increasing the dosing interval to six hours (37). This finding was compatible with the previous pharmacokinetic study of vaginal misoprostol, which showed that the plasma level was sustained for up to four hours after administration (35). This regimen of misoprostol had been shown by randomized study to be more effective when compared with the standard regimen of gemeprost (33). Vaginal misoprostol is now the preferred method of medical abortion for the second trimester because of its efficacy, low cost, and drug stability at room temperature. The long induction to abortion interval is the main disadvantage of prostaglandin-only regimen. It may take a median of 15 hours for the abortion to occur.

Mifepristone plus Prostaglandin Regimen

Mifepristone is the antiprogestogen that is approved for use clinically for induction of abortion. It increases the sensitivity of the uterus to prostaglandins. The use of oral mifepristone 36–48 hours before prostaglandin administration can increase the abortion rate, shorten the induction to abortion interval, and reduce the amount of prostaglandin required in second-trimester abortion (38–43). The recommended dose of mifepristone is 600 mg, but it has been shown in a randomized trial that the abortion rate and induction to abortion interval were the same even if the dose was reduced to 200 mg (44).

If mifepristone pretreatment was used before gemeprost (1 mg every 6 hours), the induction to abortion interval could be decreased from 15.7 to 6.6 hours, and the abortion rate in 24 hours was increased from 72% to 95% (38). The efficacy of this regimen has been confirmed in another two larger series (42,43). The dosage of gemeprost can be further decreased to 0.5 mg every 6 hours without jeopardizing the abortion rate and induction to abortion interval (45).

Mifepristone can shorten the induction to abortion interval of a regimen using misoprostol as well. A regimen using mifepristone in combination with vaginal and oral misoprostol was developed, which involved the use of 600 μg vaginal misoprostol as the first dose followed by 400 μg oral misoprostol every three hours up to a maximum of four doses. The abortion rate (97%) and the induction to abortion interval (6.5 hours) were the same as using similar doses of vaginal misoprostol (46). The results were later confirmed by a larger series of patients using a slightly higher initial dose of vaginal misoprostol (800 μg). It was believed that the use of vaginal misoprostol as the first dose could lead to more effective cervical priming, and there was no advantage in the vaginal administration of subsequent doses (41). There may be a need for surgical evacuation for retained placenta or incomplete abortion. The surgical evacuation rate is about 10%, and the rate decreases with experience (47).

Side Effects and Complications of Medical Abortion in the Second Trimester

In general, the use of prostaglandins, gemeprost, and misoprostol, with or without mifepristone, is safe and effective for medical abortion in the second trimester. Minor side effects of prostaglandins like vomiting, diarrhea, and fever are common. Diarrhea is more common in women using gemeprost, whereas fever is more common when misoprostol is used (48). Serious complications including uterine rupture, major hemorrhage, and cervical tear are rare (41–43). Cases of uterine rupture were reported to occur with both gemeprost and misoprostol, and the use of mifepristone did not exclude the possibility (49–52). The incidence of uterine rupture was estimated to be 0.5% in the second trimester using mifepristone and gemeprost (51). Risk factors of uterine rupture include previous caesarean section, grand multipara, advanced gestation, prolonged prostaglandin therapy, and the use of oxytocin in addition to prostaglandins (51,52). Cardiovascular complications are uncommon with gemeprost and misoprostol. Long-term complications associated with medical abortion in the second trimester using gemeprost and misoprostol with or without mifepristone are rarely reported. There is no known association with subsequent infertility or miscarriage after medical abortion by the noninvasive oral or vaginal route of prostaglandin analogues.

THE CHOICE OF ABORTION METHOD FOR FETAL ABNORMALITIES

If the fetal abnormality can be diagnosed with certainty in the late first trimester, surgical method is the method of choice for termination of pregnancy at this gestation. Surgical abortion by vacuum aspiration is a safe and short procedure, which usually takes <10 minutes. On the other hand, the success of medical abortion is less predictable at this gestation. It may take several hours for the abortion to occur. Surgical abortion can save the woman a procedure which is associated with pain.

The situation may not be the same if the diagnosis of fetal abnormality is made during the second trimester. In the past, it was considered that surgical abortion by D&E was safer than medical abortion. However, this was based on studies comparing D&E with medical methods, including saline instillation, intra-amniotic urea, or oxytocin infusion, that are not used anymore (8). While D&E remains as safe as it was, the techniques of medical abortion have improved, particularly with the introduction of mifepristone. There has been no proper randomized study comparing D&E with modern methods of medical abortion in the second trimester.

D&E is a quick procedure and is, therefore, less expensive. It is less painful than medical abortion since it can be done under anesthesia. The women do not have to be in contact with the abnormal fetus, and it may be more acceptable to some women who do not want to see their fetus after abortion. However, it may be less acceptable to some gynecologists who may find it distressing to perform the procedure, especially at an advanced gestation. Although complications are not common in expert hands, they may lead to serious consequences like cervical incompetence and infertility. Besides, in order to maintain the surgical skill of D&E, a sufficiently large case-load is required and it may not be possible in many of the units providing prenatal diagnosis service.

On the other hand, medical abortion is less dependent on the skills of the providers. With standard management protocol, second-trimester abortion can be carried out by a nurse under the supervision of a gynecologist. It is less traumatic when compared to surgical abortion, and the complications are usually minor. The only disadvantage of this method is the longer abortion process compared to the surgical method. However, if the time required for priming of the cervix is also included, D&E may take a longer duration than expected. With the introduction of mifepristone, the induction to abortion interval for medical abortion is much shortened. The median time taken for the abortion to occur is about six hours after the administration of prostaglandin analogue. Although mifepristone has to be taken 36–48 hours earlier, women usually experience minimal symptoms or pain after mifepristone and only start to have pain after the administration of prostaglandin analogues. The pain is usually not severe and can be controlled by analgesics. Besides, there is frequently a need for autopsy examination of the fetus to define or refine the exact pathology. This would be very important in the setting of prenatal diagnosis, for the counseling of the woman on future pregnancy as well as the education of the doctors. Obviously, medical abortion has the advantage of allowing an easier autopsy examination, especially on structural abnormalities, which are more difficult with the surgical specimen from D&E.

The abortions for fetal abnormalities are different from the abortions for the other indications. Many of these pregnancies are planned and wanted. The mother usually has established bonding with their expected baby. This is especially true for the more advanced gestation. It may take time for the mourning process and there is evidence to show that showing and holding the fetus may help the mother to cope and mourn. Seeing and holding the fetus emphasizes the reality of the loss, which is helpful in the grief process. Some of the parents may choose to take pictures of the fetus and these memories may be of great value to them (53,54). Medical abortion also provides an intact fetus for this purpose.

CONCLUSION

It is important to provide a safe abortion to the woman who is diagnosed to have an abnormal fetus. As it is not always possible to have an early prenatal diagnosis, many of these abortions take place in the second trimester. D&E as well as medical abortion using a combination of mifepristone and prostaglandin analogue are considered to be safe methods for second-trimester abortion. However, D&E requires surgical expertise and is a more technically demanding procedure especially when the fetus is at advanced gestational age. On the other hand, medical abortion is simple, noninvasive, and does not depend on the skill of the one who carries out the abortion. In the setting of abortion for fetal abnormality, medical abortion also has the additional advantage of providing an intact fetus for the coping and mourning process of the parents as well as the autopsy examination.

REFERENCES

1. Child TJ, Thomas J, Rees M, MacKenzie IZ. A comparative study of surgical and medical procedures: 932 pregnancy terminations up to 63 days gestation. Hum Reprod 2001; 16:67–71.
2. Joint study of the Royal College of General Practitioners and the Royal College of Obstetricians and Gynaecologists. Induction abortion operations and their early sequelae. J R Coll Gen Pract 1985; 35:175–180.
3. Hakim-Elahi E, Tovell HM, Burnhill MS. Complications of first trimester abortion: a report of 170,000 cases. Obstet Gynaecol 1990; 76:129–135.
4. Child TJ, Thomas J, Rees M, MacKenzie IZ. Morbidity of first trimester aspiration termination and the seniority of the surgeon. Hum Reprod 2001; 16:875–878.
5. El-Refaey H, Calder L, Wheatley DN, Templeton A. Cervical priming with prostaglandin E1 analogues, misoprostol and gemeprost. Lancet 1994; 343:1207–1209.
6. Ngai SW, Chan YM, Tang OS, Ho PC. The use of misoprostol for pre-operative cervical dilatation prior to vacuum aspiration: a randomized trial. Hum Reprod 1999; 14: 2139–2142.

7. Tang OS, Mok KH, Ho PC. A randomised study comparing the use of sublingual to vaginal misoprostol for pre-operative cervical priming prior to surgical termination of pregnancy in the first trimester. Hum Reprod 2004; 19:1101–1104.

8. Grimes DA, Cates W Jr. Complications from legally-induced abortion: a review. Obstet Gynaecol Surv 1979; 34:177–191.

9. Kulier R, Fekih A, Hofmeyr GJ, Campana A. Surgical methods for first trimester termination of pregnancy. Cochrane Database Syst Rev 2001; (4):CD002900.

10. Baird DT. Mode of action of medical methods of abortion. J Am Med Women Assoc 2000; 55(3 Suppl):121–126.

11. Van Look PFA, Bygdeman M. Antiprogesterone steroids: a new dimension in human fertility regulation. Oxford Rev Reprod Biol 1989; 11:1–60.

12. Couzinet B, Strat NL, Ulmann A. Termination of very early pregnancy by the progesterone antagonist RU 486 (mifepristone). N Engl J Med 1986; 315:1565–1570.

13. Bygdeman M, Swahn ML. Progesterone receptor blockage: effect on uterine contractility and early pregnancy. Contraception 1985; 32:45–51.

14. Cameron IT, Michie AF, Baird DT. Therapeutic abortion in early pregnancy with antiprogestogen RU 486 alone or in combination with prostaglandin analogue (gemeprost). Contraception 1986; 34:45967.

15. UK Multicentre Study Group. Oral mifepristone 600 mg and vaginal gemeprost for midtrimester induction of abortion. Contraception 1997; 56:361–366.

16. Ulmann A, Silvestre L, Chemama L, et al. Medical termination of early pregnancy with mifepristone (RU486) followed by a prostaglandin analogue. Acta Obstet Gynecol Scand 1992; 71:278–283.

17. Anon. A death associated with mifepristone/sulprostone. Lancet 1991; 337:969–970.

18. Spitz IM, Bardin CW, Benton L, Robbins A. Early termination of pregnancy with mifepristone (RU 486) and the orally active prostaglandin misoprostol. N Engl J Med 1998; 21:1509–1513.

19. El-Refaey H, Rajasekar D, Abdalla M, Calder L, Templeton A. Induction of abortion with mifepristone (RU 486) and oral or vaginal misoprostol. N Engl J Med 1995; 332:983–987.

20. Ashok PW, Penney GC, Flett GM, Templeton A. An effective regimen for early medical abortion: a report of 2000 consecutive cases. Hum Reprod 1998; 13:2962–2965.

21. Bartley J, Brown A, Elton R, Baird DT. A double blind randomized control trial between vaginal gemeprost and misoprostol in combination with mifepristone for induction of abortion in early pregnancy. Hum Reprod 2001; 16:2098–2102.

22. McKinley C, Thong KJ, Baird DT. The effect of dose of mifepristone and gestation on the efficacy of medical abortion with mifepristone and misoprostol. Hum Reprod 1993; 8:1502–1505.

23. World Health Organization Task Force on Post-Ovulatory Methods for Fertility Regulation. Termination of pregnancy with reduced doses of mifepristone. Br Med J 1993; 307:532–537.

24. Ashok PW, Flett GM, Templeton A. Termination of pregnancy at 9–13 weeks amenorrhoea with mifepristone and misoprostol. Lancet 1998; 352:542–543.

25. Grimes DA, Schulz KF, Cates WJ Jr. Prevention of uterine perforation during curettage abortion. J Am Med Assoc 1984; 251:2108–2111.

26. WHO Scientific Group on Medical Methods for Termination of Pregnancy. Methods of abortion after 14 weeks of gestation. WHO Technical Report Series on Medical Methods for Termination of Pregnancy. Geneva: WHO, 1997:42–54.

27. Lauersen NH, Den T, Iliescu C, Wilson KH, Graves ZR. Cervical priming prior to dilatation and evacuation: a comparison of methods. Am J Obstet Gynecol 1982; 144:890–894.

28. Todd CS, Soler M, Castleman L, Rogers MK, Blumenthal PD. Buccal misoprostol as cervical preparation for second trimester pregnancy termination. Contraception 2002; 65:415–418.

29. Royal College of Obstetricians and Gynaecologists. The care of women requesting induced abortion. London: RCOG, 2000.
30. WHO Prostaglandin Task Force. Termination of second trimester pregnancy with laminaria and intramuscular 15-methyl PGF2α or 16-phenoxy-ω-17,18,19,20-tetranor PGE2 methyl sulfonylamide. A randomized multicenter study. Int J Gynaecol Obstet 1988; 26:129–135.
31. Cameron IT, Michie AF, Baird DT. Prostaglandin-induced pregnancy termination: further studies using gemeprost (16, 16 dimethyl-trans-Δ²-PGE1 methyl ester) vaginal pessaries in the early second trimester. Prostaglandins 1987; 34:111–117.
32. Thong KJ, Robertson AJ, Baird DT. A retrospective study of 932 second trimester terminations using gemeprost (16, 16 dimethyl-trans-Δ²-PGE1 methyl ester). Prostaglandins 1992; 44:65–74.
33. Wong KS, Ngai CSW, Wong AYK, Tang LCH, Ho PC. Vaginal misoprostol compared with vaginal gemeprost in termination of second trimester pregnancy. Contraception 1998; 58:207–210.
34. Thong KJ, Baird DT. An open study comparing two regimens of gemeprost for the termination of pregnancy in the second trimester. Acta Obstet Gynecol Scand 1992; 71: 191–196.
35. Ziemam M, Fong SK, Benowitz NL, Banskter D, Darney PD. Absorption kinetics of misoprostol with oral or vaginal administration. Obstet Gynecol 1997; 90:88–92.
36. Ho PC, Ngai SW, Liu KL, Wong GCY, Lee SWH. Vaginal misoprostol compared with oral misoprostol in termination of second-trimester pregnancy. Obstet Gynecol 1997; 90:735–738.
37. Wong KS, Ngai CSW, Yeo ELK, Tang LCH, Ho PC. A comparison of two regimens of intravaginal misoprostol for termination of second trimester pregnancy: a randomized comparative trial. Hum Reprod 2000; 15:709–712.
38. Thong KJ, Baird DT. A study of gemeprost alone, dilapan or mifepristone in combination with gemeprost for the termination of second trimester pregnancy. Contraception 1992; 46:11–17.
39. Ho PC, Tsang SSK, Ma HK. Reducing the induction to abortion interval in termination of second trimester pregnancies: a comparison of mifepristone with laminaria tent. Br J Obstet Gynaecol 1995; 102:648–651.
40. UK Multicenter Study Group. Oral mifepristone 600 mg and vaginal gemeprost for mid-trimester induction of abortion. Contraception 1997; 56:361–366.
41. Ashok PW, Templeton A. Nonsurgical mid-trimester termination of pregnancy: a review of 500 consecutive cases. Br J Obstet Gynaecol 1999; 106:706–710.
42. Gemzell-Danielsson K, Östlund E. Termination of second trimester pregnancy with mifepristone and gemeprost. The clinical experience of 197 consecutive cases. Acta Obstet Gynecol Scand 2000; 79:702–706.
43. OS Tang, KJ Thong, DT Baird. Second trimester medical abortion with mifepristone and gemeprost: a review of 956 cases. Contraception 2001; 64:29–32.
44. Webster D, Penny GC, Templeton A. A comparison of 600 mg and 200 mg mifepristone prior to second trimester abortion with the prostaglandin misoprostol. Br J Obstet Gynaecol 1996; 103:706–709.
45. Thong KJ, Lynch P, Baird DT. A randomised study of two doses of gemeprost in combination with mifepristone for induction of abortion in the second trimester of pregnancy. Contraception 1996; 54:97–100.
46. El-Refaey H, Templeton A. Induction of abortion in the second trimester by a combination of misoprostol and mifepristone: a randomized comparison between two misoprostol regimens. Hum Reprod 1995; 10:475–478.
47. Bartley J, Baird DT. A randomised study of misoprostol and gemeprost in combination with mifepristone for induction of abortion in the second trimester of pregnancy. Br J Obstet Gynaecol 2002; 109:1290–1294.

48. Nuutila M, Toivonen J, Ylikorkala O, Halmesmäki E. A comparison between two doses of intravaginal misoprostol and gemeprost for induction of second-trimester abortion. Obstet Gynecol 1997; 90:896–900.
49. Phillips K, Berry C, Mathers AM. Uterine rupture during second trimester of pregnancy using mifepristone and a prostaglandin. Eur J Obstet Gynaecol 1996; 65:175–176.
50. Chen M, Shih JC, Chiu WT, Hsieh FJ. Separation of cesarean scar during second-trimester intravaginal misoprostol abortion. Obstet Gynecol 1999; 94:840.
51. Norman JE. Uterine rupture during therapeutic abortion in the second trimester using mifepristone and prostaglandin. Br J Obstet Gynaecol 1995; 102:332–333.
52. Wiener JJ, Evans AS. Uterine rupture in midtrimester abortion. A complication of gemeprost vaginal pessaries and oxytocin, Case report. Br J Obstet Gynaecol 1990; 97: 1061–1062.
53. Lorenzen J, Holzgreve W. Helping parents to grieve after second trimester termination of pregnancy for fetopathic reasons. Fetal Diagn Ther 1995; 10:147–156.
54. Geerinck-Vercammen CR, Kanhai HHH. Coping with termination of pregnancy for fetal abnormality in a supportive environment. Prenat Diagn 2003; 23:543–548.

29

Fetal Reduction

Mark I. Evans, David W. Britt, Doina Ciorica, and John C. Fletcher[†]
Department of Obstetrics and Gynecology, Institute for Genetics and Fetal Medicine,
St. Luke's-Roosevelt Hospital Center, New York, New York, U.S.A.

INTRODUCTION

Louise Brown, the first baby to come from in vitro fertilization (IVF) was born in 1978. In the > 25 years since that event, millions of babies have been born benefiting from infertility therapies including more than 1,000,000 IVF babies. These incredible success stories, however, have had corresponding serious side effects. The twin pregnancy rate, commonly quoted for decades to be 1 in 90, now has doubled to more than 1 in 45. About 70% of all twins in the United States have come from infertility treatments. Some IVF programs create as many multiples as singletons.

All multiple pregnancies have continued to rise and the incidence of prematurity and related sequelae clearly correlate with fetal number (Fig. 1) (Tables 1 and 2) (1). With increasing public and professional attention, some of the very high order multiples have diminished, particularly secondary to lower transfer numbers of embryos in IVF. There are some suggestions that the incidence of triplets and higher is slowly diminishing, but the incidence is still very high.

In this field, as with many others, it is often easier to appreciate the numerator than the denominator. Published pregnancy losses in multiple pregnancies are mostly a function of how early in pregnancy one establishes the denominator (2,3). Some reports by perinatologists are overly, and we believe inappropriately, optimistic because these physicians do not start "counting" until they begin to see patients at nearly 20 weeks, at which time most losses have already occurred (3,4). Many other articles have addressed these issues, and these will not be repeated here (4–6).

In the 1980s, about 75% of multifetal pregnancy patients seeking reduction had pregnancies initiated with ovulation induction agents such as pergonal (7). However, even with the first month of the lowest dose of clomid, quintuplets have occurred. Over the years, cases induced by assisted reproductive technologies (ARTs), such as IVF, have become increasingly common. Currently, about 70% of patients we see seeking reduction have pregnancies generated by ARTs (8).

[†]Deceased.

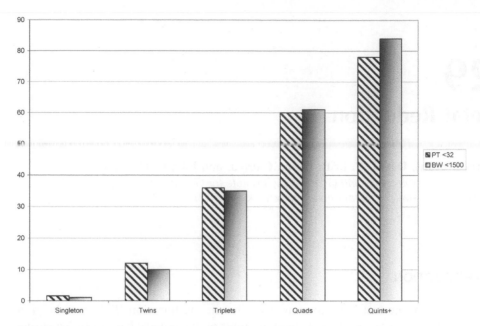

Figure 1 Risks of prematurity as a function of fetal number. *Diagonal lines*: pre-term birth <32 weeks; *shaded*: area birth weight <1500 g. *Source*: 2002 United States Centers for Disease Control Data.

Despite the increased utilization of ARTs, the proportion of cases significantly hyperstimulated and resulting in quintuplets or more, has dramatically decreased, <10% of all cases seen by us. Regardless, the 2002 report of the Society of Assisted Reproductive Technologies (SART) published in December 2004 suggested that of

Table 1 Multiple Births in the United States

Year	Twins	Triplets	Quadruplets	Quintuplets and higher multiples
2002	125,134	6898	434	69
2001	121,246	6885	501	85
2000	118,916	6742	506	77
1999	114,307	6742	512	67
1998	110,670	6919	627	79
1997	104,137	6148	510	79
1996	100,750	5298	560	81
1995	96,736	4551	365	57
1994	97,064	4233	315	46
1993	96,445	3834	277	57
1992	95,372	3547	310	26
1991	94,779	3121	203	22
1990	93,865	2830	185	13
1989	90,118	2529	229	40
% Change from 1989 to 2002	38.9%	172.8%	89.6%	72.5%

Source: Data taken from National Vital Statistics Report, 2003, Volume 52, No. 10, p. 22.

Table 2 Ratio of Observed to Expected Multiples

Births	Observed	Expected	Ratio
Twins	125,134	44,686	2.80:1
Triplets	6898	496	13.9:1
Quadruplets	434	6	72.3:1
Quintuplets and higher multiples	69	0.07	985.7:1

Note: Total births in 2002 was 4,021,726.

all pregnancies achieved by ARTs in the United States, 50.9% are singletons, 37.8% twins, 6.9% triplets or higher, and 4.4% were unknown (8–10). By birth, the percentages were 57.6% singletons, 39.6% twins, and 2.8% triplets or higher, reflecting the increased pregnancy loss rate of higher order multiples (10). In our experience with referred cases of ovulation stimulation, particularly those using follicle stimulating hormone (FSH) analogs, the proportion of cases that are quintuplets or more has fallen but not as dramatically (11).

Such data continue to reinforce the significant role of vigilance in monitoring the infertility therapies. The vast majority of multifetal cases occur to physicians with the best of equipment and with the best of intentions who have an unfortunate and reasonably unpredictable or unpreventable maloccurrence. Despite this, clearly some cases might have been prevented if increased vigilance had been used (11–13).

DEMOGRAPHICS

Over the past decade, the pattern of patients seeking multifetal pregnancy reduction (MFPR) has evolved considerably (11,12). With the rapid expansion of availability of donor eggs, the number of "older women" seeking MFPR has increased dramatically. In our experience, over 10% of all patients we see seeking MFPR are over 40 years of age, and nearly half of them are using donor eggs. As a consequence of the shift to older patients, many of whom already had previous relationships and children, there is an increased desire by these patients to have only one further child. The number of experienced centers willing to do two to one reductions is still very limited, but we believe it can be justified under the appropriate circumstances (11,13).

For patients who are "older," particularly using their own eggs, the issue of genetic diagnosis comes into play. By 2001, more than 50% of patients in the United States having ART cycles were over 35 years of age (Table 3) (1,9,10,14). In the 1980s and early 1990s, the most common approach was to offer amniocentesis at 16 to 17 weeks on the remaining twins. A 1995 paper suggested an 11% loss rate in these cases, which caused considerable concern (15). However, the issue was settled by a much larger collaborative series in 1998 that showed that loss rates were no higher than comparable controls of MFPR patients who did not have amniocentesis (16). The collaborative data show a loss rate of 5%, which was certainly no higher than the group of patients post-MFPR who did not have genetic studies.

Since the centers with the most MFPR experience were also the ones who had the same accomplishments with chorionic villus sampling (CVS), combinations of the procedures were very logical. There are two competing possibilities as to the best approach to first trimester genetic diagnosis, i.e., should it be before or after the

Table 3 Maternal Age and ART[a]

All cases	81,915
Fresh nondonor	60,780
<35	28,778
35–37	14,416
38–40	11,301
41–42	4,365
42+	2,190

[a]2001 SART data.
Abbreviations: ART, assisted reproductive technologies;
SART, Society of Assisted Reproductive Technologies.

performance of MFPR? Published data in the early 1990s doing the CVS first followed by reductions suggested a 1% to 2% error rate as to which fetus was which, particularly if the entire karyotype is obtained before going on to reduction (17). Therefore, for the first 10 to 15 years, the approach we used was to generally do the reduction first at approximately 10.5 weeks in patients reducing down to twins or triplets, followed by CVS approximately 1 week later (11,14). However, in patients going to a singleton pregnancy, essentially putting "all of their eggs in one basket," we believed the best approach was to know what was in the basket before reducing the other embryos (11,12). In these cases, we performed a CVS on usually all the fetuses or one more than the intended stopping number, and performed a fluorescent in situ hybridization (FISH) analysis with probes for chromosomes 13, 18, 21, X, and Y. Whereas about 30% of overall anomalies seen on karyotype would not be detectable by FISH with these probes (18), there is always residual risk (19). The absolute risk, given both a normal FISH and a normal ultrasound including nuchal translucency (20), is only about 1/500. We believe that risk is lower than the increased risk from the 2-week wait necessary to get the full karyotype. We have now commonly extended this approach to all patients who are appropriate candidates for prenatal diagnosis regardless of the fetal number (Fig. 2). Over the past few years, more than half our patients have combined CVS and MFPR procedures. With data now suggesting increased risks of chromosomal and other anomalies in patients conceiving by IVF and especially with ICSI (intracytoplasmic sperm injection), the utilization of prenatal diagnosis will likely increase even further (21–26).

The other approach used by another group was to perform the CVS and complete karyotype first and have the patient come back for the reduction. Although "mistakes" were common 10 years ago, the chance of error has been considerably reduced, and they believed the benefits of the full karyotype justified the wait. The issue as to the better of these two approaches is currently unsettled and would require a very large series to differentiate among small risks.

CLINICAL USES

MFPR is a clinical procedure developed in the 1980s when a small number of centers in both the United States and Europe attempted to reduce the usual and tremendously adverse sequelae of multifetal pregnancies by selectively terminating or reducing the number of fetuses to a more manageable number. The first European reports by Dumez (27), and the first American report by Evans et al. (28), followed

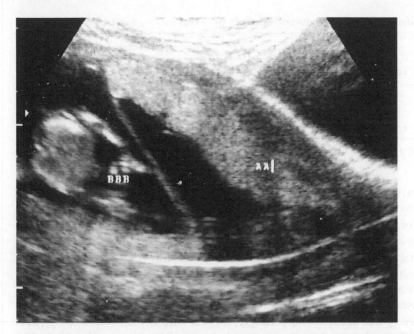

Figure 2 CVS in multiple pregnancies. CVS catheter inserted transcervically into posterior placenta. Anterior placenta could be done easily by either the transcervical or transabdominal approach. *Abbreviation*: CVS, chorionic villus sampling.

by a further report by Berkowitz et al. (29), and later Wapner et al. (30), described a surgical approach to improve the outcome in such cases.

Even these early reports appreciated the ethical dilemma faced by couples and physicians under such difficult circumstances (13). In the mid-1980s, needles were inserted transabdominally and maneuvered into the thorax for the injection of potassium chloride (KCl) or mechanical disruption of the fetus by mechanical destruction, air embolization, or KCl injections despite relatively mediocre ultrasound visualization. Transcervical aspirations were also initially tried, but with little success. Some centers also used transvaginal mechanical disruption, but data suggested a significantly higher loss rate than with the transabdominal route (31). Today, virtually all experienced operators perform the procedure inserting needles transabdominally under ultrasound guidance.

RESULTS

Over more than a decade, several centers with the world's largest experience have collaborated to leverage the power of their data. In 1993 the first collaborative report showed a 16% pregnancy loss rate through 24 completed weeks (17). While by today's standards, that was not a very satisfactory number, it did represent a major improvement for higher-order multiple pregnancies. Further collaborative papers have shown continued dramatic improvements in the overall outcomes of such pregnancies (Table 4) (11). The 2001 collaborative data demonstrated that the outcome of triplets reduced to twins, and quadruplets reduced to twins now perform essentially as if they started as twins (11). Even with the tremendous advances in neonatal

Table 4 Multifetal Pregnancy Reduction—Losses by Years

Years	Total	Losses (wk)		Deliveries (wk)			
		% < 24	% > 24	% 25–28	% 29–32	% 33–36	% 37+
1986–1990	508	13.2	4.5	10.0	21.1	15.7	35.4
1991–1994	724	9.4	0.3	2.8	5.4	21.1	61.0
1995–1998	1356	6.4	0.2	4.3	10.2	31.5	47.4

Source: From Ref. 11.

care for premature babies, the 95% take-home baby rate for triplets and the 92% take-home baby rate for quadruplets clearly represent dramatic improvements over natural statistics. Not only has the pregnancy loss rate been substantially lowered, but so has the rate of very dangerous early prematurity. Both continue to be correlated with the starting number. Data from the past few years show that the improvements are, not surprisingly, greatest from the higher starting numbers (Fig. 3).

The lowest pregnancy loss rates are for those cases reduced to twins with increasing losses for singletons followed by triplets. However, the rate of early premature delivery has been, not surprisingly, highest with triplets followed by twins and lowest with singletons. Mean gestational age at delivery was also lower for higher-order cases. Birth weights following MFPR decreased with starting and finishing numbers reflecting increasing prematurity (32).

While data in the literature are conflicting, our experiences suggest that triplets reduced to twins do much better in terms of loss and prematurity than do unreduced triplets. We believe that if a patient's primary goal is to maximize the chances of surviving children, reduction of triplets to twins achieves the best liveborn results. More recent analyses suggest that while mortality is lowest with twins, morbidity is lowest with remaining singletons.

Numerous papers have argued over the past several years whether triplets have better outcomes "reduced" or not. Yaron et al. (33) compared triplets to twins data

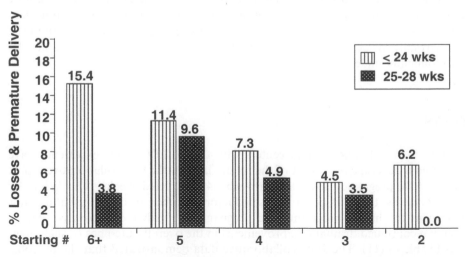

Figure 3 Multifetal pregnancy reduction losses and very prematures by starting number. *Source*: From Ref. 11.

to unreduced triplets with two large cohorts of twins. The data show substantial improvement of reduced twins as compared to triplets. The data from the most recent collaborative series suggest that pregnancy outcomes for cases starting at triplets, or even quadruplets reduced to twins, do fundamentally start as twins. These data, therefore, support some cautious aggressiveness in infertility treatments to achieve pregnancy in difficult clinical situations. However, when higher numbers occur, good outcomes clearly diminish. A 2001 paper suggested that reduced triplets did worse than continuing ones (34). However, analysis of that series showed a loss rate following MFPR twice that seen in our collaborative series (11) and poorer outcomes in every other category for remaining triplets. Several other recent papers have likewise shown higher risks for "unreduced" triplets than for reduced cases (35–38). It is clear that one must use extreme caution in choosing comparison groups (Table 5). An ever increasing situation involves the inclusion of a monozygotic (MZ) pair of twins in a higher-order multiple (39). Our experience suggests that provided the "singleton" seems healthy, that the best outcomes are achieved by reduction of the MZ twins. Obviously, if the singleton is not healthy, then keeping the twins is the next choice.

Pregnancy loss is not the only deleterious outcome. Very early preterm delivery correlates with the starting number. However, it has not been well appreciated that about 20% of babies born at <750 g develop cerebral palsy (40). In Western Australia, Peterson et al. showed that the rate of cerebral palsy was 4.6 times higher for twins than singletons per live births, but 8.3 times higher when calculated per pregnancy (41). Pharoah and Cooke calculated cerebral palsy rates per 1000 first-year survivor at 2.3 for singletons, 12.6 for twins, and 44.8 for triplets (42).

In the 2001 collaborative report, the subset of patients who reduced from two to one, (not for fetal anomalies) included 154 patients. These data suggested a loss rate comparable to three to two, but, in about one-third of the $2 \rightarrow 1$ cases, there was a medical indication for the procedure, e.g., maternal cardiac disease or prior

Table 5 Reduced vs. "Unreduced" Triplets Comparison

	MFPR cases				
		Deliveries (wk)			
Years	*Losses <24 wk*	*24–28 wk*	*29–32 wk*	*33–36 wk*	*37+ wk*
1980s	6.7%	6.1%	9.1%	36.9%	47.9%
1990–1994	5.7%	5.2%	9.9%	39.2%	45.2%
1995–1998	4.5%	3.2%	6.9%	28.3%	55.1%
1998–2002	5.1%	4.6%	10.8%	41.8%	37.6%
Mean GA 35.5 PMR (10.0/1000)					
1998–2002	8.0%	4.0%	12.0%	4.0%	72.0%
(3 to >1)		Mean GA 39.5	PMR 0/1000		
Unreduced triplets					
98 (Leondires)	9.9%	Mean GA 33.3	PMR 55/1000		
99 (Angel)	8.0%	Mean GA 32.3	PMR 29/1000		
99 (Lipitz)	25.0%	Mean GA 33.5	PMR 109/1000		
02 (Francois)	8.3%	Mean GA 31.0	PMR 57.6/1000		

Abbreviations: MFPR, multifetal pregnancy reduction; GA, gestational age; PMR.
Source: From Refs. 35–38,45a.

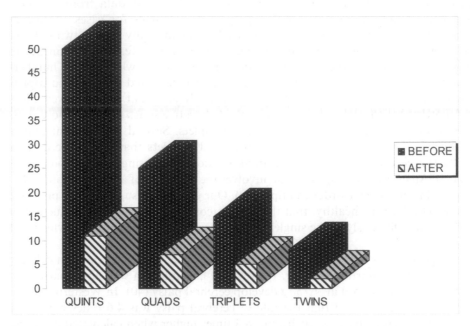

Figure 4 Risk reduction. Risk reduction as a function of starting number. Numbers on *left* are risks of spontaneous loss without reduction. Numbers on *right* are after reduction.

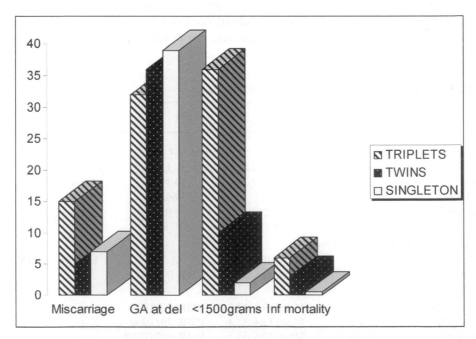

Figure 5 Risks starting with triplets. Reduction of triplets to twins has lower loss rates but higher incidence of prematurity, low birth weight, and infant mortality than reducing to a singleton. Numbers on *left* are risks with triplets, in the *middle* risks with twins, and on the *right*, risks with a remaining singleton.

twin pregnancy with severe prematurity, or uterine abnormality (11). In recent years, however, the demographics are changing, and the vast majority of such cases are from women in their 40s, or even 50s, some of whom are using donor eggs and who, more for social than medical reasons, only want a singleton pregnancy (42,43). New data suggest that twins reduced to a singleton do better than remaining as twins (13). Consistent with the aforementioned, more women are desirous to reduce to a singleton. In a recent series of triplets, we found the average age of outpatients reducing to twins to be 37 years and to a singleton 41 years (44). While the reduction in pregnancy loss risk for 3–1 is not as much as 3–2, (from 15% to 7% and from 15% to 5%, respectively), the gestational age at delivery for the resulting singleton is higher, and the incidence of births <1500 g is 10 times higher for twins than singletons (1). These data have made counseling of such patients far more complex than before (Figs. 4 and 5). Not surprisingly, there are often differences between members of the couple as to the desirability of twins or singleton (45). There are also profound public health implications to these decisions, as 2000 United States data show that of $10.2 billion spent per year on initial newborn care, 57% of the money is spent on the 9% of babies born at <37 weeks (46). This progress is much more likely to rise than fall.

SOCIETAL ISSUES

MFPR will always be controversial. Opinions on MFPR, in our experience have never followed the classic "pro-choice/pro-life" dichotomy (2,7,11,14). We believe that the real debate over the next 5 to 10 years will not be whether or not MFPR should be performed with triplets or more. A serious debate will emerge over whether or not it will be appropriate to offer MFPR routinely for twins, even natural ones for whom the outcome has commonly been considered "good enough" (44). Our data suggest that reduction of twins to a singleton actually improves the outcome of the remaining fetus (44). No consensus on appropriateness of routine 2→1 reductions, however, is ever likely to emerge. We do, however, expect the proportion of patients reducing to a singleton to steadily increase over the next several years.

The ethical issues surrounding MFPR will also always be controversial. Over the years, much has been written on the subject. Opinions will always vary substantially from outraged condemnation to complete acceptance. No short paragraph could do justice to the subject other than to state that most proponents do not believe this is a frivolous procedure, but see it in terms of the principle of proportionality, i.e., therapy to achieve the most good for the least harm (13,47–49).

How patients "hear" and internalize data and make decisions with respect to reduction have been fascinating to us over the years. Much of the literature on medical decision making has emphasized a rational choice model in which emotions, feelings, and values are treated as complications that must be considered as a second stage of an analysis that puts hard data regarding relative risks center stage (50,51). Even in the literature that talks about genuine alternative models of decision making (for example, systematic vs. heuristic), a central assumption is that these are individual differences in style that can be identified through what people say (52,53).

We have approached this problem from a different direction, arguing that where controversial, high-anxiety decisions are concerned, patients treat these decisions as an ongoing part of the social reality that they are creating to live in and raise a family (54). These realities, composed of supportive people and institutions together with complexes of supportive values, norms, and attitudes are the source of frames that the patients use to view the data (47–49). The decisions they make and how they justify those decisions may help resolve incompatible elements in the realities in which they find themselves enmeshed. It may often happen, for example, that parents who have gone through reduction to two or one live in families and/or work in communities where being engaged in reduction would be considered as something shameful. The less control they have over the selection of family, friends, and workplaces, given the prospect of such stigma, the more likely they are to simply present their pregnancies to these people as if their pregnancies had always involved twins or singleton. Where they have more control over the situation—as typically happens with friends versus family—they may be more likely to selectively share their experiences.

The one thing all such patients have in common is a very strong desire to have a family (Table 6). But there does not appear to be a single set of supportive institutions, people, and norms that is conducive to going through the pain, stress, and resource expenditure of IVF. There are three viable alternative resolutions. The first of these, a rational Medical Model, looks superficially like what one would expect from the rational analysis model. But the commitment to factual analysis comes from their having selected themselves into the hard sciences, medicine, dentistry, engineering, or the law—disciplines in which the "facts" are crucial. Such women will want to see the numbers regarding the relative risk associated with different reduction choices and will want to engage in a rigorous discussion of the data and their implications. And they will be likely to choose a final number for reduction that maximizes the chances of a "take-home" baby.

The lens of scientific objectivity is not the only frame through which women who have gone through IVF in order to have a child will examine these data.

Table 6 Frame Comparison

	Medical frame	Fundamentalist frame	Lifestyle frame
Intensity of commitment to having children	High	High	High
Intensity of training in medicine, dentistry, hard sciences, and the law	High	Low	Modest
Intensity of commitment to belief that life begins at conception	Modest	High	Modest
Intensity of commitment to career	High	Low	High
Source of moral authority for resolution	Relative survivability of fetuses	Minimization of damage to moral beliefs through a "barely sufficient" reduction	Having a "normal" life in a culture that values both careers and family for women

For those who have immersed themselves in a social reality that has a strong emphasis on norms against abortion and/or reduction—such that they themselves have such normative beliefs and are heavily involved in churches that reinforce similar beliefs—a detached examination of the "facts" is simply not possible. These "facts" hold no special moral authority. Their beliefs and those of the individuals and social institutions in which they have selected themselves have a moral authority as well. The balance that such women will likely seek is one that reduces their relative risk to acceptable limits. So, unless the consequences are dire, they will not reduce or choose to reduce only to three. We labeled such a resolution a Fundamentalist Model.

Finally, there are those for whom the demands of career and/or existing children constitute powerful elements in their constructed realities. For such women—and this includes many of the older patients we encountered—the essential balance that they seek is a more secular one, a Lifestyle Model, one that emphasizes creating a family situation in which having a family can be balanced with having a career. Such women will more than likely choose reduction to two or even one embryo, depending on the number of other children they have and the level of resources that the family has.

Where women have selected themselves into and/or been trained to accept the legitimacy of rigorously determined statistics regarding relative risk (a Medical Frame), reduction choices *can* be straightforward—or at least they can appear to be relatively straightforward. This is usually not the case, however, for women who must forge a resolution among potentially incompatible elements, as for women who are struggling to reconcile the potentially oppositional elements of religious beliefs and involvement with risks associated with higher-level pregnancies (Fundamentalist Frame) or those who are struggling to reconcile the potentially conflicting identities of home and career (Lifestyle Frame). We have been able to examine some of these issues in a few studies to date. In one we were able to trace the extreme fluctuations in anxiety and stress as women progress through IVF and then must confront the painful choice of reduction (48). In the second study, we were able to show that the meaning of detecting a fetal anomaly changes depending on the needs of the patient and her spouse for some confirmation regarding their choice (47).

SUMMARY

Over the last two decades, MFPR has become a well-established and integral part of infertility therapy and the attempts to deal with sequelae of aggressive infertility management. In the mid-1980s, the risks and benefits of the procedure could only be guessed (10–14). We now have very clear and precise data on the risks and benefits as well as an understanding that the risks increase substantially with the starting and finishing number of fetuses in multifetal pregnancies. The collaborative loss rate numbers, i.e., 4.5% for triplets, 8% for quadruplets, 11% for quintuplets, and 15% for sextuplets or more for the procedure performed by an experienced operator seem reasonable ones to present to patients. Our own experience and anecdotal reports from other groups suggest that less experienced operators have worse outcomes.

Pregnancy loss is not the only poor outcome. The other main issue with which to be concerned is very early preterm delivery and the profound consequences to such infants. Here again there is an increasing rate of poor outcomes correlated with the starting number. The finishing numbers are also critical, with twins having the best viable pregnancy outcomes for cases starting with three or more. Triplets and singletons do not do as well. However, an emerging appreciation that singletons have prematurity rates less than twins is making the counseling far more complex. We continue to hope, however, that MFPR will become obsolete as better control of ovulation agents and assisted reproductive technologies make multifetal pregnancies uncommon.

REFERENCES

1. Martin JA, Hamilton BE, Ventura SJ, et al. Births: Final Data for 2001. National Vital Statistics Reports, vol 51#2. Hyattville, MD: National Center for Health Statistics, 2002.
2. Evans MI, Rodeck CH, Stewart KS, Yaron Y, Johnson MP. Multiple gestation: genetic issues, selective termination, and fetal reduction. In: Gleisher N, Buttino L Jr, Elkayam U, Evans MI, Galbraith RM, Gall SA, Sibai BM, eds. Principles and Practices of Medical Therapy in Pregnancy. 3rd ed. Norwalk, Connecticut: Appleton and Lange Publishing Co., 1998:235–242.
3. Evans MI, Ayoub MA, Shalhoub AG, Feldman B, Yaron Y. Spontaneous abortions in couples declining multifetal pregnancy reduction. Fetal Diagn Ther 2002; 17:343–346.
4. Keith LG, Blickstein I. Triplet Pregnancies. London: Parthenon Press, 2002.
5. Luke B, Brown MB, Nugent C, Gonzalez-Quintero VH, Witter FR, Newman RB. Risk factors for adverse outcomes in spontaneous versus assisted conception twin pregnancies. Fertil Steril 2004; 81:315–319.
6. Anwar HN, Ihab MU, Johnny BR, Tarek SH, Abdallah MA, Antoine AA. Pregnancy outcomes in spontaneous twins versus twins who were conceived through in vitro fertilization. Am J Obstet Gynecol 2003; 189:513–518.
7. Evans MI, Dommergues M, Wapner RJ, et al. Efficacy of transabdominal multifetal pregnancy reduction: collaborative experience among the world's largest centers. Obstet Gynecol 1993; 82:61–67.
8. Toner JP. Progress we can be proud of: U.S. trends in assisted reproduction over the first 20 years. Fertil Steril 2002; 78:943–950.
9. Wright VC, Schieve LA, Reynolds MA, Jeng G, Kissin D. Assisted reproductive technology surveillance—United States, 2001. MMWR Surveill Summ 2004; 53:1–20.
10. US Govt Printing Office. 2002 Assisted Reproductive Technology Success Rates. National Summary and Fertility Clinic Reports. Centers for Disease Control, US Govt Printing Office, December 2004.
11. Evans MI, Berkowitz R, Wapner R, et al. Multifetal pregnancy reduction (MFPR): improved outcomes with increased experience. Am J Obstet Gynecol 2001; 184:97–103.
12. Adashi EY, Barri PN, Berkowitz R, et al. Infertility therapy-assisted multiple pregnancies (births): an on-going epidemic. Reprod Med Online 2003; 7:515–542.
13. Evans MI, Fletcher JC. Multifetal pregnancy reduction. In: Reece EA, Hobbins JC, Mahoney MJ, Petrie R, eds. Medicine of the Fetus and its Mother. Philadelphia: Lippincott Harper Publishing Co., 1992:1345–1362.
14. Evans MI, Littman L, St Louis L, et al. Evolving patterns of iatrogenic multifetal pregnancy generation: implications for aggressiveness of infertility treatments. Am J Obstet Gynecol 1995; 172:1750–1753.
15. Tabsh KM, Theroux NL. Genetic amniocentesis following multifetal pregnancy reduction twins: assessing the risk. Prenat Diagn 1995; 15:221–223.
16. McLean LK, Evans MI, Carpenter RJ, Johnson MP, Goldberg JD. Genetic amniocentesis (AMN) following multifetal pregnancy reduction (MFPR) does not increase the risk of pregnancy loss. Prenat Diagn 1998; 18:186–188.
17. Brambati B, Tului L, Baldi M, Guercilena S. Genetic analysis prior to selective termination in multiple pregnancy: technical aspects and clinical outcome. Hum Reprod 1995; 10:818–825.

18. Evans MI, Henry GP, Miller WA, et al. International, collaborative assessment of 146,000 prenatal karyotypes: expected limitations if only chromosome-specific probes and fluorescent in situ hybridization were used. Hum Reprod 1999; 14:1213–1216.

19. Homer J, Bhatt S, Huang B, Thangavelu M. Residual risk for cytogenetic abnormalities after prenatal diagnosis by interphase fluorescence in situ hybridizatio (FISH). Prenat Diagn 2003; 23:556–571.

20. Greene RA, Wapner J, Evans MI. Amniocentesis and chorionic villus sampling in triplet pregnancy. In: Keith LG, Blickstein I, Oleszcuk JJ, eds. Triplet Pregnancy. London: Parthenon Publishing Group, 73–84.

21. Zadori J, Kozinszky Z, Orvos H, Katona M, Kaali SG, Pal A. The incidence of major birth defects following in vitro fertilization. J Assist Reprod Genet 2003; 20:131–132.

22. Pinborg A, Loft A, Schmidt L, Andersen AN. Morbidity in a Danish national cohort of 472 IVF/ICSI twins, 1132 non-IVF/ICSI twins and 634 IVF/ICSI singletons: health-related and social implications for the children and their families. Hum Reprod 2003; 18:1234–1243.

23. Place I, Englert Y. A prospective longitudinal study of the physical, psychomotor, and intellectual development of singleton children up to 5 years who were conceived by intra-cytoplasmic sperm injection compared with children conceived spontaneously and by in vitro fertilization. Fertil Steril 2003; 80:1388–1397.

24. Retzloff MG, Hornstein MD. Is intracytoplasmic sperm injection safe? Fertil Steril 2003; 80:851–859.

25. Kurinczuk JJ. Safety issues in assisted reproduction technology. From theory to reality— just what are the data telling us about ICSI offspring health and future fertility and should we be concerned? Hum Reprod 2003; 18:925–931.

26. Tournaye H. ICSI: A technique too far? Int J Androl 2003; 26:63–69.

27. Dumez Y, Oury JF. Method for first trimester selective abortion in multiple pregnancy. Contrib Gynecol Obstet 1986; 15:50.

28. Evans MI, Fletcher JC, Zador IE, Newton BW, Struyk CK, Quigg MH. Selective first trimester termination in octuplet and quadruplet pregnancies: clinical and ethical issues. Obstct Gynecol 1988; 71:289–296.

29. Berkowitz RL, Lynch L, Chitkara U, et al. Selective reduction of multiple pregnancies in the first trimester. N Engl J Med 1988; 318:1043.

30. Wapner RJ, Davis GH, Johnson A. Selective reduction of multifetal pregnancies. Lancet 1990; 335:90–93.

31. Timor-Tritsch IE, Peisner DB, Monteagudo A, Lerner JP, Sharma S. Multifetal pregnancy reduction by transvaginal puncture: evaluation of the technique used in 134 cases. Am J Obstet Gynecol 1993; 168:799–804.

32. Torok O, Lapinski R, Salafia CM, Bernasko J, Berkowitz RL. Multifetal pregnancy reduction is not associated with an increased risk of intrauterine growth restriction, except for very high order multiples. Am J Obstet Gynecol 1998; 179:221–225.

33. Yaron Y, Bryant-Greenwood PK, Dave N, et al. Multifetal pregnancy reduction (MFPR) of triplets to twins: comparison with non-reduced triplets and twins. Am J Obstet Gynecol 1999; 180:1268–1271.

34. Leondires MP, Ernst SD, Miller BT, et al. Triplets: outcomes of expectant management versus multifetal reduction for 127 pregnancies. Am J Obstet Gynecol 1999; 72:257–260.

35. Lipitz S, Shulman A, Achiron R, et al. A comparative study of multifetal pregnancy reduction from triplets to twins in the first versus early second trimesters after detailed fetal screening. Ultrasound Obstet Gynecol 2001; 18:35–38.

36. Angel JL, Kalter CS, Morales WJ, et al. Aggressive prerinatal care for high-order multiple gestations: does good perinatal outcome justify aggressive assisted reproductive techniques? Am J Obstet Gynecol 1999; 181:253–259.

37. Sepulveda W, Munoz H, Alcalde JL. Conjoined twins in a triplet pregnancy: early prenatal diagnosis with three-dimensional ultrasound and review of the literature. Ultrasound Obstet Gynecol 2003; 22:199–204.

38. Francois K, Sears C, Wilson R, Elliot J. Twelve year experience of triplet pregnancies at a single institution. Am J Obstet Gynecol 2001; 185:S112.
39. Yakin K, Kahraman S, Comert S. Three blastocyst stage embryo transfer resulting in a quintuplet pregnancy. Hum Reprod 2001; 16:782–784.
40. ACOG. Neonatal Encephalopathy and Cerebral Palsy: Defining the Pathogensis and Pathophysiology. Task Force of American College of Obstetricians and Gynecologists. Washington, DC: ACOG, 2003.
41. Petterson B, Nelson K, Watson L, et al. Twins, triplets, and cerebral palsy in births in Western Australia in the 1980s. Br Med J 1993; 307:1239–1243.
42. Pharoah PO, Cooke T. Cerebral palsy and multiple births. Arch Dis Child Fetal Neonatal Edn 1996; 75:F174–F177.
43. Templeton A. The multiple gestation epidemic: the role of the assisted reproductive technologies. Am J Obstet Gynecol 2004; 190:894–898.
44. Evans MI, Kaufman MI, Urban AJ, Krivchenia EL, Britt DW, Wapner RJ. Fetal reduction from twins to a singleton: a reasonable consideration. Obstet Gynecol 2004. In press.
45. Kalra SK, Milad MP, Klock SC, Crobman, WA. Infertility patients and their partners: differences in the desire for twin gestations. Obstet Gynecol 2003; 102:152–155.
45a. Evans MI, Krivchenia EL, Kaufman M, Zador IE, Birtt DW, Wapner RJ. The optimal management of first trimester triplets: reduce. The Central Association of Obstetricians and Gynecologists. Annual Meeting, Las Vegas, Nevada, October 27–30, 2002.
46. St. John EB, Nelson KG, Oliver SP, Bishno RR, Goldenberg RL. Cost of neonatal care according to gestational age at birth and survival status. Am J Obstet Gynecol 2000; 182:170–175.
47. Britt DW, Risinger ST, Mans M, Evans MI. Devastation and relief: conflicting meanings in discovering fetal anomalies. Ultrasound Obstet Gynecol 2002; 20:1–5.
48. Britt DW, Risinger ST, Mans M, Evans MI. Anxiety among women who have undergone fertility therapy and who are considering MFPR: trends and scenarios. J Matern Fetal Neonatal Med. In press.
49. Britt DW, Evans WJ, Mehta SS, Evans MI. Framing the decision: determinants of how women considering MFPR as a pregnancy-management strategy frame their moral dilemma. Fetal Diagn Ther 2004; 19:232–240.
50. Redelmeier DA, Rozin P, Kahneman D. Understanding patients' decisions: cognitive and emotional perspectives. J Am Med Assoc 1993; 270:72–76.
51. Chapman GB, Elstein AS. Cognitive processes and biases in medical decision making. In: Chapman GB, Sonnenberg FA, eds. Decision Making in Health Care: Theory, Psychology and Applications. New York: Cambridge University Press, 2000:183–210.
52. Steginga SK, Occhipinti S. The application of the heuristic-systematic processing model to treatment decision making about prostate cancer. Med Decis Making 2004; 24.
53. Hamm RM. Theory about heuristic strategies based on verbal protocol analysis: the emperor needs a shave. Med Decis Making 2004; 24:681–686.
54. Britt DW, Campbell EQ. Assessing the linkage of norms, environments and deviance. Soc Forces 1977, December, 532–549.

30

Gene Therapy

Anna L. David and Charles H. Rodeck
Department of Obstetrics and Gynaecology, Royal Free and University College London Medical School, London, U.K.

INTRODUCTION

Gene therapy uses the intracellular delivery of genetic material for the treatment of disease (Fig. 1). A wide range of diseases including cancer, vascular and neurodegenerative disorders, and inherited genetic diseases are being considered as targets for this therapy in adults. Application of gene therapy in utero has been considered as a strategy for treatment or even prevention of early onset genetic disorders such as cystic fibrosis (CF) and Duchenne muscular dystrophy (1). Gene transfer to the developing fetus may target rapidly expanding stem cell populations that are inaccessible after birth and may allow permanent gene transfer by use of integrating vector systems. The functionally immature fetal immune system may permit induction of immune tolerance against vector and transgene and, thereby, facilitate repeated treatment after birth. Finally, and most importantly for clinicians, fetal gene therapy would give a third choice to parents following prenatal diagnosis of inherited disease, where currently termination of pregnancy or acceptance of an affected child have been the only options. Application of this therapy in the fetus must be safe, reliable, and cost-effective. Recent developments in the understanding of genetic disease, vector design, and minimally invasive delivery techniques have brought fetal gene therapy closer to clinical practice. Prenatal studies in animal models are being pursued in parallel with adult studies of gene therapy, but they remain presently at the experimental stage. This chapter explores the latest developments in the field of fetal gene therapy and its implications for future clinical application.

THE CANDIDATE DISEASES

Fetal gene therapy has been proposed to be appropriate for life-threatening disorders in which prenatal gene delivery maintains a clear advantage over cell transplantation or postnatal gene therapy and for which there are currently no satisfactory treatments available (2). Some of the diseases that may be suitable for fetal treatment are listed in Table 1. Studies on animal models of human disease such as canine

535

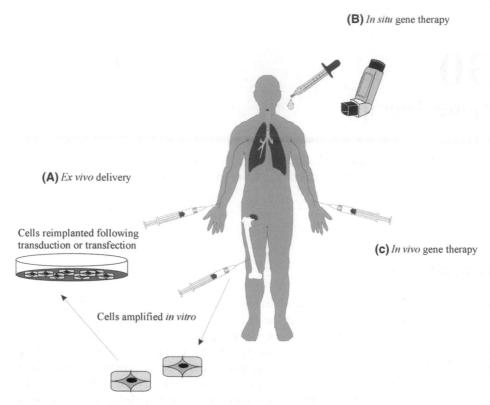

Figure 1 Diagrammatic representation of the different ways of applying gene therapy vectors. (**A**) Ex vivo delivery: genetic material is delivered to cells after their removal and culture in vitro, before subsequent reimplantation, e.g., stem cell gene therapy. (**B**) In situ gene therapy: gene therapy is delivered directly to the tissue of interest, e.g., the airways for treatment of cystic fibrosis. (**C**) In vivo gene therapy: systemic administration of gene therapy where there is insufficient targeting of vectors to the correct tissue sites, e.g., metabolic storage disorders.

hemophilia B have improved our understanding of disease processes and have shown that gene therapy treatment is possible (3). Transgenic mouse models such as for spinal muscular atrophy (4) and sickle cell disease (5) have been developed and will enable the results of gene transfer to be evaluated. Two diseases, CF and hemophilia B, are discussed in more detail in this chapter to illustrate recent progress.

Cystic Fibrosis

CF appears to be an ideal candidate for treatment with fetal gene therapy. First, it is the most common lethal autosomal recessive disorder in Caucasians with an incidence of 1 in 2000 live births in Western Europe and North America. Several mutations of the cystic fibrosis transmembrane regulator (CFTR) gene encoding the CFTR protein have been identified, and the resulting disease is characterized by abnormal electrolyte transport in the epithelia of the airways, the ducts of the sweat glands and exocrine pancreas, and the intestine. The main sites of CFTR expression in the non-CF human bronchi are the submucosal glands (6). In vitro studies, where normal and CF airway cells were mixed, suggest that as few as 6% to 10% of cells

Table 1 Examples of Candidate Diseases for Fetal Gene Therapy

Disease	Therapeutic gene product	Target cells/organ
Cystic fibrosis	CF transmembrane conductance regulator	Airway and intestinal epithelial cells
Metabolic disorders		
Ornithine transcarbamylase deficiency	Ornithine transcarbamylase	Hepatocytes
Glycogen storage disorders		
Pompe disease	α1,4-Glucosidase	Hepatocytes, myocytes, and neurons
Sphingolipid storage disorders		
Tay-Sachs disease	β-*N*-Acetylhexosaminidase	Fibroblasts, neurons
Mucopolysaccharide storage disorders		
Sly disease	β-Glucuronidase	Hepatocytes, neurons
Muscular dystrophies		
Duchenne	Dystrophin	Myocytes
Neurological disorders		
Spinal muscular atrophy	Survival motor neuron protein	Motor neurons
Hemophilias		
Hemophilia B	Human factor IX clotting factor	Hepatocytes
Hemoglobinopathies		
β-Thalassemia	β-Globin chains of hemoglobin	Hematopoietic precursor cells
Immunodeficiency disorders		
X-linked severe combined immunodeficiency	γc Cytokine receptor	Hematopoietic precursor cells
Skin disorders		
Dystrophic epidermolysis bullosa	Type VII collagen	Keratinocytes
Non-inherited perinatal diseases		
Hypoxia–ischemia	Neurotrophic factors	Cortical neurons
Placental disorders		
Severe preeclampsia	Nitric oxide synthase	Trophoblasts

Abbreviation: CF, cystic fibrosis.

expressing normal CFTR are required to correct the chloride transport defect of an epithelial cell monolayer (7), thus, successful gene therapy may require only relatively low level epithelial airway transduction.

Phase 1 gene therapy trials directed toward pulmonary disease in CF have shown equivocal results and highlight the problems of present gene therapy approaches in adults (8). The lungs may already be severely damaged or obstructed, even in young adult patients, limiting delivery of gene therapy to the airway epithelium. Fluorocarbon liquids such as perflubron have recently been shown to improve distribution of adenoviral vectors and gene expression in normal and diseased adult lungs (9,10). Pretreatment of airway with detergents (11) or agents that modulate paracellular permeability such as the fatty acid sodium caprate (12) or ethylene glycol tetraacetic acid (EGTA) (13) also improve adenovirus-mediated airway transduction. Immune responses to the vector, particularly in the case of adenoviral vectors, limit the dose that may be safely administered and reduce the duration of expression.

The CFTR gene has been proposed to play an important, albeit still unknown, physiological role in normal fetal development (14,15). Furthermore, the CF disease process appears to begin during development of CF fetuses, since by the midtrimester a proinflammatory state exists in fetal CF airways (16), and there are abnormalities of the pancreas and small bowel (17). Submucosal gland development has been studied in the rhesus monkey fetus (18) and although not characterized in the human fetal airways, submucosal gland progenitors have been identified in the human adult lung (19). Gene transfer to a human fetal lung xenograft model in severe combined immunodeficiency (SCID) mice was efficiently achieved using adenoviral vectors (20), and long-term expression in the surface epithelial and submucosal gland cells was observed up to four weeks and nine months after administration of adeno-associated and lentiviral vectors, respectively (21,22).

The early disease manifestation and poor results from gene therapy treatment of adults with CF have led to research on fetal gene therapy for this disease in animal models. Despite the multiorgan manifestation of CF, first approaches are directed toward gene delivery to the fetal airways, which has been achieved by intra-amniotic application and, in larger animals, by intratracheal injection. Other genetic diseases that could benefit from progress achieved in pulmonary gene delivery are α1-antitrypsin deficiency (23) and surfactant protein B deficiency (24).

Hemophilias

The hemophilias A and B are also particularly suitable for gene therapy in utero. Both are X-linked hereditary hemorrhagic disorders that occur in 1 in 10,000 fetuses and 1 in 25,000 males, respectively, and are caused by the absence or dysfunction of the respective human factor VIII (hFVIII) or IX (hFIX) clotting factors (25). Current treatment uses replacement therapy with hFVIII or hFIX. Unfortunately, a number of patients develop antibodies to therapy leading to ineffective treatment and occasional anaphylaxis (26). Indeed, the complications of hemophilia treatment, which include the major risk of HIV (human immunodeficiency virus) and hepatitis B infections, have in some cases been far worse than the diseases themselves, increasing their morbidity and mortality (27).

As the coagulation factors are required in the blood and can be secreted functionally from a variety of tissues, the actual site of production is not so important as long as therapeutic plasma levels are realized. Adult gene therapy strategies have, therefore, concentrated on application to the muscle or the liver. Successful delivery and expression of FIX has been achieved in adult animal models of hemophilia B following portal intravascular administration of adenoviral (28) and retroviral vectors (29). Sustained FIX expression was also observed after intramuscular injection of adult hemophiliac dogs with adeno-associated viral (AAV) vectors expressing canine FIX (3,30) and after intravascular injection of adult hemophiliac mice with AAV vectors expressing hFIX (31). These results culminated in the first clinical trial in humans that showed promising results, although only low-level hFIX expression has so far been observed (32). Recently, a study of clinical safety with the AAV vector was halted due to the development of minor liver toxicity in two patients and the suggestion that their bodies were mounting an immune response to the vector (33). Successful delivery and expression of therapeutic hFIX without formation of antibodies has been achieved following administration of retroviral vectors in neonatal animal models (34). Prenatal gene therapy could be applied to the fetus via a number of routes including muscle, peritoneal, hepatic, intravascular, or skin application. More recently, our group has demonstrated that in utero application can provide long-term postnatal correction of the hemophiliac phenotype in FIX deficient mice (35).

VECTORS FOR FETAL GENE THERAPY

The development of efficient vector systems is crucial for the success of gene therapy. The ideal vector for fetal somatic gene therapy would introduce a transcriptionally regulated therapeutic gene into all organs relevant to the genetic disorder by a single safe application. Although none of the present vector systems meets all these criteria, many of them have characteristics that may be beneficial to the fetal approach.

Nonviral Vectors

Nonviral gene delivery systems can be chemical or physical. Synthetic nonviral vector systems have many potential advantages compared with viral vectors. They have significantly lower toxicity, immunogenicity, and oncogenic potential, and there is no limit to the size of nucleic acid that may be delivered, from oligonucleotides to artificial chromosomes. In addition, the production of synthetic nonviral vectors has simpler quality control and easier pharmaceutical and regulatory requirements. Nonviral gene delivery systems, however, are not efficient at mediating gene transfer and are not particularly stable in biological fluids. Because of this, there have been few studies investigating fetal gene therapy using nonviral vector systems.

Cationic liposome/micelle-based systems are the most promising synthetic nonviral vectors (36). These liposomes bind and condense DNA spontaneously to form complexes with high affinity to cell membranes. Gene delivery occurs by endocytosis of the complexes followed by disruption of the endosomal membrane. Cationic polymers such as polyethylene glycol (PEG) that complex with nucleic acid can mediate gene transfer in a similar way. Application of the cationic polymer polyethylenimine (PEI) to the liver of late gestation fetal mice enhanced gene transfer to the liver as compared with administration of naked DNA. More importantly, the fetal liver appeared to be especially amenable to the uptake and expression of concentrated naked DNA and the gene transfer efficiency was 40 times higher than that achieved in adult liver (37).

The DNA introduced as plasmid molecules remains episomal and will be lost over time following cell division. This is a particular disadvantage in the fetus where cell populations are rapidly dividing. Transient gene transfer may be useful, however, in the management of a developmental setting in which therapy is only required for a relatively short time. For instance, short-term transgene expression has been shown to be a promising approach to maintain a patent ductus arteriosus prior to surgery for congenital heart defects in neonates (38). Liposomes containing plasmid expressing a decoy RNA designed to sequester fibronectin mRNA binding protein were delivered to the ductus arteriosus in fetal sheep at 90 days of gestation, prior to the onset of intimal cushion formation at 100 days of gestation. Fibronectin synthesis was inhibited resulting in a 60% reduction in intimal thickness and increased ductal patency at term.

More recently, nonviral systems have been developed that integrate into the host genome and could thus, in principle, provide long-term gene expression, but these vectors are still at an early stage of experimental design (39).

Physical methods of gene transfer such as electroporation, microinjection, or biolistics using gene guns would be technically difficult to achieve in the fetus because of problems with access.

Viral Vectors

Studies of gene therapy in the fetus have, therefore, concentrated on viral vectors, many of which have been designed to deliver reporter genes such as the β-galactosidase gene (lacZ). These allow tracking of the transduced cells and definition of tissue expression by biochemical staining assays. Alternatively, use of vectors carrying therapeutic genes allows the assessment of potentially curative levels of the expressed protein and, in animal models of disease, even the observation of phenotype correction. The hFIX gene, for instance, can be used both as a marker gene, allowing the analysis of blood levels of the hFIX protein over time in nonhemophiliac animals, and in the study of the correction of the blood clotting parameters in animal models of hemophilia. Postnatal readministration of hFIX protein or the hFIX vector to fetally treated animals can be used to examine whether immune tolerance has been achieved.

Retrovirus

Vectors that are able to integrate into the host genome such as retroviruses, lentiviruses, and to a lesser extent adeno-associated viruses may offer the possibility of permanent gene delivery. Figure 2 illustrates the production of attenuated therapeutic retrovirus vectors and demonstrates how these vectors are assembled and packaged in virus producer cells using only vital elements from the wild-type virus. Although only fairly low virus titers can be produced, virus gene transfer may be improved by complexing vectors with cationic agents (41), or by the administration of retrovirus producer cells in vivo to allow localized gene delivery close to the site of cell transfer (42,43).

Retroviruses require dividing cells for gene transfer (44), which suggests that they may be better suited for use in fetal tissues where cells are rapidly dividing rather than in adult applications. Other problems include reports of premature promoter shutdown (45,46) leading to transcriptional shutoff. Human serum can almost completely inactivate some retroviral particles (47), which limits their use in vivo although increased resistance to serum inactivation can be achieved by generating retroviruses from particular human packaging cells (48) or by pseudotyping, which replaces the natural envelope of the retrovirus with a heterologous envelope (49). A particular problem with in utero application is that amniotic fluid has also been shown in vitro to have a mild inhibitory effect on retrovirus infection (50). A further difficulty is the relatively short half-life of the retroviral particles in vivo, which may hinder transduction because fetal cell division is nonsynchronized and only those cells undergoing cell division at the time of infection will become transduced.

Retroviruses were used in the first successful gene therapy trial, where bone marrow stem cells transduced ex vivo with retroviral vectors expressing the correct cDNA were delivered to infants suffering from an X-linked form of SCID (51). The infants were able to leave protective isolation, discontinue treatment, and

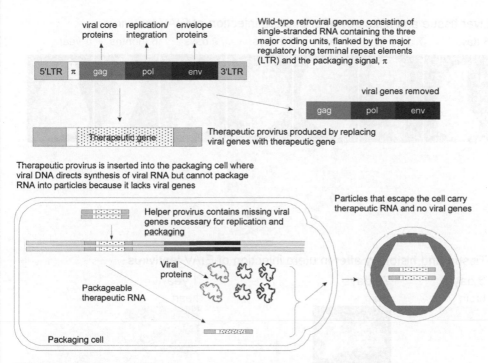

Figure 2 Diagram of safe manufacture of retrovirus vectors from wild-type retrovirus. *Source*: From Ref. 40.

appear to be developing normally (52). However, 3 of the 17 patients treated for X-linked SCID have developed acute lymphoblastic leukemia (ALL) three years after successful gene therapy treatment, which has been shown to involve insertional mutagenesis. An expanded clonal population of T cells was demonstrated to be carrying the γc transgene inserted at 11p13 in the region of LMO2, an oncogene frequently overexpressed in T-cell leukemias (53). Insertional mutagenesis is an acknowledged potential complication with retroviral-mediated gene transfer because gene integration occurs randomly into the genome. This is the first report of malignant change in humans following retroviral gene therapy, and only one example has been found in extensive animal studies using this vector (54). There is now evidence that the therapeutic γc transgene can act as an oncogene when under the control of a retroviral promoter and can collaborate with the LMO2 oncogene (55). This may explain the high incidence of leukemia observed in this study and suggests that if a therapeutic transgene does not have oncogenic potential, then the risk of cancer should be low.

Lentivirus

Because of the limitation of infection to dividing cells by retroviruses, alternative vectors such as lentiviruses have been developed to circumvent this restriction. Significant progress has been made in recent years in the development of lentiviral vectors, a retroviral subgroup based on the HIV (56) or equine infectious anemia virus (EIAV) (57). HIV vectors are capable of transferring genes into nondividing cells such as neurons (58) and quiescent hematopoietic progenitor cells (59), which will be particularly useful for these tissue targets. Lentiviral vectors integrate into the genome randomly and are, therefore, theoretically able to cause insertional mutagenesis.

Liver tissue and histology after in utero injection of EIAV lentivirus

3 days   7 days   14 days   28 days   79 days   6 months   1 year

Tissue and histology after in utero injection of EIAV lentivirus

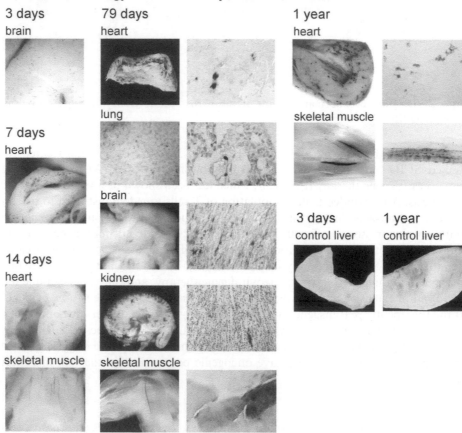

Figure 3   (*Caption on facing page*)

Lentiviruses can be made more stable by pseudotyping that allows virus titres to be improved by ultracentrifugation. This offers the opportunity of infecting a greater number of cells in vivo and different envelopes allow targeted gene transfer to specific tissues, for example, to the nervous system (60) and airways (61). Both the EIAV vector, a vector derived from nonprimate animal lentiviruses (57), and feline immunodeficiency virus (FIV) (62) have been developed in an attempt to create vectors for use in human treatment that are not associated with any human pathology. Our recent work has shown that high-level sustained transgene expression can be achieved in a variety of tissues using the EIAV vector in fetal mice after intravascular administration (Fig. 3) (63).

Adeno-Associated Viral Vectors

AAV, a common human parvovirus, is also a promising novel vector system. AAV naturally requires coinfection with adenovirus as a helper virus, but the latest AAV vectors circumvent the need for adenovirus and, therefore, make the production of pure AAV particles easier (64). AAV is also able to infect nondividing cells and to achieve long-lasting gene correction in vitro and in vivo (3,65,66). The basis for long-term transgene expression is not quite clear. Integration of the wild-type virus is predominantly at an apparently specific functionally unimportant location on human chromosome 19, reducing the theoretical risk of insertional mutagenesis; however, recombinant vector appears to integrate at low levels and nonspecifically (67). AAV vectors have a limited capacity for the insertion of foreign genes that is about 4.7 kb, although recently to increase AAV packaging capacity "split AAV vectors" have been designed where large genes are split between two AAV genomes. After concatemerization of these genomes in the host cell mRNA, splicing allows the removal of intervening ITR sequences and restoration of the split coding sequence to yield wild-type functional protein (68). Because the extent of AAV integration is still in question, this vector system may not give the permanent gene expression ideal for in utero gene therapy without repeat treatment, although long-term transgene expression after intraperitoneal delivery in mice has recently been reported (69). Some caution has also been expressed as AAV integration appears to induce chromosome deletions (70). A correlation between early abortion as well as male infertility and the presence of wild-type AAV DNA in the genital tract has been suggested (71–74). Although no causal relationship has been established, this issue stresses the

---

Figure 3 (*Facing page*) (*Upper panel*) Representative sections of fetal livers harvested at 72 hours, 7, 14, 28, 79, 168 days, and 1 year after yolk sac injection of high titer EAIV SMART2Z (equine infectious anamia virus vector expressing the β-galactosidase gene driven by the CMV promoter) lentiviral vector ($n = 1$, 1, 3, 1, and 1, respectively). Uniform hepatocyte staining is observed after 72 hours followed by the emergence of clusters of β-galactosidase-stained hepatocytes to day 79. Macroscopic appearance of liver sections (*top row*, ×10). Microscopic analyses (*bottom row*, ×400). Age-matched noninfected control livers of three-day-old and one-year-old animals are shown in the lower panel. (*Lower panel*) Representative sections of fetal tissues harvested at 72 hours, 7, 14, 79 days, and 1 year after yolk sac injection of high titer EAIV SMART2Z lentiviral vector ($n = 1/4$, 1, 1, 3, and 1, respectively). High-level staining is observed after 72 hours and 79 days in brain, 7, 14, and 79 days in heart, and 14 and 79 days in skeletal muscle. Low-level expression is shown in lung and kidney at 79 days postinjection. Macroscopic appearance of tissues (*left columns*, ×10). Microscopic analysis (*right column*, ×400). *Source*: From Ref. 63.

importance of using recombinant AAV stocks devoid of contaminating replication-competent AAV for fetal gene therapy.

Adenovirus

Adenoviral vectors have been used as attractive vectors for proof of principle studies in fetal gene therapy since they have continually achieved highly efficient gene transfer in vivo. The adenoviral coding sequences necessary for viral replication are deleted, rendering them replication defective. They are relatively stable and can be obtained at high titer making systemic administration in humans and large animal models feasible. The adenovirus genome replicates outside the chromosome, which avoids the risk of insertional mutagenesis but results in only transient gene expression. Their broad host range and tropism to most cells of the human body, including the respiratory epithelium, has made them very useful in initial pathfinder studies on vector delivery and transgene expression. They are particularly useful for exploring different technical approaches to fetal gene therapy.

Factors that determine the kinetics of transgene expression include vector elimination, since adenovirus is not an integrating vector, and promoter shutdown. Adenoviral vectors are also highly immunogenic. Major concerns about the safety of adenoviral vectors were raised following the death of Jesse Gelsinger from a systemic inflammatory response to a first generation adenovirus vector used for a phase 1 clinical trial toward gene therapy of the inherited metabolic disorder, ornithine transcarbamylase deficiency (75). Even fetal administration of adenoviral vectors has been associated with an immune response (76), particularly after postnatal repeat exposure to the vector (77). Attempts to reduce the immunogenicity and toxicity of the vector and to increase its insert capacity have led to the generation of the so-called "gutless vectors" in which essentially all adenoviral coding sequences have been eliminated (78,79).

Because adenoviruses provide highly efficient gene transfer yet transient expression, novel hybrid vectors have been developed to take advantage of adenovirus infectivity and the permanent nature of integrative vectors such as retroviruses and lentiviruses (80,81). Hybrid vectors of recombinant AAV packaged in adenovirus capsids can mediate transfer of large fragments of foreign DNA and achieve stable long-term transgene expression in rapidly proliferating cells (82). Hybrid vectors may offer efficient gene expression to fetal organs such as the lung in which it has so far proved difficult to achieve high-level gene transfer with integrating vectors.

Sendai Virus

Recently, the negative strand RNA cytoplasmically replicating Sendai virus, a member of the paramyxovirus family, was developed as a gene transfer vector. Early vectors still capable of self-propagation were found to provide very high levels of marker gene expression in a wide range of tissues including bronchial epithelium (83), skeletal muscle (84), and vascular endothelium (85). Second-generation vectors, although still capable of intracytoplasmic replication of the RNA genome, are incapable of intercellular propagation. In these vectors, genes encoding surface glycoproteins including the hemagglutinin-neuraminidase (HN) protein or the fusion (F) protein, which are responsible for cell binding and infection, have been deleted from the viral genome (86). Injection of F-deficient Sendai virus vector (87) into the fetal mouse via various routes including intravascular, intra-amniotic, intra-muscular, intraperitoneal, and intraspinal injection resulted in expression of marker gene in gut wall, lung, muscle, peritoneal mesothelia, and dorsal route ganglia, respectively. Further optimization will be needed to develop these first-generation constructs into clinically applicable vectors.

APPLICATION OF GENE THERAPY TO THE FETUS

Developments in vectorology must be accompanied by improvements in minimally invasive methods of delivering vectors to the fetus if this therapy is to be clinically applicable. Invasive surgical techniques such as maternal laparotomy or hysterotomy must be performed to access the fetus in small animal models, but have also been applied in large animal studies such as in the sheep (88,89). Surgery carries a high morbidity from wound infection and hemorrhage, and the risk of mortality is significant. Well-established minimally invasive techniques used clinically in fetal medicine are being investigated and adapted. Amniocentesis, used clinically for prenatal diagnosis, is one of the safest intrauterine procedures. Intra-amniotic application of vectors may be only of limited use in fetal gene therapy because of vector dilution by the large volume of amniotic fluid, although it would be the ideal application route for in utero gene therapy of skin diseases.

Accessing the systemic circulation has greater potential. Fetal blood is usually obtained in the second trimester under ultrasound guidance either from the placental cord insertion, the fetal heart, or more safely from the intrahepatic umbilical vein. The procedure has a good success rate clinically, is low risk, and is used commonly for rapid karyotyping or fetal blood transfusion (90). Earlier in pregnancy, intracardiac injection allows access to the fetal circulation. From 12 weeks of gestation, ultrasound-guided intracardiac puncture for fetal blood sampling has been performed on patients undergoing surgical termination of pregnancy (91). Similarly, radiolabeled fetal liver cells were successfully injected into the heart of 13-week-old fetuses under ultrasound guidance (92) prior to prostaglandin termination of pregnancy. No fetal heart rate abnormalities were detected, and all fetuses were alive at least six hours after the procedure.

Intraperitoneal injection can be used for blood transfusion before 18 weeks of gestation (93) and could be a useful route for application of gene therapy as an alternative to intravascular delivery. It has been applied for in utero stem cell transplantation in humans from 14 weeks of gestation (94,95).

Coelocentesis uses ultrasound to guide a needle into the extraembryonic coelom in the early first trimester. It has a success rate of > 95% at 6 to 11 weeks of gestation, and has been suggested as a possible technique for stem cell engraftment in early gestation (2). It may be of little use, however, for in utero gene therapy because of the limited transfer from the extraembryonic coelom via the amniotic membrane to the amniotic cavity (96). Studies on the risk of miscarriage in ongoing pregnancies beyond the first trimester following coelocentesis gave controversial results (97).

Fetoscopy has been used to instill gene therapy into the fetal trachea for targeting the fetal airways (98). Recently, adenoviral vectors have been delivered to the fetal trachea using a percutaneous transthoracic route of injection in fetal sheep (99). Other potentially useful routes for gene therapy delivery include intramuscular injection for congenital muscular dystrophies and intrahepatic injection for metabolic storage disorders.

FETAL GENE THERAPY STUDIES

Since the initial attempts in the early 1990s, fetal gene therapy has been investigated in a range of different animals using a variety of techniques. The possible routes of administration are illustrated in Figure 4. Studies in large animals have mainly used sheep, since primates are more costly and difficult to maintain. Unfortunately, there are few large animal models of human genetic disease available for testing of gene therapy. It is for this reason that small animals such as mice are commonly used, although their size precludes development of minimally invasive techniques of application.

Direct Targeting of the Fetal Circulation

Delivery of vectors to the systemic fetal circulation appears to be a highly effective route for targeting gene therapy to a range of fetal tissues and particularly to the liver for treatment of diseases such as the hemophilias and the metabolic and storage disorders. This can be accomplished in small animals such as the mouse by intracardiac injection (101,102) or by injection into the yolk sac vessels (103). Indeed, yolk sac vessel injection of adenoviral vectors containing the hFIX gene into fetal mice resulted in therapeutic levels of hFIX expression (104). Long-term transgene expression was observed in the liver, heart, brain, and muscle up to a year after delivery of lentiviral vectors containing the β-galactosidase gene into yolk sac vessels of fetal mice (63) and was then used to achieve correction of the hemophilic phenotype in FIX-deficient mice (35).

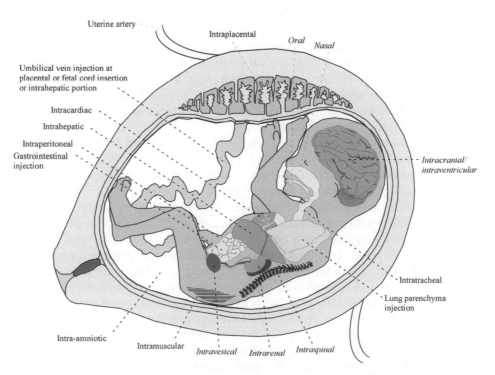

Figure 4 Routes of administration of gene therapy to the fetus. Routes in *italics* have not yet been applied in a fetal animal model using ultrasound-guided injection. *Source*: From Ref. 100.

In larger animals such as in the sheep, intravascular delivery can be achieved by injection via the umbilical vein (105). Adenoviral vectors containing the lacZ or hFIX genes were delivered into the umbilical vein of late gestation fetal sheep using ultrasound-guided percutaneous injection from 102 days gestation (term = 145 days) (106). Positive lacZ expression was seen in ~30% of fetal hepatocytes, and hFIX expression in fetal and neonatal plasma by ELISA analysis reached therapeutic levels within a week of delivery in two animals.

In early gestation, delivery of adenoviral vectors into the umbilical vein of fetal sheep at 60 days of gestation via hysterotomy resulted in widespread transduction of fetal tissues (105). Attempts to inject adenoviral vectors into the umbilical vein of fetal sheep at the earlier time of 53 days of gestation using ultrasound guidance were unsuccessful due to procedure-related mortality (107).

Ultrasound-guided intracardiac injection has been used to deliver adenoviral vectors to the late gestation fetal rabbit (102). Transgene expression was observed in up to 40% of fetal hepatocytes and was transient as expected. A fetal immune response to the vector and transgene was detected. Unfortunately, the procedure also had a 25% to 40% mortality rate, comparable to other studies on fetal blood sampling in rabbits (108). Although technically straightforward, ultrasound-guided intracardiac delivery of adenoviral vectors to fetal sheep in early gestation resulted in 100% mortality due to hemorrhage (107).

Alternative Routes for Targeting the Fetal Circulation and Liver

Due to the peculiarities of the fetal anatomy, vector delivery via the umbilical vein or yolk sac vessels will preferentially target the liver, which is an important organ for treatment of many genetic diseases. However, in early pregnancy this has not been technically possible and alternative approaches to reach the liver and the circulation have been tried.

Intrahepatic Injection

Fetal intrahepatic injection has been performed in mice using adenoviral vectors (109–112), AAV (112;113), and lentiviral vectors (114). In these studies, high levels of transgene expression in fetal hepatocytes were observed as well as gene transfer to other organs such as the heart, spleen, lung, intestine, and brain suggesting hematogenic spread.

Ultrasound-guided intrahepatic injection has been performed in a few large animal models. In the late gestation fetal rabbit, X-gal staining of the fetal hepatocytes was seen two days after ultrasound-guided intrahepatic injection of adenoviral lacZ (115). Similarly, strong expression of transgenic enhanced green fluorescent protein was observed in hepatocytes one month after ultrasound-guided intrahepatic delivery of AAV vectors to the late-gestation rhesus monkey (116). Ultrasound-guided intrahepatic injection in early gestation fetuses has also been performed with fetal survival rates of 81% in the sheep (107). Only low level hepatocyte transduction, however, was observed after adenoviral and retroviral mediated gene transfer into fetal sheep (107) and primates (117). The different results achieved in large animal models as compared with the fetal mouse may be due to a number of factors including the infectivity of the fetal hepatocytes, the ability of fetal hepatocytes to express the transgene, and vector toxicity, which is a particular problem with adenovirus.

Intraperitoneal Injection

Intraperitoneal injection has also been used for successful gene transfer to multiple tissues including the liver in fetal mice (110,118), rats (119,120), and sheep (88). Persistent peritoneal expression was observed 18 months after intraperitoneal injection of AAV serotype 2 (AAV2) vectors containing the luciferase gene in fetal mice (121). Recent studies in the fetal mouse have shown that transgene expression could be increased by intraperitoneal injection of AAV5 serotype vectors rather than AAV2 serotype vectors, and by changing the promoter (69).

In large animal models, retroviral vectors containing the α-L-iduronidase gene were delivered by ultrasound-guided injection after exteriorization of the uterus, into the peritoneal cavity or yolk sac of midgestation fetal dogs with canine α-L-iduronidase deficiency (mucopolysaccharidosis type 1). Low-level tissue transduction was observed, but transgene expression did not persist beyond the neonatal period (122). In early gestation fetal primates, ultrasound-guided intraperitoneal injection of retroviral and lentiviral vectors resulted in only low-level tissue transduction (117). In contrast, long-term transduction of hematopoietic stem cells in the bone marrow and blood could be demonstrated five years following delivery of retroviral vectors into the peritoneal cavity of early gestation fetal sheep by laparotomy (123). Delivery of adenoviral vectors containing the hFIX gene to early gestation fetal sheep by ultrasound-guided intraperitoneal injection had good fetal survival of 77% and therapeutic hFIX production was achieved, albeit transiently (Fig. 5) (107). Immunohistochemical analysis after delivery of adenoviral lacZ vectors showed positive transgene expression in the peritoneal cavity and subcapsular hepatocytes. The intraperitoneal route also gave the most comprehensive spread of vector to fetal tissues as determined by polymerase chain reaction (PCR) analysis (107). Thus, the intraperitoneal route in the fetus appears to result in widespread hematogenic spread of gene therapy vectors.

Intramuscular Injection

The main aim of intramuscular injection is to target the muscle for treatment of muscular dystrophies, but this route may also be used for ectopic production of proteins such as hFIX in the treatment of hemophilias. In the fetal mouse, injection of adenoviral vectors containing the lacZ gene into the shoulder or hindlimb musculature resulted in persistent muscle and liver transgene expression for 16 and 8 weeks, respectively, after injection (124). Intramuscular injection of lentiviral vectors led to transduction of myocytes and cardiomyocytes indicating systemic spread of the virus from the site of injection (114).

In vivo expression of hFIX can be achieved after intramuscular injection of adenovirus and AAV hFIX vectors in adult and fetal mice (125). A recent study using EIAV lentivirus containing the lacZ gene combined intrathoracic, supracostal, intraperitoneal, and intramuscular injection of three limbs and a single flank in the fetal mouse. This resulted in widespread gene expression in all injected muscles and also the diaphragm and heart, which are the essential muscle groups to be reached for successful gene therapy of Duchenne muscular dystrophy (126).

Finally, delivery of adenoviral vectors into the hindlimb musculature by ultrasound-guided injection has been explored in the early gestation fetal sheep. Fetal survival was 91% and therapeutic levels of hFIX were also obtained after injection of adenovirus hFIX vector (Fig. 5). Immunohistochemistry for β-galactosidase after injection of adenovirus lacZ vector resulted in strong transgene expression in

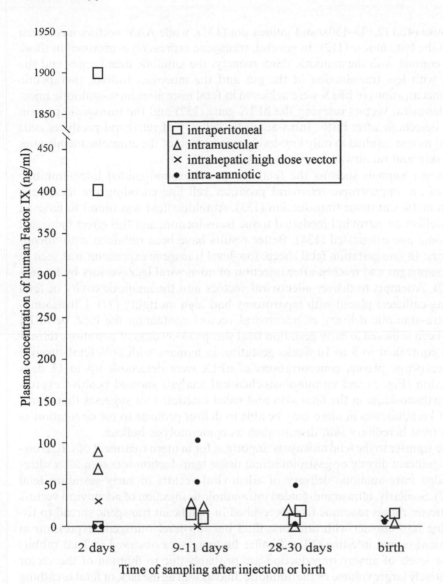

Figure 5 Time course of transgene expression after ultrasound-guided intraperitoneal, intramuscular, intrahepatic, or intra-amniotic delivery of an adenoviral vector containing the human factor IX gene to early gestation sheep fetuses. Concentrations of human factor IX in fetal or lamb plasma were determined by ELISA analysis. Fetal samples were collected at postmortem. *Source*: From Ref. 107.

the hindlimb musculature and occasional positively stained hepatocytes. PCR analysis of vector presence in fetal tissues confirmed that broad hematogenic spread of vector had occurred (107).

Targeting the Fetal Airways

Intra-Amniotic Injection

Intra-amniotic application has been investigated extensively in small animal models. Adenoviral vectors expressing the lacZ gene have been delivered to the fetal rat

(127), mouse (42,112,127–130), and guinea pig (131), while AAV vectors have been applied to the fetal mouse (112). In general, transgene expression is maximal in those tissues in contact with the amniotic fluid, namely, the amniotic membranes and the fetal skin with less transduction of the gut and the mucosae. Indeed, therapeutic plasma concentrations of hFIX were achieved in fetal mice after intra-amniotic injection of adenoviral vectors carrying the hFIX gene (132) and the transgenic protein remained detectable after birth. Intra-amniotic delivery of retroviral producer cells to the fetal mouse resulted in only low-level transduction of the amniotic membranes and fetal skin and no airway or gut transduction (42).

In larger animals such as the fetal sheep, ultrasound-guided intra-amniotic injection of an amphotropic retroviral producer cell line encoding the lacZ gene resulted in inefficient tissue transduction (133). Amniotic fluid was found to have an inhibitory effect on retroviral-mediated tissue transduction, and this effect increased as gestational age progressed (134). Better results have been obtained with adenoviral vectors. In late gestation fetal sheep, low-level transgene expression was seen in the fetal esophagus and trachea after injection of adenoviral lacZ vectors by laparotomy (130). Attempts to deliver adenoviral vectors into the amniotic cavity of fetal sheep using catheters placed with laparotomy had high mortality (77). Ultrasound-guided intra-amniotic delivery of adenoviral vectors containing the lacZ or hFIX genes has been achieved in early gestation fetal sheep (33–39 days of gestation, term = 145 days) equivalent to 8 to 10 weeks gestation in humans with 86% fetal survival (107). Therapeutic plasma concentrations of hFIX were detectable up to 11 days after injection (Fig. 5) and immunohistochemical analysis showed positive expression of β-galactosidase in the fetal skin and nasal cavities. This suggests that transduction of keratinocytes in utero may be able to deliver proteins to the circulation as well as to treat hereditary skin disease such as epidermolysis bullosa.

Gene transfer to the fetal airways is important for in utero treatment of CF. However, no significant airway or gastrointestinal tissue transduction was seen after ultrasound-guided intra-amniotic delivery of adenoviral vectors to early gestation fetal sheep (107). Similarly, ultrasound-guided intra-amniotic injection of adenoviral vectors in midtrimester rhesus macaque fetuses resulted in significant transgene spread to tissues coming into contact with amniotic fluid but low-level transgene expression in the fetal airways and intestine (135). Similar findings were observed in fetal rabbits (136). Low levels of airway transduction are probably due to dilution of the vector by the relatively larger volume of the amniotic fluid as well as the lack of fetal breathing movements or fetal swallowing at this early gestation. It may be possible to enhance fetal breathing movements in later gestation using agents such as theophylline (137) that lead to an intake of amniotic fluid to the lungs against the continuous outflow of tracheal fluid (138,139). Indeed increased intake of marker dye and some enhancement of adenovirus-mediated marker gene expression was observed in mouse fetuses after theophylline and carbondioxide administration, however the most important factor for efficient and consistent pulmonary transgene delivery was the dose of the adenovirus vector applied (140). Recent attempts to reproduce the report by Larson et al. 1997 (128), that the CF-phenotype in CFTR-knockout mice can be cured by short-term prenatal expression of CFTR from an adenovirus vector, have been unsuccessful (141).

Direct Lung Parenchymal Injection

Direct injection of the lung parenchyma has been attempted to access the fetal airways but with poor results. In midgestation fetal primates, ultrasound-guided injection of lentiviral vectors into the lung resulted in low-level transgene expression in the fetal airways (142). However, in the midgestation sheep fetus, ultrasound-guided delivery of an adenoviral vector to the lung parenchyma elicited only localized gene transfer and no spread within the airways could be detected (unpublished results).

Tracheal Injection

Direct instillation of vector into the trachea has been more successful. Placement of catheters in the fetal sheep trachea can be performed by highly invasive techniques by laparotomy (76,89,143) or fetoscopically (98,105). Low-level transduction of the proximal airways was achieved using adenoviral or retroviral vectors, and occlusion of the trachea with a balloon improved distal airway transduction. These techniques, however, carry a significant morbidity and mortality.

Recently, a percutaneous transthoracic route of injection of the fetal trachea has been developed in midgestation sheep using ultrasound guidance to target the fetal airways as illustrated in Figure 6 (99). Using this technique, good transgene expression was achieved in the fetal trachea and airways following intratracheal delivery of an adenovirus lacZ vector (144). Transgene expression was enhanced by pretreatment of the fetal airways with sodium caprate, a fatty acid that opens the tight junctions between airway epithelial cells. This allows the vector to reach the basolateral surface where the coxsackie-adenovirus receptor (CAR receptor) responsible for binding adenovirus is situated. Further enhancement of transgene expression was achieved by complexing the adenoviral vector with diethylaminoethyl (DEAE) dextran, a polycation that neutralizes the negative charge on the vector, improving vector binding to the CAR receptor (Fig. 7). Instillation of perflubron, an inert fluorocarbon, resulted in a redistribution of expression from the upper to the peripheral airways and is most likely due to flushing of the vector solution further down the airways by the water immiscible perflubron (145). These results show proof of principle for the relatively safe and minimally invasive delivery of a gene therapy vector to the fetal airways that resulted in levels of transgene expression in the airway epithelia that may be relevant to a therapeutic application in CF gene therapy.

Targeting the Fetal Gut

Intrapharyngeal delivery has been attempted once in fetal rabbits with laparotomy to target the fetal gastrointestinal system as a model for the treatment of meconium ileus due to CF (146). Gene transfer of the small bowel enterocytes was achieved but there was significant maternal and fetal loss related to anesthesia and the invasive surgery used. Ultrasound-guided injection of barium into the fetal stomach of rabbits has been performed successfully (147) and this technique could be extended to deliver gene therapy to the fetal gut. Gene delivery to the gut of fetal mice has been observed after intra-amniotic vector application and was most likely a result of fetal swallowing (42).

Delivery to the Placenta

Targeting the placenta could be used in the treatment of placental disorders such as preeclampsia or intrauterine growth restriction. Low-level gene transfer to the placenta has been achieved using angiographically guided injection of nonviral vectors into the uterine artery (148). The intraplacental route has been attempted in

(A)

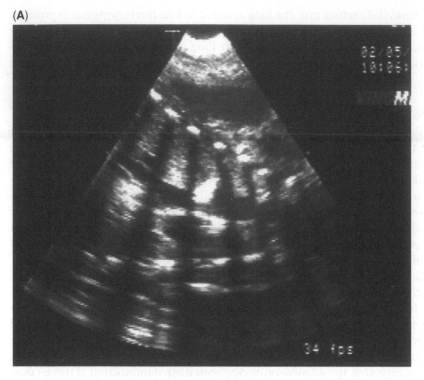

(B)

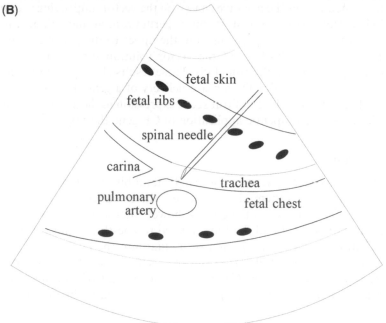

Figure 6 (**A**) Ultrasonogram and (**B**) diagram of sheep fetus at 114 days of gestation in longitudinal section. A 20-gauge spinal needle is inserted into the fetal thorax between the third and fourth rib, penetrates the lung parenchyma and enters the fetal trachea just proximal to the carina. *Source*: From Ref. 99.

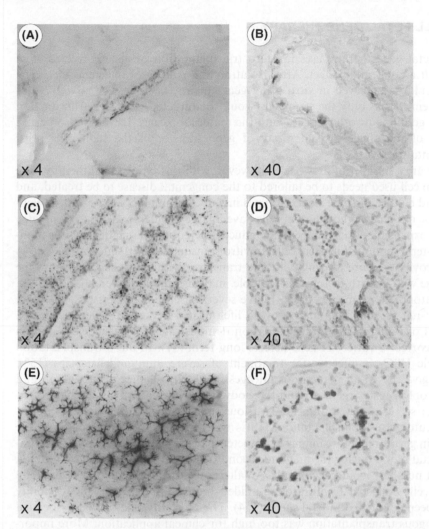

Figure 7 Adenovirus mediated β-galactosidase expression in the airways of midgestation fetal sheep after ultrasound-guided injection of an adenoviral vector containing the lacZ gene into the fetal trachea. The airways were pretreated with the fatty acid sodium caprate, and the adenoviral vector was complexed with the polycation DEAE dextran to improve transduction of airway epithelium. Widespread gene expression on X-gal staining can be seen in the small airways (**A**) and (**B**) and the trachea (**C**). There is also widespread immunohistochemical localization of β-galactosidase expression in the distal airway epithelium (**D**). (**E** and **F**) Instillation of perflubron, an inert fluorocarbon, after delivery of sodium caprate and DEAE dextran complexed adenoviral vectors to the trachea resulted in enhanced transduction of the distal airways. *Abbreviation*: DEAE, diethylaminoethyl. *Source*: Photographs courtesy of L Gregory, Gene Therapy Research Group, Imperial College, London.

mice, rats, guinea pigs, and rabbits. Somatic gene transfer to the fetal heart and liver was achieved in some studies using mice (149,150), but others have found little or no fetal gene transfer in mice and guinea pigs (131) or rats (151). Commonly, the placenta showed the most transfection, but maternal tissues also demonstrate transgene expression, which although not unexpected, is undesirable in therapy that is aimed at the fetus.

STEM CELL FETAL GENE THERAPY

Stem cell fetal gene therapy uses in utero transplantation of gene corrected stem cells to treat a congenital defect. After isolation and culture of the stem cells, gene transfer would be achieved in vitro using gene therapy vectors. The advantage of such a system is that only the stem cells would be targeted, avoiding transduction of the fetal germline or other tissues, and the maternal tissues. It would also permit assessment of the efficiency and safety of gene transfer of the stem cells prior to transplantation.

There are a number of drawbacks, however, with this type of fetal therapy. The type of stem cell used needs to be tailored to the congenital disease to be treated, and isolation and culture of some stem cell types in sufficient numbers, for example, neurons, may be difficult. Although stem cells have a large proliferative capacity, in vitro culture and expansion of cell numbers can induce differentiation that depletes the number of long-term repopulating stem cells. In vitro transduction with integrating vectors such as retrovirus requires cycling cells, and transferring quiescent stem cells into the cycling stage with growth factors, for example, may also induce differentiation (152).

Hematopoietic stem cells (HSCs) have several useful characteristics. They are able to self-renew, and thus may provide lifelong correction of a genetic defect. The success of bone marrow transplantation demonstrates that genetically normal HSCs can correct a variety of gene defects long term (51). In utero transplantation of allogeneic HSCs is effective for treatment of severe immunodeficiencies (153). HSCs can give rise to all the various lineages of blood cells in the circulation and tissue macrophages in organs around the body. Gene corrected HSCs could potentially deliver secreted gene products to various tissues and into the general circulation. For autologous transplantation, HSCs would need to be collected from the fetus early in gestation before immune competence develops. HSCs are present abundantly in fetal blood during the first and second trimesters, although their collection in sufficient numbers would be difficult. An alternative strategy would be to use fetal liver stem cells collected by ultrasound-guided biopsy and a successful feasibility study has been conducted in fetal sheep (154). The mortality rate of 73% associated with autologous transplantation was too high for clinical application. More importantly, engraftment from autologous compared with allogeneic fetal liver stem cells was comparable, suggesting that autologous transplantation did not offer an engraftment advantage when applied in early gestation (155).

The success of fetal stem cell therapy depends critically on the ability to transfer genes into stem cells in vitro. Gene transfer into murine HSCs can be achieved with high efficiency using retroviral vectors (156). Studies show retroviral gene transfer into large animal (157) and human HSCs (158) is less successful, although transduction of fetal HSCs is more efficient than that of adult cells (159). Improved gene transfer has recently been achieved by using retroviral vectors pseudotyped with different envelopes, for example, the RD114 envelope from the feline endogenous virus (160) and long-term efficient transduction of CD34+ human HSCs can be attained with lentiviral vectors (59).

Mesenchymal stem cells (MSCs) are becoming increasingly more important for transplantation therapy. In particular, they have the ability to differentiate among multiple lineages, and human MSCs show engraftment and site-specific differentiation after in utero transplantation in sheep (161). Circulating fetal MSCs are present from the first trimester and can be efficiently transduced with retroviral vectors (162).

Fetal MSCs have also been isolated from second-trimester amniotic fluid taken at amniocentesis for prenatal diagnosis, and these may provide an excellent source of cells for intrauterine fetal tissue engineering (163).

ETHICAL AND SAFETY ISSUES

There are various ethical issues in relation to fetal gene therapy that need to be addressed before such therapy could be applied clinically (164,165). One major concern is that fetal gene therapy has potential adverse effects such as injury, infection, severe immune reactions, or preterm labor on the fetus as well as on the mother. Furthermore, many parents decide to terminate an affected pregnancy, and therefore the option of in utero treatment must be at least as safe for the mother, and should also reliably treat the disease (166).

There is a theoretical risk that the therapeutic gene product or vector that is required at a certain stage during fetal development could cause oncogenesis. In addition, insertion of vector sequences may cause developmental aberrations to occur. While one of the aims of prenatal gene therapy is to achieve immune tolerance to the transgene and delivery system, vectors must be designed to be sufficiently different from the wild type so that the immune system remains able to mount an effective immune response against wild-type virus infection.

The problem of insertional mutagenesis as a potential risk of retroviral gene therapy has been debated for some years. This serious adverse event has now been identified in a trial of gene therapy for X-linked severe combined immunodeficiency syndrome in which CD34+ HSCs were transduced ex vivo with the γc gene using retroviral vectors. Further work is needed to address this issue and to devise strategies to determine and possibly direct integration sites.

Germline transmission is another risk that raises ethical concerns. Fetal somatic gene therapy does not aim to modify the genetic content of the germline, but inadvertent gene transfer to the germline could occur. Compartmentalization of the primordial germ cells in the gonads is complete by seven weeks of gestation in humans, and it is unlikely, therefore, that any therapy applied after this time would result in germ-line transduction. Examination of germ cells after delivery of retroviral vectors (88,123) or adenoviral vectors to early gestation fetal sheep has not shown any detectable transmission (107). Following intravascular administration of adenoviral vectors to late gestation fetal sheep, vector DNA was detectable by PCR in the gonads, but extensive investigation by RT-PCR could not detect any gene expression. A similar risk of germ-line transduction occurs with AAV that can integrate into the genome. No AAV sequences were detectable in the germ-line tissues of fetal mice receiving injection of AAV vectors via the intraperitoneal route nor the tissues of their progeny (121). Many of these issues are not confined to in utero or even adult gene therapy and concerns regarding germ-line transmission can be raised in particular for chemotherapy and infertility treatment (167).

Finally, there is the concern that fetal gene therapy research poses special challenges to informed consent (168). The decision to participate in a fetal gene therapy trial would occur close to the time of prenatal diagnosis of the condition. The parents may hear information in a highly biased way and not consider the risk to future pregnancies. It will be important to ensure that parents are adequately counseled and understand these issues before agreeing to take part in any future research.

The general public remains concerned that ethical discussions about issues such as gene therapy, cloning, and the Human Genome Project are falling behind the technology (169). It is, therefore, important to provide adequate information that will allow the public to understand the risks and benefits of these novel techniques and to enable an educated involvement in the decision-making process along with health professionals. This will also help individuals give informed consent as these procedures become used in clinical practice.

CONCLUSIONS

Fetal gene therapy offers the potential for obstetricians and gene therapists not only to diagnose but also to treat inherited genetic disease. However, for the treatment to be acceptable, it must offer advantages over postnatal gene therapy, be safe for both mother and fetus, and preferably avoid germ-line transmission. Currently, in utero gene therapy remains an experimental procedure. But in the future, better understanding of the development of genetic disease in the fetus and improvements in vector design and targeting of fetal tissues should allow this technology to move into clinical practice.

REFERENCES

1. Coutelle C, Douar A-M, Colledge WH, Froster U. The challenge of fetal gene therapy. Nat Med 1995; 1:864–866.
2. Wilson JM, Wivel NA. Report on the potential use of gene therapy in utero. Gene Therapy Advisory Committee. Hum Gene Ther 1999; 10:689–692.
3. Herzog RW, Yang EY, Couto LB, et al. Long-term correction of canine hemophilia B by gene transfer of blood coagulation factor IX mediated by adeno-associated viral vector. Nat Med 1999; 5:56–63.
4. Hsieh-Li HM, Chang J, Jong Y, et al. A mouse model for spinal muscular atrophy. Nat Genet 2000; 24:66–70.
5. Blouin M, Beauchemin H, Wight A, et al. Genetic correction of sickle cell disease: Insights using transgenic mouse models. Nat Med 2000; 6:177–182.
6. Engelhardt JF, Yankaskas JR, Ernst SA, et al. Submucosal glands are the predominant site of CFTR expression in the human bronchus. Nat Genet 1992; 2:240–248.
7. Johnson LG, Olsen JC, Sarkadi B, Moore KL, Swanstrom R, Boucher RC. Efficiency of gene transfer for restoration of normal airway epithelial function in cystic fibrosis. Nat Genet 1992; 2:21–25.
8. Bigger B, Coutelle C. Perspectives on gene therapy for cystic fibrosis airway disease. Biodrugs 2001; 15:615–634.
9. Weiss DJ, Strandflord TP, Liggitt D, Clark JG. Perflubron enhances adenovirus-mediated gene expression in lungs of transgenic mice with chronic alveolar filling. Hum Gene Ther 1999; 10:2287–2293.
10. Weiss DJ, Bonneau L, Liggitt D. Use of perfluorochemical liquid allows earlier detection of gene expression and use of less vector in normal lung and enhances gene expression in acutely injured lung. Mol Ther 2001; 3:734–745.
11. Parsons DW, Grubb BR, Johnson LG, Boucher RC. Enhanced in vivo airway gene transfer via transient modification of host barrier properties with a surface-active agent. Hum Gene Ther 1998; 9:2661–2672.
12. Gregory LG, Harbottle RP, Lawrence L, Knapton HJ, Themis M, Coutelle C. Enhancement of adenovirus-mediated gene transfer to the airways by DEAE dextran and sodium caprate in vivo. Mol Ther 2002; 7:1–8.

13. Wang G, Zabner J, Deering C, et al. Increasing epithelial junction permeability enhances gene transfer to airway epithelia in vivo. Am J Respir Cell Mol Biol 2000; 22:129–138.

14. Gaillard D, Ruocco S, Lallemand A, Dalemans W, Hinnrasky J, Puchelle E. Immuno-histochemical localization of cystic fibrosis transmembrane conductance regulator in human fetal airway and digestive mucosa. Pediatr Res 1994; 36:137–143.

15. Tizzano EF, O'Brodovich H, Chitayat D, Benichou JC, Buchwald M. Regional expression of CFTR in developing human respiratory tissues. Am J Respir Cell Mol Biol 1994; 10:355–362.

16. Hubeau C, Puchelle E, Gaillard D. Distinct pattern of immune cell population in the lung of human fetuses with cystic fibrosis. J Allergy Clin Immunol 2001; 108:524–529.

17. Boué A, Muller F, Nezelof C, et al. Prenatal diagnosis in 200 pregnancies with a 1-in-4 risk of cystic fibrosis. Hum Genet 1986; 74:288–297.

18. Plopper CG, Weir AJ, Nishio SJ, Cranz DL, St George JA. Tracheal submucosal gland development in the rhesus monkey, *Macaca mulatta*: ultrastructure and histochemistry. Anat Embryol 1986; 174:167–178.

19. Engelhardt JF, Schlossberg H, Yankaskas JR, Dudus L. Progenitor cells of the adult human airway involved in submucosal gland development. Development 1995; 121: 2031–2046.

20. Peault B, Tirouvanziam R, Sombardier MN, Chen S, Perricaudet M, Gaillard D. Gene transfer to human fetal pulmonary tissue developed in immunodeficient SCID mice. Hum Gene Ther 1994; 5:1131–1137.

21. Lim F-Y, Martin B, Radu A, Crombleholme TM. Adeno-associated virus (AAV)-mediated fetal gene transfer in respiratory epithelium and submucosal gland cells in human fetal tracheal organ culture. J Pediatr Surg 2002; 37:1051–1057.

22. Lim F-Y, Kobinger GP, Weiner DJ, Radu A, Wilson JM, Crombleholme TM. Human fetal trachea-SCID mouse xenografts: efficacy of vesicular stomatitis virus-G pseudo-typed lentiviral-mediated gene transfer. J Pediatr Surg 2003; 38:834–839.

23. Stecenko AA, Brigham KL. Gene therapy progress and prospects: alpha-1 antitrypsin. Gene Ther 2003; 10:95–99.

24. Cole FS, Hamvas A, Nogee LM. Genetic disorders of neonatal respiratory function. Pediatr Res 2003; 50:157–162.

25. Furie B, Limentani SA, Rosenfield CG. A practical guide to the evaluation and treatment of hemophilia. Blood 1994; 84:3–9.

26. Lusher JM. Inhibitors in young boys with haemophilia. Baillieres Best Pract Res Clin Haematol 2000; 13:457–468.

27. Soucie JM, Nuss R, Evatt B, et al. Mortality among males with hemophilia: relations with source of medical care. The Hemophilia Surveillance System Project Investigators. Blood 2000; 96:437–442.

28. Kay MA, Landen CN, Rothenberg SR, et al. In vivo hepatic gene therapy: Complete albeit transient correction of factor IX deficiency in hemophilia B dogs. Proc Natl Acad Sci USA 1994; 91:2353–2357.

29. Kay MA, Rothenberg SR, Landen CN, et al. In vivo gene therapy of hemophilia B: sustained partial correction in factor IX-deficient dogs. Science 1993; 262:117–119.

30. Chao H, Samulski RJ, Bellinger D, Monahan PE, Nichols T, Walsh CE. Persistent expression of canine factor IX in hemophilia B canines. Gene Ther 1999; 6:1695–1704.

31. Snyder RO, Miao C, Meuse L, et al. Correction of hemophilia B in canine and murine models using recombinant adeno-associated viral vectors. Nat Med 1999; 5:64–70.

32. Manno CS, Chew AJ, Hutchison S, et al. AAV-mediated factor IX gene transfer to skeletal muscle in patients with severe hemophilia B. Blood 2003; 101:2963–2972.

33. Kaiser J. Side effects sideline hemophilia trial. Science 2004; 304:1424–1425.

34. Xu L, Gao C, Sands MS, et al. Neonatal or hepatocyte growth factor-potentiated adult gene therapy with a retroviral vector results in therapeutic levels of canine factor IX for hemophilia B. Blood 2003; 101:3924–3932.

35. Waddington SN, Nivsarkar MS, Mistry AR, et al. Permanent phenotypic correction of hemophilia B in immunocompetent mice by prenatal gene therapy. Blood 2004; 104: 2714–2721.

36. Gao X, Huang L. Cationic liposome-mediated gene transfer. Gene Ther 1998; 2:710–722.

37. Gharwan H, Wightman L, Kircheis R, Wagner E, Zatloukal K. Nonviral gene transfer into fetal mouse livers (a comparison between the cationic polymer PEI and naked DNA). Gene Ther 2003; 10:810–817.

38. Mason CA, Bigras JL, O'Blenes SB, et al. Gene transfer in utero biologically engineers a patent ductus arteriosus in lambs by arresting fibronectin-dependent neointimal formation. Nat Med 1999; 5:176–182.

39. Olivares EC, Hollis RP, Chalberg TW, Meuse L, Kay MA, Calos MP. Site-specific genomic integration produces therapeutic Factor IX levels in mice. Nat Biotechnol 2002; 20:1124–1128.

40. David AL, Themis M, Cook T, Coutelle C, Rodeck CH. Fetal gene therapy. Ultrasound Rev Obstet Gynaecol 2001; 1:14–27.

41. Themis M, Forbes SJ, Chan L, et al. Enhanced in vitro and in vivo gene delivery using cationic agent complexed retrovirus vectors. Gene Ther 1998; 5:1180–1186.

42. Douar A-M, Adebakin S, Themis M, Pavirani A, Cook T, Coutelle C. Foetal gene delivery in mice by intra-amniotic administration of retroviral producer cells and adenovirus. Gene Ther 1997; 4:883–890.

43. Russel DW, Berger MS, Miller AD. The effects of human serum and cerebrospinal fluid on retroviral vectors and packaging cell lines. Hum Gene Ther 1995; 6:635–641.

44. Miller DG, Adam MA, Miller AD. Gene transfer by retrovirus vectors occurs only in cells that are actively replicating at the time of infection. Mol Cell Biol 1990; 10: 4239–4242.

45. Palmer TD, Rosman GJ, Osborne WRA, Miller D. Genetically modified skin fibroblasts persist long after transplantation but gradually inactivate introduced genes. Proc Natl Acad Sci USA 1991; 88:1330–1334.

46. Challita PM, Kohn DB. Lack of expression from a retroviral vector after transduction of murine hematopoietic stem cells is associated with methylation in vivo. Proc Natl Acad Sci USA 1994; 91:2567–2571.

47. Welsh RJ, Cooper NR, Jensen FC, Oldstone MB. Human serum lyses RNA tumor viruses. Nature 1975; 257:612–614.

48. Cosset FL, Takeuchi Y, Battini JL, Weiss RA, Collins MK. High-titer packaging cells producing recombinant retroviruses resistant to human serum. J Virol 1995; 69:7430–7436.

49. Engelstädter M, Buchholz CJ, Bobkova M, et al. Targeted gene transfer to lymphocytes using murine leukaemia virus vectors pseudotyped with spleen necrosis virus envelope proteins. Gene Ther 2001; 8:1202–1206.

50. Douar A-M, Themis M, Sandig V, Friedmann T, Coutelle C. Effect of amniotic fluid on cationic lipid mediated transfection and viral infection. Gene Ther 1996; 3:789–796.

51. Cavazzana-Calvo M, Hacein-Bey S, de Saint Basile G, et al. Gene therapy of human severe combined immunodeficiency (SCID)-X1 disease. Science 2000; 288:669–672.

52. Hacein-Bey-Abina S, Le Deist F, Carlier F, et al. Sustained correction of X-linked severe combined immunodeficiency by ex vivo gene therapy. N Engl J Med 2002; 346:1185–1193.

53. Marshall E. Gene therapy a suspect in leukemia-like disease. Science 2002; 298:34–35.

54. Li Z, Düllmann J, Schiedlmeier B, et al. Murine leukemia induced by retroviral gene marking. Science 2002; 296:497.

55. Davé UP, Jenkins NA, Copeland NG. Gene therapy insertional mutagenesis insights. Science 2004; 303:333.

56. Trono D. Lentiviral vectors: turning a deadly foe into a therapeutic agent. Gene Ther 2000; 7:20–23.

57. Mitrophanous K, Yoon S, Rohll J, et al. Stable gene transfer to the nervous system using a non-primate lentiviral vector. Gene Ther 1999; 6:1808–1818.

58. Naldini L, Blomer U, Gallay P, et al. In vivo gene delivery and stable transduction of nondividing cells by a lentiviral vector. Science 1996; 272:263–267.

59. Case SS, Price MA, Jordan CT, et al. Stable transduction of quiescent CD34(+)CD38(−) human hematopoietic cells by HIV-1-based lentiviral vectors. Proc Natl Acad Sci USA 1999; 96:2988–2993.

60. Mazarakis ND, Azzouz M, Rohll JB, et al. Rabies virus glycoprotein pseudotyping of lentiviral vectors enables retrograde axonal transport and access to the nervous system after peripheral delivery. Hum Mol Genet 2001; 10:2109–2121.

61. Kobinger GP, Weiner DJ, Yu QC, Wilson JM. Filovirus-pseudotyped lentiviral vector can efficiently and stably transduce airway epithelia in vivo. Nat Biotechnol 2001; 19:225–230.

62. Wang G, Slepushkin V, Zabner J, et al. Feline immunodeficiency virus vectors persistently transduce nondividing airway epithelia and correct the cystic fibrosis defect. J Clin Investig 1999; 104:R55–R62.

63. Waddington SN, Mitrophanous KA, Ellard F, et al. Long-term transgene expression by administration of a lentivirus-based vector to the fetal circulation of immuno-competent mice. Gene Ther 2003; 10:1234–1240.

64. Xiao X, Li J, Samulski RJ. Production of high-titer recombinant adeno-associated virus vectors in the absence of helper adenovirus. J Virol 1998; 72:2224–2232.

65. Wang L, Takabe K, Bidlingmaier SM, Ill CR, Verma IM. Sustained correction of bleeding disorder in hemophilia B mice by gene therapy. Proc Natl Acad Sci USA 1999:96.

66. Kay MA, Manno CS, Ragni MV, et al. Evidence for gene transfer and expression of factor IX in haemophilia B patients treated with an AAV vector. Nat Genet 2000; 24:257–261.

67. Monahan PE, Samulski RJ. Adeno-associated virus vectors for gene therapy: more pros than cons? Mol Med Today 2000; 6:433–440.

68. Sun L, Li J, Xiao X. Overcoming adeno-associated virus vector size limitation through viral DNA heterodimerization. Nat Med 2000; 6:599–602.

69. Lipshutz GS, Titre D, Brindle M, Bisconte AR, Contag CH, Gaensler KM. Comparison of gene expression after intraperitoneal delivery of AAV2 or AAV5 in utero. Mol Ther 2003; 8:90–98.

70. Nakai H, Montini E, Fuess S, Storm TA, Grompe M, Kay MA. AAV serotype 2 vectors preferentially integrate into active genes in mice. Nat Genet 2003; 34:297–302.

71. Burguete T, Rabreau M, Fontanges-Darriet M, et al. Evidence for infection of the human embryo with adeno-associated virus in pregnancy. Hum Reprod 1999; 14:2396–2401.

72. Tobiasch E, Rabreau M, Geletneky K, et al. Detection of adeno-associated virus DNA in human genital tissue and in material from spontaneous abortion. J Med Virol 1994; 44:215–222.

73. Rohde V, Erles K, Sattler HP, Derouet H, Wullich B, Schlehofer JR. Detection of adeno-associated virus in human semen: does viral infection play a role in the pathogenesis of male infertility? Fertil Steril 1999; 72:814–816.

74. Erles K, Rohde V, Thaele M, Roth S, Edler L, Schlehofer JR. DNA of adeno-associated virus (AAV) in testicular tissue and in abnormal semen samples. Hum Reprod 2001; 16:2333–2337.

75. Lehrman S. Virus treatment questioned after gene therapy death. Nature 1999; 401: 517–518.

76. McCray PB, Armstrong K, Zabner J, et al. Adenoviral-mediated gene transfer to fetal pulmonary epithelia in vitro and in vivo. J Clin Investig 1995; 95:2620–2632.

77. Iwamoto HS, Trapnell BC, McConnell CJ, Daugherty C, Whitsett JA. Pulmonary inflammation associated with repeated, prenatal exposure to an E1, E3-deleted adenoviral vector in sheep. Gene Ther 1999; 6:98–106.

78. Chen HH, Mack LM, Kelly R, Ontell M, Kochanek S, Clemens PR. Persistence in muscle of an adenoviral vector that lacks all viral genes. Proc Natl Acad Sci USA 1997; 94:1645–1650.
79. Schiedner G, Morral N, Parks RJ, et al. Genomic DNA transfer with a high-capacity adenovirus vector results in improved in vivo gene expression and decreased toxicity. Nat Genet 1998; 18:180–183.
80. Murphy SJ, Chong H, Bell S, Diaz RM, Vile RG. Novel integrating adenoviral/ retroviral hybrid vector for gene therapy. Hum Gene Ther 2002; 13:745–760.
81. Kubo S, Mitani K. A new hybrid system capable of efficient lentiviral vector production and stable gene transfer mediated by a single helper-dependent adenoviral vector. J Virol 2003; 77:2964–2971.
82. Gonçalves MAFV, van der Velde I, Knaän-Shanzer S, Valerio D, de Vries AAF. Stable transduction of large DNA by high-capacity adeno-associated virus/adenovirus hybrid vectors. Virology 2004; 321:287–297.
83. Yonemitsu Y, Kitson C, Ferrari S, et al. Efficient gene transfer to airway epithelium using recombinant Sendai virus. Nat Biotechnol 2000; 18:970–973.
84. Shiotani A, Fukumura M, Maeda M, et al. Skeletal muscle regeneration after insulin-like growth factor 1 gene transfer by recombinant Sendai virus vector. Gene Ther 2001; 8:1043–1050.
85. Masaki I, Yonemitsu Y, Komori K, et al. Recombinant Sendai virus-mediated gene transfer to vasculature: a new class of efficient gene transfer vector to the vascular system. FASEB J 2001; 15:1294–1296.
86. Inoue M, Tokusumi Y, Ban H, et al. Nontransmissible virus-like particle formation by F-deficient Sendai virus is temperature sensitive and reduced by mutations in M and HN proteins. J Virol 2003; 77:3238–3246.
87. Waddington SN, Buckley SMK, Berloehr C, et al. Reduced toxicity of F-deficient Sendai virus vector in the mouse fetus. Gene Ther 2004; 11:599–608.
88. Tran ND, Porada CD, Zhao Y, Almeida-Porada G, Anderson WF, Zanjani ED. In utero transfer and expression of exogenous genes in sheep. Exp Hematol 2000; 28:17–30.
89. Vincent MC, Trapnell BC, Baughman RP, Wert SE, Whitsett JA, Iwamoto HS. Adenovirus-mediated gene transfer to the respiratory tract of fetal sheep in utero. Hum Gene Ther 1995; 6:1019–1028.
90. Nicolini U, Nicolaidis P, Fisk NM, Tannirandorn Y, Rodeck C. Fetal blood sampling from the intrahepatic vein: analysis of safety and clinical experience with 214 procedures. Obstet Gynaecol 1990; 76:47–53.
91. Jauniaux E, Gulbis B, Gerloo E. Free amino acids in human fetal liver and fluids at 12–17 weeks of gestation. Hum Reprod 1999; 14:1638–1641.
92. Westgren M, Ek S, Bui T, et al. Tissue distribution of transplanted fetal liver cells in the human fetal recipient. Am J Obstet Gynecol 1997; 176:49–53.
93. Rodeck CH, Deans A. Red cell alloimmunisation. In: Rodeck CH, Whittle MJ, eds. Fetal Medicine: Basic Science and Clinical Practice. London: Churchill Livingstone, 1999:785–804.
94. Touraine JL. Induction of transplantation tolerance in humans using stem cell transplants prenatally or postnatally. Transplant Proc 1999; 31(7):2735–2737.
95. Muench MO, Rai J, Barcena A, et al. Transplantation of a fetus with paternal Thy-1(+)CD34(+) cells for chronic granulomatous disease. Bone Marrow Transplant 2001; 27:355–364.
96. Jauniaux E, Gulbis B. Fluid compartments of the embryonic environment. Hum Reprod Update 2000; 6:268–278.
97. Santolaya-Forgas J, Vengalil S, Kushwaha A, Bieniarz A, Fortman J. Assessment of the risk of fetal loss after the coelocentesis procedure using a baboon model. Fetal Diagn Ther 1998; 13:257–260.
98. Sylvester KG, Yang EY, Cass DL, Crombleholme TM, Scott Adzick N. Fetoscopic gene therapy for congenital lung disease. J Pediatr Surg 1997; 7:964–969.

99. David AL, Peebles DM, Gregory L, et al. Percutaneous ultrasound-guided injection of the trachea in fetal sheep: a novel technique to target the fetal airways. Fetal Diagn Ther 2003; 18:385–390.

100. David AL, Themis M, Waddington SN, et al. The current status and future direction of fetal gene therapy. Gene Ther Mol Biol 2003; 7:181–209.

101. Christensen G, Minamisawa S, Gruber PJ, Wang Y, Chien KR. High-efficiency, long-term cardiac expression of foreign genes in living mouse embryos and neonates. Circulation 2000; 101:178–184.

102. Wang G, Williamson R, Mueller G, Thomas P, Davidson BL, McCray Jr PB. Ultrasound-guided gene therapy to hepatocytes in utero. Fetal Diagn Ther 1998; 13: 197–205.

103. Schachtner SK, Buck CA, Bergelson JM, Baldwin HS. Temporally regulated expression patterns following in utero adenovirus-mediated gene transfer. Gene Ther 1996; 6:1249–1257.

104. Waddington SN, Buckley SMK, Nivsarkar M, et al. In utero gene transfer of human factor IX to fetal mice can induce postnatal tolerance of the exogenous clotting factor. Blood 2003; 101:1359–1366.

105. Yang EY, Cass DL, Sylvester KG, Wilson JM, Adzick NS. Fetal gene therapy: efficacy, toxicity, and immunologic effects of early gestation recombinant adenovirus. J Pediatr Surg 1999; 34:235–241.

106. Themis M, Schneider H, Kiserud T, et al. Successful expression of β-galactosidase and factor IX transgenes in fetal and neonatal sheep after ultrasound-guided percutaneous adenovirus vector administration into the umbilical vein. Gene Ther 1999; 6: 1239–1248.

107. David AL, Cook T, Waddington S, et al. Ultrasound guided percutaneous delivery of adenoviral vectors encoding the β-galactosidase and human factor IX genes to early gestation fetal sheep in utero. Hum Gene Ther 2003; 14:353–364.

108. Moise KJ, Hesketh DE, Belfort MM, et al. Ultrasound-guided blood sampling of rabbit fetuses. Lab Anim Sci 1992; 42:398–401.

109. Lipshutz GS, Flebbe-Rehwaldt L, Gaensler KML. Adenovirus-mediated gene transfer in the midgestation fetal mouse. J Surg Res 1999; 84:150–156.

110. Lipshutz GS, Flebbe-Rehwaldt L, Gaensler KML. Adenovirus-mediated gene transfer to the peritoneum and hepatic parenchyma of fetal mice in utero. Surgery 1999; 126:171–177.

111. Lipshutz GS, Flebbe-Rehwaldt L, Gaensler KML. Reexpression following readministration of an adenoviral vector in adult mice after initial in utero adenoviral administration. Mol Ther 2000; 2:374–380.

112. Mitchell M, Jerebtsova M, Batshaw ML, Newman K, Ye X. Long-term gene transfer to mouse fetuses with recombinant adenovirus and adeno-associated virus (AAV) vectors. Gene Ther 2000; 7:1986–1992.

113. Sabatino DE, MacKenzie TC, Campagnoli C, Liu Y-L, High KA, Flake AW. Long-term expression of factor IX after in utero administration of adeno-associated viral vectors in hemophilia B mice (abstract). Blood 2002; 100(11):3421.

114. MacKenzie TC, Kobinger GP, Kootstra NA, et al. Efficient transduction of liver and muscle after in utero injection of lentiviral vectors with different pseudotypes. Mol Ther 2002; 6:349–358.

115. Baumgartner TL, Baumgartner BJ, Hudon L, Moise KJ. Ultrasonographically guided direct gene transfer in utero: Successful induction of β-galactosidase in a rabbit model. Am J Obstet Gynecol 1999; 181:848–852.

116. Lai L, Davison BB, Veazey RS, Fisher KJ, Baskin GB. A preliminary evaluation of recombinant adeno-associated virus biodistribution in rhesus monkeys after intrahepatic inoculation in utero. Hum Gene Ther 2002; 13:2027–2039.

117. Tarantal AF, O'Rourke JP, Case SS, et al. Rhesus monkey model for fetal gene transfer: studies with retroviral-based vector systems. Mol Ther 2001; 3:128–138.

118. Lipshutz GS, Sarkar R, Flebbe-Rehwaldt L, Kazazian H, Gaensler KML. Short-term correction of factor VIII deficiency in a murine model of hemophilia A after delivery of adenovirus murine factor VIII in utero. Proc Natl Acad Sci USA 1999; 96:13324–13329.

119. Hatzoglou M, Lamers W, Bosch F, Wynshaw-Boris A, Clapp DW, Hanson RW. Hepatic gene transfer in animals using retrovirus containing the promoter from the gene for phosphoenolpyruvate carboxykinase. J Biol Chem 1990; 265:17285–17293.

120. Hatzoglou M, Moorman A, Lamers W. Persistent expression of genes transferred in the fetal rat liver via retroviruses. Somat Cell Mol Genet 1995; 21:265–278.

121. Lipshutz GS, Gruber CA, Cao Y, Hardy J, Contag CH, Gaensler KML. In utero delivery of adeno-associated viral vectors: intraperitoneal gene transfer produces long-term expression. Mol Ther 2001; 3:284–292.

122. Meertens L, Zhao Y, Rosic-Kablar S, et al. In utero injection of alpha-L-iduronidase-carrying retrovirus in canine mucopolysaccharidosis type I: infection of multiple tissues and neonatal gene expression. Hum Gene Ther 2002; 13:1809–1820.

123. Porada CD, Tran N, Eglitis M, et al. In utero gene therapy: transfer and long-term expression of the bacterial *neo*^{r} gene in sheep after direct injection of retroviral vectors into preimmune fetuses. Hum Gene Ther 1998; 9:1571–1585.

124. Yang EY, Kim HB, Shaaban AF, Milner R, Adzick NS, Flake. Persistent postnatal transgene expression in both muscle and liver after fetal injection of recombinant adenovirus. J Pediatr Surg 1999; 34(5):766–772.

125. Schneider H, Mühle C, Douar A-M, et al. Sustained delivery of therapeutic concentrations of human clotting factor IX—a comparison of adenoviral and AAV vectors administered in utero. J Gene Med 2002; 4:46–53.

126. Gregory LG, Waddington SN, Holder MV, et al. Highly efficient EIAV-mediated in utero gene transfer and expression in the major muscle groups affected by Duchenne muscular dystrophy. Gene Ther 2004; 11:1117–1125.

127. Sekhon HS, Larson JE. In utero gene transfer into the pulmonary epithelium. Nat Med 1995; 1:1201–1203.

128. Larson JE, Morrow SL, Happel L, Sharp JF, Cohen JC. Reversal of cystic fibrosis phenotype in mice by gene therapy in utero. Lancet 1997; 349:619–620.

129. Larson JE, Delcarpio JB, Farberman MM, Morrow SL, Cohen JC. CFTR modulates lung secretory cell proliferation and differentiation. Am J Physiol 2000; 279:L333–L341.

130. Holzinger A, Trapnell BC, Weaver TE, Whitsett JA, Iwamoto HS. Intraamniotic administration of an adenoviral vector for gene transfer to fetal sheep and mouse tissues. Pediatr Res 1995; 38:844–850.

131. Senoo M, Matsubara Y, Fujii K, et al. Adenovirus-mediated in utero gene transfer in mice and guinea pigs: tissue distribution of recombinant adenovirus determined by quantitative TaqMan-polymerase chain reaction assay. Mol Genet Metab 2000; 69:269–276.

132. Schneider H, Adebakin S, Themis M, et al. Therapeutic plasma concentrations of human factor IX in mice after gene delivery into the amniotic cavity: a model for the prenatal treatment of haemophilia B. J Gene Med 1999; 1:424–432.

133. Galan HL, Bennett ML, Tyson RW, et al. Inefficient transduction of sheep in utero after intra-amniotic injection of retroviral producer cells. Am J Obstet Gynecol 2002; 187:469–474.

134. Bennett M, Galan H, Owens G, et al. In utero gene delivery by intraamniotic injection of a retroviral vector producer cell line in a nonhuman primate model. Hum Gene Ther 2001; 12:1857–1865.

135. Larson JE, Morrow SL, Delcarpio JB, et al. Gene transfer into the fetal primate: evidence for the secretion of transgene product. Mol Ther 2000; 2:631–639.

136. Boyle MP, Enke RA, Adams RJ, Guggino WB, Zeitlin PL. In utero AAV-mediated gene transfer to rabbit pulmonary epithelium. Mol Ther 2001; 4:115–121.

137. Moss IR, Scarpelli EM. Stimulatory effect of theophylline on regulation of fetal breathing movements. Pediatr Res 1981; 15:870–873.

138. Kalache KD, Chaoui R, Marcks B, et al. Differentiation between human fetal breathing patterns by investigation of breathing-related tracheal fluid flow velocity using Doppler sonography. Prenat Diagn 2000; 20:45–50.

139. Badalian SS, Chao CR, Fox HE, Timor TI. Fetal breathing-related nasal fluid flow velocity in uncomplicated pregnancies. Am J Obstet Gynecol 1993; 169:563–567.

140. Buckley SM, Waddington SN, Jezzard S, et al. Factors influencing adenovirus-mediated airway transduction in fetal mice. Mol Ther 2005; 12:484.

141. Buckley SMK, Waddington SN, Jezzard S, Themis M, Colledge WH, Coutelle C. Intra-amniotic application of CFTR-expressing adenovirus does not reverse cystic fibrosis phenotype in inbred *Cftr*-knockout mice (abstract). Mol Ther 2003; 7:S200.

142. Tarantal AF, Lee CI, Ekert JE, et al. Lentiviral vector gene transfer into fetal rhesus monkeys (*Macaca mulatta*): lung-targeting approaches. Mol Ther 2001; 4:614–621.

143. Pitt BR, Schwarz MA, Pilewski JM, et al. Retrovirus-mediated gene transfer in lungs of living fetal sheep. Gene Ther 1995; 2:344–350.

144. Peebles D, Gregory LG, David A, et al. Widespread and efficient marker gene expression in the airway epithelia of fetal sheep after minimally invasive tracheal application of recombinant adenovirus in utero. Gene Ther 2004; 11:70–78.

145. Weiss DJ, Strandjord TP, Jackson JC, Clark JG, Liggitt D. Perfluorochemical liquid-enhanced adenoviral vector distribution and expression in lungs of spontaneously breathing rodents. Exp Lung Res 1999; 25:317–333.

146. Wu Y, Liu J, Woo S, Finegold MJ, Brandt ML. Prenatal orogastric gene delivery results in transduction of the small bowel in the fetal rabbit. Fetal Diagn Ther 1999; 14:323–327.

147. Brandt ML, Moise KJJ, Eckert JW, et al. Transuterine puncture of the fetal stomach provides access to the small bowel in the rabbit. J Investig Surg 1997; 10(1–2):41–46.

148. Heikkilä A, Hiltunen MO, Turunen MP, et al. Angiographically guided utero-placental gene transfer in rabbits with adenoviruses, plasmid/liposomes and plasmid/polyethyleneimine complexes. Gene Ther 2001; 8:784–788.

149. Woo YJ, Raju GP, Swain JL, Richmond ME, Gardner TJ, Balice-Gordon RJ. In utero cardiac gene transfer via intraplacental delivery of recombinant adenovirus. Circulation 1997; 96:3561–3569.

150. Türkay A, Saunders TL, Kurachi K. Intrauterine gene transfer: gestational stage-specific gene delivery in mice. Gene Ther 1999; 6:1685–1694.

151. Xing A, Boileau P, Caüzac M, Challier J-C, Girard J, Hauguel-de-Mouzon S. Comparative in vivo approaches for selective adenovirus-mediated gene delivery to the placenta. Hum Gene Ther 2000; 11:167–177.

152. Kittler EL, Peters SO, Crittenden RB, et al. Cytokine-facilitated transduction leads to low-level engraftment in nonablated hosts. Blood 1997; 90:865–872.

153. Flake AW, Roncarolo MG, Puck JM, et al. Treatment of X-linked severe combined immunodeficiency by in utero transplantation of paternal bone marrow. N Engl J Med 1996; 335:1806–1810.

154. Surbek DV, Young A, Danzer E, Schoeberlein A, Dudler L, Holzgreve W. Ultrasound-guided stem cell sampling from the early ovine fetus for prenatal ex vivo gene therapy. Am J Obstet Gynecol 2002; 187:960–963.

155. Schoeberlein A, Holzgreve W, Dudler L, Hahn S, Surbek DV. In utero transplantation of autologous and allogeneic fetal liver stem cells in ovine fetuses. Am J Obstet Gynecol 2004; 191:1030–1036.

156. Eglitis MA, Kantoff P, Gilboa E, Anderson WF. Gene expression in mice after high efficiency retroviral-mediated gene transfer. Science 1985; 230:1395–1398.

157. Bodine DM, Moritz T, Donahue RE, et al. Long-term in vivo expression of a murine adenosine deaminase gene in rhesus monkey hematopoietic cells of multiple lineages after retroviral mediated transfer into CD34+ bone marrow cells. Blood 1993; 82:1975–1980.

158. Ward M, Richardson C, Pioli P, et al. Transfer and expression of the human multiple drug resistance gene in human CD34+ cells. Blood 1994; 84:1408.

159. Ekhterae D, Crumbleholme T, Karson E, Harrison MR, Anderson WF, Zanjani ED. Retroviral vector-mediated transfer of the bacterial neomycin resistance gene into fetal and adult sheep and human hematopoietic progenitors in vitro. Blood 1990; 75:365–369.

160. Ward M, Sattler R, Grossman IR, et al. A stable murine-based RD114 retroviral packaging line efficiently transduces human hematopoietic cells. Mol Ther 2003; 8:804–812.

161. Liechty KW, MacKenzie TC, Shaaban AF, et al. Human mesenchymal stem cells engraft and demonstrate site-specific differentiation after in utero transplantation in sheep. Nat Med 2000; 6:1282–1286.

162. Campagnoli C, Bellantuono I, Kumar S, Fairburn LJ, Roberts I, Fisk NM. High transduction efficiency of circulating first trimester fetal mesenchymal stem cells: potential targets for in utero ex vivo gene therapy. Br J Obstet Gynaecol 2002; 109:952–954.

163. Tsai MS, Lee JL, Chang YJ, Hwang SM. Isolation of human multipotent mesenchymal stem cells from second-trimester amniotic fluid using a novel two-stage culture protocol. Hum Reprod 2004; 19:1450–1456.

164. Recombinant DNA Advisory Committee. Prenatal gene transfer; Scientific, medical, and ethical issues. Hum Gene Ther 2000; 11:1211–1229.

165. Fletcher JC, Richter G. Human fetal gene therapy: moral and ethical questions. Hum Gene Ther 1996; 7:1605–1614.

166. Coutelle C, Rodeck C. On the scientific and ethical issues of fetal somatic gene therapy. Gene Ther 2002; 9:670–673.

167. Schneider H, Coutelle C. In utero gene therapy: the case for. Nat Med 1999; 5:256–257.

168. Burger IM, Wilfond BS. Limitations of informed consent for in utero gene transfer research: implications for investigators and institutional review boards. Hum Gene Ther 2000; 11:1057–1063.

169. Brown P. Regulations not keeping up with developments in genetics, says poll. Br Med J 2000; 321:1369.

31

Maternal/Fetal Conflict: A Legal and Ethical Conundrum

Nanette Elster

Spence & Elster, P.C., Lincolnshire, Illinois, U.S.A.

INTRODUCTION

What is the status of the fetus? The answer to this question might differ depending on whether the definition sought is legal, medical, or moral. Maternal–fetal conflict raises not only medical issues but legal and ethical issues as well. It is the convergence of these three areas that create such conflict for practitioners. With recent advances in medicine and technology enabling such things as fetal surgery and the expanding time frame in which a fetus might be considered viable, maternal–fetal conflicts may become even more pronounced.

In no other medical setting is it legally or ethically appropriate to force one individual to undergo a medical treatment or procedure to benefit another. A parent, for example, cannot legally be compelled to donate blood, bone marrow, or an organ to save the life of a child (1). "The common law has consistently held to a rule which provides that one human being is under no legal compulsion to give aid or to take action to save that human being or to rescue" (1). However, it is not unprecedented that a pregnant woman might be forced to undergo a medical intervention such as a blood transfusion (2) or cesarean section (3) to save the life of the fetus she is gestating. This is an example of when moral obligations and legal obligations diverge, not only for the pregnant woman but also for the physician treating her. How such conflicts are resolved has changed over time and continues to vary from jurisdiction to jurisdiction. The political landscape, state and federal laws, and professional codes of ethics all provide some guidance albeit inconsistent at times.

POLITICAL BACKGROUND

Any legal and/or ethical analysis of the issue of maternal–fetal conflict must necessarily begin by considering the political context in which such conflicts arise. A number of political actions have been taken during the current administration, which have begun to reshape, if not redefine, the status of the fetus in our society.

Debate over the status of the fetus has been fodder for political debate for the better part of the last 30 years, since the landmark Supreme Court ruling in *Roe v. Wade* (4). The Court made it clear in this case that legally, a fetus is not considered to be a person. The Court reasoned that:

> The Constitution does not define "person" in so many words. Section 1 of the Fourteenth Amendment contains three references to "person." The first, in defining "citizens," speaks of "persons born or naturalized in the United States." The word also appears both in the Due Process Clause and in the Equal Protection Clause. "Person" is used in other places in the Constitution: in the listing of qualifications for Representatives and Senators.... But in nearly all these instances, the use of the word is such that it has application only postnatally. None indicates, with any assurance, that it has any possible pre-natal application (4).

The determination of the Court in *Roe* has been at the center of controversy since that time. In recent years, there have been a number of cases, laws, and regulations at both the state and federal level, which have sought to refute the notion that legal personhood is not established prenatally, and in fact, imbue a particular status upon the fetus from the earliest stages of development.

One example of the shift in status of the fetus is the 2002 amendment to the regulations under the State Children's Health Insurance Program (SCHIP) (5). SCHIP was enacted in 1997 as somewhat of a safety net to provide health insurance coverage for uninsured children up to 19 years of age whose family income exceeded state Medicaid eligibility standards but was still below 200% of the federal poverty level (6). The program, however, did not offer benefits for pregnant women, although the child being gestated would have been eligible for SCHIP upon birth. The Bush administration sought to remedy this problem swiftly through the rule-making process by redefining the term "child."

The Final Rule now defines "Child" as "an individual under the age of 19 including the period from conception to birth" (5). The amendment, however, does little to extend or increase the benefits available to pregnant women in need of prenatal services. "By making the fetus the legal beneficiary, the rule limits reimbursement for services during pregnancy to those that directly affect a fetus.... As a result, women may not be covered for the full range of medical services they need during the prenatal period" (7). One commentator argues that the new definition could place physicians in a difficult predicament: "The failure to follow ethical and professional standards requiring comprehensive care may constitute malpractice, yet rendering uncompensated care... could place them at substantial financial risk" (7). The rule has, therefore, been criticized as being more of a political maneuver to redefine the status of embryos rather than a means to extend health care access to those in need.

Another recent example of the politicization of the status of the fetus is the enactment of fetal homicide or "feticide" laws. Such laws are a dramatic shift from the late 1800s when the Massachusetts court in *Dietrich v. Northampton* (8) found that the fetus did not exist separate from the mother and, therefore, could not sue for injuries sustained in utero. Current fetal homicide laws make it a separate crime when an action toward a woman results in the death of the fetus she is gestating. As of June 2005, at least 34 states had some form of fetal homicide law (9), and application of these statutes is currently being put to the test in a number of jurisdictions (10). At least 15 of these state laws apply to the earliest stages of pregnancy such as Louisiana where "unborn child" is defined as "any individual of the human species from fertilization and implantation until birth" (11). This is the same definition used in the recently enacted federal Unborn Victims of Violence Act (12).

While many of these laws, including the federal law, provide an exception for abortion, other medical treatments, and actions by the woman, others do not. For example, under Virginia law:

A. Any person who unlawfully, willfully, deliberately, maliciously and with premeditation kills the fetus of another is guilty of a Class 2 felony.

B. Any person who unlawfully, willfully, deliberately and maliciously kills the fetus of another is guilty of a felony punishable by confinement in a state correctional facility for not less than five nor more than 40 years (13).

Under these fetal homicide laws such as Virginia's that do not provide an exception for physicians or the pregnant woman, the question remains whether a physician might face criminal liability for failure to perform a cesarean section or provide other recommended treatment refused by the mother/patient or if the mother's behavior in refusing treatment that results in the death of the fetus would subject her to criminal liability.

These are two significant examples of how integral politics are in shaping the social status of the fetus. The status of the fetus is quite significant in determining what, if any, legal rights must be afforded to the fetus and has been central to a number of legal disputes arising out of a woman's decisions and behaviors during her pregnancy.

LEGAL ANALYSIS

The starting point for legal analysis of the conflict between a woman and her physician over the care of her fetus is that a person has a right to maintain bodily integrity. Implicit in this right is the fact that a competent person can accept or refuse medical treatment. "Every human being of adult years and sound mind has a right to determine what shall be done with his own body" (14). This principle was reaffirmed by the Supreme Court in the seminal case, *Cruzan v. Director of Missouri Department of Health* in which the Court reasoned that "a competent person has a constitutionally protected liberty interest in refusing unwanted medical treatment" (15). A liberty interest is considered to be a fundamental right and as such, the state must prove a compelling interest in impinging on that right. "Where certain 'fundamental rights' are involved, the Court has held that regulation limiting these rights may be justified only by a 'compelling state interest,' and that legislative enactments must be narrowly drawn..." (4). This burden is a difficult one to satisfy; however, the discussion that follows illustrates how a state's interest in the potential for life may satisfy this burden. The cases also make clear that there is little consistency between jurisdictions with respect to application of this balancing test.

CESAREAN SECTION/BLOOD TRANSFUSION

Nowhere in medicine has the conflict between a woman and her physician over the care of the fetus been more pronounced than with respect to forced cesarean sections and blood transfusions. Practitioners and courts alike have come out on both sides of the issue, leaving physicians in continual professional, not to mention legal limbo.

Numerous hospitals have sought court orders to compel a particular medical treatment of a pregnant woman over her refusal. A study conducted in 1987 by Kolder et al. revealed that there were at least 21 cases in which court orders were sought for medical intervention against a pregnant woman's wishes, and 86% of the orders were granted (16). During the 1990s, however, the majority of emergency rulings permitting court ordered intervention were overturned on appeal (17). *In re A.C.* (18) and *In re Fetus Brown* (19) are two examples of this shift away from paternalism. It is important to note that in both cases, the order for intervention was granted and the intervention imposed, however, the decisions were both reversed on appeal.

The case of *In re A.C.* was brought before the District of Columbia Court of Appeals challenging a court ordered cesarean section. Angela Carder at 25 weeks of pregnancy was diagnosed with a lung tumor. A week and a half later Ms. Carder, who had chosen to fight this recurrent bout of cancer aggressively was near death and the hospital sought an emergency court order to perform a cesarean section to deliver the fetus. After a hearing in Ms. Carder's hospital room, the order was granted and the operation performed. Tragically, the baby died shortly after birth and Angela Carder died two days later (20). The decision ordering the cesarean section was appealed.

The appellate court vacated the order for the cesarean section and held "that it would be an extraordinary case indeed in which a court might ever be justified in overriding the patient's wishes and authorizing a major surgical procedure such as a cesarean section" (20). In a related action, Carder's parents sued the hospital asserting a range of claims including malpractice (21). The case was settled and part of the settlement entailed the hospital implementing policy designed to protect patients from such actions occurring in the future including adopting a hospital policy echoing the Court of Appeals decision to protect pregnant patients' rights to make health care decisions (22).

In 1997, the Illinois Appellate Court, confronted with another case involving a forced medical intervention for a pregnant woman, reached a similar conclusion to that in *In re A.C.* In *In re Fetus Brown* the court was confronted with an appeal from a court ordered blood transfusion (19). At just over 34 weeks of pregnancy, Darlene Brown underwent a surgical procedure resulting in a serious loss of blood. Ms. Brown, being a Jehovah's Witness, refused a medically recommended blood transfusion. Other measures were taken to control her bleeding but more blood loss occurred, posing a life-threatening risk to her and her fetus. Ms. Brown continued to refuse the transfusion and the State subsequently petitioned the court to appoint a temporary custodian of the fetus in order to consent to the transfusion. The order was granted, naming the hospital administrator as the "temporary custodian" of the fetus. Brown continued to refuse the transfusion and was sedated and forcibly restrained in order to perform the intervention. She delivered a healthy baby and regained her health as well. Nevertheless, Darlene Brown appealed the decision in which a temporary custodian had been appointed for her fetus.

Although the facts of this case were resolved, the appellate court found that the public policy implications of the case were of such significant importance that future guidance on such issues was necessary. In the court's opinion, this case did not involve balancing the interests of the mother against those of her fetus but rather the balancing of the mother's interest against the State's interest in the viable fetus (19). Relying on previous case law in Illinois, the court held that "the State may not override a pregnant woman's competent treatment decisions, including refusal of recommended invasive medical procedures, to potentially save the life of the viable fetus" (19).

The rulings in these cases and the strong position favoring the woman's autonomy led one commentator to suggest that, "future judicial decisions imposing invasive medical treatment on pregnant women, whether to benefit the woman, the fetus, or both, are unlikely" (17). This, however, has not been the case.

In 1999, in *Pemberton v. Tallahassee Memorial Regional Medical Center*, (23) a woman appealed a court ordered cesarean section. Ms. Pemberton had chosen to give birth at home with a midwife in attendance. After a full day in labor she needed IV fluids and presented to the emergency room at Tallahassee Memorial. It was determined at that time that she needed a cesarean section. She left the hospital against medical advice and was later returned to the hospital by ambulance against her will at which point a hearing was held and the procedure was ordered by the judge. She and the baby were both healthy following delivery. Ms. Pemberton challenged the order, nonetheless, asserting that it violated her constitutional rights. On appeal, however, the court held that "Whatever the scope of Ms. Pemberton's personal constitutional rights in this situation, they clearly did not outweigh the interests of the State of Florida in preserving the life of the unborn child" (23).

While factually not dissimilar to *In re A.C.* and *In re Fetus Brown*, the outcome in *Pemberton* was apposite. Such contrary outcomes leave physicians in a legal quagmire. The lack of uniformity in these cases makes it clear that the actions that can be taken can and do vary from state to state, and with recent legal and policy developments redefining the fetus, outcomes such as that in *Pemberton* may become more common.

A recent iteration of this issue arose in 2004 in Utah where a woman, Melissa Ann Rowland, who refused to undergo a cesarean section resulting in the death of one of her unborn twins, was charged with murder (24). The murder charges were subsequently dropped when concerns were raised about Ms. Rowland's mental health (25). This case represents an attempt to utilize fetal homicide laws to prosecute for drug use during pregnancy. With the murder charges dropped, Rowland did plead guilty to child endangerment for using cocaine during her pregnancy (25). Although a cesarean section was not forcibly performed upon Melissa Rowland, the attempt to prosecute her for murder for her refusal to undergo a cesarean section suggests a serious erosion of the autonomy rights of pregnant women to make medical decisions during their pregnancies. An important point to remember when these conflicts arise is that "the ability of a physician to secure a court order does not equate with a duty to seek one" (26).

CONDUCT DURING PREGNANCY

Coercive and, at times, punitive actions taken against women for behaviors or actions during their pregnancies is an area which has influenced and may continue to influence the physician–patient relationship by putting the physician in a potentially adversarial relationship with the pregnant patient. These types of actions, like the action taken in *Pemberton*, imply that the care of the fetus may govern the relationship between the physician and the pregnant patient. There seems to be a shift from the model of the pregnant woman as one- to the two-patient model in which the fetus is also a patient, to once again a one-patient model. However, in the shifting paradigm, now the one patient is the fetus.

Coercive or punitive action against pregnant woman for their behavior has occurred most often with respect to drug/alcohol use during pregnancy. Responses to maternal drug use during pregnancy have typically taken one of the two approaches: a punitive approach or a public health approach (27). The two approaches, however, are not mutually exclusive. The public health approach focuses on treating the substance abuse as well as its underlying causes, whereas the punitive approach involves such measures as civil commitment, criminal prosecution, sterilization, or forced Norplant use and/or termination of parental rights (28). At least 200 women in over 30 states have been arrested and criminally charged for drug use during pregnancy (28).

It was not until 1997 that any appellate court viewing the prosecution of a pregnant woman for drug use upheld such an action (28). The most common reason that these criminal prosecutions were not upheld was because the laws being applied did not recognize the fetus as a person. Around the same time, however, several states enacted or amended legislation to specifically address prenatal substance use through other types of laws. For example, South Dakota amended its definition of an abused or neglected child to include, a child "Who was subject to prenatal exposure to abusive use of alcohol or any controlled drug or substance not lawfully prescribed by a practitioner..." (29). Additionally, in 1997 The South Carolina Supreme Court in reversing the appellate court's decision to reverse a child endangerment conviction stemming from a pregnant woman's use of cocaine during pregnancy held that viable fetuses are "persons" within the meaning of the state child endangerment law (30).

Amidst this turmoil, the United States Supreme Court heard the case of *Ferguson v. City of Charleston* (31). The issue in *Ferguson* was whether a pregnant woman still maintains the constitutional right to be free from an unreasonable, nonconsensual search. In this case, the City of Charleston, the County prosecutor, and the Medical University of South Carolina, a public hospital, developed and implemented an interagency policy on cocaine abuse during pregnancy. Based on criteria such as no, late, or inadequate prenatal care; abruptio placenta; and intrauterine growth retardation of "no obvious cause," hospital staff members tested pregnant patients for cocaine use. Positive test results were then reported to the police. During the term of this policy nearly 30 women were actually arrested (32). The Court in *Ferguson* held that "performance of a diagnostic test to obtain evidence of a patient's criminal conduct for law enforcement purposes is an unreasonable search if the patient has not consented to the procedure" (31).

These cases and this issue of criminalizing or creating civil actions for maternal behavior during pregnancy become very important for the integrity of the physician–patient relationship. Physicians are mandated reporters of child abuse and neglect (33) and if prenatal substance abuse or other behavior is found to constitute child abuse and neglect, this could severely compromise the physician's relationship with the pregnant patient. That was precisely the concern of many of the "friends of the court" who submitted briefs to the Supreme Court in the *Ferguson* case. And, the Court recognized the significance of the physician–patient relationship in its rationale. In dicta, the Court said, "The reasonable expectation of privacy enjoyed by the typical patient undergoing diagnostic tests in a hospital is that the results of those tests will not be shared with nonmedical personnel without her consent" (31).

As with compelled interventions during pregnancy, punitive or coercive measures applied to deal with particular behaviors during pregnancy threaten to compromise the physician–patient relationship. In the American College of Obstetricians and Gynecologists (ACOG) Ethics Committee Opinion, "Patient Choice in the

Maternal–Fetal Relationship," the Committee recognizes that compelling treatment or involving judicial authority to protect the fetus may have broader reaching, and the potential unintended consequence of "criminalizing non-compliance with medical recommendations" (34). If the relationship is one based on trust, threats of punitive action or actions taken against a patient's wishes will do little to foster the development of such a relationship. As one commentator has suggested, "if a physician goes to court to force treatment, that physician becomes the patient's adversary rather than advocate" (17). Nevertheless, in our litigious society these conflicts continue to place physicians in what seem to be untenable situations. It will have a chilling effect on the practice of medicine if a physician were to be found liable for malpractice and/or guilty of murder for tragic consequences that may result from following the informed wishes of the patient.

ETHICAL ANALYSIS

As the previous discussion has illustrated, there is varied legal precedent with respect to addressing a range of maternal–fetal conflicts. Despite laws or legal precedent, however, the ethical dilemmas inherent in maternal–fetal conflict are not any more easily resolved. Additionally, even when the law provides a clear answer, that does not always resolve the ethical conflict because what might be legal, might not necessarily be moral or ethical.

The starting point for ethical analysis of these conflicts lies in balancing autonomy and beneficence. The three guiding principles of an ethical analysis are autonomy, beneficence, and justice (35). Autonomy in the biomedical context refers to a competent individual's right to make decisions regarding personal healthcare—respect for persons. Beneficence is to do no harm and to maximize benefits while minimizing risks; and the principle of justice is simply about treating people equally. The ACOG Committee on Ethics summarizes the principle of justice as requiring "that pregnant and nonpregnant individuals... be afforded similar rights" (34). The balancing of these three principles, however, becomes complicated when the interests of two patients are at issue that must be balanced against each other (36).

The codes of ethics of a number of professional medical societies have attempted to address the maternal–fetal conflict within the autonomy, beneficence, justice framework. The American Medical Association (AMA), ACOG, and even the American Academy of Pediatrics (AAP) have all weighed in on this issue and come to very similar ethical resolutions of such dilemmas, putting greatest weight on the autonomy of the pregnant patient.

According to the AMA:

> Judicial intervention is inappropriate when a woman has made an informed refusal of a medical treatment designed to benefit her fetus. If an exceptional circumstance could be found in which a medical treatment poses an insignificant or no health risk to the woman, entails a minimal invasion of her bodily integrity, and would clearly prevent substantial and irreversible harm to her fetus, it might be appropriate for a physician to seek judicial intervention. However, the fundamental principle against compelled medical procedures should control in all cases which do not present such exceptional circumstances. (37)

The ACOG ethical guidelines recommend that "Obstetricians should refrain from performing procedures that are unwanted by a pregnant woman. The use of judicial authority to implement treatment regimens to protect the fetus violates the pregnant woman's autonomy and should be avoided" (34). And, the AAP Committee on Bioethics identifies three conditions that must be satisfied in order to contemplate going against a woman's refusal of a recommended intervention: "1) There is reasonable certainty that the fetus will suffer irrevocable and substantial harm without the intervention, 2) the intervention has been shown to be effective, and 3) the risk to the health and well-being of the pregnant woman is negligible" (38). The AAP Committee goes on to find that "given the potential adverse consequences of forced medical or surgical procedures, court intervention should be seen only as a last resort" (38).

Unlike case law or statutory law, however, these guidelines are merely recommendations and, therefore, are not binding; nevertheless they are of tremendous importance in considering a maternal–fetal conflict. In the context of maternal–fetal conflicts, respect for persons as in any other context can be accomplished through the informed consent process. A clear and understandable description of the risks, benefits, and alternatives to a recommended course of action should enable a competent patient to render an appropriate decision. That decision may nevertheless not be what the physician recommends and believes to be the best course of action, but making a decision that goes against clinical recommendations does not mean that the patient is irrational and that her choice should be disregarded. After all, what truly is the point of informed consent if a competent patient cannot refuse the treatment for which consent is sought?

The principle of beneficence is probably the most difficult to reconcile when addressing a maternal–fetal conflict. If a woman and the fetus are found to have the same moral status and the proposed intervention or impingement on the liberty of the woman to protect the fetus is minor or of minimal risk to her, the interests of the fetus may prevail, especially if the amount of harm from the intervention is minimal in light of the risk to the fetus and if the risk of harm to the fetus is great without such intervention. On the other hand, if the moral status of the woman is greater than that of her unborn child, her informed choice must be respected. From a legal perspective, the fetus, while deserving a heightened level of respect, does not have the same status as a liveborn individual.

Finally, if justice is about treating like people similarly, allowing nonpregnant individuals to refuse treatment and prohibiting pregnant woman from doing so would not seem to promote this principle.

Personal viewpoints will undoubtedly influence a practitioner in balancing these three principles, and for this reason, the practitioner should make such treatment decisions in consideration of hospital policies, reference to existing professional society guidelines, in consultation with colleagues including the assistance of an ethics committee or ethics consultant as well as mental health professionals. In fact, the ACOG Committee recommends that "Consultation with others, including an institutional ethics committee, should be sought when appropriate to aid the pregnant woman and obstetrician in resolving the conflict" (34).

CONCLUSION

The Supreme Court in *Planned Parenthood v. Casey* summed up the unique role of a pregnant woman:

The mother who carries a child to full term is subject to anxieties, to physical constraints, to pain that only she must bear. That these sacrifices have from the beginning of the human race been endured by woman with a pride that ennobles her in the eyes of others and gives to the infant a bond of love cannot alone be grounds for the State to insist she make the sacrifice. Her suffering is too intimate and personal for the State to insist, without more, upon its own vision of the woman's role, however dominant that vision has been in the course of our history and our culture. The destiny of the woman must be shaped to a large extent on her own conception of her spiritual imperatives and her place in society. (39)

It is directly a result of this unique position of pregnant women that maternal–fetal conflicts pose such tremendous challenges. They involve a range of legal and ethical issues as well as personal and societal values that are often inextricably intertwined and at times seemingly irreconcilable. Having an understanding of what is legally required in a particular jurisdiction, knowing hospital policy, and knowing professional society guidelines as well as maintaining clear and open communication with a patient from the outset of the relationship may help to reduce these conflicts and preserve the integrity of the physician–patient relationship, even in the event of a disagreement. As with many ethical dilemmas, the ethical course of action is not necessarily the legal course of action, nor is the legal course of action necessarily the ethical one.

REFERENCES

1. See, e.g., *McFall v. Shimp*, 10 Pa.D. & C.3d 90 (1978). While this case involved two cousins, the rationale can easily be extended to the parent–child relationship as well. This case involved a court action to compel a cousin to donate bone marrow. The court refused to grant the order.
2. See, e.g., *Application of President and Directors of Georgetown College, Inc.*, 331 F.2d 1000 (D.C. Cir. 1964).
3. See, e.g., *Pemberton v. Tallahassee Memorial Regional Medical Center, Inc.*, 66 F. Supp.2d 1247 (N.D. Fla. 1999).
4. *Roe v. Wade*. 410 U.S. 113 (1973).
5. 67 *Federal Register* 61955–61974 (October 2, 2002).
6. Centers for Medicare and Medicaid Services at http://www.cms.hhs.gov/schip/about-SCHIP.asp.
7. Cynthia Dailard. New SCHIP prenatal care rule advances fetal rights at low-income women's expense. The Guttmacher Report on Public Policy 3–5 (December 2002).
8. *Dietrich v. Northampton*, 138 Mass. 14 (1884).
9. National Conference of State Legislatures. Fetal homicide, at http://www.ncsl.org/programs/health/fethom.htm. (2005).
10. See, e.g., Ashley Cook. Capital murder case tests new law. Lufkin Daily News October 15, 2004.
11. La. Rev. Stat. Ann. Sec. 14:2.
12. H.R. 1997, signed into law (April 2004).
13. Va. Code sec. 18.2–32.2 (2004).
14. *Schloendorff v. Society of New York Hospitals*, 105 N.E.2d 92 (NY 1914).
15. *Cruzan v. Director, Missouri Department of Health*, 497 US 261 (1990).
16. Kolder VE, Gallagher J, Parsons MT. Court-ordered obstetrical interventions. N Engl J Med 1987; 316:1192.
17. Goldblatt AD. Commentary: no more jurisdiction over Jehovah. J Law Med Ethics 1999; 27:190–191.

18. 572 A.2d 1235 (D.C. 1990).
19. 689 N.E. 2d 397 (Ill. App. Ct. 1997).
20. *In re A.C.*, 573 A.2d 1235 (D.C. App. 1990).
21. See, ACLU. Coercive and punitive governmental responses to women's conduct during pregnancy, at http://archive.aclu.org/issues/reproduct/coercive.html.
22. Terry E. Thornton, Lynn Paltrow. The rights of pregnant patients: Carder case brings bold policy initiatives. 8 HealthSpan 1991 at http://advocatedforpregnant women.org/articles/angela.htm.
23. 66 F. Supp.2d 1247 (N.D. Fla. 1999).
24. Sherry F. Colb. Crying murder when cesarean section refused, at http://www.cnn.com (March 19, 2004).
25. See, e.g., Kaiser Daily Reproductive Health Report. Utah prosecutors drop murder charges against woman who gave birth to stillborn infant after allegedly refusing cesarean section, April 9, 2004 at http:// www.kaisernetwork.org.
26. Levy JK. Jehovah's Witnesses, pregnancy, and blood transfusions: a paradigm for the autonomy of all pregnant women. J Law Med Ethics 1999; 27:171.
27. Schroedel JR, Fiber P. Developments and trends in the law: punitive versus public health responses to drug use by pregnant women. Yale J Health Policy Law Ethics 2001; 1:217.
28. Lynn Paltrow, David Cohen, Corinne Carey. Governmental responses to pregnant women who use alcohol or other drugs: year 2000 overview—an analysis. at http://lindesmith.org/lindesmith/library/NAPWanalysis2.html.
29. S.D. Codified Laws 26-8A-2(9) (Michie 1998).
30. 492 S.E.2d 777 (S.C. 1997), *cert. denied*, 523 U.S. 1145 (1998).
31. 532 U.S. 67 (2001).
32. Harris L, Paltrow L. The status of pregnant women and fetuses in criminal law. J Am Med Assoc 2003; 289:1697–1699.
33. See, e.g., 23 Pa. Cons. Stat. Ann. §6311.
34. American College of Obstetricians and Gynecologists Ethics Committee. Patient choice in the maternal–fetal relationship. Revised January 2004.
35. Beauchamp TL, Childress JL. Principles of Biomedical Ethics. New York: Oxford University Press, 2001.
36. Tran L. Legal rights and the maternal–fetal conflict. BioTech J 2004; 2:76.
37. American Medical Association, Policy H-420.969. Legal interventions during pregnancy. at http://www.ama-assn.org.
38. American Academy of Pediatrics, Committee on Bioethics. Fetal therapy—ethical considerations. Pediatrics 1999; 103:1061.
39. 505 U.S. 833, 852 (1992).

32
Ethical Issues

Guido de Wert and Wybo Dondorp
Health Ethics and Philosophy, Faculty of Medicine, Maastricht University, Maastricht, The Netherlands

INTRODUCTION

Fetal medicine is a highly dynamic specialty. Advances in this field promise ever-increasing opportunities for prevention and treatment, resulting in real benefits for future children, prospective parents and society as a whole. At the same time, it is widely felt that developments in fetal medicine raise all sorts of moral and societal questions that need ethical scrutiny. The aim of this chapter is to contribute to this ethical reflection, focusing on ethical debates and regulations in Europe. Clearly, there is no single "European view." While there may be a strong consensus on some of the relevant issues, regulations in European countries vary substantially. This chapter does not provide a systematic, exhaustive inventory and comparison of ethical debates and regulations regarding fetal medicine in Europe, but a selective overview, highlighting some of the major trends and controversies. We concentrate on the following topics: prenatal diagnosis (PD), preimplantation genetic diagnosis (PGD), prenatal screening, and fetal/in utero research.

PRENATAL DIAGNOSIS

PD is usually defined as testing the fetus in case of an increased risk of a handicap or disease that can be detected before birth. Ethical questions and concerns regard pre-test counseling, PD stricto sensu, and the possible selective termination of pregnancy.

Counseling
There is a strong consensus in Europe that pre-test counseling should precede PD (1). The primary goal of this counseling is to help people make well-considered decisions that correspond to their own values. According to many authors and reports, the core ethical principle of genetic counseling is non-directiveness, which reflects the principle of respect for reproductive autonomy: counseling should not aim at reducing the incidence of genetic disorders (2,3). There is an ongoing debate about the precise implications of this principle. Is it, for instance, permissible for the counselor to give his own opinion? Critics are concerned that this would threaten the client's autonomy.

575

Others, however, argue that, at least in some situations, this may well help the client make well-considered decisions—what matters, then, are the "dialogical qualities" of the counselor. A common interpretation of the principle of non-directiveness is that the counselor should give unconditional support to clients, whatever they decide or request. This interpretation, however, is untenable, as clients' requests may be ethically problematic, and giving unconditional support may be at odds with professional autonomy or standards (4,5). Some examples will be given subsequently.

In the past, it was often considered to be good clinical practice to restrict access to PD to people who planned to terminate an affected pregnancy—after all, so the argument ran, (invasive) PD is not without risk. This practice ("conditional access") is now widely regarded as paternalistic and unacceptable (5,6). Abortion is one possible outcome of PD, but there are a number of reasons why people may opt for PD even if they reject termination or have not yet made up their minds. For most women/couples, the test brings reassurance, while others, who receive an unfavorable result, may be enabled to prepare for the birth of an affected child and/or to opt for delivery at a specialized clinic.

Ethics of Selective Abortion

PD is controversial because of its link with selective abortion; after all, women usually terminate pregnancy if a serious abnormality is found. Critics have two objections. The first objection is that PD and, more particularly, selective abortion, is at odds with the rights and interests of people with the respective disorders—the so-called "disability rights critique." As this objection regards prenatal screening more particularly, it will be briefly discussed in the section "Prenatal Screening." The second objection is that abortion (whether selective or not) cannot be justified in view of the high moral status of the fetus.

Like everywhere else, there is considerable difference of opinion in Europe with regard to the moral status of the fetus. Extreme views hold either that abortion amounts to the killing of a person (murder) or that abortion is a "self-regarding," morally neutral, act. In between these (minority) views are various intermediary positions. While these differ in some important aspects, they come to a similar conclusion (a phenomenon called "overlapping consensus"): the fetus has a real, but relatively limited moral status, which may be over-ridden by other morally relevant considerations. There is, then, a strong consensus that abortion can be morally justified if there are "good reasons"—and that preventing the birth of a seriously handicapped child may be one of these good reasons.

This dominant view is reflected in legislation allowing abortion either on the woman's request (acknowledging her right not to reproduce and/or the right to self-determination) or for specifically stated reasons. Even in countries with more restrictive legislation on abortion (Portugal, Poland), legislation includes the diagnosis of a (serious) fetal disorder. In Northern Ireland, there is continuing uncertainty concerning the situations in which abortion is lawful.

In many national legislations, gestational age limits are stricter for abortion for psychosocial reasons than for abortion for medical reasons, including fetal disorders. In some countries (France, Belgium, and the United Kingdom) terminations may be performed at any gestational age to protect the woman's life/health or because of fetal disorders. Other countries, including The Netherlands, permit terminations until the fetus is "viable"; the Dutch legislature has explicitly equated the killing of a viable fetus with infanticide. The Dutch Government recently clarified that in case of lethal disorders, like anencephaly, the prohibition to terminate pregnancies in the third trimester does not apply, as fetuses thus affected will never be viable, irrespective of their stage of development.

Indications: Setting Boundaries

The main controversy concerning PD regards its indications. According to the regulations in many European countries, PD should focus on the detection of serious handicaps and disorders. These legislations, however, do not specify which handicaps and disorders are serious—this is considered to be a matter for clinical judgment and accepted practice. While some critics urge policy makers to make a list specifying which handicaps/disorders qualify for (prenatal testing and) selective abortion, there is a widespread opposition to such lists, for various reasons (2,5,6). First, a list would not do justice to the particular situation of applicants and their evaluation of the risks and problems at hand. A second, more practical, objection is that most genetic defects have a variable expression. Third, as genetics and reproductive medicine are dynamic fields, any such list would be constantly outdated. Furthermore, clinical practice makes clear that women do not terminate wanted pregnancies for trivial reasons. And finally, a list could have adverse, discriminatory, social repercussions, as it could easily be interpreted as indicating which life is "not worth living" (cf. section "Prenatal Screening"). Clearly, there are difficult cases and sometimes very uncommon requests for PD. Many clinics have regular interdisciplinary meetings in order to discuss these cases.

The Case of PD for Late-Onset Disorders

Some types of PD are especially controversial. One of these is PD for late-onset disorders. Before commenting on the normative aspects involved, it is important to put things in perspective; until now, people only rarely request PD for these disorders (7).

It is not always fully clear whether legislations that allow selective abortions as a means to prevent the birth of affected children allow terminations because of (a high risk of) late-onset disorders. Laws regarding abortion in, for instance, Belgium and France, could be interpreted as prohibiting the latter, as children carrying relevant mutations do not suffer from the disease at the moment of birth. This restrictive interpretation is, however, debatable, because it is not explicitly excluded in the law that it is sufficient that the child will probably or with certainty suffer from the disease in the future (8).

The British Medical Association (BMA) recently repeated its concerns about the routine use of PD for adult onset disorders, but at the same time accepts that, in some circumstances, after careful counseling and consideration, such testing could be appropriate (6). This may well reflect the dominant view in most European countries. In The Netherlands, the Minister of Public Health explicitly stated that politics should not impose a particular restrictive view on prospective parents who are wrestling with these highly complex decisions (9). Any general moral evaluation of PD for late-onset disorders seems to be problematic, as it is important to take into account morally relevant variables like the severity of the disorder and the suffering involved, the possible availability of therapeutic options, the age of onset, and the penetrance of the specific mutations. Needless to say, ethical balancing is not a mathematical exercise.

The paradigm case is PD of Huntington's disease (HD). While critics argue that a child carrying the mutation will have several decades of good living and that we should acknowledge the moral ambiguity of the quest for "perfect babies," many people consider this case to be justified, as HD is a midlife-onset, highly disabling, lethal disease, and the penetrance of the mutation is complete. It is insensitive, if not an insult, to disqualify termination because of the prospect of HD as symptomatic of "genetic perfectionism."

The real issue, then, is not whether we should permit PD of HD, but under what conditions (10). First, what about PD of HD "just for reassurance" of prospective parents who do not intend to terminate affected pregnancies? In the case of untreatable late-onset disorders, the policy of "unconditional access" to PD (see earlier) would be problematic, as this could easily result in a breach of the future child's right "not to know," i.e., the right to decide for himself whether or not to undergo presymptomatic testing (11). Clearly, women can and should never be forced to terminate pregnancy—but to say that the traditional guidance should be followed in all cases may well be a non sequitur. Second, what about exclusion testing, which enables people to remain ignorant of their own genetic status (to have their right not to know respected) and to prevent the transmission of the HD-mutation at the same time (12)? Critics object that aborting a fetus at 50% risk instead of performing a complete PD and trying to preserve the fetus without the HD-mutation is too high a price for protecting the at-risk person's right not to know his genetic status—but is this a convincing objection in view of both the only relative status of the fetus and the weight to be given to the right not to know? Third, how do we evaluate direct testing in the fetus of prospective parents at 50% risk? According to the international guidelines, doctors should not perform such testing as one would risk "double bad news," "unfortunately, both the fetus and you carry HD (13)." We would argue that this guidance is unjustifiably paternalistic, and that it disregards the burdens and "cons" of the alternative options, including, "no testing, just carry the pregnancy to term," "no testing, just terminate pregnancy," and exclusion testing. The international guidelines, then, should be reconsidered. Finally, how do we handle requests from women for PD of HD when their male partners are at risk and do not want to know their genetic status (14)? Which right should prevail, the right to know or the right not to know?

In most European countries, there is an ongoing debate about the morality of PD of mutations in breast (and ovarian) cancer genes (BRCA), predisposing to hereditary breast and ovarian cancer (HBOC). This is even more controversial than PD of HD, because the penetrance of these mutations is incomplete (the life-time risk is 50%–80%), and preventive interventions may effectively reduce morbidity and mortality in carriers (15). But, according to the Ethics Committees of both the Royal Dutch Society of Physicians and the Dutch Society for Clinical Genetics, premature conclusions should be resisted (16,17). First, the life-time risk is very high. Furthermore, morally relevant questions concern the effectiveness of available preventive and/or therapeutic measures, and the burdens imposed by the respective medical interventions. Unfortunately, the effectiveness of medical surveillance (mammography) is currently far from optimal. Though the effectiveness of prophylactic bilateral mastectomy appears to be high, long-term follow up studies and study of more carriers are necessary to definitely establish the protective value of this procedure (18). Furthermore, prophylactic surgery may have major implications for women's quality of life. In view of this, it may well be argued that the fear of prospective parents that their future daughter(s) may inherit a BRCA gene mutation is far from unreasonable, and that termination of pregnancy in case of a female carrier fetus is not unjustified.

Induction and Selective Reduction of Multiple Pregnancy

Like PGD (cf. para. 3), this alternative strategy aims at preventing the birth of an affected child while avoiding a termination of pregnancy (19). The procedure involves four steps: ovarian stimulation, gamete intra-fallopian transfer (GIFT), chorion villus sampling (CVS), and selective fetal reduction, and is based on the high rate of multiple pregnancies following ovulation induction and GIFT—the higher the number of conceptuses, the higher is the chance that at least one or some of them will be unaffected and a termination can be avoided. Even though in most, if not all, European countries a multifetal pregnancy reduction (MFPR) is presently lawful and ethically justified provided the circumstances match the criteria for termination, there seems to be very little support for the current strategy among professionals in Europe. This is not surprising (4). Problems and pitfalls include the following: (i) in case of a large multiple pregnancy, it will be difficult to test all the individual fetuses, so it may be necessary to perform a ("nonselective") MFPR before the CVS, (ii) there is a risk of losing the entire pregnancy after a MFPR, and (iii) overzealous ovarian stimulation does have deleterious effects even if MFPR can be performed— after the reduction, there is still a "price to be paid" in an increased risk of prematurity and associated morbidity (20).

PD of Normal Behavioral Traits

While there are presently no genetic susceptibility tests for normal behavioral traits like IQ, sexual orientation (SO), and anti-social behavior, in the future such tests may become available. Therefore, a proactive ethical reflection is needed.

Referring to the consensus in clinical genetics and in public opinion against the use of PD in order to select babies on the basis of nonclinical characteristics, the Nuffield Council on Bioethics takes the view that abortion merely on the basis of information about behavioral traits in the normal range is morally unacceptable (21). Should we really categorically reject selective abortion because of, say, SO, irrespective of the cultural context, the specific motive of the prospective parents, and the penetrance of the predisposition? Let us assume that a test with a reasonable predictive value would be developed. Clearly, a homophobic motive for PD would be morally problematic. But take the case of prospective parents who live in a homophobic society or subculture, and who want to protect their future child from harm. Critics object that selective abortion can only be justified in view of the impact of future disease/handicaps on the child's quality of life, and that abortion due to SO would reinforce and perpetuate the prejudices and discrimination against gays and lesbians (22). With regard to the first objection, one may argue that, from the future child's perspective, it makes little difference whether quality of life is diminished by prejudices and discrimination or by a handicap/disorder (23). The second objection illustrates the potential clash between a "micro"–and a socio-ethical perspective (24). Which perspective should prevail? How do you handle the potential conflict between your responsibility as a prospective parent to promote the best interests of your future child and your responsibility as a citizen to fight societal prejudices? Clearly, this moral conflict may resemble the conflict inherent in preventing the conception/birth of daughters "for their own interest" in sexist cultures (25).

PREIMPLANTATION GENETIC DIAGNOSIS

PGD was developed as an alternative to PD for couples at high risk of transmitting a genetic defect; it allows couples to start a pregnancy knowing that the child will (almost certainly) not be affected by the particular disease/handicap. There are basically two approaches to obtain material for the analysis: polar body biopsy (PBB) and blastomere biopsy. The former is informative only for disorders of maternal origin and is practiced in only a few centers, mostly in countries that prohibit blastomere biopsy (see subsequent paragraph). The following paragraphs concentrate on the ethics of the latter.

Divergent Regulations

"Postconception" PGD is prohibited in, among other countries, Germany and Italy (26,27). One of the arguments against it is that selection is at odds with the human dignity of the embryo, and that a blastomere biopsy amounts to killing a "totipotent" cell, which has the same status as an embryo. Though a majority of the German National Ethics Advisory Board is in favor of lifting the ban, the German Government seems not to be willing to do so (28).

The arguments in favor of a categorical ban are unconvincing in view of the relatively low moral status of the embryo and because PGD may be a reasonable alternative strategy to avoid serious harm. Furthermore, the ban has bizarre practical implications as it obliges applicants for in vitro fertilization (IVF), even when they are at high risk of having a severely handicapped child, to accept a non-selective transfer of all embryos available, while laws in the same countries allow women to terminate affected pregnancies.

Most European countries accept PGD on more or less restrictive medical conditions. French law states that the genetic defect must be "of a particular severity and incurable at the moment of diagnosis (29)." In the United Kingdom, the Human Fertilisation and Embryology Authority (HFEA) and the Human Genetics Commission agree that, when deciding about the appropriateness of PGD, factors to be taken into account include the degree of suffering associated with the condition, the availability of effective therapy now and in the future, and the family circumstances of the people seeking PGD (30). In The Netherlands, recent regulations state that PGD is justified when there is a high risk of serious disease/handicap (31). Later, some controversial possible applications of PGD will be briefly listed.

Controversial Cases

Cases Fitting in with the Medical Model

According to the traditional moral framework, PGD should focus on the diagnosis of genetic defects that (may) affect the health of this particular potential child—the so-called medical model. Clearly, this is not to say that possible applications that fit in with this model do not raise any moral questions. Take, for example, the case of PGD for late-onset disorders, like HD or early-onset, autosomal dominant, Alzheimer's disease (32).

First, PGD for untreatable adult-onset disorders raises questions in view of the doctor's responsibility to take into account the interests of the future child (33–35). After all, in view of the fact that a carrier will inevitably get HD or early-onset AD, competence as a parent will be lost steadily. Furthermore, serious behavioral problems, like aggression and sexual disinhibition, may develop. A case-by-case approach seems to be preferable, taking into account, among other factors, the coping skills of the (prospective) parent not at risk and the quality of the network of the family (10). Clearly, in many cases the child will be an adolescent or even an adult when the parent at risk becomes symptomatic. Decisions may become even more complex when people applying for medically assisted reproduction are already symptomatic. What about the case of a woman who denies that she already is affected by HD, and who hopes that she can conceive quickly by IVF/PGD as she considers it to be important that her child will grow up, at least for some years, with a healthy mother?

Second, there are applications of PGD for late-onset disorders, which aim at preventing the transmittance of the mutation while at the same time protecting the asymptomatic applicant's right not to know his own genetic status. One of the possible strategies is "nondisclosure" PGD (36): couples are offered PGD without ever being informed of the test results. They will be told only that embryos were tested and that only apparently disease-free embryos were replaced. Couples would not be given any information about the number of eggs and embryos obtained, the number of successful diagnoses, etc. Hence, people at risk would derive no direct or indirect information about their own genetic status, while PGD, if performed accurately, could reduce the risk for their progeny to zero. This procedure raises, however, troubling issues: can this approach effectively protect the at-risk parent's right not to know his/her personal genetic status—and if so, at what financial, medical, and psychological costs (10,37)? Let us suppose that the first PGD-cycle does not identify any carrier embryo. The statistical risk of the parent at risk may become close to zero. To tell the client this good news would constitute an indirect breach of other at-risk clients' right not to know; after all, they may draw their own conclusion if they do not receive this good news. The problem, then, becomes whether one should offer a second (and a third, fourth, etc.) IVF–PGD cycle. Another problem arises, if there are no embryos available for transfer, either because all embryos carry HD, or for other reasons, like IVF failure. The client at risk might, rightly or wrongly, infer carrier status. Should one consider a sham transfer? For these reasons, the ESHRE Ethics Task Force and IVF/PGD clinics in, among others, the United Kingdom, France, Belgium, and The Netherlands are highly skeptical about nondisclosure PGD (38).

Intermediate Cases

Some applications of PGD do not fit into the medical model stricto sensu, as (part of) the testing is not linked to health problems in the future child, whereas there still is a link to the medical model in the wider sense, in that the testing may be relevant for the health of a "third party." These cases illustrate that the traditional dichotomy between the medical model on the one hand and the autonomy model on the other hand is simplistic—these cases represent an intermediate category (39). The most well-known case is, of course, PGD/HLA-typing.

PGD/HLA-typing is highly controversial (40). Critics argue that this procedure involves the instrumentalization of the child, that it carries disproportional (psychosocial) risks, that healthy embryos that cannot be matched may be destroyed, and that this is but a first step towards the designer baby (the slipper slope argument). One may, however, seriously doubt whether these objections are convincing. What matters first and foremost is whether the parents will value the child only as a transplant source or whether they will also love the child for itself (38,41). There is no evidence whatsoever to suggest that the parents involved would be bad parents. The objection in terms of status of the embryo is weak in view of both the dominant view that this status is relatively low and the reality of the disaster hanging over the heads of the parents and the terminally ill child. Finally, the slippery slope argument disregards the "therapeutic intent" of PGD/HLA-testing.

Regulations in Europe differ widely. In The Netherlands, PGD/HLA-typing is prohibited (31)—which is remarkable, as there has hardly been any open societal debate about the issues involved. France permits PGD/HLA-typing on the condition that PGD is primarily undertaken to avoid a serious disorder in the future child—HLA-typing is "only additional." In the United Kingdom, the HFEA recently decided that PGD solely in order to provide a compatible "donor" for an existing child is permitted as well (42). The latter type of testing is accepted practice in Belgium as well.

We want to stress that it would be misleading to present PGD/HLA-typing as an easy way out of the parents' dilemma. For various reasons, including the suboptimal "take-home baby rate" of the procedure and the fact that parents may feel pressured to opt for this procedure while they cannot afford another child, it is imperative to develop alternative strategies. One future option might be PGD/HLA-typing in order to select matched embryos whose hES cells could be used in cell therapy. While creating embryos "for instrumental use" is at odds with the guidance of the European Convention (43) and is presently prohibited in most European countries, this may well be justified from a moral point of view (40,44) and is permitted, on conditions, in the United Kingdom and Belgium.

Beyond the Medical Model

Most controversial are applications of PGD for nonmedical reasons. First, there is preimplantation sex selection for social reasons. There seems to be a strong consensus in European countries that this type of sex selection is not acceptable. Objections are, among others, that children should be accepted and loved unconditionally, that sex selection might set the scene for "designer babies," and that it may reinforce sexist views. The Health Council of The Netherlands suggested some sort of a compromise, namely, to allow sex selection for "family balancing" when PGD is necessary for medical reasons anyway and no additional testing is needed (45). The Embryo Act in The Netherlands prohibits PGD aiming at sex selection for non-medical reasons (46). It is not clear whether this Act also prohibits the additional selection for sex in the context of medically indicated PGD. In the United Kingdom, the BMA is opposed to sex selection for social reasons (6). Likewise, the HFEA recently concluded that sex selection for nonmedical reasons should not be permitted in the United Kingdom (6,47). Critics of a prohibition argue, however, that reproductive freedom (and, more general, "the presumption in favor of liberty") should be respected if there is no evidence of foreseeable harm from allowing people freedom to choose. Concerns that boys would be favored if selection was permitted, and that, as a consequence, the sex-ratio would be distorted, could easily be circumvented by allowing nonmedical sex selection only for family balancing (48–50). The ESHRE Ethics Task Force has not been able to reach a unanimous decision regarding PGD for non-medical sex selection (38).

Second, there are possible future applications in the field of behavioral genetics, in particular, PGD of normal behavioral traits. While the Nuffield Council on Bioethics considers abortion merely on the basis of behavioral traits in the normal range to be morally unacceptable (cf. section "Prenatal Diagnosis"), the Council takes the view that issues raised by the use of PGD are different: "Whereas selective termination following PD is applied to a fetus that has already implanted and is developing in the womb, PGD is used to select which embryos to implant. Thus, PGD does not precede the termination of a potential human life, but precedes instead the choice as to which embryo, among those created by IVF, is to be given a chance of developing into a human being. … Whereas PD would be used to end a life, PGD is, in effect, used to choose which life to start. Hence, the moral prohibitions which apply in the case of PD, do not apply in the same way in the use of PGD (21)." While the Nuffield Council concludes that, at present, the case for permitting selection based on the identification of behavioral traits in the normal range remains to be made, the Report states that it might turn out that there are possibilities for "modest applications" of this type of PGD. Clearly, even if one accepts the Nuffield Council's view (as we do) that preimplantation embryos and fetuses have a (gradually) different moral status, it does not necessarily follow that selecting for behavioral traits in the normal range in the context of PD on the one hand and PGD on the other hand should be evaluated differently. After all, it is not just the status of the embryo/fetus that matters morally.

Affected Embryos: A Source of Human Embryonic Stem Cells

PGD, apart from being an alternative option for preventing the birth of affected children, can also be used as a novel source of (affected) embryos and hES cells for research. Although affected embryos are unsuitable for transfer, these embryos may be of better quality (developmental potential) than embryos surplus to regular IVF/intracytoplasmic sperm injection (51). Furthermore, hES cell lines derived from affected embryos could provide valuable tools to study cell–cell interactions, disease progression and the efficacy and toxicity of drug therapies at the cellular level. While critics consider such "instrumental use" of human embryos to be at odds with the status of the embryo, the dominant view in many European countries (including the United Kingdom, Belgium, and The Netherlands) seems to be that such use could be justified, as the status of preimplantation embryos is considered to be relatively low, and this research use would meet both the principle of proportionality (the aim of the research is, after all, highly important) and the principle of subsidiarity (there is no good research alternative) (52).

PRENATAL SCREENING

Screening aims at the systematic early detection or exclusion of disease or carrier status among apparently healthy individuals, through the offer of unsolicited tests. Whereas some of these are diagnostic, most are preselection tests; they identify those individuals at high enough risk to warrant the use of invasive and/or expensive diagnostic tests. An important implication of this is the generation of large numbers of "false-positives," meaning the identification of individuals as high risk who upon further testing are shown not to be affected or carriers. Screening tests may also lead to false-negative results. This is when the test fails to identify individuals affected by the disease or having the condition at which the screening is directed. Cut-offs are used to optimize the balance between false-positive and -negative results.

For the normative assessment of screening programs, a general framework of criteria has been developed (53–57). These refer to test quality and disease characteristics and require the availability of meaningful (treatment) options in case of a positive final test result. Participation must be voluntary and based on informed consent. Because of its unsolicited nature, screening is acceptable only if the balance of benefits and harms for those involved can be shown to be positive.

The Disability Rights Critique

Prenatal screening usually focuses on the early detection of serious fetal disorders. Part of the debate on its moral acceptability hinges on the general absence of treatment options in case of a positive final test result. The further development of intra-uterine therapy may lead to exceptions to this for specific conditions, possibly including spina bifida (cf. section "Fetal Therapy"). At present, however, the only meaningful option opened up by a final positive outcome of prenatal screening is a choice between termination of pregnancy and preparing for the birth of a child with the relevant disorder. Is this an acceptable reason for offering screening to pregnant women? The question can either be framed as referring to the morality of abortion per se (discussed in the section "Prenatal Diagnosis") or to that of selective abortion as a means of avoiding the birth of a child with a disorder or disability that cannot be cured.

According to what has been called "the expressivist argument," selective abortion expresses the discriminatory view that the lives of those affected by the disorder or handicap are less worth living (58–61). If taken as a claim about parental motives, this cannot be maintained (62). Prospective parents who decide to terminate an affected pregnancy may do so because they want to spare their child the burdens of a handicapped existence, or because they feel that given their circumstances, they would not be able to parent a (severely) handicapped child. Whereas these motives do presuppose a judgment of the quality of life of affected persons and their families—a judgment that may well be criticized as being too negative (63)—they do not imply the discriminatory value judgment that the lives of persons with Down syndrome, spina bifida, cystic fibrosis (CF), etc. are not worth living. Nor is such a judgment implied in the periconceptional use of folic acid to reduce the risk of having a child with a neural tube defect. Acceptance of the latter is indeed inconsistent with the claim that selective abortion is inherently discriminatory. If this invites the reply that selective abortion is different from taking folic acid because it involves ending an already existing human life, the argument leads us back to the discussion of the moral status of the fetus. If the fetus were to be regarded as a person, a parental decision to terminate an affected pregnancy would be morally unacceptable. But on that assumption, all abortions would be so. If the fetus is not a person, the unconditional respect we owe to all persons (with or without disabilities), is not at stake (64,65).

However, the expressivist argument may also be taken as referring to why prenatal screening is being offered in the first place. According to the authors of a recent British HTA-study discussing the merits of introducing prenatal carrier screening for CF, the purpose is "to reduce the birth prevalence of the disorder (. . .) by identifying carrier couples who can have PD and selective termination of pregnancy" (66). This "public health approach" to prenatal screening is morally unacceptable for two reasons. First, it sends the message that the existence of individuals with disorders such as Down syndrome, spina bifida, or CF is a burden, and society should rather try to avoid it. If that is the reason for offering prenatal screening, the practice is indeed inherently discriminatory (60,63). Second, it turns what ought to be an autonomous parental decision into a means for achieving a societal goal. This can only lead to pressuring prospective parents into making the "right" preventive decisions, and to holding them accountable if they do not. By contrast, the only morally acceptable purpose of offering prenatal screening is the provision of information and reproductive choice to the prospective parents, enabling them to determine the outcome of the pregnancy in accordance with what—from their own perspective—having a (severely) handicapped child would mean, both for the child and for themselves and their family (67,68). It is important to note that this is not a matter of enhancing reproductive autonomy as such, but of providing information and choice with respect to what constitute (serious) health problems. Without this qualification, the question arises why prenatal testing should not also be offered for sex selection, or even to enable deaf parents to abort a hearing child (69). Moreover, it is not enough that the provision of reproductive choice should be the officially stated goal of prenatal screening programs. Far more important is how the program is being delivered in practice. If the information given to (potential) participants is incomplete or unbalanced, if counseling is directive and support absent or minimal, if abortion rates rather than informed decisions are taken as a measure of success, it becomes difficult to maintain that the aim is really to provide prospective parents with meaningful reproductive options (70,71).

For there to be a genuine choice between termination or preparing oneself for the birth of a handicapped child, it is essential that facilities and conditions are guaranteed within society for the care, support, and integration of people with a handicap (55,63,72).

Prenatal Screening for Down Syndrome

In most European countries, screening for Down syndrome (and other aneuploidies) was introduced in the 1970s. This was based on an offer of invasive testing (amniocentesis from 16 weeks onward, later also CVS from 11 weeks onward) to pregnant women in a higher risk group which could at the time only be defined in terms of maternal age (38, 36, or 35 being used as age limits). These diagnostic procedures have a miscarriage risk of around 1% based on the literature (73,74), but which may be lower (0.3–0.5%) in practice (68). Upon the diagnosis of Down syndrome, a large majority of women (more than 90%) choose termination (75). Since the 1980s, the development of non-invasive preselection tests (based on biochemical markers in maternal serum, soft echo markers, or a combination of both) made it possible to individualize risk assessment and offer Down syndrome screening to all pregnant women, regardless of age, while significantly improving the detection/ miscarriage ratio (74). For those in the higher age group, individualized risk assessment means that in most cases invasive testing, with the attached risk of miscarriage, can be avoided. Conversely, younger women need no longer be excluded because of the low risk they have as a group (but not necessarily as individuals). Initially, risk assessment testing was only possible in the second trimester (triple test from 14 weeks onward), making amniocentesis the diagnostic procedure of choice. More recently, tests are being developed for risk assessment in the first trimester (around 11 weeks). Early screening is a clear preference of the majority of eligible women (76–78).

The introduction of these preselection tests has made Down syndrome screening more efficient, but also more complex, both practically and morally. The main disadvantages are the effects of false-positive and -negative test results, "unnecessary" invasive procedures and related fetal losses, the induction of "unnecessary" anxiety and false reassurance. Screening of this kind also requires complex decision making with regard to both the screening process as a whole (what seems an innocent test may present one with very difficult choices later on) and to the nature of the information provided by the test (for most people, including health professionals, risk information proves difficult to understand and handle).

There has been much debate in some European countries (Denmark, The Netherlands) about whether these disadvantages outweigh the advantages of the screening, especially for those in the younger age group with their relatively low pre-test risk. Some of the edge of this has been taken away by the gradual improvement of risk-assessment tests, leading to higher detection and lower false-positive rates. At present, the best method for risk assessment is a combined test involving maternal serum markers and ultrasound measurement of nuchal translucency [(NT), a subcutaneous fluid accumulation behind the neck of the fetus], both in the first trimester of pregnancy (79,80). According to a recent meta-analysis, this approach has a sensitivity of 82% and a false-positive rate of 2.1% at a cutoff of 1:250 (81). Theoretically, even better results could be obtained through a strategy combining risk assessment in the first and second trimesters ("integrated test"). This, however, presupposes nondisclosure of initial results, which may be difficult to achieve in actual practice, stands in opposition to the preference most women have for early testing, and may violate their right to information.

In order to guarantee the quality of the whole process, it is essential that information, testing, counseling, and follow-up all be offered as integrated services in the context of a coordinated and properly monitored screening program. However, in many European countries or regions, testing for Down syndrome is mainly left to local initiative, leading to sub-quality service and inequity of access. This is the situation in Germany (82) and Belgium, but also in The Netherlands, where the government's decision not to permit Down syndrome screening to be offered to women under 36 has led to uncoordinated testing on request (83). In the United Kingdom, all eligible women are now to be offered Down syndrome screening, as a first step in an important effort to overcome the until recently existing situation of highly fragmented and inconsistent services (74). The National Screening Committee has set the target that by 2007 all will be offered screening based on tests with a detection rate of at least 75% at a maximum false-positive rate of 3% (79). France has had a national program of offering all pregnant women Down syndrome screening since 1997 (84). Regional programs function in several other countries. In these programs, uptake rates are consistently high [97% in France (57)]. While this is in line with the finding that the majority of women hold positive attitudes toward prenatal screening for Down syndrome (with only a minority of screen-positive women expressing regret), there is reason for concern over the extent to which participation is actually based on well-informed decision making. The authors of a recent systematic review of the literature on psychosocial aspects of prenatal screening conclude that on the whole, "levels of knowledge adequate for decision making are not being achieved" (85). If the goal of offering prenatal screening is indeed the provision of reproductive choice (rather than reducing the number of Down syndrome births), this urgently deserves more systematic attention (86).

Informed Consent for Prenatal Screening

An important question is how much information should be given at what stage of the screening process. There are two dangers to be avoided here, each connected to a different understanding of what informed consent (or choice) requires (87,88). According to what has been called the "event model" of informed consent, candidate participants should right from the start be provided with all information required for making informed choices at each stage of the process they are about to enter. However, since only a small percentage of participants will eventually find themselves confronted with all those choices, this is both impractical and undesirable. The danger here is that of "information overload," frustrating rather than facilitating well-informed decision making. Following the alternative "process-model," informed consent is understood as an evolving process in itself, keeping pace with the dynamics of screening. This means that participants should be provided with only so much information as they need at each stage of the process. Here, the opposite danger emerges, that of the "screening trap," where women and their partners suddenly find themselves confronted with a choice for which they were not prepared and which they would rather not have had. In order to steer clear of both dangers, participants should be informed, not about everything that may be relevant at later stages, but about the kind of choices they may be presented with in the course of the screening process as a whole.

This information includes the possibility of unexpected or additional results, meaning the diagnosis of disorders or health-related conditions other than those the screening was offered for. In Down syndrome screening, participants should be prepared that the diagnosis of a relatively mild sex-chromosomal disorder may present them with an even more difficult decision than if a more severe disorder were detected. Because some may prefer not to be confronted with such findings at all, the question arises whether (or to what extent) prenatal screening should accommodate a "right not to know" (89). Would it be possible, at the stage of counseling for amniocentesis or CVS, to allow women and their partners to indicate what outcomes they would rather not receive (90)? Although very much in line with the aim of providing reproductive choice, limits to this clearly follow from the practical impossibility of discussing all conceivable outcomes (68). From this perspective, the introduction of new molecular techniques (quantitative fluorescent polymerase chain reaction or QF-PCR) that allow for more rapid and cheap detection of specific aneuploidies (91) has the further advantage of allowing their precise targeting.

According to a recent definition, an informed choice is not only based on relevant knowledge, but also consistent with the decision maker's values (86). Where a person's knowledge is sufficient, but her behavior (acceptance or declination of screening) does not reflect her own values, informed choice is still not achieved. The development of a scientific measure for assessing the multiple dimensions of this concept has led to new research into the impact of screening organization on informed choice (92).

Screening for Neural Tube Defects

Screening for neural tube defects (NTDs)(anencephaly, spina bifida) was introduced in the 1970s on the basis of maternal serum α-fetoprotein (MSAFP) as a risk assessment (preselection) test (from 15 weeks onward), with amniocentesis and later also advanced ultrasound as diagnostic follow up. A clear majority of women chooses termination at the diagnosis of a NTD. The combined figures of several European countries are 64% for spina bifida and 84% for anencephaly (75). As from the 1980s, risk assessment screening for NTDs and Down syndrome was usually combined, MSAFP being one of the markers in the triple test. As a result of improvement of ultrasound techniques, this approach is increasingly being abandoned for spina bifida screening as part of a routine "fetal malformation scan" around 20 weeks of pregnancy (anencephaly being usually found at an earlier "dating scan"). As a screening test for spina bifida, routine ultrasound has the advantage of a near 100% specificity (no false-positive results). The sensitivity is comparable to that of MSAFP, 80% (93).

Because routine ultrasound is used both for obstetric monitoring and for screening, there is cause for concern that women may be screened without their informed consent or even without their awareness of it. The fact that a large majority of women (and their partners) has a very positive attitude towards ultrasound as a means of "seeing the baby" (94) only adds to the challenge this poses for informed decision making (95). Moreover, women should be aware that ultrasound screening may also yield findings about other structural disorders than NTDs. Especially in case of findings with unclear clinical relevance this may lead to difficult choices, "unnecessary" medical interventions, anxiety, and undermining of confidence.

Programs for the primary prevention of NTDs through raising preconceptional folic acid status, as now exist in several European countries, should be regarded as complementary to the offer of prenatal screening. Results of these programs are still disappointing (96).

Carrier Screening for Recessive Genetic Disease: Prenatal or Preconceptional?

Carrier testing for recessive genetic disease takes the form of screening if it is actively and systematically offered to relatives of known carriers (cascade screening), or to (parts of) the general population (population screening). For pragmatic reasons, carrier screening directed at the general population is usually offered in pregnancy, as the target population (couples planning reproduction) is most easily reached through the channel of routine prenatal care. The moral drawback of this is that pregnancy is already underway, leaving couples found to be at risk only the possibility of PD and of having an abortion or preparing for the birth of a handicapped child should the fetus be affected. The alternative strategy of preconceptional screening is directed at couples of reproductive age who may consider having children. This has the advantage of providing a wider range of reproductive options in case of a positive result. In addition to PD, those found at risk preconceptionally may choose not to have children, adopt a child, conceive through IVF and PGD, or reproduce using donor gametes. This wider range also allows those to participate who reject PD and/or abortion. Moreover, decision making need not be done in the emotionally charged period of pregnancy and under the pressure of time, nor be complicated by the different logic and implications of simultaneous screening for other types of fetal disorder, such as Down syndrome. Preconceptional screening also avoids the concern that pregnant women may find it difficult to critically consider or reject options offered to them in the context of prenatal care. For all these reasons, it is not surprising that pregnant women are found to prefer preconceptional over prenatal carrier screening (97). Organizationally, however, preconceptional screening is indeed a more challenging proposal. Uptake rates will be determined by the level of motivation, which tends to be lower where pregnancy is still only a future possibility. At this point, the two perspectives of the purpose of prenatal screening discussed earlier in this section lead to opposite practical conclusions. On what was criticized as the "public health view," the greater effectiveness of offering carrier screening during pregnancy is seen to outweigh the advantages a preconceptional approach would have for participants (66). On the contrasting view defended here, pragmatic reasons for choosing a prenatal strategy cannot change the fact that preconceptional screening is the preferred approach from a moral point of view. A morally defensible strategy might also consist of a combination of both approaches, offering prenatal

carrier screening as a back-up to couples who for whatever reason did not participate in preconceptional screening.

Carrier Screening for Cystic Fibrosis

In carrier screening for CF, as for other autosomal recessive diseases (hematoglobi-
nopathies, Tay–Sachs disease, etc.), the risk of having an affected child is one in four
if both partners are carriers. Screening enables those identified as "carrier couples"
to base their reproductive decisions on that information. Adequate pre- and post-test
counseling is necessary to ensure that participants understand the implications of
possible results (85). This includes information about the disease, its pattern
of inheritance, the variability of its expression, treatment options, etc. Participants
also need to know that carriers are not themselves at an increased risk of disease
and that, because of the imperfect sensitivity of carrier tests (as is the case in screening for CF), a negative test result does not mean that one is definitely not a carrier.

There has been much debate about how carrier screening for CF is best conducted. In "sequential" or "stepwise" screening, it is only after the woman has
received a positive result that her partner also is asked to provide a sample. For some
couples, the outcome of this will be that they have a discordant status, the woman is a
carrier, and the man is not. The couple is then at a residual risk of having a child with
CF (in a recent British review, the figure given for this is 1 in 620, assuming the test
detects 85% of carriers (66)). Since this knowledge may lead to anxiety without meaningful options, the alternative of "couple screening" has been proposed (98), in which
samples of both partners are collected prior to testing and a positive result is given
only if both partners are found to be carriers (the man's sample still being tested only
if the woman is found positive). This also avoids transient high levels of anxiety in the
interval between testing, especially when screening is done in pregnancy. However, in
a randomized trial of both approaches, couple screening was found to induce more
anxiety and false reassurance (99). The variant of "couple screening with full disclosure" does not retain information about discordant results, but differs from sequential screening in that a positive result of the woman is not reported until her partner's
sample has also been tested. While refraining from a final conclusion, the authors of a
recent review of the literature suggest that the latter approach may "bring the best
possible world from the perspective of parental anxiety" (85). Meanwhile, research
of attitudes of participants has shown a clear preference for strategies offering full
disclosure (100,101). From a moral point of view, non-disclosure of individual test
results is a form of paternalism that would require stronger justification than the literature about induction of anxiety seems to provide. Moreover, the retention of test
results containing personal health information is legally questionable and at odds
with the very aim of the screening. Knowledge of discordant status changes the
risk status of the couple (making it, in fact, considerably higher than it was prior
to screening). Even if there are no options attached to this outcome (at least not when
screening is done in pregnancy), the couple may find it important to have this information. In one of the attitude studies just quoted, the main reason for rejecting non-
disclosure was that participants "did not want any information to be withheld from
them" (101). In addition to this, the information would allow them to inform the
woman's relatives, and if she were to have children in a future relationship, it would
be important for her to know that she is a carrier. On the other hand, those who do
not want to be informed about other positive results that they might have as a couple,
should have their "right not to know" respected.

In the same study, participants suggested that in addition to full disclosure they might have preferred a policy in which (the samples of) both partners would be tested ("simultaneous testing"). The researchers comment that this would not only double the cost of testing, but also lead to the identification of twice as many discordant couples (101). Here, the question arises whether the arguments against non-disclosure would also support simultaneous testing. A reason why this need not follow is that the right of participants to information collected about them as a result of screening ("right to know") should be distinguished from a supposed right to information for which extra testing would be necessary. The question to be asked is whether such extra testing could be justified by the purpose for which the screening was offered (informed decisions in reproduction). As the higher risk connected to discordant status (as compared to the situation in which one partner is negative and the other not tested) does not provide couples with extra options (neither in terms of PD nor in terms of altered childbearing decisions (102)), this fully hinges on the importance given to the potential use of individual carrier information in future relationships.

Where screening is not based on simultaneous testing, reasons for testing the woman first (and her partner only if she is found to be a carrier) are pragmatic, and stronger in prenatal than in preconceptional screening. In the latter context, a case could be made for allowing couples to determine the order of testing, based on how each of the partners would value the knowledge of being a carrier.

In the 1990s several pilots of prenatal carrier screening for CF were conducted, both in the United States and in Europe (the United Kingdom, Denmark, and Germany), all resulting in favorable conclusions as to whether such screening would satisfy general criteria. In the United Kingdom, the authors of an extensive HTA report recommended to proceed and make carrier screening for CF a routine offer in prenatal care, while having preconceptional screening available on request (66). Although the current (2004) policy of the National Screening Committee is still dismissive, the committee has announced further review of this. In The Netherlands, the outcome of a pilot showing that preconceptional screening would be feasible in the Dutch situation (103), has led to support for the view that if carrier screening for CF is to be introduced, it should be based on this approach. In France, the National Ethics Committee (CCNE) has recently issued a negative review of a protocol for a French pilot of prenatal CF-carrier screening (104). Part of the arguments of the commission are of a general nature, referring to possible social consequences of offering carrier screening to the general population (risk of stigmatization and the specter of eugenics) and would therefore also apply to preconceptional programs.

Carrier Screening for Hemoglobinopathies

Whereas CF is the most common single gene disorder among Caucasians, hemoglobinopathies [thalassaemia, sickle cell disease (SCD)] mainly affect Black, Asian, and Mediterranean populations in Europe. Carrier screening programs for hemoglobinopathies have a long history in some high-incidence regions, like Cyprus and Sardinia. This includes both prenatal and preconceptional (also premarital) strategies. In the United Kingdom, it was recommended in 1993 that universal prenatal carrier screening should be offered in districts with large ethnic minorities, and selective screening (offered to women with an non–North European ethnic background, or with a low mean corpuscular hemoglobin) elsewhere. In an effort to end inconsistent screening practices, a national program has been set up integrating prenatal and neonatal screening for hemoglobinopathies. One of the questions raised in the context of the further development of the prenatal screening policy is how equity and efficiency are to be balanced. Where efficiency dictates that universal screening cannot be offered everywhere, equity requires that couples with the same risk of an affected pregnancy receive the same prenatal services, regardless of whether they live in a universal-screening or a selective-screening district (105). Selection based on ethnic group is used as an indicator of carrier frequency. However, since the concept of ethnicity is a social rather than a biological construct, this is not a very precise instrument. Morally, an important concern is that it might contribute to ethnic stereotyping (3,106).

As compared to carrier screening for CF, very little is known about the psychosocial aspects of carrier screening for hemoglobinopathies or other disorders. In the same review quoted earlier, the authors summarize the evidence that there is a suggestion that "women do not understand the tests or their purpose." The problem is compounded by language difficulties, making it "unlikely that informed consent is routinely achieved" (85). Where an affected pregnancy has been diagnosed, the predictability of the severity of the disorder is found to be a determinant of the decision to terminate or continue the pregnancy, in combination with gestational age. For SCD, the severity of which cannot be predicted, termination is far more often requested in the first trimester than in the second (107). This underscores the need for early information and counseling, which tends to be a greater challenge with respect to the very groups (often ethnic minorities) that are at greatest risk (108). It also shows that the time window within which prenatal screening can provide meaningful reproductive choices may be even tighter than the one determined by the legal limit for selective abortion. While this is one of the reasons for preferring preconceptional screening, that approach is not considered as a serious alternative in the United Kingdom, mainly because of practical obstacles limiting expected effectiveness (105). In The Netherlands, it is felt that if introduction of carrier screening for hemoglobinopathies were to be considered, it would have to be preconceptional screening. The combined information about preconceptional screening for CF and hemoglobinopathies in the context of a broader provision of preconceptional care may also be an effective way of counteracting ethnic stereotyping.

Carrier Screening for Fragile X

A non-autosomal recessive disease for which carrier screening has been proposed, is fragile X syndrome (FXS). Because of its X-linked pattern of inheritance, the carrier status of the prospective mother alone determines the risk of having an affected child. FXS is the most common form of inherited mental retardation in males (apart from Down syndrome, which is a chromosomal disorder). Of those with a full mutation, all males and around half of all females are affected. Males are generally more severely affected, prohibiting independent living. Of females with a full mutation 25% will have intellectual disability, one or two further quarters have lesser learning difficulties (109). Unlike males, affected females may live independently.

Not only women with a full mutation (>200 CGG-repeats), but also those with a premutation (approximately 55–200 repeats) are at risk of having a child with FXS, as such premutations are unstable and may expand into a full mutation during maternal transmission (110). Identification and counseling of women at risk is complicated, firstly, by the existence of premutation-sized alleles, which are in fact stable. Secondly, there is uncertainty and controversy about the clinical importance of findings in a "gray zone" (intermediate alleles), leading to the use of different cut-offs for PD. Findings in these ranges change the nature of carrier screening for FXS from carrier screening stricto sensu into a form of risk assessment screening. As in screening for Down syndrome, this has the potential of inducing high levels of anxiety, and leads to difficult decision making. Does the fact that, for Down syndrome, prenatal risk assessment screening is widely accepted mean that this should not stand in the way of prenatal screening for FXS either? Differences are that being identified as a (supposed) FXS carrier raises concerns for all future pregnancies and may also have implications for relatives (111). Moreover, screening for Down syndrome can only be offered prenatally, whereas in the case of carrier screening for FXS, there are alternative approaches (cascade screening and preconceptional population screening) that avoid distressing pregnant women, and merit further consideration. The counseling of FXS carriers is complicated further by the fact that premutations, initially characterized as harmless for carriers themselves, may well have consequences for their health; approximately 20% of females carrying a premutation will develop premature ovarian failure (POF), while at least one-third of all male carriers will develop "fragile-X-associated tremor/ataxia syndrome" (FXTAS) (112).

A further difficulty arises with respect to decision making and counseling after PD has identified a female fetus with a full mutation. Because around half of all females with a full mutation are not affected, most of those affected are not severely retarded, and the outcome of individual cases cannot be predicted, the decision whether or not to ask for an abortion is even more complex than if the fetus (with a full mutation) were male. This has led to the recent proposal by Wald and Morris that FXS be regarded as a different disorder in males and females and that prenatal carrier screening be directed exclusively at the identification of pregnant women at risk of having a male child with the disorder (113). They argue that if it were not for the fact that "male" and "female" FXS arise from the same genotype, (prenatal) screening for the disorder in females would never have been suggested. On their proposal, screening would have to start with determination of fetal sex, offered to all pregnant women. Only those with a male fetus would then be screened for FXS. Invasive testing for fetal sex would of course not be acceptable as an initial screen. But a new test, which still requires validation, might make it possible to determine fetal sex in cell free fetal DNA in maternal serum during the first trimester (114).

The proposal has been criticized for underestimating the health impact for females with FXS, for depriving hidden carriers with a female fetus of other reproductive options in their subsequent pregnancies, including IVF/PGD, and for sidestepping the arguments favoring screening prior to pregnancy (109). Moreover, it would seem that precisely because they arise from the same genotype, "male" and "female" FXS cannot so easily be kept separate when offering screening. First, the initial step of sex determination would not be exempt from the requirement of informed choice. One would have to tell participants about the difference between "male" and "female" FXS. What if some are made anxious and ask for carrier testing regardless of the sex of the fetus? Secondly, as a consequence of screening for "male" FXS, carriers who have had a male fetus in a prior pregnancy will know about their being at risk for having a child with FXS. This will change the meaning of the initial sex determination test in their further pregnancies. In those pregnancies there is already knowledge about carrier status and related concerns should the fetus be female. Whereas it might then still be sensible to offer sex determination so as to allow carriers with a female fetus to choose not to have it tested for FXS (thereby respecting their "right not to know"), it is difficult to see how one could impose this as a condition, and offer fetal mutation testing only to carriers with a male fetus. If this makes it problematic, at least in those pregnancies, to maintain the limitation to screening for "male" FXS only, the question arises whether it is fair not to provide all participants with the same information and opportunities with regard to both "male" and "female" FXS. Finally, a morally relevant consideration is also that offering early non-invasive sex determination to all pregnant women lowers the threshold for those who might want to use the outcome for sex-selective abortion for non-medical reasons (115).

All this is not to deny that Wald and Morris have pointed to an important concern about (prenatal) carrier screening for FXS. A variant of their proposal might involve offering sex determination prior to mutation testing in the fetus (but after carrier identification among women). Further research would be needed to see whether that is an acceptable way of allowing participants to avoid being put before the dilemma of having to decide about aborting a female fetus with a full mutation. The option of IVF/PGD (requiring preconceptional carrier identification) could also provide a way of avoiding this, although not without raising potential dilemmas of its own.

Pilots of prenatal FXS screening have been conducted in Israel and Finland (116,117). Both these studies led to favorable conclusions, but also revealed the anxiety-inducing potential of the screening, especially in women with repeats in the intermediate allele group. A Spanish pilot was even stopped because of the anxiety it caused among participants (118). It is significant that after completing these pilots, the research groups involved have all recommended preconceptional rather than prenatal carrier screening for FXS (116,118,119). This reservation is shared by researchers and policy makers in The Netherlands: if carrier screening for FXS is considered, priority should be given to a further discussion of how to overcome practical barriers to a preconceptional approach (111). In the United Kingdom, the National Screening Committee decided in 2004 that prenatal FXS screening should not be introduced. This was done on the basis of three extensive HTA reports (110,120,121).

In view of the recent findings concerning the possible implications of premutations for the health of carriers themselves, both prenatal and preconceptional population FXS screening seems to be premature at best.

Wrongful Life

The proliferation of prenatal tests used in the contexts of both diagnosis and screening have led to questions about liability of doctors and other health care workers. Damage can occur if they fail to provide appropriate care, either by not acting according to the professional standards, or by not respecting patient or third party rights (122). This includes a failure to provide correct or sufficient information about testing opportunities that should have been offered either in view of a medical indication or as a routine screening test. Where this leads to the birth of a handicapped child, which the parents would otherwise have chosen to prevent, health care professionals may face "wrongful birth" and possibly also "wrongful life" claims (123). The former are relatively uncontroversial. "Wrongful birth" is an action brought by the parents against health care professionals, holding them responsible for the material and immaterial damages that they, the parents, have suffered as a result of the birth of the child. By contrast, "wrongful life" is an action brought by the child, holding health care professionals responsible for its handicapped existence resulting from their failure to offer the parents prenatal testing (124,125). Wrongful life claims are controversial. Opponents have argued that such claims imply an impossible proposition, namely that for the disabled child, life is worse than non-existence. Since the child could not possibly have had a healthy life, how to determine the prejudice? Commentators arguing from the perspective of the "disability rights critique" (cf. section "Prenatal Screening") add to this that it would be immoral to see handicapped existence as a prejudice, as that would imply a discriminatory value judgment about the lives of the disabled (125). Courts have also shown themselves sensitive to this line of argument, especially in the United States (124). Germany provides a classic European example: when explaining its rejection of a wrongful life claim in a rubella case, the German Federal Court explicitly referred to the historical shadows of Nazi justice as prohibiting a judicial pronouncement upon the worth of other people's lives (126).

Against this objection, it can be argued that wrongful life actions do not imply categorical judgments of the lives of disabled persons. Nor should they necessarily be taken to imply that, for the child in question, nonexistence would have been better (127). There are good reasons for regarding such actions from the perspective of what they aim to achieve within the framework of legal liability, rather than taking them literally as championing an impossible "right not to be born" (128). What they aim to achieve, and can only achieve in this way, is to entitle the child to indemnification for damages suffered as a consequence of professional malpractice, providing it with the financial means for its long-term care, treatment, and income needs, needs that are often insufficiently met by society. So conceived, "wrongful life" actions serve to support the social position of disabled individuals rather than discriminate against them as a group. Further objections that have been raised point to the possible societal consequences of awarding "wrongful life" claims. One concern is that defensive medicine will lead to unnecessary testing in pregnancy and to pressure on women to abort any fetuses that might be born with a handicap (72,129). Another fear is that "wrongful life" actions against health professionals may clear the way for claims raised by the child against its parents, thereby undermining parental reproductive autonomy and promoting eugenic tendencies in society (72). As is the case with most "slippery slope" arguments, their speculative nature makes it difficult to assess the weight of these objections (128). The concern about effects of defensive medicine underlines the need of having precise indications and professional guidelines in place, so as to ensure that doctors, who act in accordance with their professional standards, need not fear litigation (127).

Internationally, there are incidental cases in which "wrongful life" claims against health professionals were awarded by the courts (in Europe this involves France, Belgium, and The Netherlands), but they have been rejected elsewhere (Austria, Germany, and Portugal, the United Kingdom) (123,128). In the United Kingdom, the Court of Appeal in the McKay case stated that life cannot be an injury (123). In France, the positive ruling by the Cour de Cassation in the famous Perruche case of November 2000 led to fierce debate (125). Since 2002, new French legislation prohibits "wrongful life" actions (130). In The Netherlands, the High Court has recently (March 2005) confirmed the earlier decision by the Court of The Hague to award a wrongful life claim in "the baby Kelly case," in which a child was born with severe handicaps after a failure by the woman's obstetrician to offer prenatal testing (131). In both rulings, the court stressed that the claim brought by the child should not be understood as presupposing the view that its handicapped life is a loss, but only as a request for compensation of material and immaterial damages incurred as a result of the obstetrician's failure. Holding the hospital and the obstetrician accountable for those damages should not be seen as a failure of respect for the human dignity of the child, but rather as providing the means that would help her lead a humane existence.

FETAL THERAPY

The first therapeutic interventions in the unborn date from the 1960s. This involved treatment of fetal Rh disease and included attempts at open fetal surgery (involving hysterotomy) so as to allow complete exchange transfusions. These were abandoned because of high rates of fetal mortality and maternal complications, and also because of the development of percutaneous transfusion procedures (132). Minimally invasive treatment of fetal alloimmunization now belongs to the most successful forms of fetal therapy (133). The great improvement of diagnostic ultrasound since the 1970s made it possible to consider the notion of correcting life-threatening anatomical malformations in utero. Open fetal surgery has been performed for a range of such conditions, including obstructive uropathy, diaphragmatic hernia, cystic adenomatoid malformation, and twin-to-twin transfusion syndrome. Since the second half of the 1990s, American groups have pioneered fetal surgery also for spina bifida (134–136). This is done on the assumption, based on animal research, that in utero closure of the NTD avoids further damage as a result of prolonged exposure of the naked neural tissue to amniotic fluid. Results, in terms of improved neurological prognosis, are until now disappointing (137).

As the fetal and maternal risks of open surgery proved substantial, the tendency has been to reduce these by developing "closed" surgical procedures (138). These include endoscopic placement of shunts for obstructive uropathy and other conditions, endoscopic tracheal occlusion so as to avoid pulmonary hypoplasia in diaphragmatic hernia, and laser coagulation of communicating placental vessels in twin-to-twin transfusion syndrome (133).

Prenatal hematopoietic stem cell (HSC) transplantation has been tried for over 15 years (139–141). It was hoped that because of the specific features of the (early) fetal environment (tolerance, bone-marrow space, isolation, and proliferation) many of the limitations of postnatal bone marrow transplantation could be avoided, and that prenatal HSC transplantation would eventually provide a cure for fetuses with a variety of hematologic and metabolic diseases (140). However, the only engraftment successes so far have been in X-linked severe combined immunodeficiency, with results comparable to those of postnatal transplantation (139,140). With regard to diseases in which donor HSC have no proliferative advantage, important difficulties still need to be overcome (139,140).

Fetal gene therapy is still in the phase of preclinical research. It is thought to hold a promise as a future approach for the treatment and prevention of a wide range of genetic diseases. Present research in animal models focuses on the effectiveness and safety of fetal gene therapy in early onset monogenetic diseases, including hemophilia, CF, and Duchenne or Becker muscular dystrophy (142). Among the specific safety concerns that have to be addressed before human experiments can be considered are a range of undefined risks (insertional mutagenesis, developmental aberrations, and induction of tolerance to viral pathogens), also including the possibility of inadvertent germ-line modification (140). It is thought that these risks can be considerably reduced or even eliminated by using an ex vivo approach to fetal gene therapy (139,140,143). This would involve autologous gene-engineered HSC transplantation.

Notwithstanding the promises of this approach, it would seem that for many of those at high genetic risk, PGD is likely to remain a more acceptable reproductive option than experimental in utero gene (or stem cell) therapy (144).

The Concept of the "Fetus as a Patient"

The concept of the "fetus as a patient" has been put forward by Chervenak and McCullough as a model of maternal-fetal ethics (145,146). While this is a useful model, it should not be misunderstood as implying the "full personhood" view of the moral status of the unborn. From the fact that the fetus can, in principle, be treated, nothing follows with regard to its moral worth (147). The concept should rather be understood as referring to the implications of the fact that, whatever its actual status, the fetus is expected to eventually become a child and a person (132,146). Up to the limit of legal abortion, this expectation is conditional upon the woman's intention to carry the pregnancy to term. If that is her intention, both the woman and the health professionals involved in her care have a duty to protect the fetus from avoidable harm. This duty is not dependent on gestational age, or whether the fetus has reached viability. However, the health professional must also consider his obligations toward the pregnant woman. Since it is literally only through her that the fetus can be reached, this entails duties both of nonmalfeasance and autonomy (146,148). The woman is not obliged to risk her life or consent to treatment that may lead to serious harm to her. Only where treatment is no longer experimental and small risks for the woman stand over against important benefits for the fetus, can it be defended that she is under a moral obligation to accept treatment so as to protect the fetus from avoidable harm. For instance, this would hold for accepted treatment of fetal anemia through the intravascular placement of thin needles under ultrasound guidance. Although in such cases directive counseling may be justified, this does not amount to giving health professionals (or society) a title to force pregnant women into accepting such treatment (132,144,147). Neither would the availability of accepted in utero treatment infringe the woman's right to abortion. Where such treatment becomes available, it only serves to enlarge the range of options opened up by PD. This is of special importance for prospective parents who, for moral or religious reasons, would not want to consider abortion, but also for others, as most pregnancies preceding prenatal care and diagnosis are wanted (144).

Risks and Benefits of Experimental Fetal Therapy

There is a growing consensus that innovation in the field of prenatal therapy should be introduced and evaluated as research, with the aim of gathering evidence concerning fetal and maternal risks and benefits (148). Clinical research should be justified by the outcome of prior animal studies of the efficacy and safety of the procedure (146). In the case of in utero gene transfer, one of the many difficult questions is how to determine whether the evidence from animal models does indeed warrant the step to human experiments. And what type of disorder should then be chosen? As the presumption of benefit must be real, initial experiments will be more difficult to justify (both ethically and legally) where alternative postnatal treatment exists (149). A specific issue here is also the risk of inadvertent germ line modification, leading to changes that will then be passed on to future individuals. The chances of this happening are thought to be very small. Does that make the germ line risk acceptable, as something to be taken on as part of a comprehensive assessment of risks and benefits (142,150)? Or should it be excluded before human experiments are undertaken (139,151)?

New interventions should ideally be evaluated as soon as possible through properly conducted prospective trials, comparing outcomes with those of standard treatment (148,152). Until now, such research has been scarce. Randomized data are only available for endoscopic tracheal occlusion in diaphragmatic hernia (showing no benefit of the intervention) and for endoscopic laser coagulation in twin-to-twin transfusion syndrome (showing higher survival and a lower rate of neurologic complications) (153,154). A randomized trial of in utero surgery of spina bifida is underway (137).

For a comprehensive assessment of the fetal and maternal risk/benefit ratio, research into long-term pediatric and maternal effects will also be needed (148). Until now, the psychosocial impact of decisions concerning (experimental) intra-uterine interventions on women and their families has not been systematically evaluated.

Informed Consent for Experimental Fetal Therapy

The main challenge with regard to informed consent is to ensure that decisions to accept or forgo experimental intra-uterine intervention are indeed well informed (155). Prospective parents whose fetus was diagnosed with a serious disorder face the difficult choice between terminating a wanted pregnancy and preparing for a handicapped child. In this situation, they may be vulnerable to expecting unwarranted therapeutic benefits from experimental interventions, especially when these are offered by their doctor. Against the background of this, close attention should be given to how information about benefits, risks, and alternatives is presented (146). However, it should also be stressed that informed consent does not relieve health professionals and researchers from their obligation of protecting the fetus and the pregnant woman from undue research risks (149).

CONCLUSIONS

In view of the rapid developments in the field of fetal medicine, an ongoing ethical debate on and analysis of its premises, goals, possible benefits, dilemmas and pitfalls, both in research and in clinical practice, is of utmost importance. Ethical reflection and education should: (i) increase public awareness of the moral issues involved; (ii) improve the understanding among medical students and professionals of the moral implications of this specialty, thereby increasing their sensitivity to the dilemmas and pitfalls and facilitating good clinical practice; and (iii) contribute to the development of adequate regulations. No doubt, fetal medicine will be at least as dynamic in the future as it is today. The major challenge, therefore, is to develop a "proactive" ethics, an ethics which timely puts the moral issues of new developments on the agenda. Clearly, interdisciplinary work, with substantial input from medical professionals, is urgently needed.

REFERENCES

1. Council of Europe. Recommendation No. R(90) 3 on Prenatal Genetic Screening, Prenatal Genetic Diagnosis and Associated Genetic Counseling, 1990.
2. Group of Advisers on the Ethical Implications of Biotechnology of the European Commission. Opinion No. 6: Ethical Aspects of Prenatal Diagnosis, 1996.

3. McNally C, et al. Ethical, legal and social aspects of genetic testing: research, development and clinical applications. Brussels European Commission. Community Res. 2004.

4. De Wert GM. Reproductive technology, genetics and ethics (in Dutch). Thesis, Amsterdam, Thela, 1999.

5. Health Council of the Netherlands. Heredity: Science and Society. The Hague: Health Council of the Netherlands, 1989.

6. Medical Ethics Today. The BMA's Handbook of Ethics and Law. London: Br Med J Publishing Group, 2004.

7. Evers-Kiebooms G, Zoetewij MW, Harper PS, eds. Prenatal Testing for Late-onset Neurogenetic Disease. Oxford: BIOS, 2002.

8. Nys H, Roemo Casabona CM, Desmet C. Legal aspects of prenatal testing for late-onset neurological diseases. In: Evers-Kiebooms G, Zoetewij MW, Harper PS, eds. Prenatal Testing for Late-onset Neurogenetic Disease. Oxford: BIOS, 2002:83–106.

9. Minister of Public Health of the Netherlands. Prenatal Diagnosis. Letter to Parliament, dated March 4, 1996 (in Dutch).

10. De Wert GM. Ethical aspects of prenatal testing and preimplantation genetic diagnosis for late-onset neurogenetic disease: the case of Huntington's disease. In: Evers-Kiebooms G, Zoetewij MW, Harper PS, eds. Prenatal Testing for Late-onset Neurogenetic Disease. Oxford: BIOS, 2002:129–158.

11. Adam S, Wiggins S, Whyte P, et al. Five year study of prenatal testing for Huntington's disease: demand, attitudes, and psychological assessment. J Med Genet 1993; 30(7): 549–556.

12. Simpson SA, Harper PS. Prenatal testing for Huntington's disease: experience within the UK 1994–1998. J Med Genet 2001; 38(5):333–335.

13. International Huntington Association and World Federation of Neurology. Guidelines for the molecular genetics predictive test in Huntington's disease. Neurology 1994; 44(8):1533–1536.

14. Tassicker R, Savulescu J, Skene L, Marshall P, Fitzgerald L, Delatycki MB. Prenatal diagnosis requests for Huntington's disease when the father is at risk and does not want to know his genetic status: clinical, legal, and ethical viewpoints. Br Med J 2003; 326(7384): 331–333.

15. Lucassen AM, Houlston RS. Clinical geneticists' attitudes and practice towards testing for breast cancer susceptibility genes. J Med Genet 2000; 37(2):157–160.

16. Royal Dutch Society of Physicians. Doctors and Genes (in Dutch). Utrecht: Royal Dutch Society of Physicians, 1997.

17. Cobben JM, Broecker AHJT, Leschot NJ. Prenatale diagnostiek naar de erfelijke aanleg voor mamma-/ovariumcarcinoom—een standpuntbepaling. Ned Tijdschr Geneeskd 2002; 146:1461–1465.

18. Meijers-Heijboer H, van Geel B, van Putten WL, et al. Breast cancer after prophylactic bilateral mastectomy in women with a BRCA1 or BRCA2 mutation. N Engl J Med 2001; 345(3):159–164.

19. Brambati B, Formigli L, Mori M, Tului L. Multiple pregnancy induction and selective fetal reduction in high genetic risk couples. Hum Reprod 1994; 9(4):746–749.

20. Evans MI, Dommergues M, Wapner RJ, et al. International, collaborative experience of 1789 patients having multifetal pregnancy reduction: a plateauing of risks and outcomes. J Soc Gynecol Investig 1996; 3(1):23–26.

21. Nuffield Council on Bioethics. Genetics and Human Behaviour. London: Nuffield Council on Bioethics, 2002.

22. Stein E. Choosing the sexual orientation of children. Bioethics 1998; 12(1):1–24.

23. Ten CL. The use of reproductive technologies in selecting the sexual orientation, the race, and the sex of children. Bioethics 1998; 12(1):45–48.

24. De Wert GM. Prenatal testing and selection; proceed with caution. In: Galjaard H, Noor LHW, eds. Prenatal Testing. New Developments and Ethical Dilemmas. Amsterdam: Royal Netherlands Academy of Sciences, 2003:61–68.

25. Warren MA. Gendercide. In: The implications of sex selection. Totowa, NJ: Rowman and Allenheld, 1985.
26. Embryo Protection Act (Germany; BGBI.I S.2746). 1990.
27. Law on Medically Assisted Reproduction (Italy). 2004.
28. Nationaler Ethikrat. Stellungnahme. Genetische Diagnostik vor und während der Schwangerschaft, 2003.
29. Loi relative au don et à utilisation des elements et produits du corps humain, à l'assistance medicale à la procreation et au diagnostic prenatal (L94–654), Revisee 2004 (L2004–800), 2004.
30. Human Fertilisation and Embryology Authority. Outcome of the public consultation on preimplantation genetic diagnosis. London HGC, 2001.
31. Planningsbesluit klinisch genetisch onderzoek en erfelijkheidsadvisering, 2003.
32. Verlinsky Y, Rechitsky S, Verlinsky O, Masciangelo C, Lederer K, Kuliev A. Preimplantation diagnosis for early-onset Alzheimer disease caused by V717L mutation. J Am Med Assoc 2002; 287(8):1018–1021.
33. Human Fertilisation and Embryology Act. 1990, UK.
34. Health Council of the Netherlands. IVF related research. Pre-implantation genetic diagnosis, Research concerned with improving IVF, Research using human embryos. Evaluation. Rijswijk: Health Council of the Netherlands, 1998.
35. O'Neill O. Autonomy and trust in bioethics. Cambridge: Cambridge University Press, 2002.
36. Schulman JD, Black SH, Handyside A, Nance WE. Preimplantation genetic testing for Huntington disease and certain other dominantly inherited disorders. Clin Genet 1996; 49(2):57–58.
37. Braude PR, De Wert GM, Evers-Kiebooms G, Pettigrew RA, Geraedts JP. Nondisclosure preimplantation genetic diagnosis for Huntington's disease: practical and ethical dilemmas. Prenat Diagn 1998; 18(13):1422–1426.
38. Shenfield F, Pennings G, Devroey P, Sureau C, Tarlatzis B, Cohen J. Taskforce 5: preimplantation genetic diagnosis. Hum Reprod 2003; 18(3):649–651.
39. De Wert GM. Preimplantation genetic diagnosis: the ethics of "intermediate" cases. Hum Reprod 2005; 20(12): 3261–3266.
40. Pennings G, de Wert G. Evolving ethics in medically assisted reproduction. Hum Reprod Update 2003; 9(4):397–404.
41. Kearney W, Caplan AC. Parity for donation of bone marrow. In: Blank RH, Bonnicksen AL, eds. Emerging Issues in Biomedical Policy. An Annual Review Vol. 1. New York: Columbia University Press, 1992:262–285.
42. Human Fertilisation and Embryology Authority. HFEA agrees to extend policy on tissue typing. 21-7-2004, Press Release.
43. Council of Europe. Convention on Human Rights and Biomedicine. Directorate of Legal Affairs, Strasbourg, 1996.
44. Warnock Report. Report of the Committee of Inquiry into Human Fertilisation and Embryology. London: Her Majesty's Stationary Office, 1984.
45. Health Council of the Netherlands. Sex Selection for Non-medical Reasons. The Hague: Health Council of the Netherlands, 1995.
46. Embryo Act (The Netherlands), 2002.
47. Human Fertilisation and Embryology Authority. Sex Selection: Options for Regulation. A Report on the HFEA's 2002–2003 Review of Sex Selection Including Discussion of Legislative and Regulatory Options. London: HFEA, 2003.
48. Dahl E. The presumption in favour of liberty: a comment on the HFEA's public consultation on sex selection. Reprod Biomed Online 2004; 8(3):266–267.
49. Pennings G. Ethics of sex selection for family balancing. Hum Reprod 1996; 11:2339–2345.
50. Robertson JA. Gender variety as a valid choice: a comment on the HFEA response to Edgar Dahl's "The presumption in favour of liberty". Reprod Biomed Online 2004; 8(3):270–271.

51. Pickering SJ, Braude PR, Patel M, et al. Preimplantation genetic diagnosis as a novel source of embryos for stem cell research. Reprod Biomed Online 2003; 7(3):353–364.
52. de Wert G, Mummery C. Human embryonic stem cells: research, ethics and policy. Hum Reprod 2003; 18(4):672–682.
53. Wilson JMG, Jungner G. Principles and practice of screening for disease. Geneva: WHO, 1968.
54. Nuffield Council on Bioethics. Genetic Screening. Ethical Issues. London: Nuffield Council on Bioethics, 1993.
55. Health Council of the Netherlands. Genetic Screening. The Hague: Health Council of The Netherlands, 1994.
56. Chadwick R, ten Have HA, Husted J, et al. Genetic screening and ethics: European perspectives. J Med Philos 1998; 23(3):255–273.
57. Godard B, ten Kate LP, Evers-Kiebooms G, Ayme S. Population genetic screening programmes: principles, techniques, practices, and policies. Eur J Hum Genet 2003; 11(Suppl 2):S49–S87.
58. Van Wijnen AC. De maatschappelijke effecten van genetisch onderzoek. Over misbruik, keuzemogelijkheden en verplichtingen. Medisch Contact 1995; 50:1192–1195.
59. Reinders JS. Moeten wij gehandicapt leven voorkomen? Ethische implicaties van beslissingen over kinderen met een aangeboren of erfelijke aandoening. Utrecht: Nederlandse Vereniging voor Bioethiek, 1996.
60. Reinders JS. The Future of the Disabled in Liberal Society. An Ethical Analysis. Notre Dame: University of Notre Dame Press, 2000.
61. Parens E, Asch A. The disability rights critique of prenatal testing: reflections and recommendations. Parens E, Asch A, eds. Prenatal Testing and Disability Rights. Washington: Georgetown University Press, 2000:3–43.
62. Nelson JL. The meaning of the act: reflections on the expressive force of reproductive decision making and policies. Kennedy Inst Ethics J 1998; 8(2):165–182.
63. Asch A. Prenatal diagnosis and selective abortion: a challenge to practice and policy. Am J Public Health 1999; 89(11):1649–1657.
64. Chadwick R. The perfect baby: introduction. In: Chadwick R, ed. Ethics, Reproduction and Genetic Control. London: Routledge; 1987, :93–135.
65. Den Hartogh GA. Prenatale diagnostiek. De morele bezwaren gewogen. Medisch Contact 1997; 52:1591–1594.
66. Murray J, Cuckle H, Taylor G, Littlewood J, Hewison J. Screening for cystic fibrosis. Health Technol Assess 1999; 3(8):1–104.
67. De Wert GM. Erfelijkheidsonderzoek en ethiek: een gordiaanse knoop. Wijsgerig perspectief 2000; 40(2000):150–156.
68. Health Council of the Netherlands. Prenatale screening: Downsyndroom, neuralebuisdefecten, routine-echoscopie. The Hague: Health Council of the Netherlands, 2001: 2001/11.
69. Davis DS. Genetic dilemmas and the child's right to an open future. Hastings Center Report 1997; 27(2):7–15.
70. Clarke AJ. Prenatal genetic screening. Paradigms and perspectives. In: Harper PS, Clarke AJ, eds. Genetics, Society, and Clinical Practice. Abingdon: Bios Scientific Publishers, 1997.
71. De Wert GM, De Wachter MA. Mag ik uw genenpaspoort? Ethische aspecten van dragerschapsonderzoek bij de voortplanting. Baarn: Ambo, 1990.
72. National Consultative Ethics Committee. Congenital Handicaps and Prejudice. Paris: CCNE, 2001:68.
73. Tabor A, Philip J, Madsen M, Bang J, Obel EB, Norgaard-Pedersen B. Randomised controlled trial of genetic amniocentesis in 4606 low-risk women. Lancet 1986; 1(8493): 1287–1293.
74. Wald NJ, Kennard A, Hackshaw A, McGuire A. Antenatal screening for Down's syndrome. J Med Screen 1997; 4(4):181–246.

75. Mansfield C, Hopfer S, Marteau TM. Termination rates after prenatal diagnosis of Down syndrome, spina bifida, anencephaly, and Turner and Klinefelter syndromes: a systematic literature review. European Concerted Action: DADA (Decision-making After the Diagnosis of a fetal Abnormality). Prenat Diagn 1999; 19(9): 808–812.

76. Mulvey S, Wallace EM. Women's knowledge of and attitudes to first and second trimester screening for Down's syndrome. Br J Obstet Gynaecol 2000; 107(10):1302–1305.

77. Weinans MJ, Huijssoon AM, Tymstra T, Gerrits MC, Beekhuis JR, Mantingh A. How women deal with the results of serum screening for Down syndrome in the second trimester of pregnancy. Prenat Diagn 2000; 20(9):705–708.

78. de Graaf IM, Tijmstra T, Bleker OP, van Lith JM. Womens' preference in Down syndrome screening. Prenat Diagn 2002; 22(7):624–629.

79. Alfirevic Z, Neilson JP. Antenatal screening for Down's syndrome. Br Med J 2004; 329(7470):811–812.

80. Health Council of the Netherlands. Prenatale Screening (2): Downsyndroom, neurale-buisdefecten. The Hague: Health Council of The Netherlands; 2004:2004/06.

81. Cuckle H, Arbuzova S. Multi-marker serum screening for chromosomal abnormalities. In: Milunsky A, ed. Genetic Disorders and the Fetus. Diagnosis, Prevention, and Treatment. Baltimore, MD: Johns Hopkins University Press, 2004.

82. Droste S, Bitzer E, Perleth M. HTA des biochemischen Screenings für fetale Chromosomenanomalien und Neurahlrohrdefekte. Bundesgesundheitsbl Gesundheitsforsch Gesundheitsschutz 2001; 44:903–907.

83. Van Lith JM, Vandenbussche F. Stilte rond prenatale screening. Medisch Contact 2003; 58:136.

84. Seror V, Costet N, Ayme S. Dépistage prénatal de la trisomie 21 par marquers sériques maternels: de l'information à la prise de décision des femmes enceintes. J Gynecol Obstet Biol Reprod (Paris) 2000; 29(5):492–500.

85. Green JM, Hewison J, Bekker HL, Bryant LD, Cuckle HS. Psychosocial aspects of genetic screening of pregnant women and newborns: a systematic review. Health Technol Assess 2004; 8(33):iii, ix–iii, 109.

86. Dormandy E, Hooper R, Michie S, Marteau TM. Informed choice to undergo prenatal screening: a comparison of two hospitals conducting testing either as part of a routine visit or requiring a separate visit. J Med Screen 2002; 9(3):109–114.

87. Lidz CW, Appelbaum PS, Meisel A. Two models of implementing informed consent. Arch Intern Med 1988; 148(6):1385–1389.

88. Press N, Browner CH. Risk, autonomy, and responsibility. Informed consent for prenatal testing. Hastings Cent Rep 1995; 25:S9–S12.

89. Sheridan E, Williams J, Caine A, Morgan R, Mason G, Mueller RF. Counselling implications of chromosomal abnormalities other than trisomy 21 detected through a maternal serum screening programme. Br J Obstet Gynaecol 1997; 104(1):42–45.

90. De Wert GM. Prenatale diagnostiek en selectieve abortus. Enkele ethische overwegingen. In: ten Have HA, ed. Ethiek en recht in de gezondheidszorg. Deventer: Kluwer, 1990:121–153.

91. Cirigliano V, Voglino G, Canadas MP, et al. Rapid prenatal diagnosis of common chromosome aneuploidies by QF-PCR. Assessment on 18,000 consecutive clinical samples. Mol Hum Reprod 2004; 10(11):839–846.

92. Marteau TM, Dormandy E, Michie S. A measure of informed choice. Health Expect 2001; 4(2):99–108.

93. Vos JM, Offringa M, Bilardo CM, Lijmer JG, Barth PG. [Sensitive and specific screening for detection of spina bifida by echography in the second trimester; systematic review and meta-analysis]. Ned Tijdschr Geneeskd 2000; 144(36):1736–1741.

94. Eurenius K, Axelsson O, Gallstedt-Fransson I, Sjoden PO. Perception of information, expectations and experiences among women and their partners attending a second-trimester routine ultrasound scan. Ultrasound Obstet Gynecol 1997; 9(2):86–90.

95. Michie S, Smith D, Marteau TM. Prenatal tests: how are women deciding? Prenat Diagn 1999; 19(8):743–748.

96. Eurocat. Prevention of Neural Tube Defects by Periconceptional Folic Acid Supplementation in Europe. Newtownabbey: Eurocat Central Registry, 2003.

97. McConkie-Rosell A, Spiridigliozzi GA, Iafolla T, Tarleton J, Lachiewicz AM. Carrier testing in the fragile X syndrome: attitudes and opinions of obligate carriers. Am J Med Genet 1997; 68(1):62–69.

98. Wald NJ. Couple screening for cystic fibrosis. Lancet 1991; 338(8778):1318–1319.

99. Miedzybrodzka ZH, Hall MH, Mollison J, et al. Antenatal screening for carriers of cystic fibrosis: randomised trial of stepwise v couple screening. Br Med J 1995; 310(6976): 353–357.

100. Miedzybrodzka Z, Semper J, Shackley P, Abdalla M, Donaldson C. Stepwise or couple antenatal carrier screening for cystic fibrosis: Women's preferences and willingness to pay. J Med Genet 1995; 32(4):282–283.

101. Henneman L, ten Kate LP. Preconceptional couple screening for cystic fibrosis carrier status: couples prefer full disclosure of test results. J Med Genet 2002; 39(5):E26.

102. Denayer L, Welkenhuysen M, Evers-Kiebooms G, Cassiman JJ, Van den Berghe H. Risk perception after CF carrier testing and impact of the test result on reproductive decision making. Am J Med Genet 1997; 69(4):422–428.

103. Henneman L, Bramsen I, van der Ploeg HM, et al. Participation in preconceptional carrier couple screening: characteristics, attitudes, and knowledge of both partners. J Med Genet 2001; 38(10):695–703.

104. National Consultative Ethics Committee. Le dépistage prénatal géneralisé de la mucoviscidose. Paris: CCNE, 2004:68.

105. Zeuner D, Ades AE, Karnon J, Brown J, Dezateux C, Anionwu EN. Antenatal and neonatal haemoglobinopathy screening in the UK: review and economic analysis. Health Technol Assess 1999; 3(11):1–186.

106. Foster MW, Sharp RR. Race, ethnicity, and genomics: social classifications as proxies of biological heterogeneity. Genome Res 2002; 12(6):844–850.

107. Davies SC, Cronin E, Gill M, Greengross P, Hickman M, Normand C. Screening for sickle cell disease and thalassaemia: a systematic review with supplementary research. Health Technol Assess 2000; 4(3):1–99.

108. Neuenschwander H, Modell B. Audit of process of antenatal screening for sickle cell disorders at a north London hospital. Br Med J 1997; 315(7111):784–785.

109. Delatycki MB, Sheffield LJ, Wake S, Cohen J. Screening approach for fragile X syndrome. Prenat Diagn 2004; 24(1):67–68.

110. Song FJ, Barton P, Sleightholme V, Yao GL, Fry-Smith A. Screening for fragile X syndrome: a literature review and modelling study. Health Technol Assess 2003; 7(16):1–106.

111. de Jong A, de Wert G. Screening op dragerschap van het fragiele-X-syndroom; ethische verkenning. Ned Tijdschr Geneeskd 2002; 146(13):611–615.

112. Hagerman PJ, Hagerman RJ. The fragile-X premutation: a maturing perspective. Am J Hum Genet 2004; 74(5):805–816.

113. Wald NJ, Morris JK. A new approach to antenatal screening for fragile X syndrome. Prenat Diagn 2003; 23(4):345–351.

114. Costa JM, Benachi A, Gautier E, Jouannic JM, Ernault P, Dumez Y. First-trimester fetal sex determination in maternal serum using real-time PCR. Prenat Diagn 2001; 21(12):1070–1074.

115. Rijnders RJ, Christiaens GC, Van der Smagt J, De Haas M, Van der Schoot CE, Ralston AS. Ethical implications of early non-invasive fetal sex determination. In: Rijnders RJ, ed. Cell-free Fetal DNA in Maternal Plasma. Thesis, Utrecht University, Utrecht, 2003:111–124.

116. Pesso R, Berkenstadt M, Cuckle H, et al. Screening for fragile X syndrome in women of reproductive age. Prenat Diagn 2000; 20(8):611–614.

117. Ryynanen M, Heinonen S, Makkonen M, Kajanoja E, Mannermaa A, Pertti K. Feasibility and acceptance of screening for fragile X mutations in low-risk pregnancies. Eur J Hum Genet 1999; 7(2):212–216.
118. Tejada MI, Duran M. Screening for female fragile X premutation and full mutation carriers. Community Genet 1999; 2(1):49–50.
119. Kallinen J, Heinonen S, Mannermaa A, Ryynanen M. Prenatal diagnosis of fragile X syndrome and the risk of expansion of a premutation. Clin Genet 2000; 58(2):111–115.
120. Murray J, Cuckle H, Taylor G, Hewison J. Screening for fragile X syndrome. Health Technol Assess 1997; 1(4):i–71.
121. Pembrey ME, Barnicoat AJ, Carmichael B, Bobrow M, Turner G. An assessment of screening strategies for fragile X syndrome in the UK. Health Technol Assess 2001; 5(7):1–95.
122. Gevers JK. Toepassing van de genetica in het kader van de hulpverlening. In: Commissie genetica, ed. Toepassing van de genetica in de gezondheidszorg. Gevolgen van de ontwikkelingen voor de huidige wet- en regelgeving. Den Haag: ZonMw, 2003:11–25.
123. Howlet MJ, Avard D, Knoppers BM. Physicians and genetic malpractice. Med Law 2002; 21:661–680.
124. Ossorio PN. Prenatal genetic testing and the courts. In: Parens E, Asch A, eds. Prenatal testing and disability rights. Washington, DC: Georgetown University Press, 2000: 308–333.
125. Duguet AM. Wrongful life: the recent French Cour de Cassation decisions. Eur J Health Law 2002; 9:139–163.
126. Bundesgerichtshof VI Zivilsenat. Fundstelle: BGHZ 1983; 86:240.
127. Gevers JK, De Wert GM. De zaak Kelly: moet de wetgever grenzen stellen? Ned Tijdschr Obstet Gynaecol 2003; 116:172–174.
128. Stolker C, Sombroek-van Doorm MP. De wrongful life-vordering: schadevergoeding of euthanasie?. Ned Tijdschr Burgerlijk Recht 2003; 20:496–506.
129. Royal Commission on Civil Liability and Compensation for Personal Injury. Royal Commission on Civil Liability and Compensation for Personal Injury. Civil Liability and Compensation for Personal Injury. Report, Vol. 1. London: HSMO, 1978: Cmnd.7045-I.
130. L'Assemblée nationale et le Sénat. LOI no. 2002–303 du 4 mars 2002 relative aux droits des malades et à la qualité du système de santé, 2002.
131. Hoge Raad der Nederlanden. Uitspraak 18 maart 2005. Eerste Kamer, nr C03/206HR, 2005. (Accessed March 18, 2005, at www.rechtspraak.nl.).
132. Health Council of the Netherlands. Het ongeboren kind als patiënt. Invasieve diagnostiek en behandeling van de foetus. Den Haag: Health Council of The Netherlands, 1990:1990/05.
133. Kumar S, O'Brien A. Recent developments in fetal medicine. Br Med J 2004; 328(7446):1002–1006.
134. Adzick NS, Sutton LN, Crombleholme TM, Flake AW. Successful fetal surgery for spina bifida. Lancet 1998; 352(9141):1675–1676.
135. Bruner JP, Tulipan N, Paschall RL, et al. Fetal surgery for myelomeningocele and the incidence of shunt-dependent hydrocephalus. J Am Med Assoc 1999; 282(19): 1819–1825.
136. Sutton LN, Adzick NS, Bilaniuk LT, Johnson MP, Crombleholme TM, Flake AW. Improvement in hindbrain herniation demonstrated by serial fetal magnetic resonance imaging following fetal surgery for myelomeningocele. J Am Med Assoc 1999; 282(19):1826–1831.
137. van Heurn LW, Harrison MR. Fetal surgery: for selected patients. The experiences of the Fetal Treatment Center in San Francisco. Ned Tijdschr Geneeskd 2003; 147(19):900–904.
138. Quintero RA, Carreño C. Operative fetoscopy. In: Rodeck CH, Whittle MJ, eds. Fetal Medicine: Basic Science and Clinical Practice. London: Churchill Livingstone, 1999:755–769.

139. Surbek DV, Holzgreve W, Nicolaides KH. Haematopoietic stem cell transplantation and gene therapy in the fetus: ready for clinical use? Hum Reprod Update 2001; 7(1):85–91.

140. Flake AW. Stem cell and genetic therapies for the fetus. Semin Pediatr Surg 2003; 12(3):202–208.

141. Touraine JL, Raudrant D, Golfier F, et al. Reappraisal of in utero stem cell transplantation based on long-term results. Fetal Diagn Ther 2004; 19(4):305–312.

142. Coutelle C, Themis M, Waddington S, et al. The hopes and fears of in utero gene therapy for genetic disease—a review. Placenta 2003; 24(Suppl B):S114–S121.

143. Zanjani ED, Anderson WF. Prospects for in utero human gene therapy. Science 1999; 285(5436):2084–2088.

144. Fletcher JC, Richter G. Human fetal gene therapy: moral and ethical questions. Hum Gene Ther 1996; 7(13):1605–1614.

145. Chervenak FA, McCullough LB. The fetus as a patient: an essential ethical concept for maternal–fetal medicine. J Matern Fetal Med 1996; 5(3):115–119.

146. Chervenak FA, McCullough LB. A comprehensive ethical framework for fetal research and its application to fetal surgery for spina bifida. Am J Obstet Gynecol 2002; 187(1):10–14.

147. Bewley S. Ethical issues in maternal-fetal medicine. In: Rodeck CH, Whittle MJ, eds. Fetal Medicine: Basic Science and Clinical Practice. London: Chrchill Livingstone, 1999:265–279.

148. Lyerly AD, Gates EA, Cefalo RC, Sugarman J. Toward the ethical evaluation and use of maternal-fetal surgery. Obstet Gynecol 2001; 98(4):689–697.

149. Burger IM, Wilfond BS. Limitations of informed consent for in utero gene transfer research: implications for investigators and institutional review boards. Hum Gene Ther 2000; 11(7):1057–1063.

150. Caplan AL, Wilson JM. The ethical challenges of in utero gene therapy. Nat Genet 2000; 24(2):107.

151. Billings PR. In utero gene therapy: the case against. Nat Med 1999; 5(3):255–256.

152. Wenstrom KD. Fetal surgery for congenital diaphragmatic hernia. N Engl J Med 2003; 349(20):1887–1888.

153. Senat MV, Deprest J, Boulvain M, Paupe A, Winer N, Ville Y. Endoscopic laser surgery versus serial amnioreduction for severe twin-to-twin transfusion syndrome. N Engl J Med 2004; 351(2):136–144.

154. Harrison MR, Keller RL, Hawgood SB, et al. A randomized trial of fetal endoscopic tracheal occlusion for severe fetal congenital diaphragmatic hernia. N Engl J Med 2003; 349(20):1916–1924.

155. Sicard D. Ethical questions raised by in utero therapeutics with stem cells and gene therapy. Fetal Diagn Ther 2004; 19(2):124–126.

Index

T - #0198 - 071024 - C0 - 254/178/35 - PB - 9780367390716 - Gloss Lamination